MDPI AG
Grosspeteranlage 5
4052 Basel
Switzerland
Tel.: +41 61 683 77 34

MDPI Books Editorial Office
E-mail: books@mdpi.com
www.mdpi.com/books

www.ingramcontent.com/pod-product-compliance
Lightning Source LLC
Chambersburg PA
CBHW061609220926
51850CB00005B/466

Pharmacological Properties and Therapeutic Potential of Honey Bee Products

Pharmacological Properties and Therapeutic Potential of Honey Bee Products

Guest Editors

Michał Miłek
Dana Marcinčáková

MDPI

Basel • Beijing • Wuhan • Barcelona • Belgrade • Novi Sad • Cluj • Manchester

Guest Editors
Michał Miłek
Department of Chemistry and Food Toxicology
University of Rzeszów
Rzeszów
Poland

Dana Marcinčáková
Department of Pharmacology and Toxicology
University of Veterinary Medicine and Pharmacy in Košice
Košice
Slovakia

Editorial Office
MDPI AG
Grosspeteranlage 5
4052 Basel, Switzerland

This is a reprint of the Special Issue, published open access by the journal *Pharmaceuticals* (ISSN 1424-8247), freely accessible at: https://www.mdpi.com/journal/pharmaceuticals/special_issues/87IO620GUU.

For citation purposes, cite each article independently as indicated on the article page online and as indicated below:

Lastname, A.A.; Lastname, B.B. Article Title. *Journal Name* **Year**, *Volume Number*, Page Range.

ISBN 978-3-7258-6804-9 (Hbk)
ISBN 978-3-7258-6805-6 (PDF)
https://doi.org/10.3390/books978-3-7258-6805-6

Contents

pharmaceuticals

MDPI

Review

Bee-Inspired Healing: Apitherapy in Veterinary Medicine for Maintenance and Improvement Animal Health and Well-Being

Jevrosima Stevanović [1], Uroš Glavinić [1], Marko Ristanić [1,*], Vladimira Erjavec [2], Barış Denk [3], Slobodan Dolašević [4] and Zoran Stanimirović [1]

1 Department of Biology, Faculty of Veterinary Medicine, University of Belgrade, 11000 Belgrade, Serbia; rocky@vet.bg.ac.rs (J.S.); uglavinic@vet.bg.ac.rs (U.G.); zoran@vet.bg.ac.rs (Z.S.)
2 Small Animal Clinic, Veterinary Faculty, University of Ljubljana, 1000 Ljubljana, Slovenia; vladimira.erjavec@vf.uni-lj.si
3 Department of Biochemistry, Faculty of Veterinary Medicine, Afyon Kocatepe University, Afyonkarahisar 03204, Turkey; bdenk@aku.edu.tr
4 Institute for Animal Husbandry, Zemun, 11080 Belgrade, Serbia; dolasevicslobodan@gmail.com
* Correspondence: mristanic@vet.bg.ac.rs

Abstract: This review aims to present current knowledge on the effects of honey bee products on animals based on in vivo studies, focusing on their application in clinical veterinary practice. Honey's best-proven effectiveness is in treating wounds, including those infected with antibiotic-resistant microorganisms, as evidenced in horses, cats, dogs, mice, and rats. Propolis manifested a healing effect in numerous inflammatory and painful conditions in mice, rats, dogs, and pigs and also helped in oncological cases in mice and rats. Bee venom is best known for its effectiveness in treating neuropathy and arthritis, as shown in dogs, mice, and rats. Besides, bee venom improved reproductive performance, immune response, and general health in rabbits, chickens, and pigs. Pollen was effective in stimulating growth and improving intestinal microflora in chickens. Royal jelly might be used in the management of animal reproduction due to its efficiency in improving fertility, as shown in rats, rabbits, and mice. Drone larvae are primarily valued for their androgenic effects and stimulation of reproductive function, as evidenced in sheep, chickens, pigs, and rats. Further research is warranted to determine the dose and method of application of honey bee products in animals.

Keywords: honey; propolis; bee venom; pollen; royal jelly; drone larvae; veterinary medicine

1. Introduction

Honey bee products, used by humans for centuries, have been gathering increasing attention in the scientific and professional public due to their therapeutic potential. Their use for numerous health problems, known as apitherapy, steadily increases in humans. However, the application of bee products in veterinary medicine is much less known to the professional and general public, although evidence shows their effectiveness in treating various diseases in animals.

Apitherapy refers to the use of honey bee (*Apis mellifera*) products for the treatment or prevention of health problems in humans and animals and is considered a branch of complementary and alternative medicine. Honey bee products encompass a diverse range of substances, including those derived primarily from plants (nectar, pollen, and plant resins collected and processed by bees with their secretions into honey, bee pollen, and propolis) and those synthesized by bees from their glands (such as royal jelly and bee venom). It is less known that bee larvae, primarily drone larvae, also hold promise for health maintenance and improvement [1,2].

This work distinguishes itself through its original focus, emphasizing findings from in vivo studies, namely those conducted on animals. Furthermore, the included studies are meticulously selected, adhering to three key criteria: they must have been published within the last 15 years, reported in peer-reviewed journals, and available in full-text format.

2. Honey

Clinical trials have extensively investigated the effects of honey on a wide range of animals, including dogs, horses, cats, cattle, and pigs, with preclinical trials involving rats, mice, and rabbits [3]. Once overshadowed by antibiotics, medical-grade honey is regaining popularity due to its antimicrobial and pro-healing properties, making it valuable for cutaneous wound healing [4]. Honey's best-known and proven efficacy in animals is in the treatment of burns and wounds, especially those refractory to conventional treatments [3–7]. Among the various types of honey, mānuka honey, derived from the *Leptospermum scoparium* shrub native to southeastern Australia and New Zealand, has proven particularly effective. The advantage of mānuka honey over other honey types is attributed to its unusually high methylglyoxal (MGO) content, considered a major antibacterial compound in mānuka honey [8]. However, there are other mechanisms of antimicrobial action characteristic of most honey types: enzymatic production of hydrogen peroxide (H_2O_2), high osmolarity due to high sugar concentration, low pH level, and the presence of the bee antimicrobial peptide defensin-1 [9]. In a study on horses, contaminated wounds on the hind limbs healed faster and more successfully when treated with mānuka honey gel or just mānuka honey compared to untreated control wounds [5]. However, in an experiment on mice, chestnut honey showed better efficacy than mānuka honey in terms of angiogenesis and reepithelialization on the seventh day of treatment, while after 14 days, the effect of both kinds of honey was equally effective and significantly better compared to the control [7]. Importantly, mānuka honey may be less effective in treating wounds because its high MGO content adversely affects two of the mechanisms of antimicrobial action by modifying protein components; MGO inhibits glucose oxidase (the enzyme responsible for H_2O_2 generation), so the accumulation of H_2O_2 is disabled [10], while defensin-1, after modification by MGO, loses its antibacterial activity [11].

Interestingly, MGO concentration in mānuka honey is still considered one of its main quality factors (presented as an important potency measure) incorporated in the "Unique Mānuka Factor" (UMF™) grading system. Originally, the UMF grade reflected only the level of antibacterial activity of honey without information about the components responsible for it [9]. With the discovery of MGO and its antibacterial potency, its concentration became the key signature marker for UMF [12]; however, MGO alone cannot explain the entirety of the antimicrobial effectiveness of mānuka honey, as this honey inhibits the growth of pathogenic bacteria at concentrations well below the minimum inhibitory concentration (MIC) of MGO alone [13–16]. The relationship between the MGO content of honey and its antibacterial effect varies and depends on the bacterial species [13–17]. For example, the positive correlation was strong in cases of *Enterococcus faecalis* and *Escherichia coli* and moderate in the case of *Staphylococcus aureus*, but no relationship was recorded between MGO content and efficacy against *Pseudomonas aeruginosa* [17]. The latest is in accordance with the previous evidence that MGO is not solely responsible for the efficacy of mānuka honey against *P. aeruginosa* [13–16]. These findings explain the result of an earlier study in which manuka honey with a lower UMF value showed greater antimicrobial activity than honey with a higher UMF value [18]. Overall, neither the MGO level nor the UMF value represents a reliable indicator of the antibacterial effect.

Excellent effects in wound healing with honey were demonstrated in cats [6,19] (Figure 1—not previously published) and dogs [20,21] (Figure 2—not previously published) regardless of whether a commercial product with medical-grade honey (L-Mesitran®) was used [6,19,21] or raw honey was applied to the gauze and then to the wound [20]. L-Mesitran® showed exceptional efficacy in treating cutaneous injuries. For instance, in a case where a cat had complete skin loss across 100% of its leg with a fractured distal ulna, the leg healed entirely, including the bone, with the regrowth of new skin and hair [6] (Figure 3).

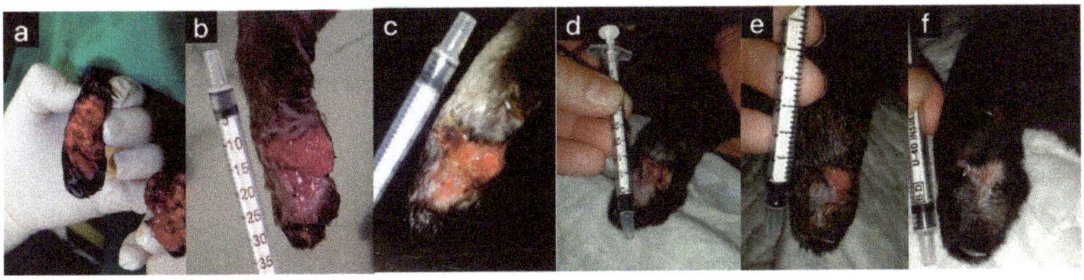

Figure 1. A part of the leg of a 1-year-old female was cat cut off by a lawnmower. The wound healed completely by the second intention with the use of medical honey. The sterile syringe was used as a scale for later wound size assessment. The leg on the day of presentation (**a**), 7 days (**b**), 11 days (**c**), 19 days (**d**), 24 days (**e**), and 30 days later (**f**). Medical grade honey was applied to the wound daily for the first 10 days and thereafter every 2–3 days (Original photo, V. Erjavec).

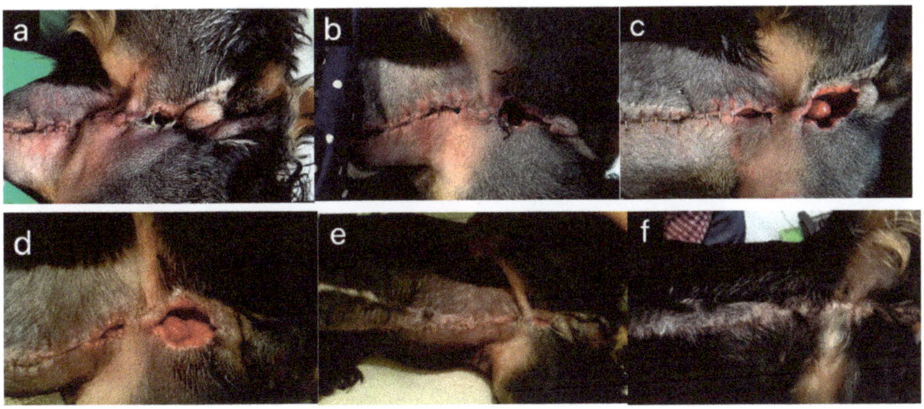

Figure 2. Dehiscence after unilateral mastectomy in a 12-year-old bitch: (**a**) on the day of presentation; (**b**) two days after presentation; (**c**) four days after presentation; (**d**) 14 days after presentation; (**e**) 21 days after presentation; (**f**) two months after presentation. Medical-grade honey was applied to the wound daily by the owner (Original photo, V. Erjavec).

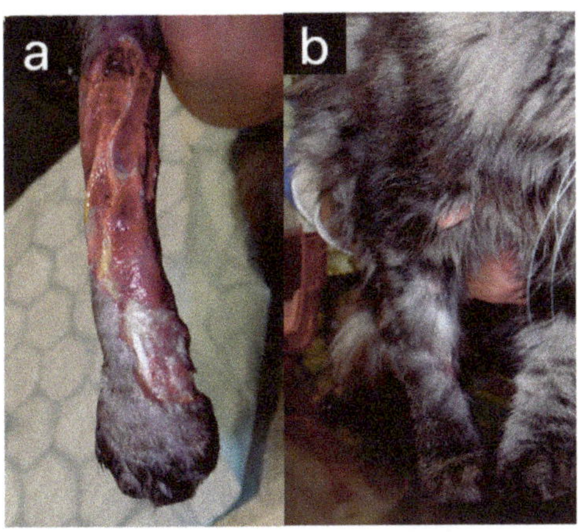

Figure 3. Complete skin loss across 100% of an 8-year-old female cat's forelimb (**a**) healed completely with minimal scarring (**b**) using medical honey [6]. (Original photo, V. Erjavec).

Full-thickness skin wounds of cats treated with medical grade honey exhibited superior outcomes (reduced edema, enhanced angiogenesis, and increased fibroblast concentration) than those treated with *Hypericum perforatum*; the latter significantly improved only tissue perfusion compared to the untreated controls [4]. This is a very important result since *H. perforatum* is traditionally used for wound healing, and it achieves healing effects through the stimulation of epithelialization and granulation [22,23], collagen accumulation [22], and the expression of genes related to tissue repair and regeneration [24].

An extensive leg wound in a 5-year-old female cattle was also successfully treated with raw honey, further proving honey's remarkable healing properties, although the wound did not fully heal due to the cow being slaughtered before complete recovery (Figure 4). The wound was rinsed with tap water, covered with raw honey, and bandaged daily for the first two weeks. Thereafter, the bandage was changed, and honey was applied every second day. No antiseptics were used during the wound healing.

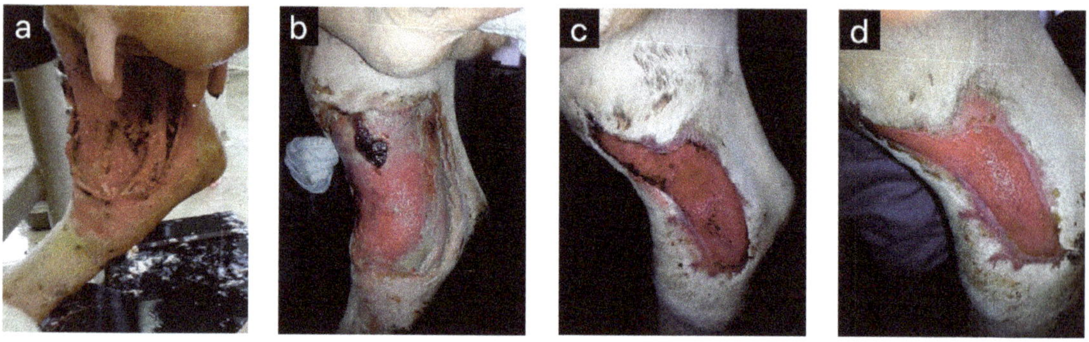

Figure 4. An extensive wound on a cow's rare leg was successfully healed with raw honey, not medical-grade honey. An infected wound with necrotic material and surrounding erythema on the first day of treatment (**a**), wound covered with some necrotic tissue and pus 14 days later (**b**), the wound is almost clean, has contracted, is covered with granulation tissue (**c**) and is epithelializing from the margins (**d**) 1.5 and 2.5 months later (Original photos donated by Clinic of ruminants, Veterinary Faculty, University of Ljubljana).

In addition to wound treatment, experiments on rats showed the efficacy of honey in the prevention and treatment of gastrointestinal problems, especially in the healing of gastric ulcers [25–28] and disorders related to metabolic syndrome, such as hyperglycemia, dyslipidemia, and hyperlipidemia [29–33].

3. Propolis

There is much evidence of the successful treatment of animals with propolis products. Propolis-based products have proven to be a good alternative to conventional antimicrobials, with ample evidence of successful treatment in animals. For example, propolis has shown an excellent antifungal effect in preclinical studies on laboratory mice with vulvovaginal candidiasis; mucoadhesive propolis-based gel demonstrated antifungal efficacy similar to clotrimazole cream [34], while propolis extract incorporated in mucoadhesive thermoresponsive systems showed antifungal action similar and even superior, depending on the propolis concentration, to those with nystatin [35].

The great attention of veterinarians has been attracted by the possibility of using propolis in the treatment of bovine mastitis caused by microorganisms resistant to conventional antibiotics because of the promising efficacy that propolis ethanolic extracts demonstrated against etiological agents of bovine mastitis, *Staphylococcus aureus* and *Escherichia coli*. However, that efficacy was demonstrated indirectly, e.g., in vitro, against standard strains and wild-types of *S. aureus* and *E. coli* isolated from mastitic milk [36], against *S. aureus* cultivated in complex media or milk [37], and against damages induced by *S. aureus* and *E-coli* in bovine mammary epithelial cells [38]. However, negative effect of propolis on mammary tissue was also reported, as it reduced the viability of bovine mammary gland explants [36]. Thus, before the introduction of propolis into the veterinary practice of mastitis treatment in cattle, clinical studies should confirm the effectiveness, dosage, and safety of propolis use in mastitis control.

The antiviral effects of propolis have been evidenced in some in vivo studies, mostly against herpes simplex viruses HSV-1 and HSV-2 [39,40]. The antiparasitic effect has been evidenced in animal models for some types of propolis. After oral administration, propolis extracts effectively decreased the infection level of the microsporidian parasite *Nosema ceranae* in honey bee intestine [41–43]. Propolis extracts were also highly effective against other protistan parasites, such as *Trypanosoma brucei* [44], *Plasmodium falciparum*, *P. berghei* [45], and *P. chabaudi* [46], as evidenced in experiments on rats applying doses 400 and 600 mg/kg against *T. brucei* [44] and much lower doses against *Plasmodium* sp. in mice [45,46]. The antiparasitic properties of propolis have also been recorded against helminths, such as against *Schistosoma mansoni*. A single dose of propolis (400 mg/kg) administered to mice significantly reduced the burden of worms and the number of eggs, both immature and those in feces [47].

Exceptional success in wound healing with propolis products has been evidenced in several animal species [48]. In rats, all tested formulations of propolis gel, containing 1.2%, 2.4%, and 3.6% *w/v* (dry matter) of propolis, showed good activity in healing skin lesions, and the best results were achieved in the group treated with a gel containing 3.6% propolis [49]. In dogs, propolis paste 30% significantly reduced the healing time of wounds due to enhanced reepithelization and contraction of wounds [50]. Healing burn wounds with ointments containing propolis was very successful in pigs [51,52]. The healing effect is explained by the prevention of fibronectin biosynthesis and its degradation in the wound area [51], as well as by the broad-spectrum antibacterial activity, acceleration of neoangiogenesis and epithelialization [52].

Interestingly, propolis, as an aqueous or ethanolic extract, was shown to be effective as an adjuvant in veterinary vaccines and even superior to traditional vaccine adjuvants [53]. For example, propolis significantly increased antibody production when added to canine parvovirus and canine coronavirus vaccines [54], a vaccine against porcine parvovirus [53], and a vaccine against the bacterium *Aeromonas salmonicida*, the cause of furunculosis in fish [55].

Hydroalcoholic extracts of red propolis have shown gastroprotective properties in rats. The basis of this effect was a significant inhibition of the development of acute ulcers, a significant decrease in the volume of gastric secretion, and a significant increase in the production of gastric mucus, as well as antioxidant, and anti-*Helicobacter pylori* activities [56].

As added to broiler feed, even at low doses (10 mg/kg), propolis effectively protected the liver and blood vessels by inhibiting the formation of pathological lesions; with an increase in the dose to 50 mg/kg, the positive effects were even better [57].

Propolis has also been found to have anticancer potential [58] and alleviate the toxic effects of chemotherapy agents [59]. The antitumor activity of propolis observed in in vivo experiments (on rats and mice) indicates its potential application in the treatment of oncological cases in veterinary medicine [58–60].

Propolis is effective in healing numerous inflammatory and painful conditions in the oral cavity, such as candidiasis, gingivitis, periodontitis, ulcers, pulp mummification, supragingival plaque, caries, herpes, wounds after surgical interventions, and cancers, as evidenced in experiments on laboratory animals [61–64]. Besides, employing propolis for tooth storage before reimplantation in healthy mixed-breed dogs proved to be effective in enhancing the success rate of the procedure [65]. It is also worth noting the excellent effectiveness of topically applied propolis ear drops in otitis externa in dogs [66] and propolis eye drops in corneal wound healing in rats [67].

When administered as a dietary supplement to alloxan-induced diabetic mice, propolis preparations mitigated hepatotoxicity and nephrotoxicity by reducing oxidative stress and minimizing the deleterious effects of free radicals on tissue [68].

Propolis achieves therapeutic properties thanks to its complex composition, but primarily to numerous phenolic compounds, of which flavonoids, phenolic acids, and esters are the most biologically active [69,70]. For propolis activities, many underlying mechanisms have been discovered and reviewed [69–71]. For example, the antimicrobial effect of propolis is based on stimulating macrophages to activate Th1 cells, which enhances the cellular immune response (release of cytokines that are essential coordinators of the immune response to intracellular pathogens); in some microorganisms, propolis disrupts the permeability of the cell membrane leading to leakage of cellular components [71]. The anti-inflammatory activity of propolis is accomplished by inhibiting cyclooxygenase and prostaglandin biosynthesis, neutralizing free radicals, reducing cytokines, nitric oxide synthesis, and immunosuppression [70]. Various mechanisms are involved in the anticancer effect of propolis, among which are those already mentioned, including its powerful antioxidant and immunomodulatory potential, as well as its ability to stimulate cell cycle arrest, induce apoptosis, inhibit angiogenesis and metastasis of tumors, inhibit specific oncogene signaling pathways, inhibit glucose uptake and metabolism in the cancer cell, and possibly participate in epigenetic regulation [71].

4. Bee Venom (Apitoxin)

Bee venom has been used since ancient times in the treatment of rheumatoid arthritis, and its success in therapy lies in its anti-inflammatory and antinociceptive effects, reducing swelling and pain, as evidenced by numerous preclinical and clinical studies [72–74]. Melittin, the dominant component of bee venom ($\geq$50% *w*/*w* of bee venom), is responsible for its anti-inflammatory effect and also exhibits anticancer potential [75,76]. For melittin, as well as other components of bee venom (phospholipase A2 and apamin), a neuroprotective effect has been demonstrated, explaining the positive effects of bee stings on neurodegenerative diseases such as Parkinson's disease, multiple sclerosis, and intervertebral disc degeneration recorded in experiments on dogs [77] and mice [78–80]. In experimental animals, bee venom was effective in the therapy of neuropathies caused by nerve injuries or chemotherapeutics [81–83].

Bee venom acupuncture has proven useful in the case of a dog diagnosed with idiopathic facial paralysis; such a therapy led to a gradual improvement of clinical signs, and complete recovery of sensory and neurological facial signs in a dog was noted after eight weeks [84].

Thanks to its antioxidant potential, bee venom improves reproductive performance, immune response, and general health status, as demonstrated in rabbits [85,86]. Antioxidant, anti-inflammatory, and anti-apoptotic mechanisms were underlying the gastroprotective effect of bee venom in an experiment on mice [87]. When added as a supplement to food or water, bee venom has improved feed conversion and increased body weight in broiler chickens without adverse side effects [88,89], while administering bee venom through a live bee sting or by injection positively affected the growth, survival, and immunity of young pigs [90]. In vivo studies on dogs [91], broiler chickens [92], mice [93], and pigs [94] have also shown that bee venom acts as an immunoprophylactic agent, as well as having antibacterial, antifungal, and antiviral effects. The positive therapeutic effect of melittin in animals infected with methicillin-resistant *Staphylococcus aureus* (MRSA) opens up the possibility of its use in treating MRSA infections [95]. Finally, the antidiabetic potential of bee venom was studied on laboratory rats [96,97]. A single-dose injection (0.5 mg/kg) can be considered an initial step in demonstrating its antidiabetic effects [97]. Additionally, the selection of solvent for the use of dry bee venom in injectable and/or topical forms is crucial. This is because the degradation/dysfunction of a specific peptide and the more complex enzymatic bioactivity of the main components in the venom should be prevented, thereby preserving the desired effectiveness of the treatment. To ensure optimal antioxidant activity, we recommend to dissolve the venom in physiological saline [98].

5. Pollen

Due to its exceptional nutritional composition, bee-collected pollen (known as "bee pollen") is considered a "functional food" and is most commonly recommended as a dietary supplement [99]. The potential of bee pollen in animal husbandry was mainly investigated in terms of its effect on growth performance, meat performance and slaughter yield. Adding bee pollen or its ethanolic extract to poultry feed in a range of 400–800 mg/kg feed effectively stimulated animal growth and improved broiler gut microflora [100]. However, this supplementation did not significantly improve meat performance and slaughter yield [101]. Even a ten-times higher concentration of bee pollen (7.5–20 g/kg feed) given to broilers did not affect slaughter yield despite significant improvement in the growth performance, the immune response [102–104], and the microbiological composition of the intestine [104].

The medicinal effects of bee pollen have been demonstrated only in treating benign prostatic hyperplasia and inflammation [105–107] and diabetes-induced testicular dysfunction [108] in experiments on rats.

From the above, one gets the impression that the evidence of the apitherapeutic effects of pollen on animals is scarce. This may be due to the poor bioavailability of pollen nutrients (due to the strong protective layers of pollen grains) and the extreme susceptibility of pollen to microbial spoilage. That is why it is necessary to work on the development of new technologies that will prevent pollen spoilage, protect sensitive pollen compounds, and ensure a higher degree of accessibility [99].

6. Royal Jelly

Very little data exists on the clinical effects of royal jelly. Here, we show only those that meet the criteria set for this review paper. In in vivo experiments (on laboratory rats), royal jelly was shown to protect the body from the toxic effects of chemotherapy, including nephrotoxicity, hepatotoxicity, and pulmonary fibrosis [109–111]. The anticancer potential of royal jelly has been demonstrated in experiments on mice [112,113]. Royal jelly is also attributed to anti-aging effects, supported by scientific evidence obtained in experiments on mice [114]. In immature rats, royal jelly has been found to promote folliculogenesis and increase ovarian hormones [115], and in ovariectomized rats, it improved bone strength [116] and showed potential in the prevention of osteoporosis [117]. It has been shown in rabbits to alleviate neurological disorders by increasing estrogen levels and the activity of the cholinergic and antioxidative systems while reducing cholesterol and restoring the autonomic nervous system [118]. Interestingly, royal jelly showed beneficial effects related to male fertility and reproductive success in rats [119–121], mice [122,123], and rabbits [124,125]. Bioactive components responsible for royal jelly biological activities are fatty acids (e.g., 10-hydroxy-2-decenoic acid), free amino acids, peptides, proteins, and phenolic compounds, among which the most numerous are flavonoids [126].

7. Drone Larvae

It is well known that animals have been eating honey bee larvae to provide significant amounts of energy and supplement their protein needs [2,127]. However, due to its importance for the bee colony, worker brood should not be taken, while drone brood can be used in cases where it is obtained as a by-product of the usual beekeeping procedure known as 'drone brood removal' aimed at controlling the *Varroa destructor* mite. This is a biotechnical procedure in which beekeepers insert a special 'trap frame' (frame with comb cells of a size corresponding to drone brood) into the hive to attract *V. destructor* mites (because drone brood is eight times more attractive to them than worker brood) [128]. When removing the 'trap frames' from the hive, the entire drone brood is discarded. This product is generally considered waste and remains unused despite its exceptional chemical composition and high nutritional value (due to the presence of proteins, fatty acids, vitamins, hormones, and antioxidants) [127], as well as pharmacological properties [2] and potential that justify its use in maintaining health. In veterinary medicine, drone larvae are primarily valued for their androgenic effects and positive impact on reproductive performance, fertility, and/or productivity. Androgenic effects have been demonstrated in various animals (laboratory and farm animals), and the studies almost always used drone larvae homogenate (DLH), either freshly made or in the form of the commercial preparation 'Apilarnil' invented by Nicolae Iliesiu in 1981 in Romania. 'Apilarnil' is made from drone larvae through a process that includes homogenization, filtration, and lyophilization [2]. For example, the androgenic effects of DLH have been demonstrated in rams when given as a dietary supplement (at doses of 10, 15, and 20 mg/kg body weight); all doses improved ram reproductive functions, reflected in increased offspring numbers. The optimal effect on sperm quality was achieved with a dose of 15 mg/kg of body weight administered once daily, which resulted in a 30.4% increase in ejaculate volume, a 14.3% increase in sperm concentration in ejaculate, and a sperm motility score of 9.2/10 points [129]. The androgenic effect of DLH in castrated laboratory rats was evidenced through a significant increase in the expression of Spot14-like androgen-inducible protein (SLAP) in rat prostate [130]. In male broilers, food supplementation with DLH during the growth period also led to androgenic effects; after 20 days of administration of DLH (4 g per broiler per day), secondary sexual characteristics (comb size, wattle size, and aggression) were more pronounced than in the control group [131]. When DLH was added to the feed of broilers aged 28 to 55 days, at doses of 2.5 and 7.5 g per individual, it also stimulated the development of secondary sexual characteristics and sexual maturation in males (increased testis weight, increased testosterone concentration, and comb size), but also led to a decrease in blood glucose and cholesterol levels and a reduction in fear [132]. Feed supplemented with DLH in doses of 2.5 and 7.5 g per individual did not stimulate the development of secondary sexual characteristics in female broilers, and anabolic effects were absent regardless of the sex of the broilers [132].

In females, the effect of DLH is different; it exhibited anabolic and actoprotective effects in young pigs when administered as a dietary supplement. Namely, given to gilts at a concentration of 25 mg of dry matter per 1 kg of food, DLH significantly increased in production parameters (live weight, average daily gain, and slaughter yield) [133]. Besides, DLH significantly affected hormone levels (increased cortisol and decreased testosterone), whereby a significantly better effect was achieved when selenopyran was introduced into the food along with DLH at a concentration of 1.2 mg per 1 kg of food [133]. An anabolic effect was also recorded in another experiment on gilts, where DLH was added to the feed (25 mg/kg of forage) for 180 days [134]; the results motivated the authors to suggest DLH as a valuable dietary additive in livestock farming for increasing meat production. However, in the same experiment, DLH significantly affected folliculogenesis in the ovaries; it stimulated the early stages of folliculogenesis but caused a decrease in the size of Graafian follicles with signs of atresia in the final stage of follicular development, along with changes in the expression of growth factors GDF9 and BMP15 responsible for proper follicle development and ovulation. In another study, supplementary feeding with 0.5 g of DLH daily enhanced the reproductive function of gilts during puberty by reducing the time to their first estrous cycle for artificial insemination [135]. Therefore, care should be taken when treating gilts with DHL (can be given to those intended for slaughter but not to those planned for reproduction).

Finally, in experimental rats, DLH showed neuroprotective potential and therapeutic potential in sepsis. Namely, it prevents the apoptosis of Purkinje cells by lowering the levels of pro-inflammatory cytokines (IL-6, TNF-α, IL-1β) that are elevated during sepsis and thus prevents sepsis-induced apoptosis in the brain [136]. It also protects the liver from lipopolysaccharide (LSP)-induced damage by reducing tissue damage, inhibiting the TLR4/HMGB-1/NF-κB signaling pathway, and protecting liver cells from DNA damage and oxidative stress [137].

8. Precautions and Final Remarks

It is important to state that products from the honey bee hive can be contaminated, both with chemicals (primarily acaricides used by beekeepers to control the honey bee mite *Varroa destructor*, but also with other pesticides commonly used in agriculture) and other environmental pollutants [138,139]. Fat-rich products such as wax and propolis, as well as hive air, are particularly prone to contamination [140–142]. Therefore, for the protection of health, strength, and immunity of honeybee colonies, it is advisable to either utilize products derived from natural sources, such as plants, algae, and fungi [143–153], or employ traditional beekeeping methods that minimize stress, reduce pathogens exposure, and negate the need for chemical treatments [154,155].

Finally, it should be emphasized that apitherapy in veterinary practice can only be applied after examination by a licensed veterinarian. Additionally, when using any bee product, care should be taken regarding the possibility of allergic reactions, though they are less commonly reported compared to humans. If an allergic reaction such as envenomation with honey bee venom is suspected, prompt veterinary attention should be sought to manage symptoms and prevent further complications [156,157].

Apitherapy has great potential for application in veterinary medicine, but officially, it can only be used as a complementary method of treatment. Growing evidence underscores the value of apitherapy in promoting animal health and vitality (Table 1). This leads to an increasing interest of animal owners and veterinarians in using bee products. However, they must recognize the potential risks associated with apitherapy, including potentially fatal anaphylactic reactions in certain cases [158,159]. However, further preclinical and clinical trials are necessary to comprehensively understand the basic mechanisms of action of bee products and determine the optimal doses and methods of their application in animals.

Table 1. The effects of honey bee products are demonstrated in vivo.

Honey Bee Product	Animal	Effect	Reference(s)
Honey	Horses	Wound healing	[5]
	Cats	Wound healing	[4,6,19]
	Dogs	Wound healing	[20,21]
	Mice	Wound healing	[7]
	Rats	Gastroprotective effect	[25]
		Gastric ulcer healing	[26–28]
		Hypoglycemic and antioxidant effects	[29]
		Protection of pancreas	[30]
		Cardioprotective effects	[31]
		Antidiabetic effect	[32]
		Anti-atherogenic effect	[33]
Propolis	Mice	Antifungal efficacy on vulvovaginal candidiasis	[34,35]
		Antiparasitic (antimalarial activity) against *Plasmodium chabaudi*	[46]
		Antiparasitic (antimalarial) effect against *Plasmodium falciparum* and *P. berghei*	[45]
		Antiparasitic properties against *Schistosoma mansoni*	[47]
		Anticarcinogenic potentials	[60]
		Mitigating hepatotoxicity and nephrotoxicity by reducing oxidative stress	[68]
	Honey bees	Antiparasitic effect against *Nosema ceranae*	[41–43]
	Rats	Antiparasitic effect against *Trypanosoma brucei* and *T. congolense*	[44]
		Wound healing	[49]
		Anticarcinogenic potential	[58]
		Gastroprotective properties due to anti-oxidant and anti-*Helicobacter pylori* activities	[56]

Table 1. *Cont.*

Honey Bee Product	Animal	Effect	Reference(s)
		Protective role during the initial phases of lingual carcinogenesis	[61]
		Antimicrobial activity against mutans streptococci, Caries prevention	[62]
		Anticaries effects	[63]
		Chemopreventive and gastroprotective effects	[64]
		Corneal wound healing	[67]
	Dogs	Wound healing	[50]
		Storage medium (on teeth replantation)	[65]
		Antimicrobial effects in otitis externa	[66]
	Pigs	Burn wounds healing	[51,52]
	Chickens	Protective effect on liver and kidney	[57]
Bee venom	Dogs	Anti-inflammatory and analgesic effects	[77]
		Healing effect on *Malassezia*-related otitis externa	[91]
		Healing effect on facial paralysis	[84]
	Mice	Neuroprotective effect in Parkinson's disease	[78]
		Neuroprotective effect in multiple sclerosis	[79]
		Antiviral efficacy against a broad panel of viruses	[93]
		Neuroprotective effects	[80,81]
	Rabbits	Positive impact on reproductive performance and immune response of male individuals	[85]
		Improvement of reproductive traits (sexual-stimulant), immune response, and health	[86]
	Chickens	Growth promoter	[88,89]
		Immunoprophylactic effects	[92]
	Pigs	Promotion of antibody production and viral clearance in PRRS virus infection	[94]
		Positive impact on growth, survival, and immunity	[90]
	Rats	Gastroprotective effect	[87]
		Antidiabetic effect	[96,97]
		Analgesic effect	[83]
		Antibacterial activity against *Staphylococcus aureus*	[82]
Pollen	Rats	Anti-inflammatory and protective effects in prostatitis treatment	[105]
		Healing effects in prostate hyperplasia and inflammation	[106,107]
		Protective role in diabetes-related glycemic control problems and sexual dysfunctions in male individuals	[108]
	Chickens	Positive effect on gut microflora colonization	[100]
		Growth promoter	[101]
		Improvement of growth performance and immune status	[102]
		Improvement in weight gain and food conversion rate	[103]
		Positive effect on daily gain, feed conversion, and microbiological composition of intestine	[104]
Royal jelly	Rats	Protection of liver and kidneys during chemotherapy	[109]
		Nephroprotective effect	[110]
		Anti-fibrotic effect against pulmonary fibrosis	[111]
		Stimulation of folliculogenesis and secretion of steroid hormones	[115]
		Improvement of bone strength after ovariectomy	[116]
		Prevention of osteoporosis after ovariectomy	[117]
		Improvement of fertility and reproductive success in males	[119–121]

Table 1. *Cont.*

Honey Bee Product	Animal	Effect	Reference(s)
	Mice	Antioxidant, immunomodulatory and anticancer effects	[112]
		Apoptotic, antioxidant, anti-inflammatory and anticancer effects	[113]
		Anti-aging effect	[114]
		Improvement of fertility and reproductive success in males	[122,123]
	Rabbits	Alleviation of neurological disorders after ovariectomy	[118]
		Improvement of fertility and reproductive success in males	[124,125]
Drone larvae	Sheep	Stimulation of reproductive function in rams	[129]
	Rats	Androgenic effect in castrated males	[130]
		Liver-protective effects	[137]
		Neuroprotective effect	[136]
	Broilers	Androgenic effects	[131]
		Androgenic effects, Decrease in blood glucose and cholesterol levels	[132]
	Pigs	Anabolic effects (increase in production parameters) in females	[133]
		Anabolic effect in females	[134]
		Improvement of fertility; stimulation of reproductive function (by reducing the time to the first estrous cycle for artificial insemination)	[135]

Author Contributions: J.S. and Z.S. conceived the idea for the manuscript and led the article. All authors performed the bibliographic research, revised critically different versions of the manuscript, and added intellectual content. V.E. provided photos that were reported in this paper for the first time. All authors have read and agreed to the published version of the manuscript.

Funding: The research was supported by the Science Fund of the Republic of Serbia, project no. 5455, Utilization of the food industry waste for improving honey bee health and protecting the environment–Waste2ProtectBees and by the Ministry of Science, Technological Development, and Innovation of the Republic of Serbia (Contract No. 451-03-66/2024-03/200143) for the activities led by Zoran Stanimirović.

Institutional Review Board Statement: The formal written consent of the owner was obtained before the animal entered the study. All procedures complied with the relevant Slovenian governmental regulations (Animal Protection Act, Official Gazette of the Republic of Slovenia, 43/2007).

Conflicts of Interest: The authors declare no conflict of interest.

References

1. Weis, W.A.; Ripari, N.; Conte, F.L.; da Silva Honorio, M.; Sartori, A.A.; Matucci, R.H.; Sforcin, J.M. An overview about apitherapy and its clinical applications. *Phytomedicine Plus* **2022**, *2*, 100239. [CrossRef]
2. Sawczuk, R.; Karpinska, J.; Miltyk, W. What do we need to know about drone brood homogenate and what is known. *J. Ethnopharmacol.* **2019**, *245*, 111581. [CrossRef] [PubMed]
3. Vogt, N.A.; Vriezen, E.; Nwosu, A.; Sargeant, J.M. A scoping review of the evidence for the medicinal use of natural honey in animals. *Front. Vet. Sci.* **2021**, *7*, 618301. [CrossRef] [PubMed]
4. Chatzimisios, K.; Tsioli, V.; Brellou, G.D.; Apostolopoulou, E.P.; Angelou, V.; Pratsinakis, E.D.; Cremers, N.A.J.; Papazoglou, L.G. Evaluation of the effectiveness of medical-grade honey and *Hypericum perforatum* ointment on second-intention healing of full-thickness skin wounds in cats. *Animals* **2023**, *14*, 36. [CrossRef] [PubMed]
5. Bischofberger, A.S.; Dart, C.M.; Horadagoda, N.; Perkins, N.R.; Jeffcott, L.B.; Little, C.B.; Dart, A.J. Effect of Manuka honey gel on the transforming growth factor β1 and β3 concentrations, bacterial counts and histomorphology of contaminated full-thickness skin wounds in equine distal limbs. *Aust. Vet. J.* **2016**, *94*, 27–34. [CrossRef] [PubMed]
6. Lukanc, B.; Potokar, T.; Erjavec, V. Complete skin regeneration with medical honey after skin loss on the entire circumference of a leg in a cat. *J. Tissue Viability* **2020**, *29*, 148–152. [CrossRef] [PubMed]
7. Budak, Ö.; Çakıroğlu, H. Examination the effects of chestnut and Manuka honey for wound healing on mice experimental model. *Med. Sci. Discov.* **2022**, *9*, 170–174. [CrossRef]

8. Blair, S.E.; Cokcetin, N.N.; Harry, E.J.; Carter, D.A. The unusual antibacterial activity of medical-grade *Leptospermum* honey: Antibacterial spectrum, resistance and transcriptome analysis. *Eur. J. Clin. Microbiol. Infect. Dis.* **2009**, *28*, 1199–1208. [CrossRef] [PubMed]
9. Kwakman, P.H.; Zaat, S.A. Antibacterial components of honey. *IUBMB Life* **2012**, *64*, 48–55. [CrossRef]
10. Majtan, J.; Bohova, J.; Prochazka, E.; Klaudiny, J. Methylglyoxal may affect hydrogen peroxide accumulation in manuka honey through the inhibition of glucose oxidase. *J. Med. Food* **2014**, *17*, 290–293. [CrossRef]
11. Majtan, J.; Klaudiny, J.; Bohova, J.; Kohutova, L.; Dzurova, M.; Sediva, M.; Bartosova, M.; Majtan, V. Methylglyoxal-induced modifications of significant honeybee proteinous components in manuka honey: Possible therapeutic implications. *Fitoterapia* **2012**, *83*, 671–677. [CrossRef] [PubMed]
12. Unique Mānuka Factor, the Golden Standard in Mānuka Honey, the Rating System. Available online: https://www.umf.org.nz/unique-manuka-factor/ (accessed on 29 April 2024).
13. Lu, J.; Carter, D.A.; Turnbull, L.; Rosendale, D.; Hedderley, D.; Stephens, J.; Gannabathula, S.; Steinhorn, G.; Schlothauer, R.C.; Whitchurch, C.B.; et al. The effect of New Zealand kanuka, manuka and clover honeys on bacterial growth dynamics and cellular morphology varies according to the species. *PLoS ONE* **2013**, *8*, e55898. [CrossRef] [PubMed]
14. Lu, J.; Turnbull, L.; Burke, C.M.; Liu, M.; Carter, D.A.; Schlothauer, R.C.; Whitchurch, C.B.; Harry, E.J. Manuka-type honeys can eradicate biofilms produced by *Staphylococcus aureus* strains with different biofilm-forming abilities. *PeerJ* **2014**, *2*, e326. [CrossRef] [PubMed]
15. Lu, J.; Cokcetin, N.N.; Burke, C.M.; Turnbull, L.; Liu, M.; Carter, D.A.; Whitchurch, C.B.; Harry, E.J. Honey can inhibit and eliminate biofilms produced by *Pseudomonas aeruginosa*. *Sci. Rep.* **2019**, *9*, 18160. [CrossRef] [PubMed]
16. Bouzo, D.; Cokcetin, N.N.; Li, L.; Ballerin, G.; Bottomley, A.L.; Lazenby, J.; Whitchurch, C.B.; Paulsen, I.T.; Hassan, K.A.; Harry, E.J. Characterizing the mechanism of action of an ancient antimicrobial, Manuka honey, against *Pseudomonas aeruginosa* using modern transcriptomics. *MSystems* **2020**, *5*, e00106-20. [CrossRef] [PubMed]
17. Green, K.J.; Lawag, I.L.; Locher, C.; Hammer, K.A. Correlation of the antibacterial activity of commercial manuka and *Leptospermum* honeys from Australia and New Zealand with methylglyoxal content and other physicochemical characteristics. *PLoS ONE* **2022**, *17*, e0272376. [CrossRef] [PubMed]
18. Girma, A.; Seo, W.; She, R.C. Antibacterial activity of varying UMF-graded Manuka honeys. *PLoS ONE* **2019**, *14*, e0224495. [CrossRef] [PubMed]
19. Lukanc, B.; Potokar, T.; Erjavec, V. Observational study of the effect of L-mesitran® medical honey on wound healing in cats. *Vet. Arhiv* **2018**, *88*, 59–74. [CrossRef]
20. Peteoaca, A.; Istrate, A.; Goanta, A.; Girdan, G.; Stefanescu, A.; Tanase, A. Therapeutic approach in managing degloving injuries of the front limbs in a dog—A case report. *Sci. Work. Ser. C Vet. Med.* **2019**, *65*, 70–78.
21. Lukanc, B.; Šteh, T.; Erjavec, V. The effect of medical honey on second intention wound healing in dogs. *Vet. Arh.* **2023**, *93*, 569–580. [CrossRef]
22. Yalcınkaya, E.; Basaran, M.M.; Tunckasık, M.E.; Yazici, G.N.; Elmas, Ç.; Kocaturk, S. Efficiency of *Hypericum perforatum*, povidone iodine, tincture benzoin and tretinoin on wound healing. *Food Chem. Toxicol.* **2022**, *166*, 113209. [CrossRef] [PubMed]
23. Vatnikov, Y.; Shabunin, S.; Kulikov, E.; Karamyan, A.; Lenchenko, E.; Sachivkina, N.; Bobkova, N.; Bokov, D.; Zhilkina, V.; Tokar, A.; et al. Effectiveness of biologically active substances from *Hypericum perforatum* L. in the complex treatment of purulent wounds. *Int. J. Pharm. Res.* **2020**, *12*, 1108–1117.
24. Sotirova, Y.; Kiselova-Kaneva, Y.; Vankova, D.; Tasinov, O.; Ivanova, D.; Popov, H.; Hristova, M.; Nikolova, K.; Andonova, V. Tissue regeneration and remodeling in rat models after application of *Hypericum perforatum* L. extract-loaded bigels. *Gels* **2024**, *10*, 341. [CrossRef] [PubMed]
25. Bukhari, M.H.; Khalil, J.; Qamar, S.; Qamar, Z.; Zahid, M.; Ansari, N.; Bakhshi, I.M. Comparative gastroprotective effects of natural honey, *Nigella sativa* and cimetidine against acetylsalicylic acid induced gastric ulcer in albino rats. *JCPSP J. Coll. Physici.* **2011**, *21*, 151–156.
26. Almasaudi, S.B.; El-Shitany, N.A.; Abbas, A.T.; Abdel-Dayem, U.A.; Ali, S.S.; Al Jaouni, S.K.; Harakeh, S. Antioxidant, anti-inflammatory, and antiulcer potential of manuka honey against gastric ulcer in rats. *Oxid. Med. Cell Longev.* **2016**, *2016*, 3643824. [CrossRef] [PubMed]
27. Almasaudi, S.B.; Abbas, A.T.; Al-Hindi, R.R.; El-Shitany, N.A.; Abdel-Dayem, U.A.; Ali, S.S.; Saleh, R.M.; Al Jaouni, S.K.; Kamal, M.A.; Harakeh, S.M. Manuka honey exerts antioxidant and anti-inflammatory activities that promote healing of acetic acid-induced gastric ulcer in rats. *J. Evid. Based Complement. Altern. Med.* **2017**, *2017*, 5413917. [CrossRef]
28. Harakeh, S.; Saber, S.H.; Akefe, I.O.; Shaker, S.; Hussain, M.B.; Almasaudi, A.S.; Saleh, S.M.; Almasaudi, S. Saudi honey alleviates indomethacin-induced gastric ulcer via improving antioxidant and anti-inflammatory responses in male albino rats. *Saudi. J. Biol. Sci.* **2022**, *29*, 3040–3050. [CrossRef] [PubMed]
29. Erejuwa, O.O.; Gurtu, S.; Sulaiman, S.A.; Wahab, M.S.; Sirajudeen, K.N.; Salleh, M.S. Hypoglycemic and antioxidant effects of honey supplementation in streptozotocin-induced diabetic rats. *Int. J. Vitam. Nutr. Res.* **2010**, *80*, 74. [PubMed]
30. Erejuwa, O.O.; Sulaiman, S.A.; Wahab, M.S.; Sirajudeen, K.N.; Salleh, M.M.; Gurtu, S. Antioxidant protection of Malaysian tualang honey in pancreas of normal and streptozotocin-induced diabetic rats. *Ann. Endocrinol. Paris* **2010**, *71*, 291–296. [CrossRef]

31. Erejuwa, O.O.; Nwobodo, N.N.; Akpan, J.L.; Okorie, U.A.; Ezeonu, C.T.; Ezeokpo, B.C.; Nwadike, K.I.; Erhiano, E.; Abdul Wahab, M.S.; Sulaiman, S.A. Nigerian honey ameliorates hyperglycemia and dyslipidemia in alloxan-induced diabetic rats. *Nutrients* **2016**, *8*, 95. [CrossRef]
32. Arabmoazzen, S.; Sarkaki, A. Antidiabetic effect of honey feeding in noise induced hyperglycemic rat: Involvement of oxidative stress. *Iran. J. Basic Med. Sci.* **2015**, *18*, 745–751. [PubMed]
33. Hemmati, M.; Karamian, M.; Malekaneh, M. Anti-atherogenic potential of natural honey: Anti-diabetic and antioxidant approaches. *J. Pharm. Pharmacol.* **2015**, *3*, 278–284. [CrossRef]
34. Berretta, A.A.; de Castro, P.A.; Cavalheiro, A.H.; Fortes, V.S.; Bom, V.P.; Nascimento, A.P.; Marquele-Oliveira, F.; Pedrazzi, V.; Ramalho, L.N.; Goldman, G.H. Evaluation of mucoadhesive gels with propolis (EPP-AF) in preclinical treatment of candidiasis vulvovaginal infection. *J. Evid. Based Complement. Altern. Med.* **2013**, *2013*, 641480. [CrossRef] [PubMed]
35. Bonfim, A.P.; Sakita, K.M.; Faria, D.R.; Arita, G.S.; Vendramini, F.A.; Capoci, I.R.; Braga, A.G.; Dos Santos, R.S.; Bruschi, M.L.; Becker, T.C.; et al. Preclinical approaches in vulvovaginal candidiasis treatment with mucoadhesive thermoresponsive systems containing propolis. *PLoS ONE* **2020**, *15*, e0243197. [CrossRef] [PubMed]
36. Fiordalisi, S.A.; Honorato, L.A.; Loiko, M.R.; Avancini, C.A.; Veleirinho, M.B.; Machado Filho, L.C.; Kuhnen, S. The effects of Brazilian propolis on etiological agents of mastitis and the viability of bovine mammary gland explants. *J. Dairy. Sci.* **2016**, *99*, 2308–2318. [CrossRef]
37. Santana, H.F.; Barbosa, A.A.; Ferreira, S.O.; Mantovani, H.C. Bactericidal activity of ethanolic extracts of propolis against *Staphylococcus aureus* isolated from mastitic cows. *World J. Microbiol. Biotechnol.* **2012**, *28*, 485–491. [CrossRef] [PubMed]
38. Wang, K.; Jin, X.L.; Shen, X.G.; Sun, L.P.; Wu, L.M.; Wei, J.Q.; Marcucci, M.C.; Hu, F.L.; Liu, J.X. Effects of Chinese propolis in protecting bovine mammary epithelial cells against mastitis pathogens-induced cell damage. *Mediat. Inflamm.* **2016**, *2016*, 8028291. [CrossRef]
39. Shimizu, T.; Takeshita, Y.; Takamori, Y.; Kai, H.; Sawamura, R.; Yoshida, H.; Watanabe, W.; Tsutsumi, A.; Park, Y.K.; Yasukawa, K.; et al. Efficacy of Brazilian propolis against herpes simplex virus type 1 infection in mice and their modes of antiherpetic efficacies. *J. Evid. Based Complement. Altern. Med.* **2011**, *2011*, 976196. [CrossRef]
40. Sartori, G.; Pesarico, A.P.; Pinton, S.; Dobrachinski, F.; Roman, S.S.; Pauletto, F.; Rodrigues, L.C.; Prigol, M. Protective effect of brown Brazilian propolis against acute vaginal lesions caused by herpes simplex virus type 2 in mice: Involvement of antioxidant and anti-inflammatory mechanisms. *Cell Biochem. Funct.* **2012**, *30*, 1–10. [CrossRef]
41. Arismendi, N.; Vargas, M.; López, M.D.; Barría, Y.; Zapata, N. Promising antimicrobial activity against the honey bee parasite *Nosema ceranae* by methanolic extracts from Chilean native plants and propolis. *J. Apicult. Res.* **2018**, *57*, 522–535. [CrossRef]
42. Burnham, A.J.; De Jong, E.; Jones, J.A.; Lehman, H.K. North American propolis extracts from upstate New York decrease *Nosema ceranae* (Microsporidia) spore levels in honey bees (*Apis mellifera*). *Front. Microbiol.* **2020**, *11*, 1719. [CrossRef] [PubMed]
43. Naree, S.; Ellis, J.D.; Benbow, M.E.; Suwannapong, G. The use of propolis for preventing and treating *Nosema ceranae* infection in western honey bee (*Apis mellifera* Linnaeus, 1787) workers. *J. Apicult. Res.* **2021**, *60*, 686–696. [CrossRef]
44. Nweze, N.E.; Okoro, H.O.; Al Robaian, M.; Omar, R.M.; Tor-Anyiin, T.A.; Watson, D.G.; Igoli, J.O. Effects of Nigerian red propolis in rats infected with. *Comp. Clin. Pathol.* **2017**, *26*, 1129–1133. [CrossRef]
45. Afrouzan, H.; Zakeri, S.; Mehrizi, A.A.; Molasalehi, S.; Tahghighi, A.; Shokrgozar, M.A.; Es-Haghi, A.; Djadid, N.D. Anti-plasmodial assessment of four different Iranian propolis extracts. *Arch. Iran. Med.* **2017**, *20*, 270–281. [PubMed]
46. AlGabbani, Q.; Mansour, L.; Elnakady, Y.A.; Al-Quraishy, S.; Alomar, S.; Al-Shaebi, E.M.; Abdel-Baki, A.A. In vivo assessment of the antimalarial and spleen-protective activities of the Saudi propolis methanolic extract. *Parasitol. Res.* **2017**, *116*, 539–547. [CrossRef] [PubMed]
47. Silva, M.P.; Silva, T.M.; Mengarda, A.C.; Salvadori, M.C.; Teixeira, F.S.; Alencar, S.M.; Luz Filho, G.C.; Bueno-Silva, B.; de Moraes, J. Brazilian red propolis exhibits antiparasitic properties in vitro and reduces worm burden and egg production in an mouse model harboring either early or chronic *Schistosoma* mansoni infection. *J. Ethnopharmacol.* **2021**, *264*, 113387. [CrossRef] [PubMed]
48. Oryan, A.; Alemzadeh, E.; Moshiri, A. Potential role of propolis in wound healing: Biological properties and therapeutic activities. *Biomed. Pharmacother.* **2018**, *98*, 469–483. [CrossRef]
49. Berretta, A.A.; Nascimento, A.P.; Bueno, P.C.; Leite, M.M.; Marchetti, J.M. Propolis standardized extract (EPP-AF®), an innovative chemically and biologically reproducible pharmaceutical compound for treating wounds. *Int. J. Biol. Sci.* **2012**, *8*, 512–521. [CrossRef]
50. Abu-Seida, A.M. Effect of propolis on experimental cutaneous wound healing in dogs. *Vet. Med. Int.* **2015**, *2015*, 672643. [CrossRef]
51. Olczyk, P.; Komosinska-Vassev, K.; Wisowski, G.; Mencner, L.; Stojko, J.; Kozma, E.M. Propolis modulates fibronectin expression in the matrix of thermal injury. *BioMed Res. Int.* **2014**, *2014*, 748101. [CrossRef]
52. Staniczek, J.; Jastrzębska-Stojko, Ż.; Stojko, R. Biological activity of propolis ointment with the addition of 1% nanosilver in the treatment of experimentally-evoked burn wounds. *Polymers* **2021**, *13*, 2312. [CrossRef] [PubMed]
53. Ma, X.; Guo, Z.; Shen, Z.; Wang, J.; Hu, Y.; Wang, D. The immune enhancement of propolis adjuvant on inactivated porcine parvovirus vaccine in guinea pig. *Cell Immunol.* **2011**, *270*, 13–18. [CrossRef]
54. Ferreira, L.N.; Fonseca, F.P.; Caetano de Castro, C.; Sica Siedler, B.; Silveira Munhoz, L.; D'Avila Vargas, G.; Fischer, G.; Oliveira Hubner, S. Effect of the etanolic extract from green propolis on production of antibodies after immunization against Canine Parvovirus (CPV) and Canine Coronavirus (CCoV). *Braz. J. Vet. Res. Anim. Sci.* **2012**, *49*, 116–122. [CrossRef]

55. Liu, S.; Wang, D.; Cao, Y.; Lu, T.; Liu, H.; Li, S. Effects of propolis on the immune enhancement of the formalin-inactivated *Aeromonas salmonicida* vaccine. *Aquac. Res.* **2020**, *51*, 4759–4770. [CrossRef]
56. de Mendonça, M.A.A.; Ribeiro, A.R.S.; de Lima, A.K.; Bezerra, G.B.; Pinheiro, M.S.; de Albuquerque-Júnior, R.L.C.; Gomes, M.Z. Padilha, F.F.; Thomazzi, S.M.; Novellino, E.; et al. Red propolis and its dyslipidemic regulator formononetin: Evaluation of antioxidant activity and gastroprotective effects in rat model of gastric ulcer. *Nutrients* **2020**, *12*, 2951. [CrossRef] [PubMed]
57. Babińska, I.; Kleczek, K.; Makowski, W.; Szarek, J. Effect of feed supplementation with propolis on liver and kidney morphology in broiler chickens. *Pak. Vet. J.* **2013**, *33*, 1–4.
58. Salehi, A.; Hosseini, S.M.; Kazemi, S. Antioxidant and anticarcinogenic potentials of propolis for dimethylhydrazine-induced colorectal cancer in Wistar rats. *BioMed Res. Int.* **2022**, *2022*, 8497562. [CrossRef]
59. Rizk, S.M.; Zaki, H.F.; Mina, M.A. Propolis attenuates doxorubicin-induced testicular toxicity in rats. *Food Chem. Toxicol.* **2014**, *67*, 176–186. [CrossRef]
60. Sameni, H.R.; Yosefi, S.; Alipour, M.; Pakdel, A.; Torabizadeh, N.; Semnani, V.; Bandegi, A.R. Co-administration of 5FU and propolis on AOM/DSS induced colorectal cancer in BALB-c mice. *Life Sci.* **2021**, *276*, 119390. [CrossRef]
61. Cavalcante, D.R.R.; de Oliveira, P.S.; Góis, S.M.; Soares, A.F.; Cardoso, J.C.; Padilha, F.F.; de Albuquerque Júnior, R.L.C. Effect of green propolis on oral epithelial dysplasia in rats. *Rev. Bras. Otorrinolaringol.* **2011**, *77*, 278–284. [CrossRef]
62. Arslan, S.; Silici, S.; Percin, D.; Koç, A.N.; Er, Ö. Antimicrobial activity of poplar propolis on mutans streptococci and caries development in rats. *Turk. J. Biol.* **2012**, *36*, 65–73. [CrossRef]
63. Bueno-Silva, B.; Koo, H.; Falsetta, M.L.; Alencar, S.M.; Ikegaki, M.; Rosalen, P.L. Effect of neovestitol–vestitol containing Brazilian red propolis on accumulation of biofilm in vitro and development of dental caries in vivo. *Biofouling* **2013**, *29*, 1233–1242 [CrossRef] [PubMed]
64. Ribeiro, D.R.; Alves, A.V.; dos Santos, E.P.; Padilha, F.F.; Gomes, M.Z.; Rabelo, A.S.; Cardoso, J.C.; Massarioli, A.P.; de Alencar, S.M.; de Albuquerque-Junior, R.L. Inhibition of DMBA-induced oral squamous cells carcinoma growth by Brazilian red propolis in rodent model. *Basic. Clin. Physiol. Pharmacol.* **2015**, *117*, 85–95. [CrossRef] [PubMed]
65. Darweesh, F.A.; Zaher, A.R.; Zaghlool, A.E.; Helal, M.E.; El-Sabaa, H.M. Honey bee propolis as a storage medium on teeth replantation in dogs (histological, histochemical and radiographic study). *Mansoura J. Dent.* **2014**, *1*, 1–6.
66. Lozina, L.A.; Peichoto, M.E.; Boehringer, S.I.; Koscinczuk, P.; Granero, G.E.; Acosta, O.C. Efficacy of Argentine propolis formulation for topical treatment of canine otitis externa. *Arq. Bras. Med. Vet. Zootec.* **2010**, *62*, 1359–1366. [CrossRef]
67. Martin, L.F.; Rocha, E.M.; Garcia, S.B.; Paula, J.S. Topical Brazilian propolis improves corneal wound healing and inflammation in rats following alkali burns. *BMC Complement. Altern. Med.* **2013**, *13*, 337. [CrossRef] [PubMed]
68. Oršolić, N.; Sirovina, D.; Končić, M.Z.; Lacković, G.; Gregorović, G. Effect of Croatian propolis on diabetic nephropathy and liver toxicity in mice. *BMC Complement. Altern. Med.* **2012**, *12*, 117. [CrossRef] [PubMed]
69. Farooqui, T.; Farooqui, A.A. Molecular mechanism underlying the therapeutic activities of propolis: A critical review. *Curr. Nutr. Food Sci.* **2010**, *6*, 186–199. [CrossRef]
70. Araujo, M.A.; Libério, S.A.; Guerra, R.N.; Ribeiro, M.N.; Nascimento, F.R. Mechanisms of action underlying the anti-inflammatory and immunomodulatory effects of propolis: A brief review. *Rev. Bras. Farmacogn.* **2012**, *22*, 208–219. [CrossRef]
71. Oršolić, N.; Jazvinšćak Jembrek, M. Molecular and cellular mechanisms of propolis and its polyphenolic compounds against cancer. *Int. J. Mol. Sci.* **2022**, *23*, 10479. [CrossRef]
72. Zhang, S.; Liu, Y.; Ye, Y.; Wang, X.R.; Lin, L.T.; Xiao, L.Y.; Zhou, P.; Shi, G.X.; Liu, C.Z. Bee venom therapy: Potential mechanisms and therapeutic applications. *Toxicon* **2018**, *148*, 64–73. [CrossRef]
73. Kocyigit, A.; Guler, E.M.; Kaleli, S.; Kocyigit, A.; Guler, E.M.; Kaleli, S. Anti-inflammatory and antioxidative properties of honey bee venom on Freund's Complete Adjuvant-induced arthritis model in rats. *Toxicon* **2019**, *161*, 4–11. [CrossRef] [PubMed]
74. Lin, T.Y.; Hsieh, C.L. Clinical applications of bee venom acupoint injection. *Toxins* **2020**, *12*, 618. [CrossRef] [PubMed]
75. Oršolić, N. Bee venom in cancer therapy. *Cancer Metastasis Rev.* **2012**, *31*, 173–194. [CrossRef] [PubMed]
76. Aufschnaiter, A.; Kohler, V.; Khalifa, S.; Abd El-Wahed, A.; Du, M.; El-Seedi, H.; Büttner, S. Apitoxin and its components against cancer, neurodegeneration and rheumatoid arthritis: Limitations and possibilities. *Toxins* **2020**, *12*, 66. [CrossRef] [PubMed]
77. Tsai, L.C.; Lin, Y.W.; Hsieh, C.L. Effects of bee venom injections at acupoints on neurologic dysfunction induced by thoracolumbar intervertebral disc disorders in canines: A randomized, controlled prospective study. *BioMed Res. Int.* **2015**, *2015*, 363801. [CrossRef] [PubMed]
78. Alvarez-Fischer, D.; Noelker, C.; Vulinović, F.; Grünewald, A.; Chevarin, C.; Klein, C.; Oertel, W.H.; Hirsch, E.C.; Michel, P.P.; Hartmann, A. Bee venom and its component apamin as neuroprotective agents in a Parkinson disease mouse model. *PLoS ONE* **2013**, *8*, e61700. [CrossRef] [PubMed]
79. Mohammadi-Rad, M.; Ghasemi, N.; Aliomrani, M. Evaluation of apamin effects on myelination process in C57BL/6 mice model of multiple sclerosis. *Res. Pharm. Sci.* **2019**, *14*, 424. [PubMed]
80. Nguyen, C.D.; Lee, G. Neuroprotective activity of melittin—The main component of bee venom—Against oxidative stress induced by Aβ25–35 in in vitro and in vivo models. *Antioxidants* **2021**, *10*, 1654. [CrossRef]
81. Khalil, W.K.; Assaf, N.; ElShebiney, S.A.; Salem, N.A. Neuroprotective effects of bee venom acupuncture therapy against rotenone-induced oxidative stress and apoptosis. *Neurochem. Int.* **2015**, *80*, 79–86. [CrossRef]
82. Choi, J.; Jeon, C.; Lee, J.H.; Jang, J.U.; Quan, F.S.; Lee, K.; Kim, W.; Kim, S.K. Suppressive effects of bee venom acupuncture on paclitaxel-induced neuropathic pain in rats: Mediation by spinal α2-adrenergic receptor. *Toxins* **2017**, *9*, 351. [CrossRef] [PubMed]

83. Li, D.; Chung, G.; Kim, S.K. The involvement of central noradrenergic pathway in the analgesic effect of bee venom acupuncture on vincristine-induced peripheral neuropathy in rats. *Toxins* **2020**, *12*, 775. [CrossRef] [PubMed]
84. Sung, H.J.; Park, H.M. Therapeutic trial of bee venom acupuncture for idiopathic facial paralysis in a dog. *J. Vet. Clin.* **2013**, *30*, 107–110.
85. El-Hanoun, A.; El-Komy, A.; El-Sabrout, K.; Abdella, M. Effect of bee venom on reproductive performance and immune response of male rabbits. *Physiol. Behav.* **2020**, *223*, 112987. [CrossRef] [PubMed]
86. Elkomy, A.; El-Hanoun, A.; Abdella, M.; El-Sabrout, K. Improving the reproductive, immunity and health status of rabbit does using honey bee venom. *J. Anim. Physiol. Anim. Nutr.* **2021**, *105*, 975–983. [CrossRef] [PubMed]
87. Mohamed, W.A.; Abd-Elhakim, Y.M.; Ismail, S.A. Involvement of the anti-inflammatory, anti-apoptotic, and anti-secretory activity of bee venom in its therapeutic effects on acetylsalicylic acid-induced gastric ulceration in rats. *Toxicology* **2019**, *419*, 11–23. [CrossRef]
88. Han, S.M.; Lee, K.G.; Yeo, J.H.; Oh, B.Y.; Kim, B.S.; Lee, W.; Baek, H.J.; Kim, S.T.; Hwang, S.J.; Pak, S.C. Effects of honeybee venom supplementation in drinking water on growth performance of broiler chickens. *Poult. Sci.* **2010**, *89*, 2396–2400. [CrossRef] [PubMed]
89. Kim, D.H.; Han, S.M.; Keum, M.C.; Lee, S.; An, B.K.; Lee, S.R.; Lee, K.W. Evaluation of bee venom as a novel feed additive in fast-growing broilers. *Brit. Poult. Sci.* **2018**, *59*, 435–442. [CrossRef]
90. Han, S.M.; Lee, K.G.; Yeo, J.H.; Hwang, S.J.; Jang, C.H.; Chenoweth, P.J.; Pak, S.C. Effects of bee venom treatment on growth performance of young pigs. *Am. J. Chin. Med.* **2009**, *37*, 253–260. [CrossRef]
91. Shin, J.C.; Kim, S.H.; Park, H.J.; Seo, K.W.; Song, K.H. Effect of aromatherapy and apipuncture on Malassezia-related otitis externa in dogs. *J. Vet. Clin.* **2012**, *29*, 470–473.
92. Jung, B.G.; Lee, J.A.; Park, S.B.; Hyun, P.M.; Park, J.K.; Suh, G.H.; Lee, B.J. Immunoprophylactic effects of administering honeybee (*Apis melifera*) venom spray against *Salmonella gallinarum* in broiler chicks. *J. Vet. Med. Sci.* **2013**, *75*, 1287–1295. [CrossRef] [PubMed]
93. Uddin, M.B.; Lee, B.H.; Nikapitiya, C.; Kim, J.H.; Kim, T.H.; Lee, H.C.; Kim, C.G.; Lee, J.S.; Kim, C.J. Inhibitory effects of bee venom and its components against viruses in vitro and in vivo. *J. Microbiol.* **2016**, *54*, 853–866. [CrossRef] [PubMed]
94. Lee, J.; Kim, Y.M.; Kim, J.H.; Cho, C.W.; Jeon, J.W.; Park, J.K.; Lee, S.H.; Jung, B.G.; Lee, B.J. Nasal delivery of chitosan/alginate nanoparticle encapsulated bee (*Apis mellifera*) venom promotes antibody production and viral clearance during porcine reproductive and respiratory syndrome virus infection by modulating T cell related responses. *Vet. Immunol. Immunop.* **2018**, *200*, 40–51. [CrossRef] [PubMed]
95. Choi, J.H.; Jang, A.Y.; Lin, S.; Lim, S.; Kim, D.; Park, K.; Han, S.M.; Yeo, J.H.; Seo, H.S. Melittin, a honeybee venom derived antimicrobial peptide, may target methicillin resistant *Staphylococcus aureus*. *Mol. Med. Rep.* **2015**, *12*, 6483–6490. [CrossRef] [PubMed]
96. Mousavi, S.M.; Imani, S.; Haghighi, S.; Mousavi, S.E.; Karimi, A. Effect of Iranian honey bee (*Apis mellifera*) venom on blood glucose and insulin in diabetic rats. *J. Arthropod-Borne Dis.* **2012**, *6*, 136–143. [PubMed]
97. Denk, B.; Fidan, A.F. Effects of honeybee (*Apis mellifera*) venom on redox balance, biochemical and hematological profile in diabetic rats: A preliminary study. *Turk. J. Vet. Anim. Sci.* **2021**, *45*, 257–265.
98. Denk, B. Exploring *Apis mellifera* L. venom's antioxidant power in various solvents: Unveiling its in vitro potential. *Kocatepe Vet. J.* **2023**, *16*, 420–431. [CrossRef]
99. Kostić, A.Ž.; Milinčić, D.D.; Barać, M.B.; Ali Shariati, M.; Tešić, Ž.L.; Pešić, M.B. The application of pollen as a functional food and feed ingredient—The present and perspectives. *Biomolecules* **2020**, *10*, 84. [CrossRef] [PubMed]
100. Kročko, M.; Čanigová, M.; Bezeková, J.; Lavová, M.; Haščík, P.; Ducková, V. Effect of nutrition with propolis and bee pollen supplements on bacteria colonization pattern in gastrointestinal tract of broiler chicken. *Sci. Pap. Anim. Sci. Biotechnol.* **2012**, *45*, 63–67.
101. Haščík, P.; Trembecká, L.; Tkáčová, J.; Kročko, M.; Čuboň, J.; Kačániová, M. Effect of bee pollen dietary supplementation on meat performance of Ross 308 broiler chickens. *J. Microb. Biotec. Food* **2015**, *4*, 55–58. [CrossRef]
102. Fazayeli-Rad, A.R.; Afzali, N.; Farhangfar, S.H.; Asghari, M.R. Effect of bee pollen on growth performance, intestinal morphometry and immune status of broiler chicks. *Eur. Poult. Sci.* **2015**, *79*, 1–9. [CrossRef]
103. Abood, S.S.; Ezzat, H.N. Effect of adding different levels from bee pollen in diet on productive performance of broiler chickens. *Plant Arch.* **2018**, *18*, 2435–2438.
104. Petričević, V.; Lukić, M.; Škrbić, Z.; Rakonjac, S.; Stanojković, A.; Nikšić, D.; Živković, V. Production parameters, microbiological composition of intestines and slaughter performance of broilers fed with bee pollen. *Züchtungskunde* **2022**, *94*, 36–46.
105. Locatelli, M.; Macchione, N.; Ferrante, C.; Chiavaroli, A.; Recinella, L.; Carradori, S.; Zengin, G.; Cesa, S.; Leporini, L.; Leone, S.; et al. Graminex pollen: Phenolic pattern, colorimetric analysis and protective effects in immortalized prostate cells (PC3) and rat prostate challenged with LPS. *Molecules* **2018**, *23*, 1145. [CrossRef] [PubMed]
106. Chen, X.; Wu, R.Z.; Zhu, Y.Q.; Ren, Z.M.; Tong, Y.L.; Yang, F.; Dai, G.H. Study on the inhibition of Mfn1 by plant-derived miR5338 mediating the treatment of BPH with rape bee pollen. *BMC Complement. Altern. Med.* **2018**, *18*, 38. [CrossRef] [PubMed]
107. Chen, X.; Wu, R.Z.; Ren, Z.M.; Tong, Y.L.; Chen, S.; Yang, F.; Dai, G.H. Regulation of microRNAs by rape bee pollen on benign prostate hyperplasia in rats. *Andrologia* **2020**, *52*, e13386. [CrossRef]

108. Mohamed, N.A.; Ahmed, O.M.; Hozayen, W.G.; Ahmed, M.A. Ameliorative effects of bee pollen and date palm pollen on the glycemic state and male sexual dysfunctions in streptozotocin-induced diabetic Wistar rats. *Biomed. Pharmacother.* **2018**, *97*, 9–18. [CrossRef] [PubMed]
109. Karadeniz, A.; Simsek, N.; Karakus, E.; Yildirim, S.; Kara, A.; Can, I.; Kisa, F.; Emre, H.; Turkeli, M. Royal jelly modulates oxidative stress and apoptosis in liver and kidneys of rats treated with cisplatin. *Oxid. Med. Cell Longev.* **2011**, *2011*, 981793. [CrossRef] [PubMed]
110. Ibrahim, A.; Eldaim, M.A.; Abdel-Daim, M.M. Nephroprotective effect of bee honey and royal jelly against subchronic cisplatin toxicity in rats. *Cytotechnology* **2016**, *68*, 1039–1048. [CrossRef]
111. Zargar, H.R.; Hemmati, A.A.; Ghafourian, M.; Arzi, A.; Rezaie, A.; Javad-Moosavi, S.A. Long-term treatment with royal jelly improves bleomycin-induced pulmonary fibrosis in rats. *Can. J. Physiol. Pharm.* **2017**, *95*, 23–31. [CrossRef]
112. Albalawi, A.E.; Althobaiti, N.A.; Alrdahe, S.S.; Alhasani, R.H.; Alaryani, F.S.; BinMowyna, M.N. Antitumor activity of royal jelly and its cellular mechanisms against Ehrlich solid tumor in mice. *BioMed Res. Int.* **2022**, *2022*, 7233997. [CrossRef] [PubMed]
113. Zhang, S.; Shao, Q.; Geng, H.; Su, S. The effect of royal jelly on the growth of breast cancer in mice. *Oncol. Lett.* **2017**, *14*, 7615–7621. [CrossRef]
114. Okumura, N.; Toda, T.; Ozawa, Y.; Watanabe, K.; Ikuta, T.; Tatefuji, T.; Hashimoto, K.; Shimizu, T. Royal jelly delays motor functional impairment during aging in genetically heterogeneous male mice. *Nutrients* **2018**, *10*, 1191. [CrossRef]
115. Ghanbari, E.; Khazaei, M.R.; Khazaei, M.; Nejati, V. Royal jelly promotes ovarian follicles growth and increases steroid hormones in immature rats. *Int. J. Fertil. Steril.* **2018**, *11*, 263–269. [PubMed]
116. Shimizu, S.; Matsushita, H.; Minami, A.; Kanazawa, H.; Suzuki, T.; Watanabe, K.; Wakatsuki, A. Royal jelly does not prevent bone loss but improves bone strength in ovariectomized rats. *Climacteric* **2018**, *21*, 601–606. [CrossRef] [PubMed]
117. Hattori, S.; Omi, N. The effects of royal jelly protein on bone mineral density and strength in ovariectomized female rats. *Phys. Act. Nutr.* **2021**, *25*, 33. [CrossRef]
118. Pan, Y.; Xu, J.; Jin, P.; Yang, Q.; Zhu, K.; You, M.; Hu, F.; Chen, M. Royal jelly ameliorates behavioral deficits, cholinergic system deficiency, and autonomic nervous dysfunction in ovariectomized cholesterol-fed rabbits. *Molecules* **2019**, *24*, 1149. [CrossRef] [PubMed]
119. Hassan, A.A. Effect of royal jelly on sexual efficiency in adult male rats. *Iraqi J. Vet. Sci.* **2009**, *23*, 155–160.
120. Mahdivand, N.; Najafi, G.; Nejati, V.; Shalizar-Jalali, A.; Rahmani, F. Royal jelly protects male rats from heat stress-induced reproductive failure. *Andrologia* **2019**, *51*, e13213. [CrossRef]
121. Asadi, N.; Kheradmand, A.; Gholami, M.; Saidi, S.H.; Mirhadi, S.A. Effect of royal jelly on testicular antioxidant enzymes activity, MDA level and spermatogenesis in rat experimental Varicocele model. *Tissue Cell* **2019**, *57*, 70–77. [CrossRef]
122. Zahmatkesh, E.; Najafi, G.; Nejati, V.; Heidari, R. Protective effect of royal jelly on the sperm parameters and testosterone level and lipid peroxidation in adult mice treated with oxymetholone. *Avicenna J. Phytomedi.* **2014**, *4*, 43.
123. Azad, F.; Nejati, V.; Shalizar-Jalali, A.; Najafi, G.; Rahmani, F. Royal jelly protects male mice against nicotine-induced reproductive failure. *Vet. Res. Forum.* **2018**, *9*, 231–238. [PubMed]
124. El-Hanoun, A.M.; Elkomy, A.E.; Fares, W.A.; Shahien, E.H. Impact of royal jelly to improve reproductive performance of male rabbits under hot summer conditions. *World Rabbit. Sci.* **2014**, *22*, 241–248. [CrossRef]
125. Khadr, A.H.; Abdou, A.; El-Sherbiny, A.M. Age of puberty and fertility of male New Zealand white rabbits orally administered with royal jelly or/and bee honey. *J. Anim. Poult. Prod. Mansoura Univ.* **2015**, *6*, 201–217. [CrossRef]
126. Guo, J.; Wang, Z.; Chen, Y.; Cao, J.; Tian, W.; Ma, B.; Dong, Y. Active components and biological functions of royal jelly. *J. Funct. Foods* **2021**, *82*, 104514. [CrossRef]
127. Ghosh, S.; Jung, C.; Meyer-Rochow, V.B. Nutritional value and chemical composition of larvae, pupae, and adults of worker honey bee, *Apis mellifera ligustica* as a sustainable food source. *J. Asia Pac. Entomol.* **2016**, *19*, 487–495. [CrossRef]
128. Odemer, R.; Odemer, F.; Liebig, G.; de Craigher, D. Temporal increase of Varroa mites in trap frames used for drone brood removal during the honey bee season. *J. Appl. Entomol.* **2022**, *146*, 1207–1211. [CrossRef]
129. Shoinbayeva, K.B.; Omirzak, T.; Bigara, T.; Abubakirova, A.; Dauylbay, A. Biologically active preparation and reproductive function of stud rams. *Asian J. Pharm.* **2017**, *11*, 184–191.
130. Seres, A.B.; Ducza, E.; Báthori, M.; Hunyadi, A.; Béni, Z.; Dékány, M.; Hajagos-Tóth, J.; Verli, J.; Gáspár, R. Androgenic effect of honeybee drone milk in castrated rats: Roles of methyl palmitate and methyl oleate. *J. Ethnopharmacol.* **2014**, *153*, 446–453. [CrossRef]
131. Yucel, B.; Acikgoz, Z.; Bayraktar, H.; Seremet, C. The effect of apilarnil (drone bee larvae) administration on growth performance and secondary sex characteristics of male broilers. *J. Anim. Vet. Adv.* **2011**, *10*, 2263–2266.
132. Altan, O.; Yucel, B.; Açikgoz, Z.; Seremet, C.; Kosoglu, M.; Turgan, N.; Ozgonul, A.M. Apilarnil reduces fear and advances sexual development in male broilers but has no effect on growth. *Brit. Poult. Sci.* **2013**, *54*, 355–361. [CrossRef] [PubMed]
133. Zdorovjova, J.V.; Boryayev, G.I.; Nosov, A.V.; Katayev, O.G.; Meloyan, G.M.; Zemljanova, J.V.; Kistanova, J.K. Hormonal status and productive qualities of young pigs at inclusion in a diet feeding homogenate drone brood. *Agrar. Sci. J.* **2018**, *2*, 3–7. (In Russian)
134. Kistanova, E.; Zdoroveva, E.; Nevitov, M.; Nosov, A.; Vysokikh, M.; Sukhanova, I.; Vishnyakova, P.; Abadjieva, D.; Ankova, D.; Rashev, P.; et al. Drone brood fed supplement impacts on the folliculogenesis in growing gilts. *Vet. Arh.* **2020**, *90*, 583–592. [CrossRef]

135. Yemets, Y.M. Dietary effects of drone larves homogenate on the homeostatic constants and the reproductive capacity of Large White gilts. *Transl. Res. Vet. Sci.* **2020**, *3*, 27–39. [CrossRef]
136. Hamamci, M.; Doganyigit, Z.; Silici, S.; Okan, A.; Kayma, E.; Yilmaz, S.; Tokpina, A.; Inan, L.E. Apilarnil: A novel neuroprotective candidate. *Acta Neurol. Taiwan.* **2020**, *29*, 33–45.
137. Doğanyiğit, Z.; Okan, A.; Kaymak, E.; Pandır, D.; Silici, S. Investigation of protective effects of apilarnil against lipopolysaccharide induced liver injury in rats via TLR 4/HMGB-1/NF-κB pathway. *Biomed. Pharmacother.* **2020**, *125*, 109967. [CrossRef] [PubMed]
138. Stevanovic, J.; Stanimirović, Z.; Aleksić, N.; Simeunović, P.; Vučićević, M. The influence of natural and synthetic substances applied in honey bee health care on the quality of bee products (invited paper). In Proceedings of the Apimondia Symposium "Apiecotech Serbia 2012", Belgrade, Serbia, 18–19 February 2012; pp. 9–34.
139. Kasiotis, K.M.; Zafeiraki, E.; Manea-Karga, E.; Anastasiadou, P.; Machera, K. Pesticide residues and metabolites in Greek honey and pollen: Bees and human health risk assessment. *Foods* **2023**, *12*, 706. [CrossRef] [PubMed]
140. Végh, R.; Csóka, M.; Mednyánszky, Z.; Sipos, L. Pesticide residues in bee bread, propolis, beeswax and royal jelly–a review of the literature and dietary risk assessment. *Food Chem. Toxicol.* **2023**, *176*, 113806. [CrossRef]
141. Simsek, I.; Kuzukiran, O.; Yurdakok-Dikmen, B.; Sireli, U.T.; Beykaya, M.; Filazi, A. Comparison of selected lipophilic compound residues in honey and propolis. *J. Food Compos. Anal.* **2021**, *102*, 104068. [CrossRef]
142. Ilić, D.; Brkić, B.; Sekulić, M.T. Biomonitoring: Developing a beehive air volatiles profile as an indicator of environmental contamination using a sustainable in-field technique. *Sustainability* **2024**, *16*, 1713. [CrossRef]
143. Stanimirović, Z.; Glavinić, U.; Lakić, N.; Radović, D.; Ristanić, M.; Tarić, E.; Stevanović, J. Efficacy of plant-derived formulation "Argus Ras" in control. *Acta Vet. Beogr.* **2017**, *67*, 191–200. [CrossRef]
144. Stanimirovic, Z.; Glavinic, U.; Jovanovic, N.M.; Ristanic, M.; Milojković-Opsenica, D.; Mutic, J.; Stevanovic, J. Preliminary trials on effects of lithium salts on *Varroa destructor*, honey and wax matrices. *J. Apicult. Res.* **2022**, *61*, 375–391. [CrossRef]
145. Stanimirović, Z.; Glavinić, U.; Ristanić, M.; Jelisić, S.; Vejnović, B.; Niketić, M.; Stevanović, J. Diet supplementation helps honey bee colonies in combat infections by enhancing their hygienic behaviour. *Acta Vet. Beogr.* **2022**, *72*, 145–166. [CrossRef]
146. Jovanovic, N.M.; Glavinic, U.; Delic, B.; Vejnovic, B.; Aleksic, N.; Mladjan, V.; Stanimirovic, Z. Plant-based supplement containing B-complex vitamins can improve bee health and increase colony performance. *Prev. Vet. Med.* **2021**, *190*, 105322. [CrossRef]
147. Jovanovic, N.M.; Glavinic, U.; Ristanic, M.; Vejnovic, B.; Stevanovic, J.; Cosic, M.; Stanimirovic, Z. Contact varroacidal efficacy of lithium citrate and its influence on viral loads, immune parameters and oxidative stress of honey bees in a field experiment. *Front. Physiol.* **2022**, *13*, 1000944. [CrossRef] [PubMed]
148. Jovanovic, N.M.; Glavinic, U.; Ristanic, M.; Vejnovic, B.; Ilic, T.; Stevanovic, J.; Stanimirovic, Z. Effects of plant-based supplement on oxidative stress of honey bees (*Apis mellifera*) infected with *Nosema ceranae*. *Animals* **2023**, *13*, 3543. [CrossRef]
149. Dolasevic, S.; Stevanovic, J.; Aleksic, N.; Glavinic, U.; Deletic, N.; Mladenovic, M.; Stanimirovic, Z. The effect of diet types on some quality characteristics of artificially reared *Apis mellifera* queens. *J. Apicult. Res.* **2020**, *59*, 115–123. [CrossRef]
150. Glavinic, U.; Stankovic, B.; Draskovic, V.; Stevanovic, J.; Petrovic, T.; Lakic, N.; Stanimirovic, Z. Dietary amino acid and vitamin complex protects honey bee from immunosuppression caused by *Nosema ceranae*. *PLoS ONE* **2017**, *12*, e0187726.
151. Glavinic, U.; Stevanovic, J.; Ristanic, M.; Rajkovic, M.; Davitkov, D.; Lakic, N.; Stanimirovic, Z. Potential of fumagillin and *Agaricus blazei* mushroom extract to reduce *Nosema ceranae* in honey bees. *Insects* **2021**, *12*, 282. [CrossRef]
152. Glavinic, U.; Rajkovic, M.; Vunduk, J.; Vejnovic, B.; Stevanovic, J.; Milenkovic, I.; Stanimirovic, Z. Effects of *Agaricus bisporus* mushroom extract on honey bees infected with *Nosema ceranae*. *Insects* **2021**, *12*, 915. [CrossRef]
153. Glavinic, U.; Blagojevic, J.; Ristanic, M.; Stevanovic, J.; Lakic, N.; Mirilovic, M.; Stanimirovic, Z. Use of thymol in *Nosema ceranae* control and health improvement of infected honey bees. *Insects* **2022**, *13*, 574. [CrossRef] [PubMed]
154. Taric, E.; Glavinic, U.; Vejnovic, B.; Stanojkovic, A.; Aleksic, N.; Dimitrijevic, V.; Stanimirovic, Z. Oxidative stress, endoparasite prevalence and social immunity in bee colonies kept traditionally vs. those kept for commercial purposes. *Insects* **2020**, *11*, 266. [CrossRef]
155. Taric, E.; Glavinic, U.; Stevanovic, J.; Vejnovic, B.; Aleksic, N.; Dimitrijevic, V.; Stanimirovic, Z. Occurrence of honey bee (*Apis mellifera* L.) pathogens in commercial and traditional hives. *J. Apicult. Res.* **2019**, *58*, 433–443. [CrossRef]
156. Rostaher, A.; Mueller, R.S.; Meile, L.; Favrot, C.; Fischer, N.M. Venom immunotherapy for Hymenoptera allergy in a dog. *Vet. Dermatol.* **2021**, *32*, 206-e52. [CrossRef]
157. Moore, A.; Burrows, A.K.; Rosenkrantz, W.S.; Ghubash, R.M.; Hosgood, G. Modified rush venom immunotherapy in dogs with Hymenoptera hypersensitivity. *Vet. Dermatol.* **2023**, *34*, 532–542. [CrossRef] [PubMed]
158. Vazquez-Revuelta, P.; Madrigal-Burgaleta, R. Death due to live bee acupuncture apitherapy. *J. Investig. Allerg. Clin.* **2018**, *28*, 45–46. [CrossRef]
159. Chen, J.; Lariviere, W.R. The nociceptive and anti-nociceptive effects of bee venom injection and therapy: A double-edged sword. *Prog. Neurobiol.* **2010**, *92*, 151–183. [CrossRef]

pharmaceuticals

MDPI

Review

The Efficacy of Honey for the Treatment of Perineal Wounds Following Vaginal Birth: A Narrative Review

Isa S. Schaap [1,†], Céline M. J. G. Lardenoije [1,†], Senna J. J. M. van Riel [1,2,3] and Niels A. J. Cremers [1,4,*]

1 Department of Gynecology and Obstetrics, Maastricht University Medical Centre+, P. Debyelaan 25, 6229 HX Maastricht, The Netherlands; isaschaap.research@gmail.com (I.S.S.); celine.lardenoije@mumc.nl (C.M.J.G.L.); sjjmvanriel@gmail.com (S.J.J.M.v.R.)

2 VieCuri Medical Centre, Tegelseweg 210, 5912 BL Venlo, The Netherlands

3 GROW Research Institute for Oncology and Reproduction, Universiteitssingel 40, 6229 ER Maastricht, The Netherlands

4 Triticum Exploitatie BV, Sleperweg 44, 6222 NK Maastricht, The Netherlands

* Correspondence: niels@mesitran.com or niels.cremers@mumc.nl; Tel.: +31-(0)43-325-1773

† These authors contributed equally to this work.

Abstract: Background/Objectives: During vaginal delivery, the perineum can be damaged either by episiotomy or by a spontaneous perineal tear, leading to several complications. The wound healing process should proceed as quickly and properly as possible without an infection. Medical grade honey (MGH) may be a potent treatment option due to its antimicrobial and pro-healing activities. This literature study investigated the role of honey in the treatment of vaginal wounds after delivery. **Methods**: Studies published before 17 July 2024 in the PubMed, Web of Science, Embase, Scopus, EBSCO host/CINAHL, Cochrane Library, and Google Scholar databases about honey, episiotomy wounds, and perineal tears, as well as those investigating wound healing and/or pain, were assessed. **Results**: Ten studies were included (six RCTs, of which three were double-blind, one was quasi-experimental with a posttest only, and three were observational studies without a control group), with 723 participants in total. Six of the seven controlled studies showed honey significantly improved various outcome measures, such as improved wound healing, and reduced need for pain medication. The three non-controlled studies also had a positive outcome, improving wound healing and decreasing pain intensity and prickling sensation. However, the overall quality of available evidence is limited. Different types of honey concentrations, origins, and additives were used in the included studies. Using a standardized MGH formulation may help to maintain consistent and potent effects. Therefore, additional research is needed to determine the efficacy of MGH in perineal trauma and to establish guidelines for clinical use. **Conclusions**: Honey potentially has a great effect on wound healing of perineal trauma; however, more research is necessary to substantiate the findings in the current literature.

Keywords: birth; perineal trauma; episiotomy; perineal tears; honey; medical grade honey; wound healing; pain

1. Introduction

During vaginal delivery, the perineum can be damaged either by episiotomy or by a spontaneous perineal tear. At least 85% of women undergoing vaginal delivery suffer from perineal trauma of varying degrees [1,2]. In the UK, only 8.6% of the nulliparous women who give birth in the hospital have an intact perineum, and 28.5% of the multiparous women [3]. The episiotomy rate in vaginal deliveries varies worldwide, from 91% in

Thailand to 4% in Denmark [4]. In the Netherlands, 16% of women who gave birth received an episiotomy in 2020 [5].

An episiotomy is a surgical procedure in which an incision is made in the perineum in the final stage of labor to dilate the vaginal orifice [6,7]. Various types of incisions are performed. In Europe, the mediolateral incision is the most common, and in the United States, the midline episiotomy is [6,7]. Indications for an episiotomy are fetal distress and shoulder dystocia [7,8]. Perineal tears can be divided into four grades: Grade 1 is a laceration limited to the vaginal mucosa or perineal skin; grade 2 involves the perineal muscles; grade 3 also includes the anal sphincter muscles; and grade 4 extends through the rectal mucosa [9,10]. In the literature, it remains unclear whether episiotomies could be used to prevent third- and fourth-degree tears, as the studies supporting this claim are observational and may be affected by confounding [9,11]. Routine use of episiotomies is not recommended by the World Health Organization [12] and the American College of Obstetrics and Gynecologists [13].

Perineal trauma is associated with both short- and long-term complications, such as pain and increased infection rates, which can lead to wound dehiscence [2,13–17]. Up to 80% of the dehiscence of episiotomy wounds are due to infection [18]. The incidence of infection after perineal trauma varies from 0.1% to 23.6% and wound dehiscence occurs between 0.21% to 24.6% [19]. Some studies show that severe perineal trauma is associated with anal incontinence, dyspareunia, and delays in resuming sexual activity [16,17,20–22]. Additionally, there might be an association between postpartum physical symptoms, such as pain and infection, and postnatal depression, anxiety, or posttraumatic stress symptoms [2]. Proper treatment is crucial to prevent an infection and accelerate recovery.

Honey may be a potent treatment to accelerate healing and has been used as therapy for wounds and local infections for thousands of years. It is an easily accessible, affordable option with good healing properties [23,24]. Honey is a thick, viscous substance composed of water, sugars, proteins, amino acids, enzymes (e.g., glucose oxidase), beeswax, minerals, pigments, and pollen [25]. Medical-grade honey (MGH) differs from regular honey because it is carefully assessed to ensure the quality of the honey, its safety, and efficacy. MGH is free of pollutants like pesticides, herbicides, heavy metals, and antibiotics [26].

MGH has antimicrobial and pro-healing properties. MGH promotes wound healing by multiple mechanisms, often related to its physicochemical composition. Its physical viscous state creates a moist wound environment, ensuring faster healing than dry or wet wounds. Autolytic debridement is stimulated by the low pH, the activation of proteases, and the lymphatic outflow generated by the osmotic activity. Granulation tissue formation, angiogenesis, and epithelialization are enhanced by the high sugar content serving as a nutrient source for the proliferation and migration of skin cells. Edema is reduced by honey's anti-inflammatory properties and osmotic activities attracting lymph fluid from beneath the wound bed [23,24,27].

Honey's antimicrobial mechanisms are also mediated by a multitude of mechanisms. Honey has a strong osmotic effect due to the high amount of sugar in honey, causing bacterial dehydration and inhibiting bacterial growth and cell division [23]. Glucose oxidase gradually converts glucose into gluconic acid and hydrogen peroxide. Gluconic acid causes the acidity of honey to reach a pH between 3.5 and 4.0, creating an environment inhospitable for bacterial growth [23]. Hydrogen peroxide aids in eliminating bacteria and sterilizes the wound site [24,25,27]. Phytomolecules in honey, such as flavonoids and polyphenols (e.g., methylglyoxal, B-defensin, chrysin), can have direct antimicrobial activity against planktonic bacteria and those existing in biofilms [23], or against viruses, fungi, and protozoa [27]. No resistance to honey has been reported to date because of the multitude of antimicrobial mechanisms [28]. Moreover, MGH possesses an immunomodulatory activity, having a dual role in controlling inflammation and infection [29]. In the inflammatory phase, honey can stimulate pro-inflammatory cytokines such as TNF-α, IL-1β, and IL-6, and activate B-, T-lymphocytes, and neutrophils that subsequently help to resolve infections. Contiguously, honey can downregulate NF-$\kappa\beta$ and MAPK pathways and exert anti-inflammatory and antioxidant effects, stimulating wound healing and reducing scar formation [23,24,27,29]. MGH is considered safe in wound care, with minimal adverse effects. Honey allergy is very rare, with an estimated incidence of 1:100,000 people consuming honey [30]. Topical application of honey may be even less harmful than consuming it; however, it is not advised to use honey in people with a known allergy. Another side effect of honey may be experiencing a stinging or burning sensation upon application to injured tissue. This pain is thought to be caused by a strong osmotic effect, especially when high concentrations of honey are used. However, honey has also been reported to decrease pain levels during wound evolution [31]. Therefore, MGH may be a good therapy option for perineal wounds.

This study aims to conduct a literature search to investigate the clinical efficacy and the effects on experienced pain and wound healing of honey on episiotomy wounds or perineal tears.

2. Results

2.1. Study Selection

A systematic literature search was performed in databases PubMed, Embase, Cochrane, EBSCO host/CINAHL, Web of Science, and Scopus, followed by a free-text search on Google Scholar. More details on the search strategy, study selection, and data extraction can be found in the methods section. A total of 55 studies were identified from different databases, as demonstrated in the flowchart (Figure 1). The duplicates (n = 26) were removed before screening, and 29 articles remained. These remaining articles were screened, and 17 were excluded based on title and abstract when it was clear that the topic of the publication was unrelated. The full text of twelve reports was sought, of which two could not be retrieved (no full text available). In the end, 10 studies were included in this article.

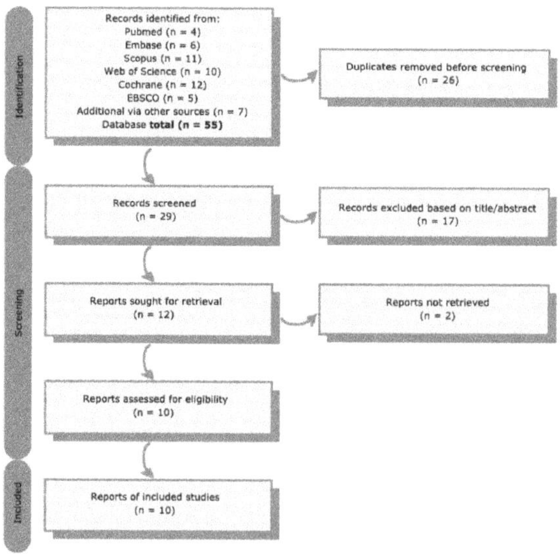

Figure 1. Flowchart study selection.

2.2. Study Characteristics

The ten studies have a total of 723 participants who received an episiotomy or had a perineal tear. The number of participants per study ranged from 20 to 120. In three studies it remains unclear whether participants had perineal tears or episiotomies (n = 86). In the other studies, a total of 579 participants received an episiotomy and 50 participants had perineal tears. Due to the loss of follow-up in one of these studies [32], the perineal trauma status for eight participants remains unknown. Different outcome measures were examined; the majority of studies had episiotomy wound healing as the primary outcome measure, assessed through the REEDA-score (see Table 1). This scale can be used to evaluate the wound healing process by describing the following five parameters: redness, edema, ecchymosis, discharge, and approximation of perineal tissue [33,34]. A lower total score indicates better wound healing.

Table 1. REEDA scoring system. Total score of 0 = healed; 1–5 = moderately healed; 6–10 = mildly healed; 11–15 = not healed. S = significant improvement in at least one interval, NS = non-significant effect.

Score	Redness	Edema	Ecchymosis	Discharge	Approximation
0	None	None	None	None	Closed
1	<0.25 cm of incision bilaterally	Perineal <1 cm from incision	<0.25 cm bilaterally or 0.5 cm unilaterally of incision	Serous	Skin separation <3 mm
2	<0.5 cm of incision bilaterally	Perineal and/or 1–2 cm from incision	<0.25–1 cm bilaterally or 0.5–2 cm unilaterally of incision	Serosanguineous	Skin and subcutaneous fat separation
3	>0.5 cm of incision bilaterally	Perineal and/or vulvar >2 cm from incision	>1 cm bilaterally or 2 cm unilaterally of incision	Bloody purulent	Skin, subcutaneous fat, and fascial layer separation

Five studies investigated the effect of honey on perineal pain intensity, assessed through the Visual Analogue Scale (VAS) for instance. Other outcome measures were pricking or burning sensation and tenderness (VAS), the number and dosage of pain relief drugs used, and the size of the wound (cm). Six study designs are randomized controlled trials (RCTs). Also, two comparative clinical study designs are used, a quasi-experimental posttest-only control group design and a one-group pretest–posttest design. Of all the studies, four took place in Iran, three in India, two in Indonesia, and one in Switzerland.

A clear overview of the included studies is provided in Table 2. Here, more detailed study characteristics such as the year of publication, country, study design, number of participants, inclusion and exclusion criteria, intervention and treatment details, control group, outcomes, and main conclusions are presented.

2.3. Data Synthesis

A meta-analysis could not be conducted due to the heterogeneity of studies. There are large variations in study design and intervention, e.g., honey formulation, dosing, application route, frequency of administration, and treatment duration, and differences in other study parameters, such as the use and composition of the control group, assessed outcome parameters, and evaluated time points (see Table 2). Due to the extensivity and diversity of the included studies, we created a new table to provide a quick overview of the results and enable a direct visual comparison of the studies (Table 3). The results can be divided into four key outcomes: wound healing, pain intensity, use of drugs to relieve pain, and pricking sensation. The significance level was included in the table depending on the study type having a control group.

Table 2. Overview of study characteristics and findings.

Selected Study, Year of Publication and Country	Trial Design and Sample Size	In- and Exclusion Criteria	Intervention	Control	Dosage/ Frequency of Treatment	Outcomes	Results/ Conclusion
Dompas et al. (2022), Indonesia [35]	One-group pretest–posttest design, $n = 20$	Not mentioned.	Group 1: 5 sheets of betel leaves boiled with 1000 mL water for 30 min to 600 mL, with pure honey.	No control group	Consuming twice a day (morning and evening) after bathing, for one week	**Wound healing *n* (%) Week 1:** Healed: 12/20 (60) Not healed: 8/20 (40)	There is an effect of green betel leaf water and pure honey on perineal wound healing in postpartum women.
Gerosa et al. (2022), Switzerland [32]	Randomized Controlled Trial (RCT), $n = 68$	**Inclusion:** >18 years, undergoing vaginal birth, speaking French, episiotomies or first- or second-degree perineal tears. **Exclusion:** third- or fourth-degree tears, postpartum hemorrhage >500 mL, allergy to honey or bee venom.	Group 1 (H): Medihoney (80% manuka honey, 20% wax) and standard maternity care.	Group 2 (C): only standard maternity care	Application on episiotomy wound after toileting practices, at least twice a day for 5 days postpartum.	**H vs. C** **Pain intensity, Mean VAS (SD)** Day (D)1: VAS 3.34 (2.35) vs. 3.38 (2.14), $p = 0.65$ D4: VAS 1.41 (1.49) vs. 2.28 (1.96), $p = 0.09$ **Qualitative pain: Questionnaire de Douleur Saint-Antoine. Mean intensity score (SD)** D1: 9.55 (7.03) vs. 8.63 (7.64), $p = 0.42$ D4: 3.93 (3.90) vs. 6.3 (7.94), $p = 0.46$ **Burning sensation during urination Mean VAS (SD)** D1: 2.64 (2.52) vs. 2.42 (2.18), $p = 0.99$ D4: 1.32 (1.93) vs. 1.73 (2.07), $p = 0.31$ **Woman who used pain relief drugs *n* (%)** D1: 23/29 (79.31) vs. 26/31 (83.87), $p = 0.75$ D4: 13/28 (46.43) vs. 17/31 (54.84), $p = 0.61$ **Mean ibuprofen use mg (SD)** D1: 707.14 (614.59) vs. 646.67 (537.38), $p = 0.79$ D4: 192.59 (339.60) vs. 466.67 (539.05), $p = 0.049$	There was no significant difference regarding pain intensity on day 1. On day 4, the VAS was 1.41 in the honey group versus 2.28 in the control group. However, this was also not significant ($p = 0.09$). A total of 93% of the women were (very) satisfied with the use of honey. There was a significant decrease in the use of ibuprofen on day 4 in favor of the honey group.

Table 2. *Cont.*

Selected Study, Year of Publication and Country	Trial Design and Sample Size	In- and Exclusion Criteria	Intervention	Control	Dosage/ Frequency of Treatment	Outcomes	Results/ Conclusion
Ghaderbasti (2022), Iran [36]	Double-blind RCT $n = 165$	**Inclusion:** primiparous women with a singleton pregnancy, gestational age of 37–42 weeks, cephalic presentation, BMI of 19.8–26, spontaneous vaginal delivery, and mediolateral episiotomy. No history of previous injury or surgery and visible lesions of the perineum, no continuous attachment, no rupture of the water sac for >18 h, no abnormal bleeding after delivery, no manual removal of the placenta, no perineal hematoma. **Exclusion:** unwillingness to continue participating in the study, incorrect use of creams, allergy to honey or olive oil, sexual intercourse in the first 10 days after delivery, history of diabetes, hypertension, cardiovascular or respiratory diseases, or any chronic illness affecting wound healing.	Group 1 (H): natural honey cream, with 0.2 paraben added as a preservative. Group 2 (O): pure olive oil Lanolin alcohol was used as the base of the creams.	Group 3 (C): placebo cream with the same weight, color, shape, and smell as the intervention groups.	Application on episiotomy wound every 12 h, up to 10 days postpartum.	**H vs. O vs. C** **Wound healing. Mean REEDA (SD)** Baseline: 4.76 (0.94) vs. 4.78 (1.03) vs. 4.82 (0.81), p = 0.955 D5: 2.64 (0.88) vs. 2.98 (1.01) vs. 5.27 (1.19), $p = 0.0001$ D10: 0.64 (0.63) vs. 1.04 (1.25) vs. 2.90 (0.74), $p = 0.0001$	The honey group had a significantly greater reduction in mean REEDA score, compared to the olive oil group. However, olive oil also showed positive effects.
Jaiswal et al. (2019), India [37]	Single-blind comparative clinical study. $n = 30$	**Inclusion:** both primiparous and multiparous women aged 18–40 years, undergoing normal vaginal delivery with an episiotomy wound. **Exclusion:** abnormal labor, third- or fourth-degree perineal tear, any complications like cervical tear or postpartum hemorrhage, systemic illness like diabetes mellitus, hypertension, etc.	Group 1 (H): Sharapunkha Moola twak kalka with honey (cream). Group 2 (J): Jatyadi taila (herb oil).	No control group	Application on episiotomy wound for three days. Dosage and frequency of application were not mentioned.	**Perineal pain (D3):** H: Mean negative rank (MR) = 7.5. Sum of negative ranks (SR) = 105, $p = 0.000$ J: MR = 7.0 SR = 91, $p = 0.000$ **Pricking sensation (D3):** H: MR = 3 SR = 15, $p = 0.034$ J: MR = 1.5. SR = 3, $p = 0.157$ **Tenderness (D3):** H: MR = 5 SR = 45, $p = 0.006$ J: MR = 7.65. SR = 99.5, $p = 0.002$ Wound healing (REEDA scale) **Redness (D3):** H: MR = 3.5. SR = 21, $p = 0.024$ J: MR = 3. SR = 15, $p = 0.038$ **Edema (D3):** H: MR = 3.5. SR = 21. $p = 0.014$ J: MR = 2. SR = 6. $p = 0.102$	In group 1, before- and after treatment, statistically significant results were obtained regarding pain ($p = 0.000$), pricking sensation ($p = 0.034$), tenderness ($p = 0.006$), redness ($p = 0.034$) and edema ($p = 0.014$). In group 2, before and after treatment, statistically significant results were obtained regarding pain ($p = 0.000$), tenderness ($p = 0.002$) and redness ($p = 0.038$), but not for pricking sensation (0.157) and edema (p = 0.102).

Table 2. *Cont.*

Selected Study, Year of Publication and Country	Trial Design and Sample Size	In- and Exclusion Criteria	Intervention	Control	Dosage/ Frequency of Treatment	Outcomes	Results/ Conclusion
Lavaf et al. (2017), Iran [38]	Double blind-three group RCT $n = 120$	**Inclusion:** among others, Iranian nationality, nulliparity, age 18–35 years, pregnancy with singleton live fetus and cephalic presentation, newborn weight of 2500–4000 gr, BMI 19.8–30, not taking medications and psychotropic drugs, not developing wound healing disruptive disorders, and no previous damages from operations in perineal region, no rupture of amniotic membrane for >18 h. **Exclusion:** using healing medications, lack of regular cream-usage according to prescription, allergy to cream, refusal of participation, having sexual intercourse in the first 5 days postpartum, refusing to attend the hospital on the 7th and 15th day.	Group 1 (H): natural honey from the Qamsar region. Concentration of 30%. Group 2 (Ph): sodium Phenytoin cream 1%.	Group 3 (C): placebo in a metal 30 g tube	Application of one knuckle of cream on episiotomy wound, once, at night, for 10 days.	**H vs. Ph vs. CE pisiotomy wound healing. (Total REEDA score), *n* (%), D7:** (score 0): 16 (48.4) vs. 14 (38.8) vs. 10 (26.3) (score 1–2): 15 (45.5) vs. 19 (52.7) vs. 20 (52.6) (score 3–5): 2 (6.1) vs. 3 (8.5) vs. 8 (21.1) $p = 0.011$ H vs. C with Mann–Whitney U test and Bonferroni correction: $p = 0.005$ **Wound discharge. *n* (%), D7:** No discharge: 28 (84.8) vs. 30 (83.3) vs. 21 (55.2) Serous: 5 (15.2) vs. 6 (16.7) vs. 15 (39.4) Bloody plasma: 0 vs. 0 vs. 1 (2.7) Septic–bloody: 0 vs. 0 vs. 1 (2.7) $p = 0.004$ Mann–Whitney U test H vs. C: $p = 0.008$ **Pain intensity [numeric scale], *n* (%), D7:** No pain [0]: 10 (30.5) vs. 4 (11.1) vs. 7 (18.4) Mild pain [1–3]: 11 (33.3) vs. 20 (55.5) vs. 14 (36.8) Middle pain [4–7]: 6 (18.1) vs. 10 (27.7) vs. 13 (34.3) Severe pain [8–10]: 6 (18.1) vs. 2 (5.7) vs. 4 (10.5) $p = 0.8$ **D14:** No pain [0]: 25 (75.7) vs. 28 (81.3) vs. 21 (55.2) Mild pain [1–3]: 4 (12.1) vs. 5 (10.8) vs. 10 (26.4) Middle pain [4–7]: 4 (12.1) vs. 3 (8.3) vs. 7 (18.4) Severe pain [8–10]:0 vs. 0 vs. 0 $p = 0.19$	There was a significant difference in total REEDA score between honey and the control group on the 7th day. There was also a significant difference in episiotomy wound discharge between honey and the control group. There was no significant difference between the three groups regarding pain intensity on the 7th or 14th day. There was no significant difference between the three groups regarding times of consumption of pain relief drugs.

Table 2. *Cont.*

Selected Study, Year of Publication and Country	Trial Design and Sample Size	In- and Exclusion Criteria	Intervention	Control	Dosage/ Frequency of Treatment	Outcomes	Results/ Conclusion
Manjula et al. (2012), India [39]	Unblinded RCT $n = 61$	**Inclusion:** postnatal women aged >18 years with right or left mediolateral episiotomy. **Exclusion:** not mentioned.	Group 1 (H): pure, natural honey without added sugar.	Group 2 (B): betadine	Application 5 mL of honey soaked in gauze to the episiotomy wound every 12 h until 5 days postpartum.	**H vs. B** **Wound healing. Mean episiotomy wound assessment score 0–18 (SD).** Baseline: 8.07 (2.27) vs. 8.23 (1.31), $p = 0.729$ D2: 4.53 (2.15) vs. 6.63 (1.94), $p = 0.000$ D3: 2.50 (1.82) vs. 3.93 (1.76), $p = 0.003$ D4: 0.90 (0.92) vs. 2.37 (1.59), $p = 0.000$ D5: 0.27 (0.64) vs. 1.40 (1.33), $p = 0.000$	There is a statistically significant difference between the healing pace of the honey group (faster) and the betadine group.
Mulyaningsih et al. (2021), Indonesia [40]	Quasi-experimental design, posttest-only control group design. $n = 36$	Not mentioned.	Group 1 (H): pineapple juice and honey.	Group 2 (C): no treatment	Consuming 150 mL pineapple juice and honey twice a day for 7 days.	**H vs. C** **Frequency healed wounds *n* (%)** Healed: 15/18 (83.3) vs. 3/18 (16.7) **Wound healing mean (SD)** (outcome measurement not specified) 24.50 (507) vs. 12.50 (507) Mann–Whitney U test $p = 0.000$	Pineapple juice and honey had a significant effect on the acceleration of perineal wound healing.
Nikpour et al. (2019), Iran [41]	Double-blind three-group RCT. $n = 120$	**Inclusion:** age of 17–35 years, gestational age of 37–42 weeks, no smoking or drug abuse, no health conditions or medications that could negatively affect wound healing, no perineal hematoma, no abnormal vaginal bleeding, no third- or fourth-degree perineal tear, and no infantile hospitalization for >7 days. **Exclusion:** using the allocated treatment irregularly, failing to refer to the study setting for follow-up visits and assessments.	Group 1 (H): 35% honey. Group 2 (Cu): Curcumin 2%.	Group 3 (C): placebo containing glycerin, Carbopol, Eucerin triethanolamine, propylparaben, distilled water, and food dye.	Application on episiotomy wound twice daily for 10 postpartum days.	**H vs. Cu vs. C** **Pain intensity. Mean (SD)** 2 h: 4.20 (2.42) vs. 3.80 (2.04) vs. 4.14 (2.27), $p = 0.762$ D5: 2.83 (1.72) vs. 3.90 (2.40) vs. 3.69 (2.17), $p = 0.121$ D10: 1.36 (1.24) vs. 2.06 (2.06) vs. 1.96 (1.42), $p = 0.202$ Group: $p = 0.253$ **Wound healing. Mean REEDA (SD)** 2 h: 2.30 (1.60) vs. 2.47 (1.40) vs. 2.79 (1.84) $p = 0.498$ D5: 2.00 (1.50) vs. 2.47 (1.25) vs. 2.21 (1.17) $p = 0.395$ D10: 1.73 (1.41) vs. 1.63 (1.27) vs. 1.83 (1.10) $p = 0.842$ Group: $p = 0.547$	There was no significant difference among the three groups regarding wound healing or pain intensity.

Table 2. *Cont.*

Selected Study, Year of Publication and Country	Trial Design and Sample Size	In- and Exclusion Criteria	Intervention	Control	Dosage/ Frequency of Treatment	Outcomes	Results/ Conclusion
Pal et al. (2017), India [42]	Comparative clinical study. $n = 30$	**Inclusion:** women aged 20–35 years, who underwent normal vaginal delivery with episiotomy or first- or second-degree perineal tear, patients who had regular antenatal checkups and previous routine investigations performed regularly. **Exclusion:** severe anemia, third degree perineal tear, any skin disease, allergic reaction, positive VDRL (Venereal Disease Research Laboratory test), HIV, HbsAg, systemic illness like diabetes mellitus, tuberculosis, thyroid dysfunction, hypertension, etc.	Group 1 (H): Nimbadi ointment, containing Nimba, Daruharidra, Yastimadhu, and Tila; the base is honey and ghee. Group 2 (Y): Yastyadi ointment, containing Yastimadhu, and Tila; the base is ghee.	No control group.	Application on the episiotomy wound twice a day for 14 days.	**Before treatment vs. after treatment** **Pain. Mean (SD)** H: 1.53 vs. 0.666 (0.833), $p = 0.002$ Y: 1.46 vs. 1.00 (0.51), $p = 0.15$ **Pricking sensation. Mean (SD)** H: 0.53 vs. 0.13 (0.50), $p = 0.031$Y: 0.73 vs. 0.26 (0.51), $p = 0.15$ **Tenderness Mean (SD)** H: 1.13 vs. 0.533 (0.632), $p = 0.07$ Y: 1.4 vs.1.0 (0.507), $p = 0.0313$ **Redness. Mean (SD)** H: 0.896 vs. 0.466 (0.56), $p = 0.002$ Y: 1.26 vs. 0.733 (0.51), $p = 0.007$ **Edema. Mean (SD)** H: 0.6 vs. 0.06 (0.83), $p = 0.031$ Y: 0.6 vs. 0.2 (0.63), $p = 0.062$ **Ecchymosis. Mean (SD)** H: 0.93 vs. 0.33 (0.50), $p = 0.003$ Y: 1.26 vs. 0.80 (0.51), $p = 0.01$ **Discharge. Mean (SD)** H: 0.46 vs. 0.06 (0.56), $p = 0.5$ Y: 0.33 vs. 0.066 (0.70), $p = 0.05$ **Approximation Mean (SD)** H: 0.20 vs. 0.06 (0.35), $p = 0.50$ Y: 0.26 vs. 0.13 (0.35), $p = 0.50$ The average improvement was 66.6% (group 1), compared to 49,8% (group 2) (all parameters)	Group 1 and 2 are not compared. In group 1, before- and after treatment, highly significant results were obtained regarding the relief of pain, tenderness, redness, and ecchymosis, and significant results were obtained regarding pricking sensation and edema. Discharge and approximation were insignificant. The average improvement was better in the Nimbadi-group than the Yastyadi-group.
Torkashvand et al. (2021), Iran [43]	RCT $n = 73$	**Inclusion:** among others, Iranian nationality, primiparous, age of 18–35 years, live term singleton pregnancy with vertex presentation, mediolateral episiotomy with no rupture, no chronic systemic diseases, no history of previous injury, surgery and visible lesions in the perineum. **Exclusion:** among others, reluctance to further participate in the study, use of other supplements for wound healing, incorrect usage of the ointment for >2 nights, sensitivity to Olea ointment.	Group 1 (H): olea ointment: herbal mixture of honey. (33.4%), olive oil (33.3%), and sesame oil (33.3%).	Group 2 (C): only routine hospital care as washing with normal saline twice per day until the 10th postpartum day.	Application on episiotomy wound at 4 h post-episiotomy and afterwards every 8 h until the 10th postpartum day.	**H vs. C** **Wound healing. Mean REEDA (SD)** Baseline: 2.72 (0.46) vs. 2.71 (0.46), $p = 0.91$ 2 h: 2.31 (0.47) vs. 2.65 (0.49), $p = 0.004$ 24 h: 1.67 (0.62) vs. 2.29 (0.46), $p < 0.001$ D5: 0.05 (0.22) vs. 0.35 (0.49), $p = 0.001$ D10: 0.00 vs. 0.29 (0.46), $p < 0.001$	There was a significant difference in episiotomy wound healing at four intervals between the Olea ointment and control group.

The effect of honey on wound healing was investigated in nine of the ten included studies. Eight studies reported beneficial effects of honey, five of these studies were with a control group [35–40,42,43]. Torkashvand et al. [43] demonstrated a significantly lower mean REEDA score in the Olea ointment group (honey) compared to the control group at four intervals. The same applies to the honey group in the RCT by Lavaf et al. [38] on the 7th day postpartum. The RCT by Manjula et al. [39] showed a significantly faster healing pace with honey compared to betadine, and the RCT of Ghaderbasti et al. [36] proved that there was a significantly greater reduction in REEDA score in the honey group compared to the olive oil group. Mulyaningsih et al. [40] conducted a quasi-experimental, posttest-only control group study, in which the consumption of pineapple juice and honey had a significant effect on the acceleration of perineal wound healing. Nikpour et al. did not find a significant difference in wound healing when comparing the mean REEDA scores of the different treatment groups (honey, curcumin, and placebo) [41]. Jaiswal et al. and Pal et al. performed comparative clinical studies in which the outcome after treatment was compared to baseline levels [37,42]. Jaiswal found significant improvements in redness and edema, while Pal found significant improvements in redness, edema, and ecchymosis, both supporting a positive effect in wound healing. The one-group pretest–posttest study by Dompas et al. [35] referred to 'an effect'. In this study, honey was consumed, combined with boiled water and betel leaves. This study did not examine whether the results were significant.

Regarding the intensity of pain, no significant differences were found in the RCTs of Gerosa et al., Nikpour et al., and Lavaf et al. [32,38,41]. However, 93% of the women in the study of Gerosa et al. were (very) satisfied with the use of honey. They found a significant decreases in the use of ibuprofen on day 4 in favor of the honey group despite the effects on pricking sensation being statistically non-significant. Lavaf did not find differences in the intake of pain relief drugs. However, Jaiswal et al. found significantly lower mean pain scores and less tenderness in the honey group after treatment when compared to before treatment [37]. In line with these findings, Pal et al. also demonstrated significantly reduced perineal pain, and less tenderness by honey [42].

Table 3. Summary of key outcomes per study. S = significant effect in favor of honey; NS = no significant difference; + = positive effect reported without significance mentioned (no control group).

Study	Wound Healing	Pain Intensity	Pain Relief Drugs Used	Pricking Sensation
Dompas, R. [35]	+			
Gerosa, D. [32]		NS	S	NS
Ghaderbasti, S. [36]	S			
Jaiswal, N. [37]	+	+		+
Lavaf, M. [38]	S	NS	NS	
Manjula, P. [39]	S			
Mulyaningsih, S. [40]	S			
Nikpour, M. [41]	NS	NS		
Pal, S. [42]	+	+		
Torkashvand, S. [43]	S			

3. Discussion

Many studies support the effectiveness of honey in wound management, for instance, in burns, diabetic foot ulcers, and chronic wounds [31,44,45]. Some studies indicate that honey can help reduce pain after tonsillectomy and in cold sores [46,47]. In this review,

10 studies were included, with a total of $n = 723$ participants who received an episiotomy or had a perineal tear. These studies have provided insight into the efficacy of honey on perineal trauma. Nine of the ten included studies found a positive effect of honey in at least one of the outcome measures. Wound healing was improved in eight out of nine studies, pain intensity was improved in two out of five studies, and pricking sensation and use of pain relief drugs improved in one out of two studies. Thus, it is found to accelerate recovery and improve the patient's quality of life. In line with the conclusions of most of the included studies, the use of honey for the treatment of perineal wounds can be recommended.

Despite the consistent findings in wound healing and sometimes positive outcomes in other parameters, it is hard to draw an overarching conclusion, and the results should be interpreted with caution. There are many variables in the study setup, intervention, control groups, evaluated time points, and outcome parameters. Two studies investigated the effect of consuming honey [35,40], while the other studies investigated the effect of local application. Not only does the application of honey vary, but the composition of honey does as well. For example, pure honey [39], a mixture of honey with olive oil and sesame oil [43], 80% Manuka honey with 20% wax [32], 30–35% honey [38,41], honey in combination with boiled betel leaves [35], and pineapple juice with honey [40] were used in the studies considered. A higher percentage of honey does not necessarily lead to a more significant improvement in wound healing. Even with lower concentrations of honey, such as 30%, significant improvements in wound healing are observed. Honey is a natural product and, due to differences in composition and quality, the biological activity of honey varies. In addition, there might have been some interaction between honey and other supplements; however, these comprehensive medical preparations can have an additive effect. More research into the chemical composition and identification of the bioactive compounds of honey or other supplements and their molecular targets may further improve the therapeutic action on vaginal trauma in the future. In contrast to regular honey, (supplemented) MGH is, at least, standardized and carefully checked to ensure its quality, safety, and efficacy, and it is considered more consistent in its activity [26,48]. Therefore, it is recommended that MGH be used in future studies.

Moreover, the overall quality of available evidence is limited. Many studies lack transparency in their presentation of the results and methods. For instance, in the results section of the study by Jaiswal et al. [37], several tables are presented without captions or clear explanations, which complicates the interpretation of the results. Some studies are less reliable due to the lack of clearly formulated inclusion and exclusion criteria, for instance in the studies of Mulyaningsih et al. [40] and Dompas et al. [35] In addition, only three RCTs were double-blinded [36,38,41]. The other studies were (probably) not blinded, or single-blind, because no information was given about blinding. Also, unreliable study designs are included, such as the one-group pretest–posttest design [35], and the quasi-experimental design [40]. Quasi-experimental designs are susceptible to confounding variables as there is a lack of randomization, which can lead to bias. The findings of these study designs have a higher chance of being influenced by external factors.

Also, multiple studies lacked a proper control group. For example, when comparing the findings after treatment to the baseline level (before treatment) [35,37,42]. For wound healing, pain, and other outcomes, maturation effects are probable, because of expected improvement over time. In addition, the control group of the included studies varied from no intervention to placebo, standard hospital care, or another non-conventional treatment. Standard care can differ between hospitals. Because there is no consistent control group across all studies, no overarching conclusions can be drawn. The studies conducted by Nikpour et al., Lavaf et al., and Ghaderbasti et al. compared honey with a placebo [36,38,41].

However, it is very challenging to create a placebo for honey, due to its distinctive texture and scent. This raises questions about the integrity of the blinding process, potentially introducing bias. In addition, a placebo can also have some activity, e.g., by creating a moist wound environment. This might be a possible explanation as to why no significant differences were found in the study by Nikpour et al.

In most studies where honey was applied topically, it was used twice daily for a duration of 3 to 14 days, mostly for 10 days. Only in the study of Torkashvand et al. [43] was it used every 8 h, and in the study of Lavaf et al. [38] honey is applied once daily. It cannot be concluded that applying honey more frequently leads to a greater significant improvement. Only two studies reported the dosing (5 mL and one knuckle of cream). The use of clear application protocols and standardized honey formulations should help to ensure consistent results in future studies.

Some studies used a small sample size of 20 or 30 participants [35,37,42]. Small sample sizes can lead to less precise, less powerful, and more biased results. The ten studies were conducted in only four countries: Iran, Switzerland, Indonesia, and India. Four of these studies were performed in Iran, and three in India. This can negatively impact the reliability of the findings because of potential cultural and socioeconomic biases.

Many of the included studies did not distinguish between perineal tears versus episiotomies. Therefore, it is not possible to draw reliable conclusions about the differential effects of honey on the type of perineal trauma. It is important to draw this distinction, because there may be a difference in healing between perineal tears and episiotomy wounds.

The strength of this review is that it offers a comprehensive overview of the current literature concerning the use of honey for episiotomy wounds and perineal tears regarding wound healing and perineal pain. This patient group is considered homogeneous, as all individuals are postpartum women within a similar age range. This review includes a wide range of recent studies, with different study designs. Due to the systematic approach of our search, the extensivity of the search terms, and the search being performed in six different databases (and using additional sources), we expect that all relevant papers were found and included in this review.

To our knowledge, no previous literature review has specifically focused on perineal trauma and honey. However, Barbosa et al. conducted a systematic review recently (2024) investigating the effects of honey on wound healing and pain relief in obstetric wounds, including cesarean sections, episiotomies, and perineal tears, based exclusively on randomized controlled trials [49]. Surprisingly, they included only two RCTs with perineal wounds. Our review included six RCTs and other study designs. In addition, this review focused on perineal trauma, as cesarean sections and perineal injuries are not comparable, particularly due to differences in location, structure, and the microbiome. Barbosa et al. [49] concluded that honey has no significant improvement in wound healing, but that it is effective in reducing pain and decreasing the use of pain control medication.

This study is a good foundation for further research. Future studies are recommended to use MGH in (double)blinded randomized controlled trials. A power calculation is required to determine the sample size. Also, more research about adverse events, patient satisfaction, and overall experiences with honey treatment is warranted. Other outcome measures that should be examined include the effect of honey on scar formation, dyspareunia, infection and dehiscence, psychological well-being, and healthcare costs. MGH has been found effective in preventing infections previously in other studies, e.g., for the treatment of lacerations and C-sections [50–52]. It would be interesting to investigate the prophylactic activity of MGH for perineal wounds in the future.

4. Materials and Methods

4.1. Search Strategy

A literature search was performed on 17 July 2024 in databases PubMed, Embase, Cochrane, EBSCO host/CINAHL, Web of Science, and Scopus. Additionally, a search was performed on Google Scholar, and the reference lists of all the included studies were reviewed manually for studies that were eligible for inclusion ("snowballing"). The literature search included all studies investigating the effect of honey on episiotomy wounds or perineal tears. MeSH-terms and free-text terms that were used are, for example, (episiotomy) [MeSH] OR (episiotomy*) OR (perineotom*) OR ("perineal tear*") OR ("perineal laceration*") OR ("vaginal tear*") AND (honey) [MeSH]. The full searches conducted in the different databases can be seen in 'Appendix A'. Filters were not added regarding language or date of publication.

4.2. Study Selection

After obtaining all references, duplicates were removed. The first selection was based on the title and abstract. Next, the full texts were retrieved and assessed to see if they met the inclusion and exclusion criteria. The inclusion criteria were as follows: (1). studies with postpartum women who had a vaginal delivery and received an episiotomy, or had a perineal tear; (2). treatment with honey, compared to (no) control group or placebo; (3). the outcome measure being pain or wound healing. Exclusion criteria were as follows: (1). no episiotomy or perineal tear; (2). no intervention with honey; (3). there is no possibility of extracting data. The search included studies and articles published in any language. Whenever necessary, studies not written in English were translated with 'Google Translate'. All articles were reviewed by one reviewer.

4.3. Data Extraction

The following data are extracted from the included studies: author, year of publication, research country, trial design, sample size, the inclusion-and-exclusion criteria, intervention and type of honey that was used, control group, dosage and frequency of treatment, outcome measures, results, and conclusion. Standardization of the study characteristics is difficult due to the diversity of research aims, study setup, and differences in reported outcome measures. However, we have unbiased and concisely presented as much relevant information as possible.

5. Conclusions

The findings of this review suggest that honey potentially has a great effect on wound healing and pain intensity of perineal trauma, as several studies show promising outcomes. However, the overall quality of available evidence is limited. Therefore, additional research, preferably in well-described large RCTs using MGH, is needed to determine the efficacy of honey in perineal trauma and to establish guidelines for clinical use. Performing cost-efficacy studies and investigating the prophylactic activity of MGH would be of additional interest.

Author Contributions: Conceptualization, S.J.J.M.v.R. and N.A.J.C.; methodology, all authors; writing—original draft preparation, I.S.S. and C.M.J.G.L.; writing—review and editing, all authors; visualization, I.S.S. and C.M.J.G.L.; supervision, C.M.J.G.L., S.J.J.M.v.R. and N.A.J.C.; project administration, N.A.J.C. All authors have read and agreed to the published version of the manuscript.

Funding: This research received no external funding.

Data Availability Statement: No new data were created or analyzed in this study. Data sharing is not applicable to this article.

Conflicts of Interest: N.A.J.C. is employed by Triticum Exploitatie BV. Triticum Exploitatie BV is the manufacturer of the MGH-based formulation L-Mesitran. This review focuses on honey, in general, and not on the range of L-Mesitran products. We ensure that we have maintained the highest standards of integrity and presented the work in an unbiased manner. The remaining authors declare that the research was conducted in the absence of any commercial or financial relationships that could be construed as a potential conflict of interest.

Appendix A Full Literature Searches

The search was performed on 17 July 2024 on five different databases.

Pubmed:

((((((((((((episiotomy[MeSH Terms]) OR (episiotom* [tiab])) OR (perineotom* [tiab])) OR (perineal tear* [tiab])) OR (perineal laceration* [tiab])) OR (perineal injur* [tiab])) OR (perineal trauma* [tiab])) OR (obstetric tear* [tiab])) OR (obstetric laceration* [tiab])) OR (vaginal tear* [tiab])) OR (vaginal laceration* [tiab])) OR (childbirth tear* [tiab])) OR (childbirth laceration* [tiab])) AND ((((((((((((((medical grade honey [tiab]) OR (therapeutic honey [tiab])) OR (medicinal honey [tiab])) OR (honey therap* [tiab])) OR (honey treatment [tiab])) OR (antibacterial honey [tiab])) OR (antimicrobial honey [tiab])) OR (medihoney [tiab])) OR (mesitran [tiab])) OR (manuka honey [tiab])) OR (leptospermum honey [tiab])) OR (tualang honey [tiab])) OR (honey [tiab])) OR (surgihoney [tiab])) OR (activon [tiab]))

Total hits: 5.

Cochrane Library:

1. ((episiotom*) OR (perineotom*) OR (perineal NEXT tear*) OR (perineal NEXT laceration*) OR (perineal NEXT injur*) OR (perineal NEXT trauma*) OR (obstetric NEXT laceration*) OR (vaginal NEXT tear*) OR (vaginal NEXT laceration*) OR (childbirth NEXT tear*) OR (childbirth NEXT laceration*)) (Word variations have been searched)
2. ((“medical grade honey”) OR (“medicinal honey”) OR (honey NEXT therap*) OR (“honey treatment”) OR (“antibacterial honey”) OR (“antimicrobial honey”) OR (“medihoney”) OR (“mesitran”) OR (“manuka honey”) OR (“leptospermum honey”) OR (“tualang honey”) OR (“honey”) OR (“surgihoney”) OR (“activon”)) (Word variations have been searched)
3. #1 AND #2

Total hits: 12.

Scopus:

((TITLE-ABS-KEY (“medical grade honey”)) OR (TITLE-ABS-KEY (“therapeutic honey”)) OR (TITLE-ABS-KEY (“medicinal honey”)) OR (TITLE-ABS-KEY (“honey therap*”)) OR (TITLE-ABS-KEY (“honey treatment”)) OR (TITLE-ABS-KEY (“antibacterial honey”)) OR (TITLE-ABS-KEY (“antimicrobial honey”)) OR (TITLE-ABS-KEY (medihoney)) OR (TITLE-ABS-KEY (mesitran)) OR (TITLE-ABS-KEY (“manuka honey”)) OR (TITLE-ABS-KEY (“tualang honey”)) OR (TITLE-ABS-KEY (“honey”)) OR (TITLE-ABS-KEY (surgihoney)) OR (TITLE-ABS-KEY (“leptospermum honey”)) OR (TITLE-ABS-KEY (activon))) AND ((TITLE-ABS-KEY (“childbirth laceration*”)) OR (TITLE-ABS-KEY (“childbirth tear*”)) OR (TITLE-ABS-KEY (“vaginal laceration*”)) OR (TITLE-ABS-KEY (“vaginal tear*”)) OR (TITLE-ABS-KEY (“obstetric laceration*”)) OR (TITLE-ABS-KEY (“obstetric tear*”)) OR (TITLE-ABS-KEY (“perineal trauma*”)) OR (TITLE-ABS-KEY (“perineal injur*”)) OR (TITLE-ABS-KEY (“perineal laceration*”)) OR (TITLE-ABS-KEY (“perineal tear*”)) OR (TITLE-ABS-KEY (perineotom*)) OR (TITLE-ABS-KEY (episiotom*)))

Total hits: 11.

Web of Science:

4. (TS = (episiotom*)) OR (TS = (perineotom*)) OR (TS = ("perineal tear*")) OR (TS = ("perineal laceration*")) OR (TS = ("perineal injur*")) OR (TS = ("perineal trauma*")) OR (TS = ("obstetric tear*")) OR (TS = ("obstetric laceration*")) OR (TS = ("vaginal tear*")) OR (TS = ("vaginal laceration*")) OR (TS = ("childbirth laceration*"))
5. (TS = ("therapeutic honey")) OR (TS = ("medical grade honey")) OR (TS = ("medicinal honey")) OR (TS = ("honey therap*")) OR (TS = ("honey treatment")) OR (TS = ("antibacterial honey")) OR (TS = ("antimicrobial honey")) OR (TS = (medihoney)) OR (TS = (mesitran)) OR (TS = ("manuka honey")) OR (TS = ("leptospermum honey")) OR (TS = ("honey")) OR (TS = ("tualang honey")) OR (TS = (surgihoney)) OR (TS = (activon))
6. #1 AND #2

   Total hits: 10.

EBSCO host/CINAHL:

7. (TI episiotom* OR AB episiotom* OR MH episiotom*) OR (TI perineotom* OR AB perineotom* OR MH perineotom*) OR (TI "perineal tear*" OR AB "perineal tear*" OR MH "perineal tear*") OR (TI "perineal trauma*" OR AB "perineal trauma*" OR MH "perineal trauma*") OR (TI "perineal laceration*" OR AB "perineal laceration*" OR MH "perineal laceration*") OR (TI "perineal injur*" OR AB "perineal injur*" OR MH "perineal injur*") OR (TI "obstetric tear*" OR AB "obstetric tear*" OR MH "obstetric tear*") OR (TI "obstetric laceration*" OR AB "obstetric laceration*" OR MH "obstetric laceration*") OR (TI "vaginal tear*" OR AB "vaginal tear*" OR MH "vaginal tear*") OR (TI "vaginal laceration*" OR AB "vaginal laceration*" OR MH "vaginal laceration*") OR (TI "childbirth tear*" OR AB "childbirth tear*" OR MH "childbirth tear*") OR (TI "childbirth laceration*" OR AB "childbirth laceration*" OR MH "childbirth laceration*")
8. (TI "medical grade honey" OR AB "medical grade honey" OR MH "medical grade honey") OR (TI "therapeutic honey" OR AB "therapeutic honey" OR MH "therapeutic honey") OR (TI "medicinal honey" OR AB "medicinal honey" OR MH "medicinal honey") OR (TI "honey therap*" OR AB "honey therap*" OR MH "honey therap*") OR (TI "honey treatment" OR AB "honey treatment" OR MH "honey treatment") OR (TI "antibacterial honey" OR AB "antibacterial honey" OR MH "antibacterial honey") OR (TI "antimicrobial honey" OR AB "antimicrobial honey" OR MH "antimicrobial honey") OR (TI medihoney OR AB medihoney OR MH medihoney) OR (TI mesitran OR AB mesitran OR MH mesitran) OR (TI "manuka honey" OR AB "manuka honey" OR MH "manuka honey") OR (TI "leptospermum honey" OR AB "leptospermum honey" OR MH "leptospermum honey") OR (TI "tualang honey" OR AB "tualang honey" OR MH "tualang honey") OR (TI honey OR AB honey OR MH honey) OR (TI surgihoney OR AB surgihoney OR MH surgihoney) OR (TI activon OR AB activon OR MH activon)
9. S1 AND S2

   Total hits: 5.

Embase:

10. episiotom*.ti,ab,kf.
11. perineotom*.ti,ab,kf.
12. "perineal tear*".ti,ab,kf.
13. "perineal laceration*".ti,ab,kf.
14. "perineal trauma*".ti,ab,kf.
15. "obstetric tear*".ti,ab,kf.

16. "obstetric laceration*".ti,ab,kf.
17. "vaginal tear*".ti,ab,kf.
18. "childbirth tear*".ti,ab,kf.
19. "childbirth laceration*".ti,ab,kf.
20. 1 or 2 or 3 or 4 or 5 or 6 or 7 or 8 or 9 or 10
21. "medical grade honey".ti,ab,kf.
22. "therapeutic honey".ti,ab,kf.
23. "medicinal honey".ti,ab,kf.
24. "honey therap*".ti,ab,kf.
25. "honey treatment".ti,ab,kf.
26. "antibacterial honey".ti,ab,kf.
27. "antimicrobial honey".ti,ab,kf.
28. medihoney.ti,ab,kf.
29. mesitran.ti,ab,kf.
30. "manuka honey".ti,ab,kf.
31. "leptospermum honey".ti,ab,kf.
32. "tualang honey".ti,ab,kf.
33. honey.ti,ab,kf.
34. surgihoney.ti,ab,kf.
35. activon.ti,ab,kf.
36. 12 or 13 or 14 or 15 or 16 or 17 or 18 or 19 or 20 or 21 or 22 or 23 or 24 or 25 or 26
37. 11 and 27

Total hits: 6.

Google Scholar:

"Episiotomy wounds" AND "honey".
Total hits: 938.
Until page 41.

References

1. Frohlich, J.; Kettle, C. Perineal care. *BMJ Clin. Evid.* **2015**, *2015*, 1401. [PubMed]
2. Opondo, C.; Harrison, S.; Sanders, J.; Quigley, M.A.; Alderdice, F. The relationship between perineal trauma and postpartum psychological outcomes: A secondary analysis of a population-based survey. *BMC Pregnancy Childbirth* **2023**, *23*, 639. [CrossRef] [PubMed]
3. Smith, L.A.; Price, N.; Simonite, V.; Burns, E.E. Incidence of and risk factors for perineal trauma: A prospective observational study. *BMC Pregnancy Childbirth* **2013**, *13*, 59. [CrossRef] [PubMed]
4. Seijmonsbergen-Schermers, A.; Thompson, S.; Feijen-de Jong, E.; Smit, M.; Prins, M.; van den Akker, T.; de Jonge, A. Understanding the perspectives and values of midwives, obstetricians and obstetric registrars regarding episiotomy: Qualitative interview study. *BMJ Open* **2021**, *11*, e037536. [CrossRef] [PubMed]
5. Perined. *Perinatale Zorg in Nederland Anno 2020: Duiding Door Landelijke Perinatale Audit en Registratie*; Perined: Utrecht, The Netherlands, 2021.
6. ACOG Practice Bulletin No. 198: Prevention and Management of Obstetric Lacerations at Vaginal Delivery. *Obstet. Gynecol.* **2018**, *132*, e87–e102. [CrossRef]
7. Barjon, K.; Vadakekut, E.S.; Mahdy, H. Episiotomy. In *StatPearls*; StatPearls Publishing: Treasure Island, FL, USA, 2024.
8. Carroli, G.; Mignini, L. Episiotomy for vaginal birth. *Cochrane Database Syst. Rev.* **2009**, *1*, CD000081. [CrossRef]
9. Goh, R.; Goh, D.; Ellepola, H. Perineal tears—A review. *Aust. J. Gen. Pract.* **2018**, *47*, 35–38. [CrossRef]
10. Okeahialam, N.A.; Sultan, A.H.; Thakar, R. The prevention of perineal trauma during vaginal birth. *Am. J. Obstet. Gynecol.* **2024**, *230*, S991–S1004. [CrossRef]
11. Richtlijnendatabase. Routinematig Episiotomie Bij Kunstverlossing. Available online: https://richtlijnendatabase.nl/richtlijn/totaalruptuur/preventie_van_een_ruptuur/routinematige_episiotomie_bij_kunstverlossing_2024.html (accessed on 12 August 2024).

12. World Health Organization. *WHO Recommendations: Intrapartum Care for a Positive Childbirth Experience*; WHO/RHR/18.12; World Health Organization: Geneva, Switzerland, 2018; ISBN-13: 978-92-4-155021-5.
13. Ramar, C.N.; Vadakekut, E.S.; Grimes, W.R. Perineal Lacerations. In *StatPearls*; StatPearls Publishing: Treasure Island, FL, USA, 2024.
14. Andrews, V.; Thakar, R.; Sultan, A.H.; Jones, P.W. Evaluation of postpartum perineal pain and dyspareunia--a prospective study. *Eur. J. Obstet. Gynecol. Reprod. Biol.* **2008**, *137*, 152–156. [CrossRef]
15. Macarthur, A.J.; Macarthur, C. Incidence, severity, and determinants of perineal pain after vaginal delivery: A prospective cohort study. *Am. J. Obstet. Gynecol.* **2004**, *191*, 1199–1204. [CrossRef]
16. Klein, M.C.; Gauthier, R.J.; Robbins, J.M.; Kaczorowski, J.; Jorgensen, S.H.; Franco, E.D.; Johnson, B.; Waghorn, K.; Gelfand, M.M.; Guralnick, M.S.; et al. Relationship of episiotomy to perineal trauma and morbidity, sexual dysfunction, and pelvic floor relaxation. *Am. J. Obstet. Gynecol.* **1994**, *171*, 591–598. [CrossRef] [PubMed]
17. Vieira, F.; Guimaraes, J.V.; Souza, M.C.S.; Sousa, P.M.L.; Santos, R.F.; Cavalcante, A. Scientific evidence on perineal trauma during labor: Integrative review. *Eur. J. Obstet. Gynecol. Reprod. Biol.* **2018**, *223*, 18–25. [CrossRef] [PubMed]
18. Kamel, A.; Khaled, M. Episiotomy and obstetric perineal wound dehiscence: Beyond soreness. *J. Obstet. Gynaecol.* **2014**, *34*, 215–217. [CrossRef]
19. Jones, K.; Webb, S.; Manresa, M.; Hodgetts-Morton, V.; Morris, R.K. The incidence of wound infection and dehiscence following childbirth-related perineal trauma: A systematic review of the evidence. *Eur. J. Obstet. Gynecol. Reprod. Biol.* **2019**, *240*, 1–8. [CrossRef] [PubMed]
20. Fenner, D.E.; Genberg, B.; Brahma, P.; Marek, L.; DeLancey, J.O. Fecal and urinary incontinence after vaginal delivery with anal sphincter disruption in an obstetrics unit in the United States. *Am. J. Obstet. Gynecol.* **2003**, *189*, 1543–1549; discussion 1549–1550. [CrossRef]
21. LaCross, A.; Groff, M.; Smaldone, A. Obstetric anal sphincter injury and anal incontinence following vaginal birth: A systematic review and meta-analysis. *J. Midwifery Womens Health* **2015**, *60*, 37–47. [CrossRef]
22. Andreucci, C.B.; Bussadori, J.C.; Pacagnella, R.C.; Chou, D.; Filippi, V.; Say, L.; Cecatti, J.G.; Brazilian, C.S.G.; Group, W.H.O.M.M.W. Sexual life and dysfunction after maternal morbidity: A systematic review. *BMC Pregnancy Childbirth* **2015**, *15*, 307. [CrossRef]
23. Saikaly, S.K.; Khachemoune, A. Honey and Wound Healing: An Update. *Am. J. Clin. Dermatol.* **2017**, *18*, 237–251. [CrossRef]
24. Scepankova, H.; Combarros-Fuertes, P.; Fresno, J.M.; Tornadijo, M.E.; Dias, M.S.; Pinto, C.A.; Saraiva, J.A.; Estevinho, L.M. Role of Honey in Advanced Wound Care. *Molecules* **2021**, *26*, 4784. [CrossRef]
25. Minden-Birkenmaier, B.A.; Bowlin, G.L. Honey-Based Templates in Wound Healing and Tissue Engineering. *Bioengineering* **2018**, *5*, 46. [CrossRef]
26. Hermanns, R.; Mateescu, C.; Thrasyvoulou, A.; Tananaki, C.; Wagener, F.A.D.T.G.; Cremers, N.A.J. Defining the standards for medical grade honey. *J. Apic. Res.* **2020**, *59*, 125–135. [CrossRef]
27. Oryan, A.; Alemzadeh, E.; Moshiri, A. Biological properties and therapeutic activities of honey in wound healing: A narrative review and meta-analysis. *J. Tissue Viability* **2016**, *25*, 98–118. [CrossRef] [PubMed]
28. Pleeging, C.C.F.; Coenye, T.; Mossialos, D.; de Rooster, H.; Chrysostomou, D.; Wagener, F.; Cremers, N.A.J. Synergistic Antimicrobial Activity of Supplemented Medical-Grade Honey against Pseudomonas aeruginosa Biofilm Formation and Eradication. *Antibiotics* **2020**, *9*, 866. [CrossRef] [PubMed]
29. Pleeging, C.C.F.; Wagener, F.; de Rooster, H.; Cremers, N.A.J. Revolutionizing non-conventional wound healing using honey by simultaneously targeting multiple molecular mechanisms. *Drug Resist. Updates* **2022**, *62*, 100834. [CrossRef] [PubMed]
30. Aguiar, R.; Duarte, F.C.; Mendes, A.; Bartolome, B.; Barbosa, M.P. Anaphylaxis caused by honey: A case report. *Asia Pac. Allergy* **2017**, *7*, 48–50. [CrossRef]
31. Holubova, A.; Chlupacova, L.; Krocova, J.; Cetlova, L.; Peters, L.J.F.; Cremers, N.A.J.; Pokorna, A. The Use of Medical Grade Honey on Infected Chronic Diabetic Foot Ulcers-A Prospective Case-Control Study. *Antibiotics* **2023**, *12*, 1364. [CrossRef]
32. Gerosa, D.; Santagata, M.; Martinez de Tejada, B.; Guittier, M.-J. Application of Honey to Reduce Perineal Laceration Pain during the Postpartum Period: A Randomized Controlled Trial. *Healthcare* **2022**, *10*, 1515. [CrossRef]
33. Alvarenga, M.B.; Francisco, A.A.; de Oliveira, S.M.; da Silva, F.M.; Shimoda, G.T.; Damiani, L.P. Episiotomy healing assessment: Redness, Oedema, Ecchymosis, Discharge, Approximation (REEDA) scale reliability. *Rev. Lat. Am. Enferm.* **2015**, *23*, 162–168. [CrossRef]
34. Armata, N.N. REEDA: Episiotomy Healing Assessment Acronym. Available online: https://www.osmosis.org/answers/reeds-episiotomy-healing-assessment-acronym (accessed on 12 August 2024).
35. Dompas, R.; Montolalu, A.; Koloay, T.G. Green Betel Leaf Water with Pure Honey Against Healing Perineum's Wounds Mother Postpartum. *J. Midwifery* **2022**, *8*, 13. [CrossRef]
36. Ghaderbasti, S.; Kabuli, K.S.; Farhadifar, F.; Shahavi, R. Comparative study of the effect of honey cream and olive oil cream on the healing rate of episiotomy. *Iran. J. Women Midwifery Infertil* **2022**, *25*, 81–93.

37. Jaiswal, N.; Ramadevi, G. A Comparative Clinical Study Of Sharapunkha Moola Twak Kalka With Jatyadi Taila Application On Episiotomy Wound. *World J. Pharm. Res.* **2019**, *8*, 1011–1022.
38. Lavaf, M.; Simbar, M.; Mojab, F.; Alavi Majd, H.; Samimi, M. Comparison of honey and phenytoin (PHT) cream effects on intensity of pain and episiotomy wound healing in nulliparous women. *J. Complement. Integr. Med.* **2017**, *15*, 20160139. [CrossRef] [PubMed]
39. Manjula, P.; Rao, A.C.; Ranjani, P. Effectiveness of Honey Versus Betadine on Episiotomy Wound Healing. *I-Manag. J. Nurs.* **2012**, *2*, 32–37.
40. Mulyaningsih, S.; Dunggio, R.; Susanti, K.A. The Effect of Pineapple Juice and Honey on the Acceleration of Perineal Wound Healing in Post-Partum Mothers in the Work Area of Dr. M.M. Dunda Limboto Hospital. *J. Community Health Provis.* **2020**, *1*, 9–16. [CrossRef]
41. Nikpour, M.; Delavar, M.A.; Khafri, S.; Ghanbarpour, A.; Moghadamnia, A.A.; Esmaeilzadeh, S.; Behmanesh, F. The Use of Honey and Curcumin for Episiotomy Pain Relief and Wound Healing: A Three-Group Double-Blind Randomized Clinical Trial. *Nurs. Midwifery Stud.* **2019**, *8*, 64–69. [CrossRef]
42. Pal, S.; Pushpalatha, B.; Bharathi, K. A comparative clinical study of nimbadi and yastyadi ointment on episiotomy wound W.S.R. to wound healing. *Ayushdhara* **2017**, *4*, 1151–1158.
43. Torkashvand, S.; Jafarzadeh-Kenarsari, F.; Donyaei-Mobarrez, Y.; Gholami Chaboki, B. Effectiveness of Olea Herbal Ointment on Episiotomy Wound Healing Among Primiparous Women: A Randomized Clinical Trial. *Jundishapur J. Nat. Pharm. Prod.* **2021**, *16*, e104570. [CrossRef]
44. Al-Waili, N.; Salom, K.; Al-Ghamdi, A.A. Honey for wound healing, ulcers, and burns; data supporting its use in clinical practice. *Sci. World J.* **2011**, *11*, 766–787. [CrossRef]
45. Papanikolaou, G.E.; Gousios, G.; Cremers, N.A.J. Use of Medical-Grade Honey to Treat Clinically Infected Heel Pressure Ulcers in High-Risk Patients: A Prospective Case Series. *Antibiotics* **2023**, *12*, 605. [CrossRef]
46. Hwang, S.H.; Song, J.N.; Jeong, Y.M.; Lee, Y.J.; Kang, J.M. The efficacy of honey for ameliorating pain after tonsillectomy: A meta-analysis. *Eur. Arch. Oto-Rhino-Laryngol.* **2016**, *273*, 811–818. [CrossRef]
47. Naik, P.P.; Mossialos, D.; Wijk, B.V.; Novakova, P.; Wagener, F.; Cremers, N.A.J. Medical-Grade Honey Outperforms Conventional Treatments for Healing Cold Sores-A Clinical Study. *Pharmaceuticals* **2021**, *14*, 1264. [CrossRef] [PubMed]
48. Lardenoije, C.; van Riel, S.; Peters, L.J.F.; Wassen, M.; Cremers, N.A.J. Medical-Grade Honey as a Potential New Therapy for Bacterial Vaginosis. *Antibiotics* **2024**, *13*, 368. [CrossRef] [PubMed]
49. Ferraz Barbosa, B.; de Moraes, F.C.A.; Araujo Alves da Silva, B.; Bordignon Barbosa, C.; Pereira da Silva, I.; da Silva, E.R.; Barros, J.C.M.; Rebouças, L.W.C.; dos Santos, N.P.C.; Fernandes, M.R. The Use of Honey for Cicatrization and Pain Control of Obstetric Wounds: A Systematic Review and Meta-Analysis of Randomized Controlled Trials. *Nutrients* **2024**, *16*, 185. [CrossRef] [PubMed]
50. Mandel, H.H.; Sutton, G.A.; Abu, E.; Kelmer, G. Intralesional application of medical grade honey improves healing of surgically treated lacerations in horses. *Equine Vet. J.* **2020**, *52*, 41–45. [CrossRef]
51. Bocoum, A.; Riel, S.; Traore, S.O.; Ngo Oum Ii, E.F.; Traore, Y.; Thera, A.T.; Fane, S.; Dembele, B.T.; Cremers, N.A.J. Medical-Grade Honey Enhances the Healing of Caesarean Section Wounds and Is Similarly Effective to Antibiotics Combined with Povidone-Iodine in the Prevention of Infections-A Prospective Cohort Study. *Antibiotics* **2023**, *12*, 92. [CrossRef]
52. Dryden, M.; Goddard, C.; Madadi, A.; Heard, M.; Saeed, K.; Cooke, J. Using antimicrobial surgihoneyto prevent caesarean wound infection. *Br. J. Midwifery* **2014**, *22*, 111–115. [CrossRef]

pharmaceuticals

MDPI

Article

Long-Term Supplementation of Royal Jelly (Raydel®) Improves Zebrafish Growth, Embryo Production and Survivability, Blood Lipid Profile and Functionality of Vital Organs: A 72-Weeks' Consumption Study

Kyung-Hyun Cho *, Hyo-Seon Nam, Ashutosh Bahuguna and Ji-Eun Kim

Raydel Research Institute, Medical Innovation Complex, Daegu 41061, Republic of Korea
* Correspondence: chok@raydel.co.kr; Tel.: +82-53-964-1990; Fax: +82-53-965-1992

Abstract: Royal jelly is a honeybee product with substantial pharmacological and health promotional activities. Nevertheless, the health implications associated with the prolonged dietary supplementation of royal jelly have yet to be elucidated extensively. Herein, 72 weeks of dietary supplementation of royal jelly at 5% and 10% (*w*/*w*) were investigated to assess the impact on zebrafish survivability, body weight, liver, testis, ovary functionality, and blood lipid profile. The results revealed no adverse effect of 72 weeks of royal jelly supplementation on zebrafish survivability. Conversely, a noteworthy enhancement in the zebrafish body weight was observed in royal-jelly-supplemented zebrafish in a concentration-dependent manner [5% and 10% (*w*/*w*)]. Interestingly, female zebrafish were found to be more biased, with a significant 17% ($p < 0.001$) and 23% ($p < 0.001$) higher body weight enhancement after 72 weeks of consumption of 5% and 10% (*w*/*w*) royal jelly, compared to the male zebrafish. The histological outcome revealed no sign of hepatotoxicity; moreover, diminished reactive oxygen species (ROS) and apoptosis were observed in the hepatic tissue of the royal-jelly-supplemented group. Consistent with the histological outcomes, the liver function biomarkers, aspartate aminotransferase (AST) and alanine aminotransferase (ALT), exhibited a significant decrease of 1.9-fold ($p = 0.006$) and 1.4-fold ($p = 0.003$) in zebrafish supplemented with royal jelly compared to those on a normal diet (ND) and zebrafish given supplements. Also, no sign of ovary and testis-related toxicity was observed in the royal-jelly-supplemented group during the 72-week period. Furthermore, the 10% (*w*/*w*) royal-jelly-consuming zebrafish exhibited a notable 2.1-fold increase ($p = 0.018$) in egg-laying ability compared to the ND-supplemented zebrafish. The 10% (*w*/*w*) royal jelly supplementation also effectively maintained the blood lipid profile by curtailing serum triglycerides (TG) and elevating high-density lipoprotein cholesterol (HDL-C). Conclusively, royal jelly dietary supplementation for a prolonged time found royal jelly to be safe to consume, to efficiently improve hepatic function, reproduction, and sexual health, and to augment the serum HDL-C level.

Keywords: royal jelly; antioxidant; high-density lipoprotein; liver; lipidemia; oxidative stress; ovary; testis; zebrafish

1. Introduction

Royal jelly is a milky white color, slightly pungent, mildly acidic (pH 3.6–4.2) viscous solution produced by the hypopharyngeal and mandibular glands of worker honeybees that are extensively consumed by the queen honeybee [1,2]. Typically, royal jelly is composed of water (50–60%), proteins (18%), carbohydrates (15%), lipids (3–6%), vitamins, trace elements, and free amino acids [3,4]. However, the composition may vary slightly according to the environmental conditions, harvesting season, floral source, etc., [5]. Proteins are the predominant constituent of royal jelly. The principal proteins present in royal jelly are known as major royal jelly proteins (MRJPs). The MRJPs are water-insoluble (49–87 kDa average molecular weight proteins) that are broadly categorized into nine distinct groups

(MRJP1–MRJP9) [1,6]. Among the nine different MRJPs, MRJP1 is the principal protein, constituting 31–66% of total MRJPs [5,7]. In addition to diverse proteins, royal jelly is a rich natural source of essential free amino acids [4]. Lipids are another vital constituent of royal jelly, accounting for 3–6% of the total royal jelly composition. Among the distinct lipids present in the royal jelly, the majority of the lipids are composed of saturated and unsaturated fatty acids (8–12 carbon chains) with mono- or dicarboxylic acid groups that account for 80% of the total lipids in royal jelly. The most noteworthy fatty acid that is exclusively present in royal jelly is 10-hydroxy-2 decanoic acid (10-HDA), which is responsible for imparting several beneficial properties to royal jelly [4,8]. Besides fatty acids, the lipid content of royal jelly is constituted of wax (5–6%), phenolic acid (4–10%), and sterol (3–4%) [5]. The royal jelly also harbors a variety of trace metals, notably serving as an abundant reservoir of potassium (2462–3120 mg/kg) [9].

Royal jelly is well known to exert numerous pharmacological effects owing to its antioxidant, anti-inflammatory, and antimicrobial properties [5]. The noteworthy role of royal jelly as an antitumor, antiallergic, antiaging, wound-healing, and immunomodulatory agent is well documented in the literature [5,8,10,11]. Also, royal jelly is substantially used in the cosmetic industry due to its inhibitory effect on sebum secretion and, consequently, its impact on acne formation, acne-induced lesions, and small wounds [12]. Several preclinical and clinical studies demonstrated royal jelly's therapeutic role against multiple sclerosis [13], traumatic brain injury [14], and infertility [15]. Nevertheless, the culminating effect of royal jelly was noted to alleviate premenstrual syndrome and menopause in females [16,17] and maintain the blood lipid profile [18].

Most of the studies conducted on royal jelly are confined to its therapeutic use, and limited sudies are available documenting a high amount of royal jelly consumption for a long duration. Also, certain regulatory authorities, such as the European Food Safety Authority, have demarcated that existing evidence does not support the claim of health benefits obtained by consuming royal jelly [19].Therefore, in the present study, a high amount (5% and 10%) of royal jelly was supplemented with the normal diet and consumed for a long duration [72 weeks (~1.5 years)] by zebrafish to examine the impact on health, aiming to explore the true potential of royal jelly as a functional food.

Zebrafish was selected as a model organism owing to its shared genomic similarity with humans [20], which recognized zebrafish as a suitable organism for preclinical studies. Several reports have documented zebrafish as a canonical animal model for fertility research [21], dyslipidemia and associated disorders [22], toxicology, and drug discovery [23] due to its higher mechanistic resemblance to humans. Moreover, zebrafish have well-developed innate and acquired immune systems like vertebrates [24]. Also, zebrafish embryos are transparent, developed externally, and of a relatively large size, thus facilitating easy insertion of the compound of interest through microinjection and an evaluation of the developmental changes. Furthermore, the outcome of the many preclinical investigations conducted on zebrafish gathered substantial information that can help to design further human trials [25], underscoring the significance and suitability of zebrafish as a model organism.

The present study aims to evaluate the effect of a prolonged (over 72 weeks) dietary supplementation of royal jelly on zebrafish survivability, body weight, liver, ovaries, testis morphology, and blood lipid profile, in addition to the egg-laying behavior of the female zebrafish with a normolipidemic diet.

2. Results

2.1. *In Vitro Antioxidant Activity of Royal Jelly*

The antioxidant activity of royal jelly was assessed via DPPH free radical scavenging and FRAP assay. As depicted in Figure 1A, royal jelly efficiently scavenges DPPH free radicals in a time- and concentration-dependent manner. At 20 min incubation, 18.8%, 23.4%, and 36.2% DPPH free radical scavenging activity was observed at 3, 6, and 12 mg/mL royal jelly concentrations, respectively. The 18.2 mg/mL royal jelly concentration was found to be the inhibitory concentration fifty (IC_{50}) for the DPPH free radicals.

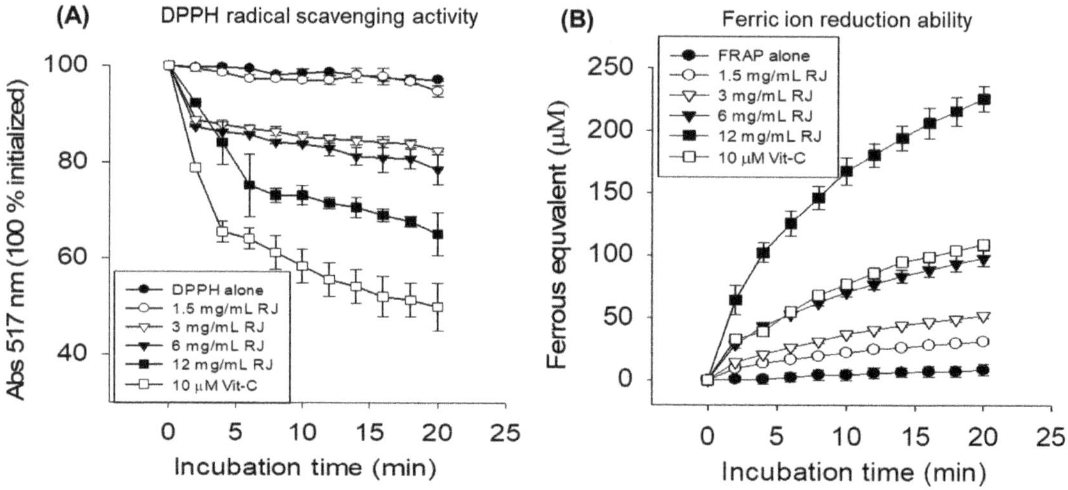

Figure 1. In vitro antioxidant activity of royal jelly. (**A**) DPPH free radical scavenging assay. (**B**) Ferric-ion-reducing antioxidant assay. Each value represents the mean ± SD of three independent experiments. RJ represents royal jelly, and Vit-C represents vitamin C (a positive control). RJ and Vit-C were dissolved in water. The indicated concentration represents the final amount of RJ and Vit-C treatment.

Royal jelly also displayed a substantial ferric ion reduction ability in both a time- and concentration-dependent manner (Figure 1B). At 20 min incubation 31.4 ± 1.4 μM, 52.1 ± 2.1 μM, 97.8 ± 6.4 μM and 225.7 ± 10.0 μM ferrous ion equivalent was observed at 1, 3, 6 and 12 mg/mL of royal jelly concentrations. The outcome of the DPPH and FRA assay suggested a substantial antioxidant potential of royal jelly.

2.2. *Protective Effect of Royal Jelly against H_2O_2 Exposure in Zebrafish Embryos*

As depicted in Figure 2A,B, the embryo's survivability in response to hydrogen peroxide (H_2O_2) exposure was severely affected in a time-dependent manner. At 5 h post-exposure to H_2O_2, the embryos' survivability declined to 82%, and finally, the death of all embryos was observed at 24 h post-exposure to H_2O_2. On the contrary, royal jelly effectively mitigated H_2O_2-induced toxicity in a dose-dependent manner. The embryos treated with 0.25 and 0.5 mg/mL royal jelly showed 22% and 32% embryo survivability at 24 h post-treatment (Figure 2A,B). At the 1 and 2 mg/mL royal jelly concentration, 66% and 70% embryo survivability was observed, signifying the protective role of royal jelly against the external stress H_2O_2 causes in zebrafish embryos.

The outcome of the dihydroethidium (DHE) and acridine orange (AO) fluorescent staining revealed massive reactive oxygen species (ROS) production and a large extent of apoptosis in the embryos exposed to H_2O_2. The treatment of embryos with royal jelly effectively prevents the H_2O_2-derived ROS generation in a dose-dependent manner (Figure 2C,D). The zebrafish embryos treated with 0.5, 1, and 2 mg/mL royal jelly displayed a significantly reduced production of ROS, by 1.7-, 3.2-, and 2.6-fold ($p < 0.001$) lower than the ROS production observed in zebrafish embryos exposed to only H_2O_2. In line with ROS production, heightened apoptosis was observed in the embryos exposed to H_2O_2, which was significantly altered by the treatment with royal jelly in a dose-dependent manner (Figure 2C,D). A significantly lower apoptosis, by 1.2-fold ($p < 0.05$) and 1.7-fold ($p < 0.001$), was observed in the embryos treated with 0.25 and 0.5 mg/mL royal jelly compared to the H_2O_2-exposed embryos. Consistent with this, a 4.6-fold ($p < 0.001$) lower apoptosis was observed in 1 and 2 mg/mL royal-jelly-treated embryos than the only H_2O_2-exposed embryos.

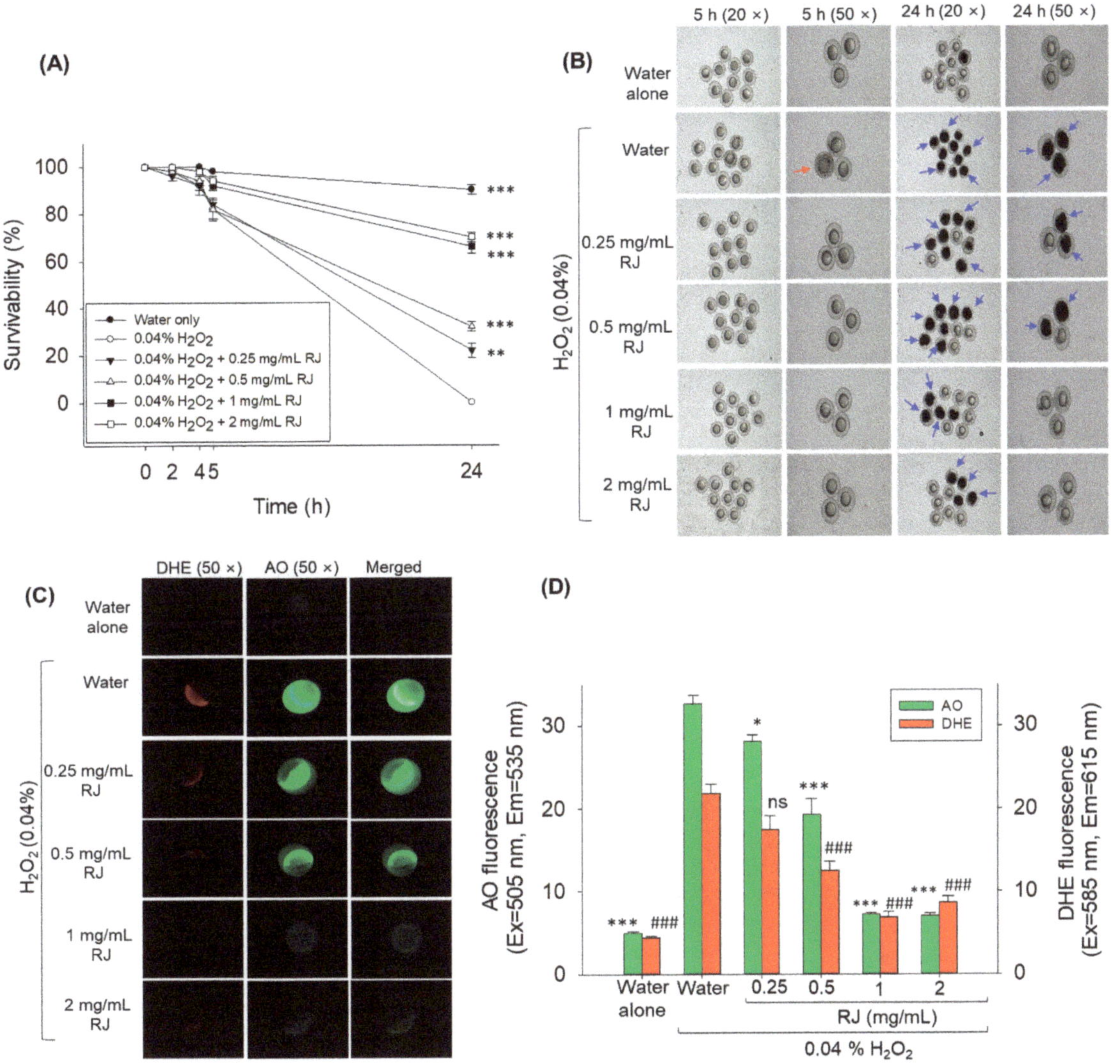

Figure 2. The effect of royal jelly on the hydrogen peroxide (H_2O_2)-induced stress in zebrafish embryos. (**A**) Kinetics of zebrafish embryo survivability 24 h post-treatment. (**B**) Images of zebrafish embryos at 5 and 24 h post-treatment (red arrow indicates swollen embryo as a sign of dying; blue arrow indicates dead embryos). (**C**) Fluorescent images of dihydroethidium (DHE)- and acridine orange (AO)-stained embryos (at 5 h post-treatment). (**D**) Image J-based quantification of DHE and AO fluorescent intensities. *, **, and *** represent the statistical difference at $p < 0.05$, $p < 0.01$, and $p < 0.001$ for AO fluorescent intensity, while ### represents the statistical difference at $p < 0.001$ for DHE fluorescent intensity compared to the water + H_2O_2-treated group; ns represents the non-significant difference between the groups. RJ stands for royal jelly.

2.3. Royal Jelly Prevents Carboxymethyllysine (CML)-Induced Acute Embryo Death

The embryo survivability, as depicted in Figure 3A,B, was severely affected by the microinjection of carboxymethyllysine (CML, 500 ng). At 24 h post-injection, the highest embryo survivability (60%) was observed in the PBS-injected group. In contrast with this, embryo survivability declined periodically and reached zero (100% mortality) at 24 h post-injection in the CML-injected group (Figure 3A,B). The royal jelly treatment of precisely 60 ng displayed a substantial protective role in embryos against the toxicity caused by CML. The 60 ng royal-jelly-injected group exhibited a significantly higher survivability, at 49% ($p < 0.001$), than the only CML-injected group. However, the 60 ng, 15 and 30 ng royal jelly injections were found to be least effective in countering CML-posed adversity in embryos. In 15 and 30 ng royal-jelly-injected groups, embryo survivability declined periodically up to 5 h post-injection, which is nearly similar to the embryo survivability pattern observed in the CML-injected group. However, after 5 h post-injection, embryo survivability becomes stable in the 15 and 30 ng royal-jelly-injected group, which is substantially higher than the embryo survivability detected in the only CML-injected group.

Most of the surviving embryos in the 60 ng royal-jelly-injected group displayed typical hatching without any sign of developmental deformities at 48 h post-injection (Figure 3B). Unlike this, normal embryo hatching was severely compromised in the 15 and 30 ng royal-jelly-injected groups. No embryo hatching was observed in the 15 and 30 ng royal-jelly-injected group at 48 h post-injection. The result signifies that the injection of royal jelly at a higher concentration (60 ng) effectively prevents CML-induced toxicity and developmental deformities in zebrafish embryos.

The results of DHE fluorescent staining observed at 5 h post-injection suggest a massive ROS production in the CML-injected group that is efficiently curtailed by the treatment of royal jelly in a dose-dependent manner (Figure 3C,D). Significantly lower ROS production, at 1.4 ($p < 0.05$), 1.9 ($p < 0.01$), and 4.3-fold ($p < 0.05$), was observed in 15, 30, and 60 ng royal-jelly-injected groups as compared to the CML+PBS-injected group. Consistent with the findings of DHE staining, the AO staining showed that royal jelly effectively prevents CML-induced apoptosis. The embryos that received 15, 30, and 60 ng royal jelly injection showed a 1.4 ($p < 0.05$), 1.9 ($p < 0.01$), and 4.3-fold ($p < 0.05$) lower AO fluorescent intensity than the CML-injected group, signifying the substantial anti-apoptotic role of royal jelly.

2.4. Body Weight and Survivability of Zebrafish

As depicted in Figure 4A, the body weight increased with time in all the groups, though the most noteworthy changes were observed in the 10% royal-jelly-supplemented groups. At 24 weeks of feeding, 332.8 ± 16.9 mg bodyweight was observed in the 10% royal-jelly-supplemented group, which is 39.2% higher than the body weight observed at the beginning (238.0 ± 6.7 mg). Contrary to this, in 5% royal-jelly- and ND-supplemented groups, a ~20% body weight enhancement was observed compared to the initial body weight. At 48 weeks, the 10% royal-jelly-supplemented groups achieved the maximum weight (406.6 ± 24.1 mg), i.e., 9.3% and 27.7% higher than the body weight observed in 5% royal-jelly- and ND-supplemented groups. At the final 72 weeks, the highest body weight was observed in the 10% royal-jelly-supplemented group, followed by the 5% royal-jelly-supplemented group, 35.1% ($p < 0.001$) and 16.7% ($p = 0.02$) higher than the body weight observed in the ND-supplemented group.

The effect of royal jelly consumption on female and male zebrafish body weight was individually determined over 72 weeks (Figure 4B,C). An enhancement in body weight was observed among all the groups; however, the royal-jelly-supplemented female zebrafish displayed a vigorous body weight enhancement in a dose- and time-dependent manner (Figure 4B). At 72 weeks, a 1.5-fold, 1.8-fold, and 2.1-fold higher body weight was observed in ND, 5%, and 10% royal-jelly-supplemented female zebrafish, respectively, compared to the initial weight. However, over the 72 weeks, the maximum body weight was noticed in female zebrafish supplemented with 10% royal jelly, i.e., weight was 1.2-fold ($p = 0.031$)

and1.4-fold ($p < 0.001$) higher than the body weight of 5% royal-jelly- and ND-supplemented groups (Figure 4B).

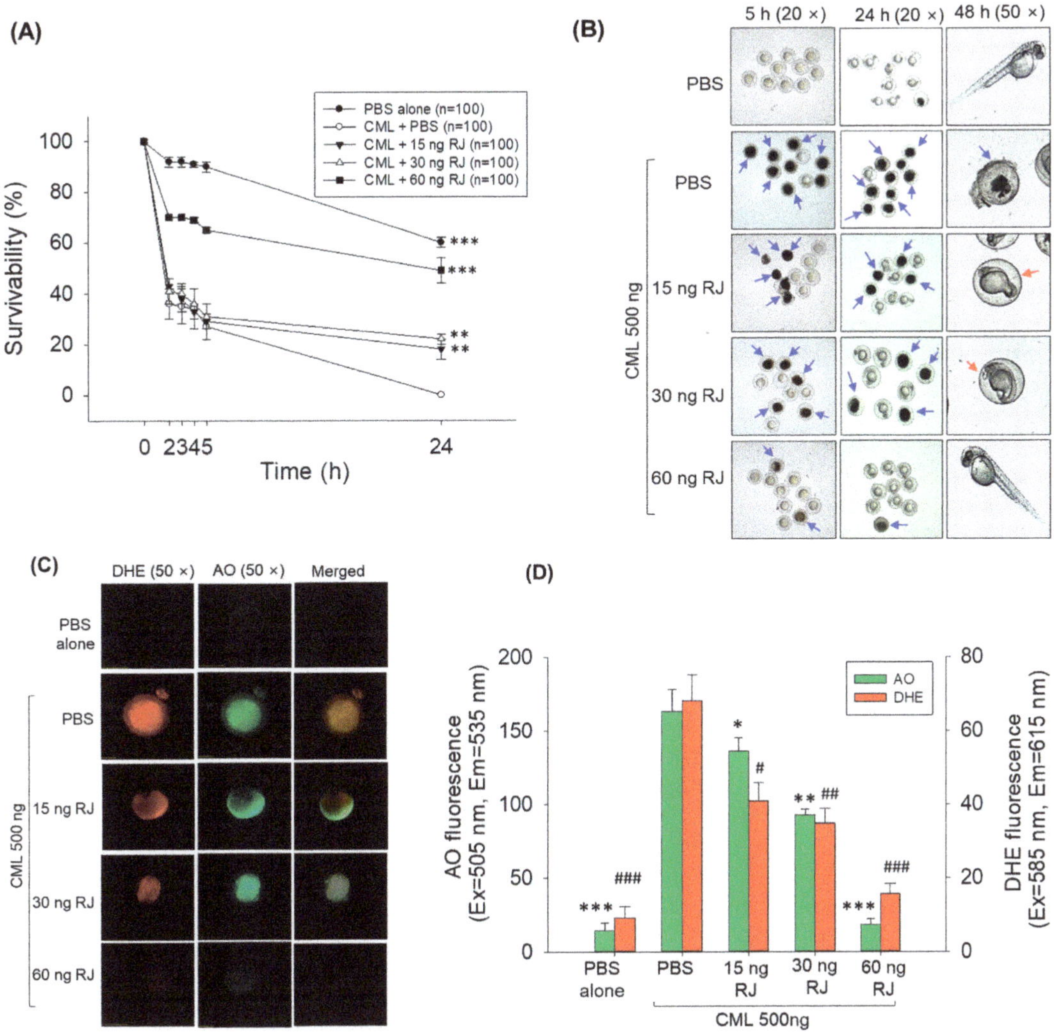

Figure 3. The effect of royal jelly on the survivability of zebrafish embryos when exposed to the acute toxicity posed by the microinjection of carboxymethyllysine (CML). (**A**) Survival kinetics of zebrafish embryos up to 24 h post-injection. (**B**) Images representing the zebrafish embryo survivability and developmental stage at 5, 24, and 48 h post-injection. The blue arrow indicates dead embryos, while the red arrow indicates unhatched embryos. (**C**) Fluorescent images of zebrafish embryos (at 5 h post-injection) stained with dihydroethidium (DHE) and acridine orange (AO). (**D**) Quantifying DHE and AO fluorescence levels in zebrafish embryos using Image J software 1.53r. Symbols *, ** and *** denote statistical significance at $p < 0.05$, $p < 0.01$, and $p < 0.001$, respectively, for AO fluorescent. Similarly, #, ## and ### represent statistical significance at $p < 0.05$, $p < 0.01$, and $p < 0.001$ for DHE fluorescent intensity compared to the CML+PBS-treated group; ns indicates a non-significant difference between the groups. RJ refers to royal jelly.

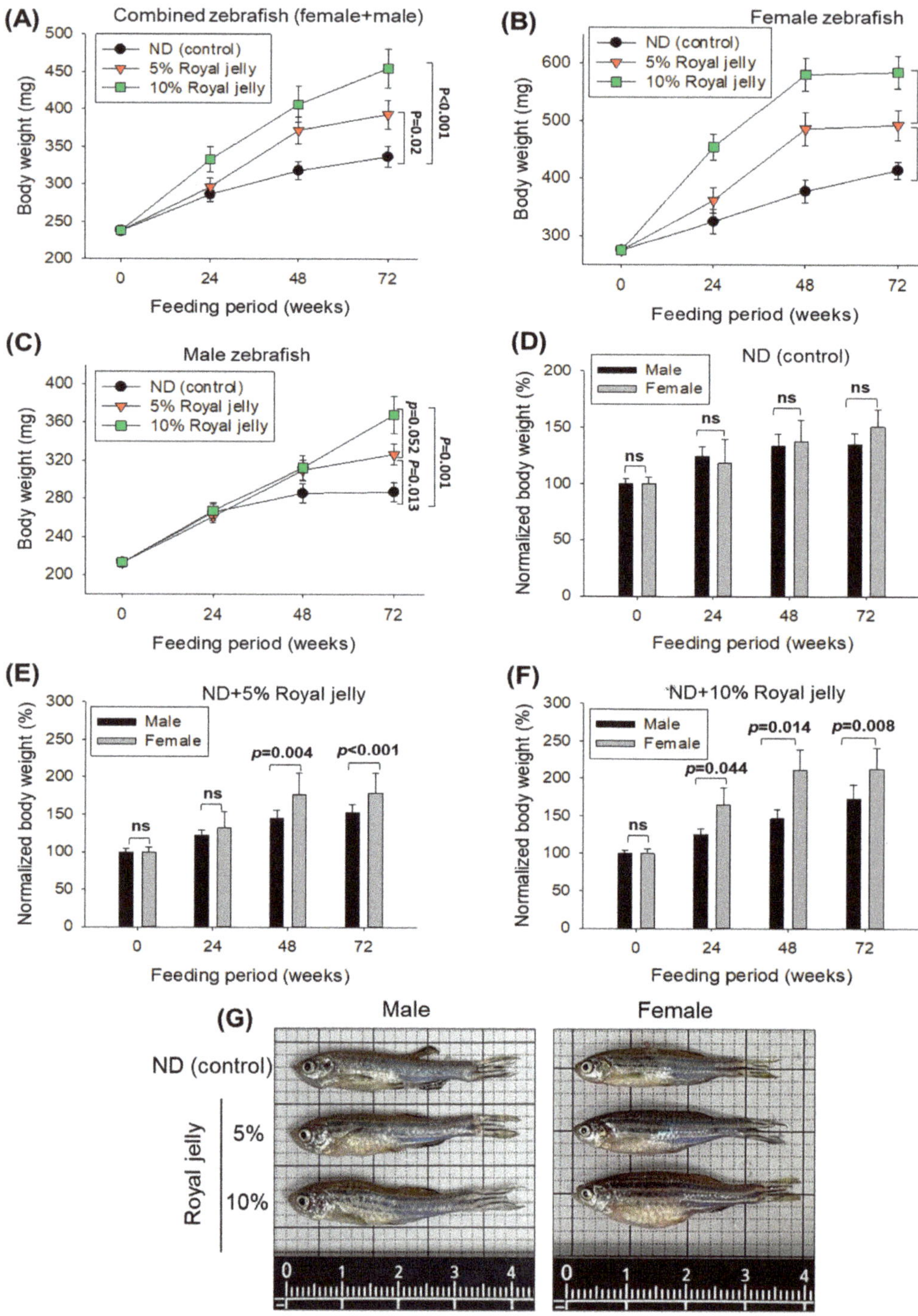

Figure 4. Long-term consumption of royal jelly on body weight of zebrafish. (**A**) A time-dependent (0–72 weeks) effect of 5% and 10% consumption of royal jelly on the body weight of zebrafish (female

and male combined). (**B**,**C**) Time-dependent (0–72 weeks) effect of 5% and 10% consumption of royal jelly on the body weight of female and male zebrafish, respectively. (**D**–**F**) Comparative time-dependent body weight changes between female and male in control, and 5% and 10% royal-jelly-supplemented groups, respectively. The normalized body weight at different time points was calculated with respect to 0-day body weight (considering this as 100%). (**G**) Representative images of male and female zebrafish from control, 5%, and 10% royal jelly consumption for 72 weeks. ND zebrafish received normal diet (ND), while zebrafish in 5% and 10% royal jelly groups received ND supplemented with 5% and 10% royal jelly. The *p*-value denotes the one-way ANOVA following Tukey's Post Hoc analysis based on statistical differences between the groups; ns indicates non-significant differences between the groups.

In contrast to the female zebrafish, the body weight of male zebrafish across the three groups remained almost similar up to 24 weeks (Figure 4C). Further, a slight increase in body weight was observed in both 5% and 10% royal-jelly-supplemented groups compared to the ND-supplemented group at 48 weeks. However, a significant enhancement of 1.3-fold ($p = 0.001$) and 1.2-fold ($p = 0.013$) in body weight in the 10% royal-jelly- and 5% royal-jelly-supplemented groups was observed compared to the ND-supplemented group at 72 weeks.

Furthermore, a comparative study between female and male body weight changes during the supplementation of ND, 5%, and 10% royal jelly revealed a non-significant effect of ND supplementation on the body weight of males and females during the 72 weeks (Figure 4D). In contrast to this, the 5% royal-jelly-supplemented group showed a 21.6% ($p = 0.004$) and 16.9% ($p < 0.001$) higher body weight in females compared to the males at 48 weeks and 72 weeks of consumption (Figure 4E). The most noteworthy effect on the female body weight enhancement was observed in the 10% royal-jelly-supplemented group (Figure 4F). At 24, 48 and 72 weeks supplementation of 10% royal jelly, the female body weight enhanced significantly, by 31.8% ($p = 0.004$), 44.1% ($p = 0.014$), and 23.2% ($p = 0.008$), compared to the male body weight at the respective time points. The results signify that royal jelly has a substantial effect on body weight enhancement, and female zebrafish are more vulnerable to this than male zebrafish.

Importantly, no adverse effect of royal jelly at the tested concentrations of 5% and 10% was observed on the survivability of zebrafish. A total of 77.5% survivability was observed in 5% and 10% royal-jelly-supplemented groups at 72 weeks, which was similar to the survivability observed in the ND-supplemented group, attesting to the safe nature of royal jelly consumption for the prolonged time.

2.5. Evaluation of the Liver

The H&E staining of the hepatic tissue extracted from ND- and royal-jelly-supplemented groups showed no sign of hepatic degeneration (Figure 5A). In all the groups, no visible signs of hepatic ballooning, lipid accumulation, and hepatic fibrosis were observed. Also, the results demonstrated no sign of excessive neutrophil infiltration around the portal vein across all the groups; however, as compared to the 5% and 10% royal jelly supplemented groups, a slightly higher neutrophil around the portal vein was observed in the ND-supplemented group. As depicted in Figure 5D, 22% and 18% H&E-stained areas were quantified in the 5% and 10% royal-jelly-supplemented groups which are 1.6-fold ($p < 0.001$) and 1.9-fold ($p < 0.001$) lower than the H&E-stained area observed in the ND-supplemented group, signifying the influence of royal jelly on hepatic health.

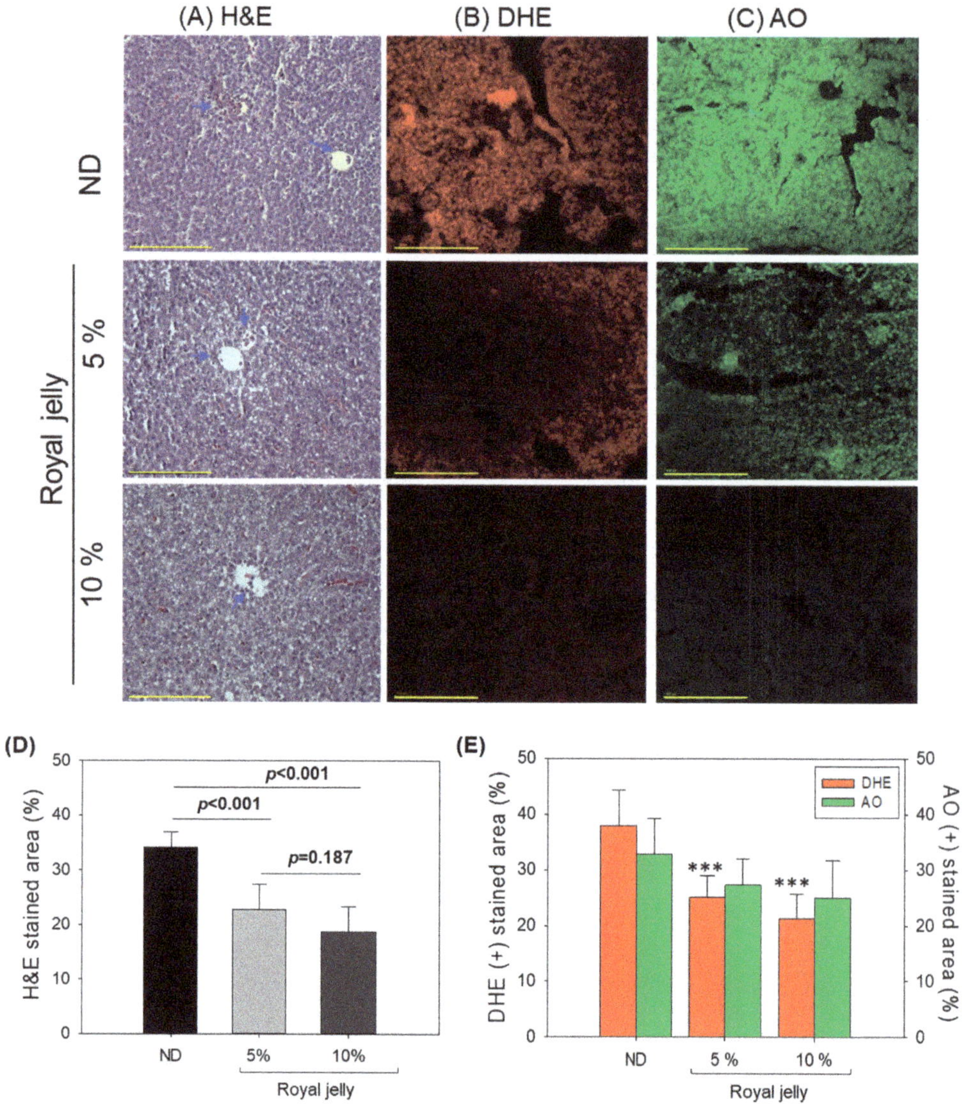

Figure 5. Effect of 72 weeks' consumption of royal jelly on hepatic tissue of zebrafish. (**A**) Hematoxylin and eosin (H&E) staining images. Blue arrow indicate the infiltration of neutrophils. (**B**) Dihydroethidium (DHE) and (**C**) acridine orange (AO) fluorescent staining, respectively. [Scale bar, 100 µm]. (**D**,**E**) DHE- and AO-stained area quantification using Image J software (http://rsb.info.nih.gov/ij/, assessed on 30 January 2023). ND zebrafish received normal diet (ND), while zebrafish in 5% and 10% royal jelly groups received ND supplemented with 5% and 10% royal jelly. The p-value denotes the one-way ANOVA following Tukey's post hoc analysis based on statistical differences between the groups. *** represents the statistical difference at $p < 0.001$ compared to the ND-supplemented group.

The ROS level in the hepatic tissue of the zebrafish after 72 weeks' consumption of royal jelly was evaluated by DHE fluorescent staining (Figure 5B,E). The results revealed a significantly higher ROS level in the ND-supplemented group, i.e., 1.5-fold ($p < 0.001$) and 1.8-fold ($p < 0.001$) higher than the DHE-stained area in the 5% and 10% royal-jelly-supplemented groups. Comparing the 5% and 10% royal-jelly-supplemented groups, a non-significant effect on the ROS level was observed.

The AO fluorescent staining did not indicate any harmful impact of royal jelly (at the tested concentrations of 5% and 10%) on the extent of hepatic apoptosis when compared to the ND-supplemented group (Figure 5C,E). Nevertheless, a marginal decrease in the AO-stained area was noted in the 5% and 10% royal-jelly-supplemented groups in comparison to the AO-stained area measured in the ND-supplemented group, although this difference between the groups was not statistically significant ($p > 0.05$).

The histology results attest no adverse effect of prolonged royal jelly consumption on the liver; furthermore, royal jelly was found to be effective in minimizing the hepatic ROS level.

2.6. Hepatic Function Biomarkers

The hepatic function was assessed after 72 weeks of the consumption of ND and royal jelly by measuring serum AST and ALT levels. Figure 6A illustrates that the ND-supplemented group exhibited the highest AST levels, 1.7-fold ($p = 0.009$) and 1.9-fold ($p = 0.006$) higher than the AST levels quantified in the 5% and 10% royal-jelly-supplemented groups. In comparison to the 5% royal-jelly-supplemented group, the 10% royal-jelly-supplemented group exhibited a 12.4% lower AST level, though the difference was statistically non-significant ($p > 0.05$).

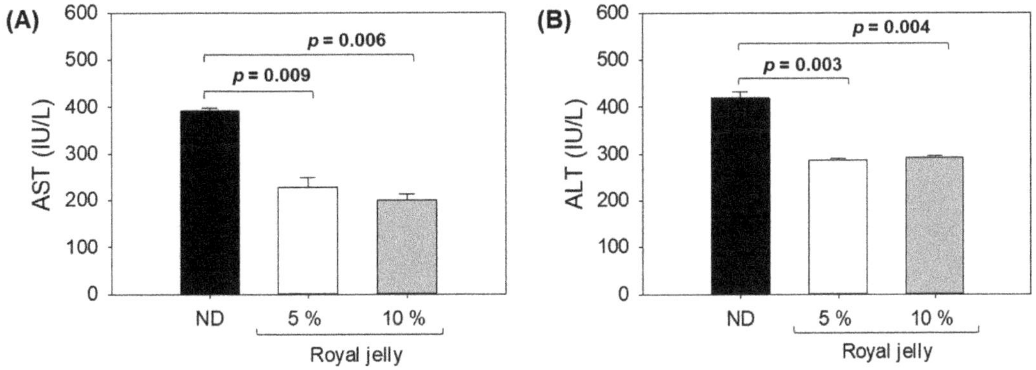

Figure 6. Effect of 72 weeks consumption of royal jelly on (**A**) aspartate aminotransferase (AST) and (**B**) alanine aminotransferase (ALT) hepatic function biomarkers. ND zebrafish received normal diet (ND), while zebrafish in 5% and 10% royal jelly groups received ND supplemented with 5% and 10% royal jelly. The *p*-value denotes the one-way ANOVA following Tukey's Post Hoc analysis based on statistical differences between the groups.

Consistent with the AST level, the maximum ALT level was detected in the ND-supplemented group, which is significantly (1.4-fold ($p = 0.003$)) higher than the ALT level detected in the 5% and 10% royal-jelly-supplemented groups.

The outcome of the hepatic function biomarkers is aligned with the hepatic histology results attesting to the non-hepatotoxic nature of royal jelly. The results strongly advocate a positive effect of royal jelly on the functionality of the liver.

2.7. Effect of Royal Jelly Consumption on Ovaries

The ovary's histology, as depicted in Figure 7, showed the different oocyte populations in the ND, 5%, and 10% royal-jelly-supplemented groups. In the ND-supplemented group, a higher prevalence of previtellogenic oocyte was determined, significantly (1.2-fold and 1.2-fold_ higher than the previtellogenic oocyte observed in the 5% and 10% royal-jelly-supplemented groups. Contrary to this, in the royal-jelly-supplemented group, a higher population of early and mature vitellogenic oocytes were noticed. As compared to the ND-supplemented group, 4-fold and 11-fold higher early vitellogenic oocytes were observed in the 5% and 10% royal-jelly-supplemented groups. Likewise, ~1.9-fold higher mature vitellogenic oocytes were observed in the 5% and 10% royal-jelly-supplemented groups as compared to the ND-supplemented group.

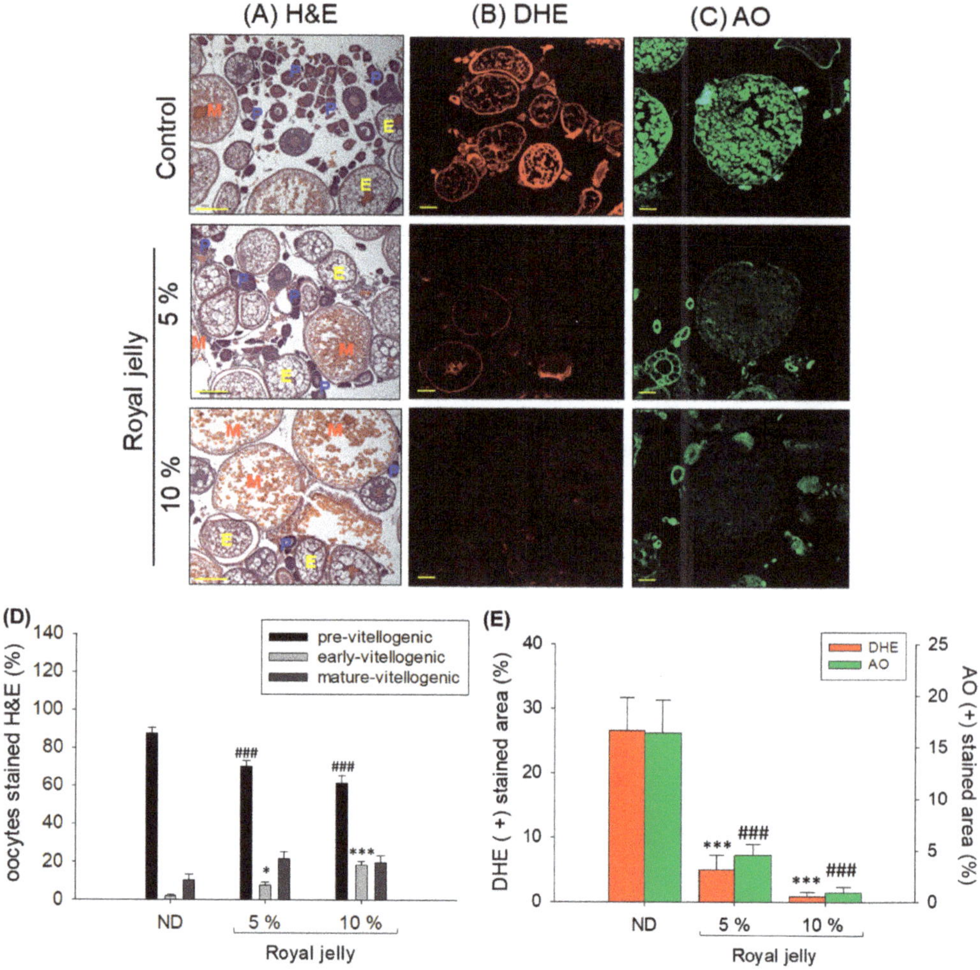

Figure 7. Effect of 72 weeks' consumption of royal jelly on the ovary of zebrafish. (**A**) Hematoxylin and eosin (H&E)-stained images (P, E, and M indicating pre-vitellogenic, early-vitellogenic, and mature-vitellogenic stages, respectively). (**B**,**C**) dihydroethidium (DHE) and acridine orange (AO) fluorescent staining, respectively. [Scale bar, 100 μm]. (**D**) Quantification of different developmental stages of oocytes. (**E**) Quantification of DHE- and AO-stained area using Image J software. ND zebrafish received normal diet (ND), while zebrafish in 5% and 10% royal jelly groups received ND supplemented with 5% and 10% royal jelly. The *p*-value denotes the one-way ANOVA following Tukey's Post Hoc analysis based on statistical differences between the groups. ### represent $p < 0.001$ for pre-vitellogenic compared to ND, while * represent $p < 0.05$ and *** represent $p < 0.001$ for early-vitellogenic compared to ND. *** and ### in (**E**) represents $p < 0.001$ compared to ND for DHE- and AO-stained areas, respectively.

The DHE staining of the ovary section revealed a diminished ROS level in the royal-jelly-supplemented group compared to the ND-supplemented group (Figure 7B,D). A significantly, 5-fold and 25-fold, lower ROS production was detected in the 5% and 10% royal-jelly-supplemented groups than the ND-supplemented group. The ovary ROS levels were affected by royal jelly supplementation in a dose-dependent manner, as is evident in the 5-fold lower ROS level in the 10% royal-jelly-supplemented group than the ROS levels observed in the 5% royal-jelly-supplemented group.

Consistent with the DHE staining, a lower extant of apoptosis as examined by AO staining was observed in the royal-jelly-supplemented groups than the ND-supplemented group (Figure 7C,D). A significant 3.6-fold and 16-fold lower apoptosis was detected in 5% and 10% royal-jelly-supplemented groups compared to the ND. As compared to the 10% royal-jelly-supplemented group, a 4.5-fold higher apoptosis was observed in 5% royal-jelly-supplemented group, suggesting the dose-dependent effect of royal jelly on diminishing apoptosis.

Combined histology and fluorescent staining outcomes showed a markable effect of royal jelly consumption on the morphology, as well as diminishing ROS levels and apoptosis.

2.8. Effect of Royal Jelly Consumption on Testis

The H&E staining, as depicted in Figure 8A, showed the testicular histology of zebrafish supplemented with ND and royal jelly. The ND-supplemented group showed a loosely arranged tubular structure with sparsely populated spermatocytes and spermatogonia. Also, a broad gap between seminiferous tubules was observed across the testis section (Figure 8A,B,E). In contrast to this, in the royal jelly, mainly in 10% supplemented groups, a tightly arranged tubular structure with densely packed spermatocytes and spermatozoa was detected. Compared to the ND-supplemented group, in the 5% and 10% royal-jelly-supplemented groups, 1.2-fold ($p < 0.001$) and 1.4-fold ($p < 0.001$) lower interstitial space was observed between seminiferous tubules. Compared to the 5% group, the 10% royal-jelly-supplemented group showed a well-defined and densely packed spermatocyte and spermatozoa, along with a 1.2-fold ($p < 0.001$) reduced interstitial space between the seminiferous tubules, signifying the dose dependent effect of royal jelly on the testis.

The DHE staining showed 1.4-fold and 2.6-fold reduced ROS levels in the testicular section of the 5% and 10% royal-jelly-supplemented groups compared to the ND-supplemented group (Figure 8C,F). Compared to the 5% group, the 10% royal-jelly-supplemented group showed an effective 1.9-fold reduction in the ROS level, testifying to the dose-dependent effect of royal jelly on alleviating the ROS level. Similar to the DHE staining, the AO staining suggested a 2.1-fold reduction in apoptosis in the 10% royal-jelly-supplemented groups (Figure 8D,F). The results of the testicular histology support the beneficial effect of royal jelly consumption on testis morphology and the elimination/prevention of ROS generation and apoptosis.

2.9. Effect of Royal Jelly Consumption on Egg-Laying Ability

As depicted in Figure 9A, royal jelly supplementation at 5% and 10% has a modulatory effect on the egg-laying behavior of zebrafish. The egg-laying ability of the 5% royal-jelly-supplemented group was enhanced by 1.6-fold compared to the ND-supplemented groups. However, the 10% royal-jelly-supplemented group showed the most noteworthy effect on the egg-laying activity, evident by the 2.1-fold ($p = 0.018$) increase in the number of laid eggs compared to the ND-supplemented group. Compared to the 5% group, the 10% royal-jelly-supplemented group showed a 1.3-fold increase in the number of laid eggs. Furthermore, royal jelly also displayed a substantial effect on the survivability of the fertilized eggs (embryos). As depicted in Figure 9B, 83% and 88% embryo survivability was observed in the 5% and 10% royal-jelly-supplemented groups compared to the 77% survivability observed in the ND-supplemented group. Among all the groups, no significant changes were observed in embryonic developmental deformities; however, the majority of embryos obtained for the 5% and 10% royal-jelly-supplemented groups displayed a deep black pigmentation on the head and the neck area (Figure 9C). The results demonstrate that royal jelly consumption has no adverse effect on the egg-laying activity of zebrafish; furthermore, royal jelly can positively modulate the egg-laying behavior and survivability of zebrafish embryos.

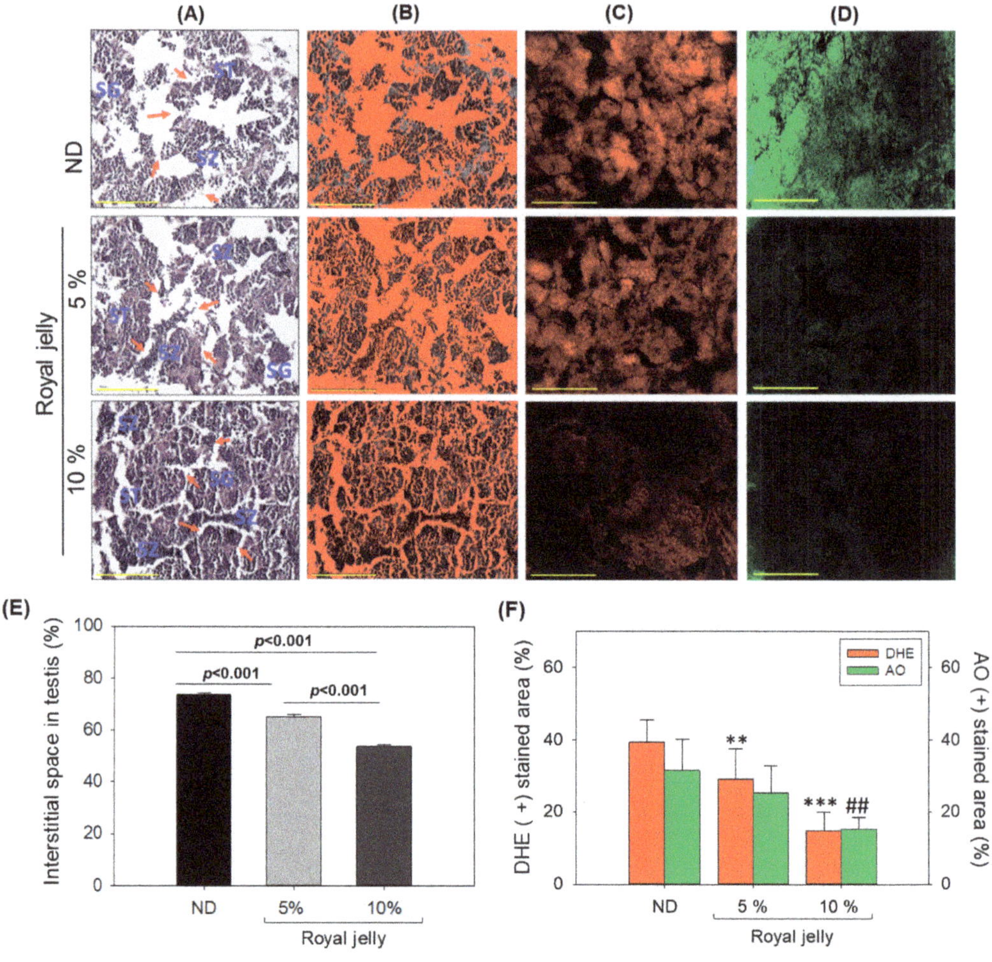

Figure 8. Effect of 72 weeks' consumption of royal jelly on testis of zebrafish. (**A**) Hematoxylin and eosin (H&E)-stained images (ST, SG and SZ denote spermatocytes, spermatogonia, and spermatozoa). The red arrow indicates the void space between seminiferous tubules. (**B**) White area (void space) appeared in H&E staining, interchanged with red color at the 220–225 threshold value for the white color using Image J software). (**C**,**D**) dihydroethidium (DHE) and acridine orange (AO) fluorescent staining, respectively. [Scale bar, 100 μm]. (**E**,**F**) quantification of DHE- and AO-stained areas using Image J software. ND zebrafish received normal diet (ND), while zebrafish in 5% and 10% royal jelly groups received ND supplemented with 5% and 10% royal jelly. The *p*-value denotes the one-way ANOVA following Tukey's Post Hoc analysis based on statistical differences between the groups. ** represent $p < 0.01$ and *** represent $p < 0.001$ compared to ND for DHE-stained area, while ## represent $p < 0.01$ compared to ND for AO-stained area.

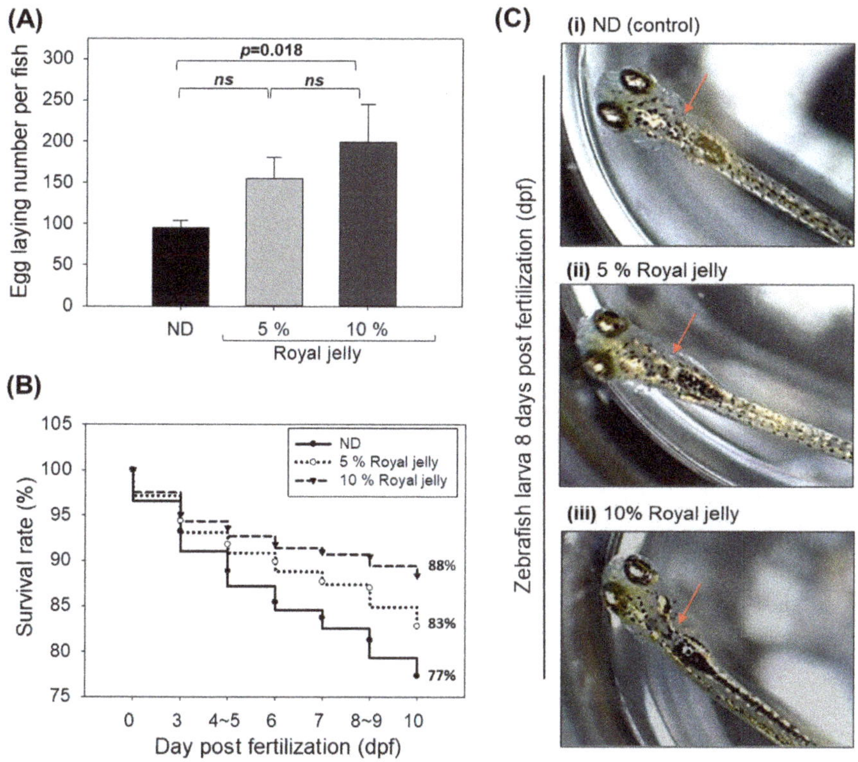

Figure 9. Effect of 72 weeks' royal jelly consumption on the egg-laying activity of zebrafish. (**A**) Quantification of the laid eggs. ns, non-significant. (**B**) Survivability of the embryos 10 days post-fertilization (dpf). (**C**) Images of zebrafish larva at 8 days post-fertilization (dpf). The red arrow indicates the pigment formation. ND zebrafish received normal diet (ND), while zebrafish in 5% and 10% royal jelly groups received ND supplemented with 5% and 10% royal jelly. The *p*-value denotes the one-way ANOVA following Tukey's Post Hoc analysis based on statistical differences between the groups.

2.10. Blood Lipid Profile

As shown in Figure 10, no significant change in TC levels was observed between the ND group and the group supplemented with royal jelly. In contrast to this, the HDL-C level was significantly changed between the groups. The maximum HDL-C level was detected in the 10% royal-jelly-supplemented group, which is 1.2-fold higher than the HDL-C level quantified in the 5 ND-supplemented group. The TG level significantly varied between the ND-, 5% royal-jelly- and 10% royal-jelly-supplemented groups. The lowest TG level was detected in the 10% royal-jelly-supplemented group, which was 36.8% and 32.2% lower than the TG levels quantified in the ND- and 5% royal-jelly-supplemented groups, respectively. Consistent with TG, the TG/HDL-C level was found to be the lowest in the 10% royal-jelly-supplemented group, which is 46.1% and 52.8% lower than the TG/HDL-C levels detected in the ND- and 5% royal-jelly-supplemented groups. No significant change in non-HDL-C levels was observed in ND-, 5%, and 10% royal-jelly-supplemented groups; however, the minimum amount was quantified in the 10% royal-jelly-supplemented group. The combined results reveal that the extended dietary supplementation of royal jelly does not exert any negative impact on the blood lipid profile; in fact, royal jelly was found to be effective in fostering the blood lipid profile of zebrafish, in spite of the body weight increase.

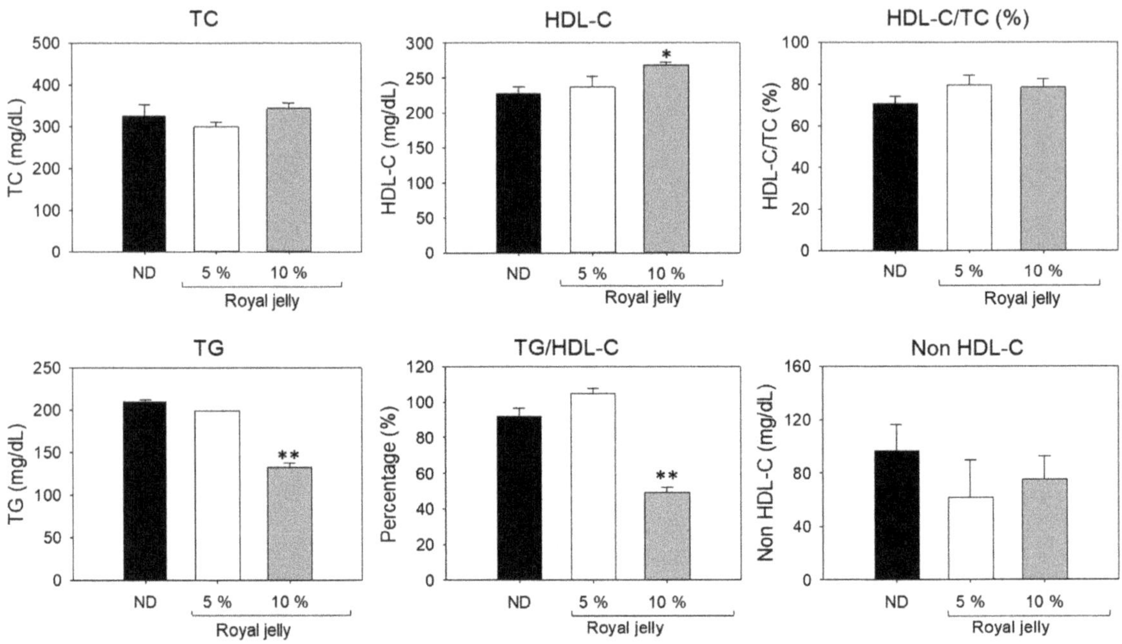

Figure 10. Impact of royal jelly consumption for 72 weeks on blood lipid profile of zebrafish. Total cholesterol (TC), triglycerides (TG), and high-density lipoprotein cholesterol (HDL-C). ND zebrafish received normal diet (ND), while zebrafish in 5% and 10% royal jelly groups received ND supplemented with 5% and 10% royal jelly. The *p*-value denotes the one-way ANOVA following Tukey's Post Hoc analysis based on statistical differences between the groups. * and ** represents $p < 0.05$ and $p < 0.01$ for early vitellogenic compared to ND.

3. Discussion

Royal jelly is a rich source of various nutrients and pharmacologically important substances and is often used as a traditional medicine [7]. Several previous reports documented royal jelly's therapeutic effect and functionality as an antioxidant, anti-inflammatory, anti-aging, antimicrobial, and wound-healing agent [5,8,10,11], making it a viable commercial product. Despite its numerous uses, the health impact of the prolonged dietary intake of royal jelly needs to be extensively documented. In view of the above, royal jelly dietary supplementation in zebrafish for 72 weeks was tested to determine the health implications.

Prior to evaluating the dietary supplementation, the in vitro antioxidant activity and the protective effect of royal jelly on zebrafish embryos were determined upon exposure to external stress induced by exposure to H_2O_2 and the injection of CML. CML, classified as an advanced glycation end product (AGE), is widely recognized for its toxicity, resulting from the initiation of ROS/oxidative stress [26,27], ultimately leading to apoptosis. The outcomes suggested a substantial DPPH free radical scavenging and ferric ion reduction activity, signifying the antioxidant activity of royal jelly. The results align with a previous study deciphering the DPPH free radical scavenging activity of royal jelly [28–31]. In another recent study, the free radical scavenging activity of major royal jelly proteins (MRJPs) was also detected, substantially protecting against DNA damage from oxidative stress [32]. In the present work, we also observed the protective role royal jelly can play n zebrafish embryos against H_2O_2- and CML-induced oxidative stress. The protective effect of zebrafish embryos is strengthened by the antioxidant properties of royal jelly, which can effectively counter the ROS-induced oxidative stress and prevent apoptotic cell death in zebrafish embryos. The findings agree with a previous report suggesting the effective role of royal jelly in improving the cellular antioxidant, consequently enhancing the survivability of *Drosophila melanogaster* [33]. Similar to this, royal jelly displayed a protective role against sodium-fluoride-induced oxidative stress in mice by upregulating the cellular antioxidants superoxide dismutase (SOD) and catalase [34]. These earlier reports [32–34] strengthen the current findings and establish the important antioxidant role of royal jelly, which not only directly scavenges the free radicals but also has a substantial effect on the cellular antioxidant, and thus has a preventive effect against oxidative-stress-induced detrimental effects.

Further, the outcome of the long-term royal jelly consumption study revealed no adverse effect of royal jelly on the survivability of zebrafish, underscoring the royal jelly's safety for consumption. Interestingly a substantial effect of royal jelly consumption on body weight enhancement was observed. The findings also revealed that females are more inclined towards weight gain compared to male zebrafish. The exact reason behind the body weight gain and its more notable effects in female zebrafish is not known. The most probable explanation for the body weight enhancement may be royal jelly's effect on improving zebrafish's metabolic process, similar to that in a bee colony to stimulate and increase larva growth [35]. However, further study is required to determine the exact reason behind the body weight enhancement achieved by the consumption of royal jelly and its bias toward female zebrafish.

The consumption of royal jelly was not shown to lead to signs of hepatotoxicity. Moreover, the outcome regarding hepatic morphology and hepatic function biomarkers (AST and ALT) revealed a beneficial effect of royal jelly consumption on the hepatic health of zebrafish. The most probable reason behind the decrease in the AST and ALT levels in the royal-jelly-fed group compared to the ND-fed group is the variation in the TG levels in these groups (Figure 9). The consumption of royal jelly is associated with decreased TG levels, which could potentially influence the reduction in AST and ALT levels. An earlier published report [36] indicated a correlation between higher TG levels and elevated AST and ALT levels, further supporting this notion. However, further study is required to reach any conclusions. In addition to hepatic morphology and hepatic function biomarkers, royal jelly consumption substantially inhibited ROS generation and apoptosis in the hepatic tissue. The major reason behind the better hepatic health that was seen in response to royal jelly consumption lies in its antioxidant nature, which minimizes the cellular ROS and consequently impacts oxidative-stress-induced apoptosis and the functionality of the liver. This notion is strongly supported by previous studies documenting the antioxidant nature of royal jelly as a key event in preventing hepatic damage against varied forms of external stress [37]. The regulatory impact of royal jelly on the expression of liver antioxidants such as glutathione S-transferase (GST) and glutathione peroxidase (GSH-px) has been documented [37,38], which helps in hepatoprotection against oxidative-stress-induced damage. Royal jelly's impact on upregulating nuclear factor erythroid 2-related factor 2 (Nrf2) has been documented, and royal jelly can consequently impact the expression of the important antioxidant enzymes that prevent hepatic damage [37,39].

We also observed low hepatic apoptosis in royal-jelly-supplemented zebrafish, attributed to the antioxidant properties of royal jelly, which can scavenge harmful ROS, which are key contributors to cellular apoptosis [40] Furthermore, the influence of royal jelly on the upregulation of the antiapoptotic Bcl-2 and downregulation of proapoptotic Bax and caspase 3 has been documented to inhibit apoptosis in the liver [39]. These findings also support the present findings regarding royal-jelly-supplemented zebrafish under similar conditions, where supplementation was found to inhibit apoptosis, and improve hepatic health.

Like the liver, no toxicity from royal jelly consumption (for 72 weeks) was noticed regarding the morphology and functionality of the ovaries and testes. Furthermore, it was observed that royal jelly enhances the functionality of the testes and ovaries, exerting a distinct influence on egg-laying behavior. The histological results suggest a diminished ROS and apoptosis in the testes and ovaries of the royal-jelly-supplemented zebrafish due to the antioxidant nature of royal jelly, improves the functionality of the testes and ovaries. This aligns well with previous findings suggesting a beneficial role of royal jelly in reproductive health [10] due to its ability to counter oxidative stress [41] Also, it has been reported that royal jelly impacts oxidative stress and modulates Bax and Bcl-2, leading to the protection of oocytes. Additionally, the impact of royal jelly (mainly imparted by 10-HDA) on reducing the follicle-stimulating hormone (FSH) and luteinizing hormone (LH) is another important reason for the improvements in ovarian health [10].

Royal jelly consumption was found to enhance body weight, which is often associated with dyslipidemia. In the present study, we found no adverse effect of prolonged royal jelly consumption on the disturbed blood lipid profile despite the significant impact on body weight. Moreover, royal jelly supplementation enhanced the HDL-C levels and reduced the TG levels. As oxidative stress and inflammation are the major culprits that disturb the lipid profile and cause dyslipidemia [42], we believe that the enhancement of the HDL-C levels and reductions in the TG levels might be linked with the antioxidant and anti-inflammation activity of royal jelly. A previously conducted study also suggested an impact of royal jelly consumption (150 mg/day) for 3 months (~12 weeks) on reducing TC, TG and LDL-C, and the elevation of HDL-C levels [18], strengthening the present findings.

4. Materials and Methods

4.1. Materials

Royal jelly was processed and analyzed by Raydel® (Raydel Australia Pty, Ltd., Thornleigh, Sydney, NSW, Australia). A detailed specification of the royal jelly is provided in Supplementary Table S1. To prepare a royal-jelly-enriched diet, normal tetrabit (Tetrabit Gmhb D49304, Melle, Germany), a regular zebrafish diet, was mixed individually with 5% and 10% (*w*/w) royal jelly. The royal-jelly-supplemented normal tetrabit was blended vigorously to ensure the proper distribution of royal jelly among normal tetrabit.

Methylene blue (Cat#M4195), diphenyl-1-picrylhydrazyl (Cat#9286), 2 phenoxyethanol (Cat#P1126), acridine orange (Cat#A9231), dihydroethidium (Cat#A37291), and *N*-ε-carboxymethyllysine (Cat#114580-5g) were purchased from Sigma Aldrich (St. Louis, MO, USA). Unless otherwise stated, all the other chemicals and reagents were of analytical grade and used as supplied.

4.2. In Vitro Antioxidant Activity

The antioxidant activity of royal jelly was evaluated by diphenyl-1-picrylhydrazyl (DPPH) [43] and ferric ion reducing (FRA) assay [44], as described previously. For the DPPH free radical scavenging assay, 10 μL of varied concentrations of royal jelly (dissolved in water) was mixed with 190 μL of diphenyl-1-picrylhydrazyl solution (DPPH, 24 mg/L in methanol) to obtain the final concentration of 1.5, 3, 6, and 12 mg/mL royal jelly. Simultaneously, a control DPPH solution devoid of royal jelly was prepared. The absorbance of 517 nm was recorded using a Spectrophotometer (UV-2600i-Shimadzu, Kyoto, Japan).

For the FRA assay, 20 μL of varying concentrations of royal jelly were combined separately with 180 μL of FRA reagent. The FRA reagent was prepared by mixing sodium acetate (0.3 M, pH 3.6) with 2,4,6-tripyridyl-S triazin (0.01 M) and ferric chloride (0.02 M) in a 10:1:1 (*v*/*v*). The final concentrations of royal jelly that were tested were 1.5, 3, 6, and 12 mg/mL. Additionally, a control FRA solution was also prepared without the inclusion of royal jelly. The FRA was determined by taking absorbance at 593 nm using a Spectrophotometer (UV-2600i-Shimadzu, Kyoto, Japan).

4.3. Zebrafish Husbandry

Zebrafish were maintained at a constant water temperature (28 °C), with a periodic light and dark cycle of 14 h and 10 h, respectively, in the automated water circulation system (Bioengineering Company, Daejeon, Republic of Korea), adhered to the criteria regarding the care and use of laboratory animals [45,46] implemented by the Animal Care

Committee and the Use of Raydel Research Institute (approval code RRI-20-003). Normal tetrabit was used to nourish the zebrafish.

4.4. Zebrafish Embryo Collection and Evaluation of Embryo-Protective Effect of Royal Jelly

Zebrafish embryos were produced following a previously described method [47]. In brief, male, and female zebrafish were segregated in the water tank using a perforated physical divider. After 16 h segregation, mating was allowed via removal of the physical barrier. The produced embryos were collected, washed, and randomly divided into 6 groups (n = 100/group) in each petri dish (100 mm diameter). The embryos in group I were suspended in the 5 mL sea salt solution (3 g sea salt suspended in 100 mL of 1 μg/mL methylene blue) (control). In contrast, the embryos in group II were suspended in a 5 mL sea salt solution containing 0.04% hydrogen peroxide (H_2O_2). Embryos in groups III, IV, V, and VI were suspended in 5 mL of 0.04% H_2O_2 containing sea salt solution supplemented with 0.25, 0.5, 1, and 2 mg/mL royal jelly, respectively. Embryos in the distinct groups were visualized under a microscope (Motic SMZ 168; Hong Kong) to evaluate embryo mortality.

4.5. Microinjection of Zebrafish Embryos

As outlined in Section 4.4, the collected embryos were randomly distributed into 5 distinct groups (n = 100 in each group). Embryos in group I received a microinjection of 8 nL PBS (vehicle). Embryos in group II were injected with 500 ng carboxymethyl lysine (CML) suspended in 8 nL PBS. Embryos in groups III, IV, and IV were co-injected with 8 nL of 500 ng CML containing 15, 30, and 60 ng of royal jelly (final), respectively. Microinjection was performed under a microscope using microcapillary pipettes attached with a pneumatic pump (PV830; World Precision Instruments, Sarasota, FL, USA) and a magnetic manipulator (MM33; Kantec, Bensenville, Chicago, IL, USA). The microinjection targeted nearly the same position on the embryo yolk to mitigate bias. The microinjected embryos across all the groups were periodically (0–48 h) visualized under the microscope to assess embryo mortality and developmental defects.

4.6. Fluorescent Staining for ROS and Apoptosis

ROS levels in the embryos were determined by dihydroethidium (DHE) fluorescent staining, as in the previously described method [47]. In brief, 10 embryos (5 h post-treatment) were washed with water and immersed in 500 μL of 30 μM DHE solution. After 30 min incubation, embryos were visualized under a fluorescent microscope (Nikon Eclipse TE2000, Tokyo, Japan) at the excitation and emission wavelengths of 585 nm and 615 nm, respectively. The extent of apoptosis was measured via acridine orange (AO) staining, as in a previously described method [47]. In brief, 10 embryos were suspended in 500 μL of 5 μg/mL AO solution. After 1 h incubation, the stained embryos were observed under a fluorescent microscope at 505 nm and 535 nm excitation and emission wavelengths, respectively. The fluorescent intensity of DHE- and AO-stained areas corresponding to ROS and apoptosis was quantified using Image J software (version 1.53r, http://rsb.info.nih.gov/ij/ accessed on 30 January 2023).

4.7. Zebrafish Fed with Royal Jelly

Zebrafish (15 weeks aged) were randomly divided into 3 distinct groups (n = 40 in each group). The group I zebrafish were fed with normal tetrabit (considered as control). In contrast, zebrafish in groups II and III were fed normal tetrabit supplemented with 5% and 10% royal jelly, respectively. The zebrafish in all groups were nurtured in the same environmental conditions for up to 72 weeks. The survivability and body weight of the zebrafish in all groups were observed periodically (0, 24, 48, and 72 weeks). The body weight was evaluated after anaesthetizing zebrafish using 2-phenoxyethanol (final 0.1%).

4.8. Effect of Royal Jelly Supplementation on Egg-Laying and Embryo Survivability of Zebrafish

After 72 weeks, the egg-laying capacity and survivability of the embryos produced from the control, 5% and 10% royal-jelly-supplemented groups were determined. The zebrafish mating in separate groups was performed using a method described in Section 2.4. All the eggs laid in the three groups were suspended in sea salt solution for embryo development. The embryo development and survivability 10 days post-fertilization (dpf) were quantified by visualizing the embryos under the microscope (Motic SMZ 168; Hong Kong).

4.9. Histological Analysis

At the end of the 72 weeks' supplementation, zebrafish (n = 10/group) were sacrificed using hypothermic shock [47] and immediately dissected to recover the liver, testis, and ovary. The dissected tissues were preserved in a 10% formalin solution. For the histological analysis, the tissue was dehydrated using ethanol and embedded in paraffin wax following tissue sectioning (7 μm thick) using microtome (Leica, CM1510s, Heidelberg, Germany). The tissue sections from the liver, ovary, and testis were processed for hematoxylin and eosin staining (H&E) [48,49] to evaluate the morphological changes.

4.10. Fluorescent Imaging for Reactive Oxygen Species (ROS) and Apoptosis

The reactive oxygen species (ROS) levels in the tissue section were evaluated by dihydroethidium (DHE) fluorescent staining, as in the previously described method [50]. In brief, the tissue section (7 μm thick) was covered with 250 μL of DHE (30 μM). After 30 min incubation in the dark, the stained section was washed with water and visualized under fluorescent microscopy (Nikon Eclipse TE2000, Tokyo, Japan) at the excitation and emission wavelengths of 588 nm and 605 nm, respectively.

The acridine orange (AO) fluorescent staining was utilized to determine the extent of apoptosis, as in a previously described method [51,52]. In brief, the tissue section (7 μm thick) was covered with 250 μL of AO solution (5 μg/mL) following 30 min incubation in the dark; the stained section was washed with water and visualized at the excitation and emission wavelengths of 502 nm and 525 nm, respectively, using a fluorescent microscope (Nikon Eclipse TE2000, Tokyo, Japan).

4.11. Blood Lipid Profile and Hepatic Function Biomarker Analysis

Two microliters of the blood were withdrawn from the zebrafish's heart and collected in the tubes containing 3 μL of ethylenediaminetetraacetic acid (EDTA, final concentration 1 mM). The serum was collected and processed for the quantification of total cholesterol (TC), triglycerides (TG), and high-density lipoprotein (HDL-C) using a commercial lipid profile diagnostic kit (cholesterol, T-CHO, and TGs, Cleantech TS-S; Walko Pure Chemical, Osaka, Japan). For TC and TG quantification, 5 μL serum was mixed individually with 200 μL of TC- and TG-specific reaction mixture (provided with the kit); after 10 min incubation at 37 °C, TC and TG levels were quantified by measuring absorbance at 490 nm. The HDL-C level was determined by mixing an equal volume of serum and separation solution (provided with the kit). After centrifugation (3000 rpm for 10 min), 20 μL supernatant was mixed with 200 μL of the reaction mixture (provided with the kit), and the HDL-C was quantified by taking absorbance at 490 nm.

The commercial assay kit (Asan Pharmaceutical, Hwasung, Republic of Korea) was utilized to quantify the serum level of aspartate transaminase (AST) and alanine transaminase (ALT), following the methodology advised by the manufacturers.

4.12. Statistical Analysis

The experiments were conducted in triplicate, and the outcomes are expressed as the mean ± standard deviation. Statistical significance among the groups was assessed through a one-way analysis of variance (ANOVA), following Tukey's post hoc analysis, employing the Statistical Package for the Social Sciences (SPSS, Chicago, IL, USA, version 29).

5. Conclusions

Royal jelly was found to have a substantial antioxidant activity that rescues zebrafish embryos from oxidative injury. The dietary consumption of royal jelly for a prolonged period (72 weeks) was found to be safe, without any visible sign of toxicity to the hepatic, ovary, and testis. Furthermore, royal jelly displayed a positive impact on hepatic and sexual health and improved blood lipid profile via elevating HDL-C levels. The most noteworthy effect of royal jelly supplementation was observed on female zebrafish's weight; however, a detailed mechanism of the body weight gain and change in adipose tissue during the consumption needs to be performed in a future study. The antioxidant nature of royal jelly was regarded as a critical mediator in improving the health-beneficial effects (Figure 11). The findings support the use of royal jelly as a safe dietary supplement, with weight enhancement occurring during long-term supplementation, particularly in the female zebrafish.

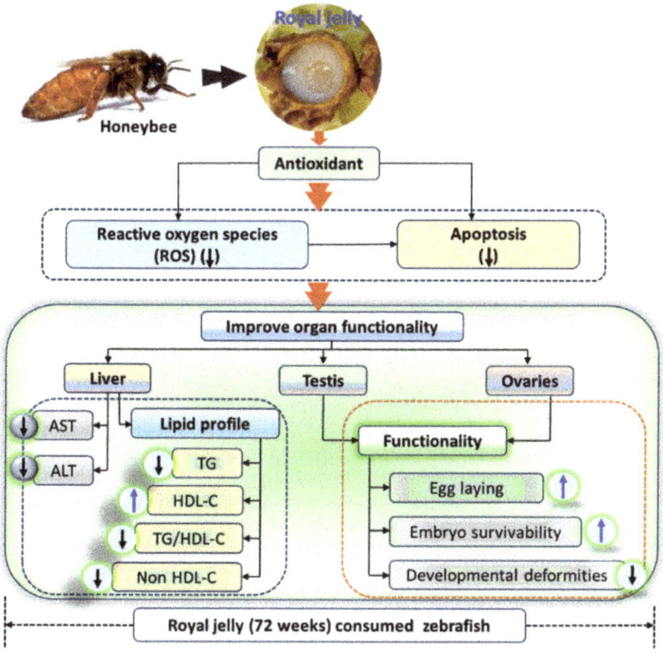

Figure 11. Summary of the various events in zebrafish after 72 weeks of royal jelly consumption. AST, aspartate aminotransferase; ALT, alanine aminotransferase; HDL-C, high-density lipoprotein-cholesterol; ROS, reactive oxygen species; TC, total cholesterol; TG, triglyceride.

Supplementary Materials: The following supporting information can be downloaded at: https://www.mdpi.com/article/10.3390/ph17030324/s1, Table S1: Ingredients composition analysis of the royal jelly (Raydel®).

Author Contributions: Conceptualization, K.-H.C.; methodology, H.-S.N., A.B. and J.-E.K.; data curation, writing—original draft preparation, K.-H.C.; writing—review and editing, K.-H.C.; supervision, K.-H.C. All authors have read and agreed to the published version of the manuscript.

Funding: This research received no external funding.

Institutional Review Board Statement: The animal study protocol was approved by Committee of Animal Care and Use of Raydel Research Institute (approval code RRI-20-004).

Informed Consent Statement: Not applicable.

Data Availability Statement: Data is contained within the article and Supplementary Material.

Conflicts of Interest: The authors declare no conflicts of interest.

References

1. Ramanathan, A.N.K.G.; Nair, A.J.; Sugunan, V.S. A review on royal jelly proteins and peptides. *J. Funct. Foods* **2018**, *44*, 255–264. [CrossRef]
2. Kocot, J.; Kiełczykowska, M.; Luchowska-Kocot, D.; Kurzepa, J.; Musik, I. Antioxidant potential of propolis, bee pollen, and royal jelly: Possible medical application. *Oxid. Med. Cell. Longev.* **2018**, *2*, 7074209. [CrossRef]
3. Nagai, T.; Inoue, R. Preparation and functional properties of water extract and alkaline extract of royal jelly. *Food Chem.* **2004**, *84*, 181–186. [CrossRef]
4. Yeung, Y.T.; Argüelles, S. *Bee Products: Royal Jelly and Propolis*; Elsevier Inc.: Amsterdam, The Netherlands, 2018; ISBN 9780128124918.
5. Ali, A.M.; Kunugi, H. Apitherapy for age-related skeletal muscle dysfunction (sarcopenia): A review on the effects of royal jelly, propolis, and bee pollen. *Foods* **2020**, *9*, 1362. [CrossRef]
6. Kunugi, H.; Ali, A.M. Royal Jelly and Its Components Promote Healthy Aging and Longevity: From Animal Models to Humans. *Int. J. Mol. Sci.* **2019**, *20*, 4662. [CrossRef]
7. Mureşan, C.I.; Dezmirean, D.S.; Marc, B.D.; Suharoschi, R.; Pop, O.L.; Buttstedt, A. Biological properties and activities of major royal jelly proteins and their derived peptides. *J. Funct. Foods* **2022**, *98*, 105286. [CrossRef]
8. Yu, X.; Tu, X.; Tao, L.; Daddam, J.; Li, S.; Hu, F. Royal Jelly fatty acids: Chemical composition, extraction, biological activity, and prospect. *J. Funct. Foods* **2023**, *111*, 105868. [CrossRef]
9. Botezan, S.; Baci, G.-M.; Bagameri, L.; Paşca, C.; Dezmirean, D.S. Current status of the bioactive properties of royal jelly: A comprehensive review with a focus on Its anticancer, anti-Inflammatory, and antioxidant effects. *Molecules* **2023**, *28*, 1510. [CrossRef]
10. Pasupuleti, V.R.; Sammugam, L.; Ramesh, N.; Gan, S.H. Honey, propolis and royal jelly: A comprehensive review of their biological actions and health benefits. *Oxid. Med. Cell. Longev.* **2017**, *2017*, 1259510. [CrossRef]
11. Maleki, V.; Jafari-Vayghan, H.; Saleh-Ghadimi, S.; Adibian, M.; Kheirouri, S.; Alizadeh, M. Effects of royal jelly on metabolic variables in diabetes mellitus: A systematic review. *Complement. Ther. Med.* **2019**, *43*, 20–27. [CrossRef]
12. Kurek-Górecka, A.; Górecki, M.; Rzepecka-Stojko, A.; Balwierz, R.; Stojko, J. Bee products in dermatology and skin care. *Molecules* **2020**, *25*, 556. [CrossRef]
13. Oshvandi, K.; Aghamohammadi, M.; Kazemi, F.; Masoumi, S.Z.; Mazdeh, M.; Molavi, V.M. Effect of royal jelly capsule on quality of life of patients with multiple sclerosis: A double-blind randomized controlled clinical trial. *Iran. Red Crescent Med. J.* **2020**, *22*, e74.
14. Shafiee, Z.; Hanifi, N.; Rashtchi, V. The effect of royal jelly on the level of consciousness in patients with traumatic brain injury: A double-blind randomized clinical trial. *Nurs. Midwifery Stud.* **2022**, *11*, 96–102.
15. Peivandi, S.; Khalili, S.S.; Abbasi, Z.; Zamaniyan, M.; Gordani, N.; Moradi, S. Effect of Royal Jelly on Sperm Parameters and Testosterone Levels in Infertile Men. *J. Maz. Univ. Med. Sci.* **2022**, *31*, 43–52.
16. Sharif, S.N.; Darsareh, F. Effect of royal jelly on menopausal symptoms: A randomized placebo-controlled clinical trial. *Complement. Ther. Clin. Pract.* **2019**, *37*, 47–50. [CrossRef] [PubMed]
17. Taavoni, S.; Barkhordari, F.; Goushegir, A.; Haghani, H. Effect of Royal Jelly on premenstrual syndrome among Iranian medical sciences students: A randomized, triple-blind, placebo-controlled study. *Complement. Ther. Med.* **2014**, *22*, 601–606. [CrossRef] [PubMed]
18. Lambrinoudaki, I.; Augoulea, A.; Rizos, D.; Politi, M.; Tsoltos, N.; Moros, M.; Chinou, I.; Graikou, K.; Kouskouni, E.; Kambani, S.; et al. Greek-origin royal jelly improves the lipid profile of postmenopausal women. *Gynecol. Endocrinol.* **2016**, *32*, 835–839. [CrossRef] [PubMed]
19. EFSA Panel on Dietetic Products, Nutrition and Allergies (NDA). Scientific Opinion on the substantiation of health claims related to: Anthocyanidins and proanthocyanidins (ID 1787, 1788, 1789, 1790, 1791); sodium alginate and ulva (ID 1873); vitamins, minerals, trace elements and standardised ginseng G115 extract (ID 8, 1673, 1674); vitamins, minerals, lysine and/or arginine and/or taurine (ID 6, 1676, 1677); plant-based preparation for use in beverages (ID 4210, 4211); *Carica papaya* L. (ID 2007); "fish protein" (ID 651); acidic water-based, non-alcoholic flavoured beverages containing calcium in the range of 0.3 to 0.8 mol per mol of acid with a pH not lower than 3.7 (ID 1170); royal jelly (ID 1225, 1226, 1227, 1228, 1230, 1231, 1326, 1328, 1329, 1982, 4696, 4697); foods low in cholesterol (ID 624); and foods low in trans-fatty acids (ID 672, 4333) pursuant to Article 13(1) of Regulation (EC) No 1924/2006. *EFSA J.* **2011**, *9*, 2083.
20. Gupta, H.R.; Patil, Y.; Singh, D.; Thakur, M. Embryonic zebrafish model-A well-established method for rapidly assessing the toxicity of homeopathic drugs: Toxicity evaluation of homeopathic drugs using zebrafish embryo model. *J. Pharmacopunct.* **2016**, *19*, 319–328. [CrossRef]
21. Hoo, J.Y.; Kumari, Y.; Shaikh, M.F.; Hue, S.M.; Goh, B.H. Zebrafish: A versatile animal model for fertility research. *BioMed Res. Int.* **2016**, *2016*, 9732780. [CrossRef]

22. Ka, J.; Jin, S.-W. Zebrafish as an emerging model for dyslipidemia and associated diseases. *J. Lipid Atheroscler.* **2021**, *10*, 42–56. [CrossRef]
23. Zhang, C.; Willett, C.; Fremgen, T. Zebrafish: An animal model for toxicological studies. In *Current Protocols in Toxicology*; Unit 1.7; John Wiley & Sons: Hoboken, NJ, USA, 2003.
24. Trede, N.S.; Zapata, A.; Zon, L.I. Fishing for lymphoid genes. *Trends Immunol.* **2001**, *22*, 302–307. [CrossRef]
25. Patton, E.E.; Zon, L.I.; Langenau, D.M. Zebrafish disease models in drug discovery: From preclinical modelling to clinical trials. *Nat. Rev. Drug Discov.* **2021**, *20*, 611–628. [CrossRef] [PubMed]
26. Cho, K.-H.; Nam, H.-S.; Kim, J.-E.; Na, H.-J.; del Carmen Dominguez-Horta, M.; Martinez-Donato, G. CIGB-258 exerts potent anti-inflammatory activity against carboxymethyllysine-induced acute inflammation in hyperlipidemic zebrafish via the protection of apolipoprotein AI. *Int. J. Mol. Sci.* **2023**, *24*, 7044. [CrossRef]
27. Lee, B.H.; Hsu, W.H.; Hsu, Y.W.; Pan, T.M. Suppression of dimerumic acid on hepatic fibrosis caused from carboxymethyl-lysine (CML) by attenuating oxidative stress depends on Nrf2 activation in hepatic stellate cells (HSCs). *Food Chem. Toxicol.* **2013**, *62*, 413–419. [CrossRef] [PubMed]
28. Nabas, Z.; Haddadin, M.S.; Haddadin, J.; Nazer, I.K. Chemical composition of royal jelly and effects of synbiotic with two different locally isolated probiotic strains on antioxidant activities. *Pol. J. Food Nutr. Sci.* **2014**, *64*, 171–180. [CrossRef]
29. Liu, J.R.; Yang, Y.C.; Shi, L.S.; Peng, C.C. Antioxidant properties of royal jelly associated with larval age and time of harvest. *J. Agric. Food Chem.* **2008**, *56*, 11447–11452. [CrossRef]
30. Guo, H.; Kouzuma, Y.; Yonekura, M. Structures and properties of antioxidative peptides derived from royal jelly protein. *Food Chem.* **2009**, *113*, 238–245. [CrossRef]
31. Watanabe, S.; Suemaru, K.; Takechi, K.; Kaji, H.; Imai, K.; Araki, H. Oral mucosal adhesive films containing royal jelly accelerate recovery from 5-fluorouracil-induced oral mucositis. *J. Pharmacol. Sci.* **2013**, *121*, 110–118. [CrossRef]
32. Park, M.J.; Kim, B.Y.; Deng, Y.; Park, H.G.; Choi, Y.S.; Lee, K.S.; Jin, B.R. Antioxidant capacity of major royal jelly proteins of honeybee (*Apis mellifera*) royal jelly. *J. Asia Pac. Entomol.* **2020**, *23*, 445–448. [CrossRef]
33. Xin, X.X.; Chen, Y.; Chen, D.; Xiao, F.; Parnell, L.D.; Zhao, J.; Liu, L.; Ordovas, J.M.; Lai, C.-Q.; Shen, L.-R. Supplementation with major Royal-Jelly proteins increases lifespan, feeding, and fecundity in *Drosophila*. *J. Agric. Food Chem.* **2016**, *64*, 5803–5812. [CrossRef]
34. Kanbur, M.; Eraslan, G.; Silici, S.; Karabacak, M. Effects of sodium fluoride exposure on some biochemical parameters in mice: Evaluation of the ameliorative effect of royal jelly applications on these parameters. *Food Chem. Toxicol.* **2009**, *47*, 1184–1189. [CrossRef]
35. Bogdanov, S. Royal Jelly, Bee Brood: Composition, Health, Medicine. *J. Bee Prod. Sci.* **2011**, *3*, 8–19.
36. Deb, S.; Puthanveetil, P.; Sakharkar, P. A population-based cross-sectional study of the association between liver enzymes and lipid levels. *Int. J. Hepatol.* **2018**, *2018*, 1286170. [CrossRef]
37. Guo, J.; Wang, Z.; Chen, Y.; Cao, J.; Tian, W.; Ma, B.; Dong, Y. Active components and biological functions of royal jelly. *J. Funct. Foods* **2021**, *82*, 104514. [CrossRef]
38. Kamakura, M.; Moriyama, T.; Sakaki, T. Changes in hepatic gene expression associated with the hypocholesterolaemic activity of royal jelly. *J. Pharm. Pharmacol.* **2006**, *58*, 1683–1689. [CrossRef] [PubMed]
39. Almeer, R.S.; Alarifi, S.; Alkahtani, S.; Ibrahim, S.R.; Ali, D.; Moneim, A. The potential hepatoprotective effect of royal jelly against cadmium chloride-induced hepatotoxicity in mice is mediated by suppression of oxidative stress and upregulation of nrf2 expression. *Biomed. Pharmacother.* **2018**, *106*, 1490–1498. [CrossRef]
40. Redza-Dutordoir, M.; Averill-Bates, D.A. Activation of apoptosis signalling pathways by reactive oxygen species. *Biochim. Biophys. Acta Mol. Cell Res.* **2016**, *1863*, 2977–2992. [CrossRef] [PubMed]
41. El-Hanoun, A.M.; Elkomy, A.E.; Fares, W.A.; Shahien, E.H. Impact of royal jelly to improve reproductive performance of male rabbits under hot summer conditions. *World Rabbit Sci.* **2014**, *22*, 241–248. [CrossRef]
42. Aparisi, Á.; Martín-Fernández, M.; Ybarra-Falcón, C.; Gil, J.F.; Carrasco-Moraleja, M.; Martínez-Paz, P.; Cusácovich, I.; Gonzalo-Benito, H.; Fuertes, R.; Marcos-Mangas, M.; et al. Dyslipidemia and inflammation as hallmarks of oxidative stress in COVID-19: A follow-up study. *Int. J. Mol. Sci.* **2022**, *23*, 15350. [CrossRef]
43. Mokaya, H.O.; Njeru, L.K.; Lattorff, H.M.G. African honeybee royal jelly: Phytochemical contents, free radical scavenging activity, and physicochemical properties. *Food Biosci.* **2020**, *37*, 100733. [CrossRef]
44. Cho, K.-H.; Kang, D.-J.; Nam, H.-S.; Kim, J.-H.; Kim, S.-Y.; Lee, J.-O.; Kim, B.-J. Ozonated sunflower oil exerted protective effect for embryo and cell survival via potent reduction power and antioxidant activity in HDL with strong antimicrobial activity. *Antioxidants* **2021**, *10*, 1651. [CrossRef] [PubMed]
45. Nusslein-Volhard, C.; Dahm, R. *Zebrafish: A Practical Approach*, 1st ed.; Oxford University Press: Oxford, UK, 2002.
46. (NRC) National Research Council of the National Academy of Sciences. *Guide for the Care and Use of Laboratory Animals*; National Academy Press: Washington, DC, USA, 2010.
47. Cho, K.-H.; Kim, J.-E.; Bahuguna, A.; Kang, D.-J. Long-Term Supplementation on of ozonated sunflower oil improves dyslipidemia and hepatic inflammation in hyperlipidemic zebrafish: Suppression of oxidative stress and inflammation against carboxymethyllysine toxicity. *Antioxidants* **2023**, *12*, 1240. [CrossRef] [PubMed]
48. Fischer, A.H.; Jacobson, K.A.; Rose, J.; Zeller, R. Hematoxylin and eosin staining of tissue and cell sections. In *Basic Methods in Microscopy*; Cold Spring Harbor Laboratory Press: New York, NY, USA, 2006; Chapter 4.

49. Cho, K.-H.; Kim, J.-E.; Bahuguna, A.; Kang, D.-J. Ozonated sunflower oil exerted potent anti-inflammatory activities with enhanced wound healing and tissue regeneration abilities against acute toxicity of carboxymethyllysine in zebrafish with improved blood lipid profile. *Antioxidants* **2023**, *12*, 1625. [CrossRef] [PubMed]
50. Cho, K.-H.; Kim, J.-E.; Baek, S.H. Cuban policosanol (Raydel®) potently protects the liver, ovary, and testis with an improvement in dyslipidemia in hyperlipidemic zebrafish: A comparative study with three Chinese policosanols. *Molecules* **2023**, *28*, 6609. [CrossRef]
51. Umali, J.; Hawkey-Noble, A.; French, C.R. Loss of foxc1 in zebrafish reduces optic nerve size and cell number in the retinal ganglion cell layer. *Vision Res.* **2019**, *156*, 66–72. [CrossRef]
52. Cho, K.-H.; Kim, J.-E.; Nam, H.-S.; Baek, S.-H.; Bahuguna, A. Consumption of policosanol (Raydel®) improves hepatic, renal, and reproductive functions in zebrafish: In Vivo comparison study among Cuban, Chinese, and American policosanol. *Pharmaceuticals* **2024**, *17*, 66. [CrossRef]

pharmaceuticals

MDPI

Article

Bee Venom-Loaded Niosomes as Innovative Platforms for Cancer Treatment: Development and Therapeutical Efficacy and Safety Evaluation

Maria Beatriz Pinto [1], Patrícia C. Pires [1,2,3,*], Ricardo C. Calhelha [4,5], Ana Rita Silva [4,5], Maria João Sousa [4,5], Miguel Vilas-Boas [4,5], Soraia I. Falcão [4,5], Francisco Veiga [1,2], Pooyan Makvandi [6,7,8] and Ana Cláudia Paiva-Santos [1,2,*]

1 Department of Pharmaceutical Technology, Faculty of Pharmacy of the University of Coimbra, University of Coimbra, Azinhaga de Santa Comba, 3000-548 Coimbra, Portugal
2 REQUIMTE/LAQV, Group of Pharmaceutical Technology, Faculty of Pharmacy of the University of Coimbra, University of Coimbra, 3000-548 Coimbra, Portugal
3 Health Sciences Research Centre (CICS-UBI), University of Beira Interior, Av. Infante D. Henrique, 6200-506 Covilhã, Portugal
4 Centro de Investigação de Montanha (CIMO), Instituto Politécnico de Bragança, Campus de Santa Apolónia, 5300-253 Bragança, Portugal; mvboas@ipb.pt (M.V.-B.); sfalcao@ipb.pt (S.I.F.)
5 Laboratório Associado para a Sustentabilidade e Tecnologia em Regiões de Montanha (SusTEC), Instituto Politécnico de Bragança, Campus de Santa Apolónia, 5300-253 Bragança, Portugal
6 The Quzhou Affiliated Hospital of Wenzhou Medical University, Quzhou People's Hospital, Quzhou 324000, China
7 Centre of Research Impact and Outreach, Chitkara University, Rajpura 140417, India
8 Department of Biomaterials, Saveetha Dental College and Hospitals, SIMATS, Saveetha University, Chennai 600077, India
* Correspondence: patriciapires@ff.uc.pt (P.C.P.); acsantos@ff.uc.pt (A.C.P.-S.)

Abstract: Despite past efforts towards therapeutical innovation, cancer remains a highly incident and lethal disease, with current treatments lacking efficiency and leading to severe side effects. Hence, it is imperative to develop new, more efficient, and safer therapies. Bee venom has proven to have multiple and synergistic bioactivities, including antitumor effects. Nevertheless, some toxic effects have been associated with its administration. To tackle these issues, in this work, bee venom-loaded niosomes were developed, for cancer treatment. The vesicles had a small (150 nm) and homogeneous (polydispersity index of 0.162) particle size, and revealed good therapeutic efficacy in in vitro gastric, colorectal, breast, lung, and cervical cancer models (inhibitory concentrations between 12.37 ng/mL and 14.72 ng/mL). Additionally, they also revealed substantial anti-inflammatory activity (inhibitory concentration of 28.98 ng/mL), effects complementary to direct antitumor activity. Niosome safety was also assessed, both in vitro (skin, liver, and kidney cells) and ex vivo (hen's egg chorioallantoic membrane), and results showed that compound encapsulation increased its safety. Hence, small, and homogeneous bee venom-loaded niosomes were successfully developed, with substantial anticancer and anti-inflammatory effects, making them potentially promising primary or adjuvant cancer therapies. Future research should focus on evaluating the potential of the developed platform in in vivo models.

Keywords: anti-inflammatory; anticancer; antitumor; bee venom; in vitro; nanosystems; natural compounds; niosomes

1. Introduction

Cancer remains one of the most incident diseases globally with high mortality rates, having been estimated to affect almost 2,000,000 people just in the United States of America in the year of 2023, with more than 600,000 related deaths, and having similar incidence rates all over the world [1–3]. This not only leads to substantial out-of-pocket costs for patients and caregivers, due to necessary in-hospital care, medication, and medical consultations, making up to 16 to 42% of their annual income, but also relevant global economic burden, being estimated to cost up to $25.2 trillion in international dollars in 2050 [4–6]. Furthermore, while life-expectancy keeps increasing, age itself becomes an important risk factor for cancer development, due to the aging process bringing about several relevant biological changes linked to cancer pathogenesis, leading to a reduction of late-life quality, increased disability, and overall rise in health costs [7–9].

Although the fast-paced advances in medicine are today able to prolong the life of these patients, and even cure them in some cases, most common cancer therapies, such as chemotherapy, radiotherapy, immunotherapy, and surgery, are linked with poor prognosis and/or severely debilitating side effects, such as nausea and vomiting, pain, fatigue, depression, hair loss, and immune system debilitation, which can lead to opportunistic infections due to the body's higher vulnerability and low defenses [10–12]. Additionally, although novel technologies have recently emerged, with recent advances including various targeted therapies, and even robotics and artificial intelligence, there is still a long way towards the effective clinical testing, and, subsequently, commercialization of these potential treatments, as well as guaranteeing that they are cost-effective [13–17]. Hence, there is an urgent need for new, more effective, and safer therapies.

In this context, natural-derived products might be the answer [18–20]. Bee venom, also known as apitoxin, is a substance produced in the venom gland under the abdominal cavity of female worker bees, and it is a colorless and odorless liquid, with an acid pH between 4.5 and 5.5. It is used by these insects to defend the hive against external threats [21]. In its composition, we can find peptides like melittin, apamin, adolapin, and scapin, and enzymes such as phospholipase A2, hyaluronidase, and lysophospholipase, as well as other substances, including amino acids, carbohydrates, pheromones, and minerals. Among all these compounds, melittin is the main active ingredient in bee venom, comprising 40% to 60% of its dry weight, followed by the enzyme phospholipase A2, present in 10–12% [22]. The complex chemical composition of bee venom, and the potential synergy surrounding the interaction between its compounds, assures a vast range of biological activities, capable of targeting different diseases. These biological properties include anti-inflammatory, antioxidant, antiviral, antimicrobial and antitumor properties (Figure 1) [23,24]. All these bioactivities could be potentially beneficial for a series of different diseases, from skin diseases, such as acne, wounds, psoriasis, or atopic dermatitis, to neurodegenerative diseases, such as Parkinson's disease, due to proven neuroprotective effects, and, of course, cancer [25,26]. Nevertheless, while bee venom can be tolerated by the human body, it can cause some allergic reactions, as well as systemic and local inflammatory responses, other immune reactions, and anticoagulant effects, which are the main drawbacks for its use as a potential therapeutic agent [22]. Bee venom toxicity has been reported to be concentration-dependent on blood cells, namely in human lymphocytes, leading to the induction of oxidative stress-related DNA damage, and, consequently, cellular instability, and overall genotoxicity, making this one of the most relevant barriers to its use for therapeutic purposes [27–29]. In this context, new strategies are needed in order to increase the safety of bee venom administration and its incorporation into nanotechnological platforms to enhance its properties, avoid degradation, and reduce the potential side effects [30].

The use of nanotechnology for drug delivery can not only protect the drug from chemical and metabolic degradation, but also allow increased permeation through biological barriers, and enable a controlled, sustained, and targeted drug delivery, hence leading to more localized therapeutic effects, and thus reduced systemic toxicity [31–33]. Several types of nanosystems have been developed over the years, namely nanoemulsions, micelles, polymeric nanoparticles, and lipid nanoparticles, such as liposomes, and their more recent and innovative alternatives, ethosomes, transfersomes and niosomes [34–36]. Niosomes are vesicular nanosystems capable of self-assembly, composed of amphiphilic molecules, such as non-ionic surfactants, which form an outer bilayered membrane, and an aqueous core [37,38]. This structure makes them highly versatile nanosystems for therapeutic application since they can deliver both hydrophobic molecules, within the bilayered membrane, and hydrophilic molecules, encapsulated within their aqueous core. Other molecules, such as cholesterol or similar lipids, can also be part of the niosomal membrane, giving them better properties, such as higher stability and deformability [39,40]. Thanks to their composition, niosomes are biodegradable and biocompatible, on account of the similarity between the lipids used for niosome production and the ones found in the human body, especially on the cellular membranes [41,42]. Additionally, when compared to their ancestors, liposomes, niosomes possess higher stability and longer shelf-life, a better capacity for controlled drug release, and lead to higher drug bioavailability [43].

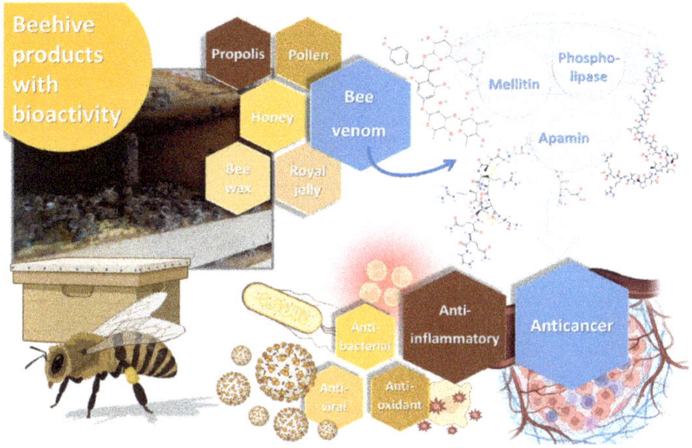

Figure 1. Schematic representation of beehive derived compounds, including a photograph of the beehive at Polytechnic Institute of Bragança's apiary, Bragança, Portugal (produced with Biorender, melittin, phospholipase and apamin molecular structures originated from PubChem).

Hence, given the great therapeutic potential of bee venom, and the promising properties of niosomes for increased therapeutic efficacy and safety, the purpose of the present study was to develop and characterize bee venom-loaded niosomes, for potential anticancer therapy. Their physicochemical, therapeutic and safety profiles were assessed, including particle size and polydispersity index determination, in vitro cytotoxicity, and anti-inflammatory potential assessment, and in vitro and ex vivo safety evaluation. Limitations regarding these assays (including the assessment of the optimum hydration temperature for niosome production, determination of the ideal dilution for particle size measurement, and the determination of the adequate positive and negative controls for the cell assays) were thoroughly assessed and resolved.

2. Results and Discussion

2.1. Niosomal Formulation Development and Characterization

The bee venom samples went through chemical characterization, by quantification of its major constituents (Table 1) [44]. An example of the obtained chromatogram using UHPLC is shown in Figure 2. Three main compounds were quantified, with melittin being the most abundant compound present in the sample (63%), followed by phospholipase A2 (12%), and apamin (1.2%), which is in agreement with the reported previous works [21,45].

Table 1. Chemical characterization of the bee venom encapsulated within the developed niosomes, or solubilized within the produced compound solution, performed by UHPLC analysis. Major compounds are presented, with values corresponding to the amount present in each analyzed sample (µg/mL).

Compounds	Bee Venom Solution (300 µg/mL)	Bee Venom-Loaded Niosomes (2 µg/mL)	Correspondent Percentage (%)
Melittin	193.43	1.29	63
Phospholipase A2	37.52	0.25	12
Apamin	3.61	0.024	1.2

UHPLC—ultra-high-performance liquid chromatography.

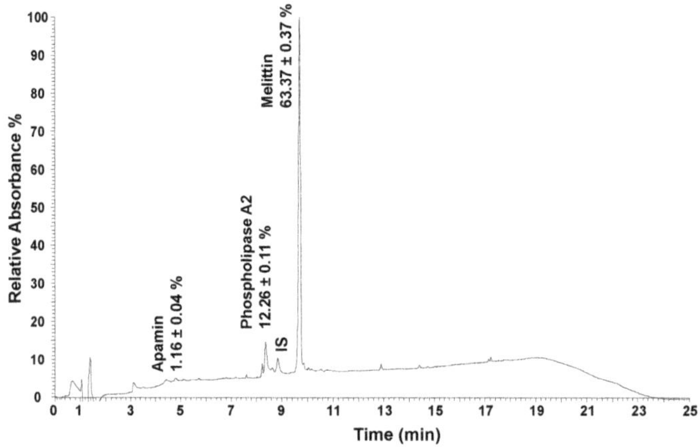

Figure 2. Example chromatogram after UHPLC analysis of the bee venom sample, at 220 nm. IS—internal standard (cytochrome C, 25 µg/mL); UHPLC—ultra-high-performance liquid chromatography.

Tween® 20, a hydrophilic non-ionic surfactant, was used to form the niosomes, with the addition of cholesterol and cetyl alcohol (1:1) as the lipidic components. It has been reported that non-ionic surfactants with HLB values above 6 require the addition of a lipidic component to correctly produce niosomes [38]. Additionally, adding cholesterol to a niosomal formulation improves the cohesion of the niosomal membrane [46], enhances membrane stability, decreases membrane fluidity, eliminates the gel-to-liquid phase transition temperature, allows better loading of hydrophilic drugs [47], and improves entrapment efficiency by filling empty spaces in the bilayer vesicle [42]. The addition of cholesterol and cetyl alcohol has also been reported to improve the overall stability of the produced niosomal structures [48].

As the main composition of bee venom is proteins, these can denature at high temperatures, hence during production, an effort should be made to use the lowest temperatures possible [49]. For this reason, multiple hydration temperatures were tested, namely 40 °C, 45 °C, 50 °C, 55 °C, and 60 °C. The results showed that after extrusion, similar particle size and PDI values were obtained for all hydration temperatures (Figure 3), and hence the lowest temperature, 40 °C, was selected. Additionally, although there was a statistically significant difference in particle size and PDI before extrusion and after extrusion ($p < 0.0001$, R^2 0.9991, one-way ANOVA with Tukey's multiple comparisons test), all extrusion cycles originated a particle size below 200 nm, which is suitable for all kinds of administration routes, making the formulation highly versatile in what concerns potential application. PDI values were also always below 0.3, for all extrusion cycles and temperatures, and in most cases also below or equal to 0.2, making the formulations highly homogeneous [50–52]. Therefore, for the selected temperature, 40 °C, the number of extrusion cycles which originated the lowest particle size and PDI values was selected, being equal to 31 extrusion cycles. These niosomes were hence selected for compound encapsulation and had a particle size of 151.2 ± 1.8 nm and a PDI of 0.091 ± 0.018 (Table 2). As for the zeta potential of the optimized formulation, it was between −30 and −40 mV, which could have a contribution in formulation stabilization through electrostatic repulsion.

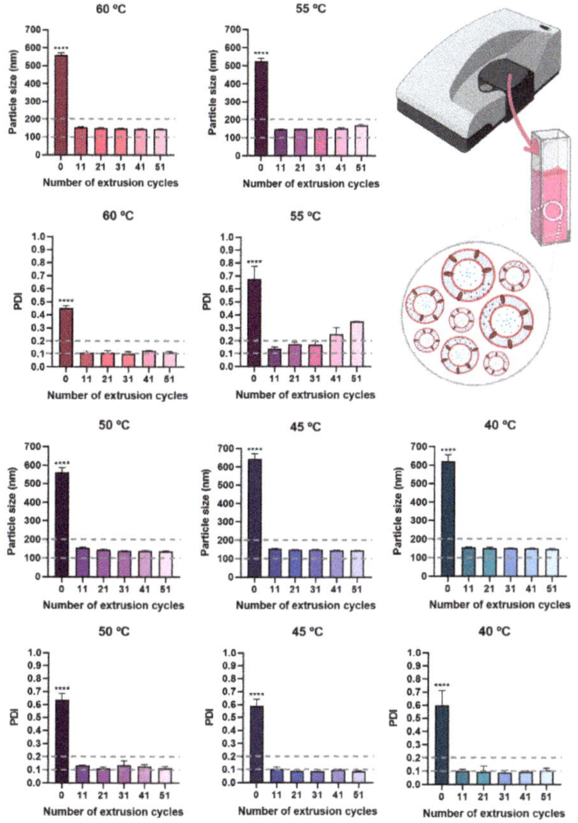

Figure 3. Particle size and PDI values of the developed niosomes (formulation vehicle), at all tested temperatures, and with a varying number of performed extrusion cycles; data is presented as mean ± standard deviation; **** $p < 0.0001$ and corresponds to the comparison of no extrusion with all extrusion cycles (R^2 0.9991, one-way ANOVA with Tukey's multiple comparisons test); PDI—polydispersity index.

Table 2. Particle size (nm) and PDI of empty and bee venom-loaded niosomes, after optimization (31 cycles of extrusion).

Formulations	Bee Venom Concentration	Particle Size (nm)	PDI
Empty niosomes (formulation vehicle)	0	151.2 ± 1.8	0.091 ± 0.018
Bee venom-loaded niosomes	2 µg/mL	150.4 ± 3.7	0.162 ± 0.008

PDI—polydispersity index.

Once the niosomes were optimized (formulation vehicle, still no encapsulated compound), bee venom was added to the vesicles' aqueous core, to be encapsulated at a concentration of 2 μg/mL. This concentration was selected based on previous studies, for it to be enough to have bioactivity, but not so much that it would be potentially toxic. According to previous studies, when using concentrations of bee venom of 3.125 μg/mL or 5 μg/mL, a substantial decrease in healthy cells' viability was observed, with values ranging from only around 50 to 60% [53]. Hence, a lower value was selected, to help guarantee formulation safety.

After the encapsulation of bee venom, the mean particle size was equal to 150.4 ± 3.7 nm, remaining the same as without compound encapsulation, and the PDI was equal to 0.162 ± 0.008, hence having a slight increase (as had been reported by previous studies [54]), but still being below 0.2, and therefore still constituting a quite homogeneous nanosystem (Table 2).

2.2. *In Vitro Cytotoxic Potential*

The in vitro cytotoxic potential of the developed bee venom-loaded niosomes was tested, at different concentrations, in different cell lines, with the cytotoxicity being evaluated using a sulforhodamine B colorimetric assay, in five human tumor cell lines, namely AGS (gastric adenocarcinoma), Caco-2 (colorectal adenocarcinoma), MCF-7 (breast adenocarcinoma), NCI-H460 (lung carcinoma) and HeLa (cervical carcinoma). Two non-tumor cell lines were also used, Vero (African green monkey kidney) and PLP2 (primary pig liver culture), to assess for potential systemic toxicity. Results are shown in Figure 4.

A substantial anticancer potential has been previously reported for bee venom, related to its capacity to inhibit cancer cell growth, and induce apoptosis, and more specifically related to its major components melittin and phospholipase A2 [55,56]. Other studies have demonstrated that bee venom can trigger regional cellular immune reactions in lymph nodes, exerting its effects through not only apoptosis, but also lysis mechanisms and tumor cell necrosis [57,58]. Our results show that the bee venom solution had the most significant cytotoxic effect, both against the studied cancer cell lines, and the healthy cell lines, attributed to its lower GI_{50} values, ranging from 5.05 to 5.87 ng/mL ($p < 0.0001$, R^2 0.9991, one-way ANOVA with Tukey's multiple comparisons test). Although this means that the bee venom solution has a higher anticancer potential while unencapsulated, it also means that it has a higher potential for toxicity in healthy tissues, hence being connected to a higher propensity for systemic side effects. Hence, compound encapsulation will reduce its potentially harmful effects in healthy cells, while still having substantial anticancer potential in tumor cell lines. Hence, when encapsulated into the niosomes, a higher targeting potential to cancer cells can be obtained, while being able to avoid destroying healthy cells.

Regarding the AGS cell line, the bee venom-loaded niosomes present a GI_{50} value of 13.19 ng/mL, still demonstrating a good cytotoxic potential after bee venom encapsulation. A previous study [59] has shown that melittin present in bee venom can stop AGS cell proliferation even at low concentrations. Concerning the Caco-2 cell line, the bee venom-loaded niosomes present a GI_{50} value of 13.82 ng/mL, thereby retaining the cytotoxic potential of bee venom after encapsulation. This anticancer activity against the Caco-2 cell line was also demonstrated in a previous study [60], where the developed nanoparticles were able to deliver the active compound to the correct target, the cancer cells. In what concerns the MCF-7 cell line, the bee venom-loaded niosomes presented a GI_{50} value of 14.05 ng/mL, thereby being substantially cytotoxic for this cell line as well. Bee venom has been proven to inhibit the growth of breast cancer cells even in small concentrations, as observed in previous studies [61]. For the NCIH460 cell line, the bee venom-loaded niosomes showed a GI_{50} value of 14.72 ng/mL, hence demonstrating good anticancer potential for this cell line too. Bee venom has also been proven to inhibit cell proliferation of NCIH460 cells in a concentration-dependent manner in prior studies [62]. Regarding the HeLa cell line, the bee venom-loaded niosomes presented a GI_{50} value of 12.37 ng/mL, still demonstrating a considerable cytotoxic potential even after compound encapsulation.

Bee venom has also demonstrated anticancer properties in these cells previously, in a concentration-dependent manner [63].

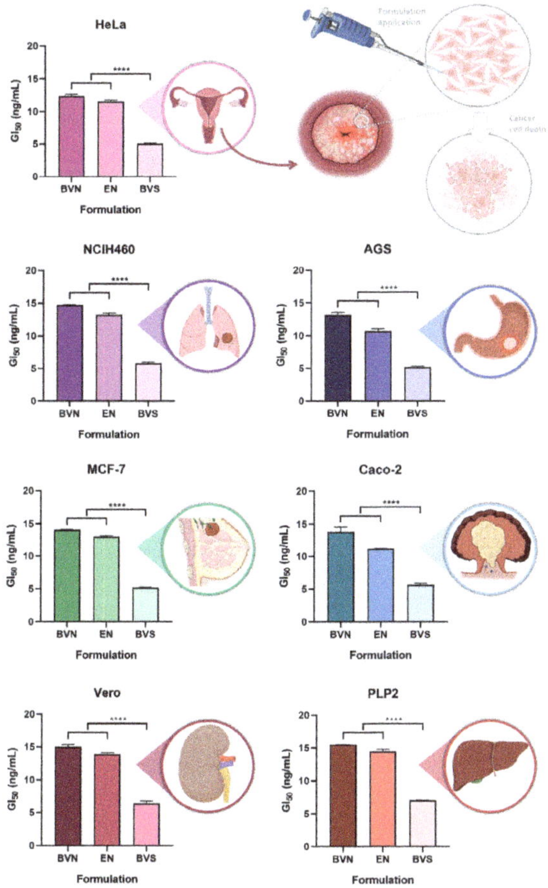

Figure 4. Cytotoxic potential of the developed bee venom-loaded niosomes, compared to the empty niosomes (formulation vehicle) and bee venom solution, in several different cancer cell lines; GI_{50} corresponds to the formulation concentration required to inhibit cell growth by 50%; data is represented as mean ± standard deviation; **** $p < 0.0001$ (R^2 0.9991, one-way ANOVA with Tukey's multiple comparisons test); AGS—gastric adenocarcinoma cell line; Caco-2—colorectal adenocarcinoma cell line; HeLa—cervical carcinoma cell line; MCF-7—breast adenocarcinoma cell line; NCI-H460—lung carcinoma cell line; PLP2—primary pig liver culture cell line; and Vero—African green monkey kidney cell line.

As for previous similar studies, regarding nanosystem development for therapeutic purposes containing bee venom, a prior study where a nanoliposome was designed to encapsulate bee venom with similar concentrations was tested in some cancer cell lines, in which a cytotoxicity assay was also performed [64]. In comparison, for our study, smaller concentrations of bee venom were necessary to inhibit the growth of cancer cells by 50%. Hence, overall, the obtained results showed that the developed bee venom-loaded niosomes could serve as a potential adjuvant treatment for several types of cancer, including cervical, breast, lung, stomach, and colorectal carcinomas. Bee venom can be used as a therapeutic agent for cancer thanks to its complex chemical composition, and even when encapsulated into niosomes, bee venom has presented good cytotoxic properties against various cancer cells, in this case enhancing its anticancer potential by providing a controlled and sustained release of the compound, ideal for a prolonged therapeutic effect.

2.3. *In Vitro Anti-Inflammatory Activity*

In recent years, the link between inflammation and cancer has been extensively studied, both in what concerns pathogenesis and therapeutics [65–67]. Inflammation has been proven to increase the chances of cancer development, promoting all stages of tumorigenesis, and not only regulating cancer development but also therapeutic responses, with chronic inflammation having an important role in both stimulating tumor progression and leading to treatment resistance [68–70]. Cancer cells and inflammatory cells have been proven to interact to form an inflammatory tumor microenvironment, with inflammatory factors and metabolites such as several cytokines (tumor necrosis factor (TNF)), interleukins (IL), interferons (IFN)), chemokines, growth factors, inflammasomes, leukotrienes, prostaglandins, and thromboxane being identified as having important roles in the initiation and regulation of cancer-related inflammatory processes [68,69,71]. Additionally, inflammation has been linked to DNA damage in cancer stem-like cells, leading not only to the development of cancer, but to more aggressive forms of the disease, and also being connected to increased oxidative stress, with the generation of reactive oxygen and nitrogen species which will also damage and lead to dysfunctional lipids and proteins [72–74]. For these reasons, compounds with anti-inflammatory action have been studied as alternative or adjuvant treatments for all types of cancers [75–77].

Hence, to assess the anti-inflammatory properties of the developed bee venom-loaded niosomes, for potential synergistic effects with the non-inflammatory related anticancer potential of the formulation, the pro-inflammatory response was evaluated in the mouse macrophage cell line RAW 264.7 (Figure 5). The developed bee venom-loaded formulation was compared with the free compound (bee venom solution), and the formulation vehicle. The IC_{50} (concentration of the formulation required to inhibit 50% of nitric oxide production) was determined and calculated, as a demonstration of its anti-inflammatory activity.

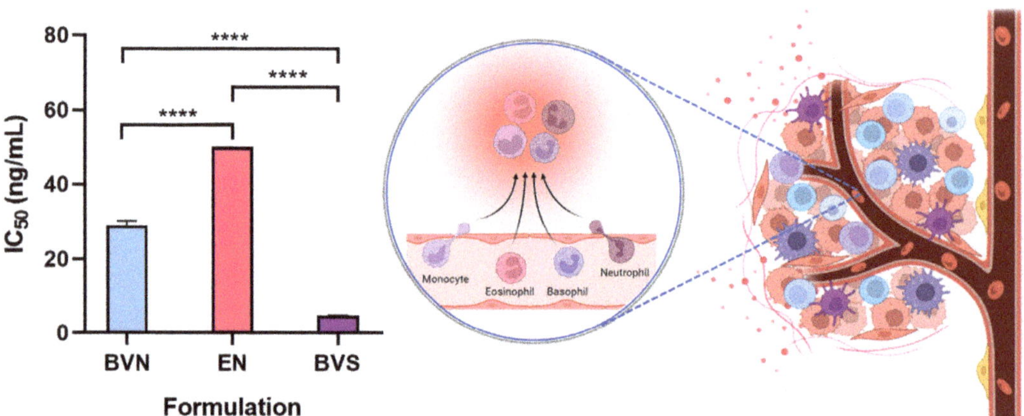

Figure 5. Anti-inflammatory potential of the developed bee venom-loaded niosomes (BVN), compared to the free compound (bee venom solution, BVS), and the formulation vehicle (empty niosomes, EN), evaluated in a mouse macrophage cell line (RAW 264.7); IC_{50} values are depicted, and correspond to formulation concentrations providing 50% of inhibition of nitric oxide production; data is represented as mean ± standard deviation; **** $p < 0.0001$ (schematic representation produced with Biorender).

The bee venom solution demonstrated an IC_{50} of 4.77 ng/mL, the lowest out of the compared formulations ($p < 0.0001$, R^2 0.9991, one-way ANOVA with Tukey's multiple comparisons test), which is indicative of an extensive anti-inflammatory potential, and in line with previous results from the research team [78]. Additionally, this potential has been further confirmed by other past publications, where similar bee venom concentrations depicted similar anti-inflammatory properties, with its main constituent, melittin, being responsible for the majority of such effects [79–81]. In what concerns specific action mechanisms, in previous studies, bee venom proved to have significant anti-inflammatory effects not only by inhibiting phospholipase A, but also by decreasing pro-inflammatory cytokines IL-1β, IL-6, and IFN-γ, and chemokines CCL22 and CCL17 levels, in in vitro assays [82–84]. Moreover, in an in vivo model of atopic dermatitis, bee venom proved to significantly reduce IL-1β, IL-4, IL-6, IL-13, immunoglobulin E (IgE) and TNF-α levels, also leading to a reduction in the number of inflammatory cells (neutrophils, eosinophils, monocytes), and cyclooxygenase-2 (COX-2) inhibition [84–86]. Also in vivo, in an arthritis animal model, bee venom has proven to have anti-inflammatory effects by inhibiting IL-1β, IL-6, TNF-α and TGF-β1 levels, as well as having complementary antioxidant effects, with a reduction in total antioxidant status, and leading to a reduction in DNA damage [21,87]. Further supporting these in vitro and in vivo results, several clinical trials with bee venom administration to inflammatory-based diseases' patients, such as rheumatoid arthritis, adhesive capsulitis, and pelvic inflammatory disease, have demonstrated promising outcomes, with substantial improvement of clinical symptoms and disease markers, after topical or intravenous administration [88–91]. Although specific molecular mechanisms are still in need of deeper exploration, these results have been suggested to be connected to COX-2 and prostaglandin E2 inhibition, among other mechanisms [88,92].

Furthermore, as expected, the formulation vehicle (empty niosomes) showed no substantial anti-inflammatory potential, with an IC_{50} value of >50 ng/mL, the highest out of the studied formulations ($p < 0.0001$, R^2 0.9991, one-way ANOVA with Tukey's multiple comparisons test), confirming that none of the components used in niosome composition depict intrinsic anti-inflammatory effects. As for the bee venom-loaded niosomes, the formulation presented an IC_{50} of 28.98 ng/mL, which albeit is higher than that obtained for the bee venom solution ($p < 0.0001$, R^2 0.9991, one-way ANOVA with Tukey's multiple comparisons test), can still be considered a relevant anti-inflammatory effect, meaning that when encapsulated into the nanometric structures the bee venom does not lose its anti-inflammatory potential. Additionally, the higher IC_{50} value of the bee venom-loaded niosomes when compared to the free compound is likely related to the controlled release of the molecule from within the nanosystems, potentially leading to a sustained and prolonged therapeutic effect, which has been shown to produce enhanced bioavailability in previous studies, using similar delivery systems and compounds [93–95].

2.4. *In Vitro Safety Assessment—Cytotoxicity Evaluation on HaCaT and HFF-1 Cell Lines*

Assays evaluating formulation safety in skin cellular models have long been applied to predict potential toxicity issues, being especially relevant for intended transdermal or topical administration [96–98]. Hence, to evaluate the safety of the developed bee venom-loaded niosomes and compare them to the vehicle formulation (empty niosomes), and free compound (bee venom solution), a sulforhodamine B colorimetric assay was conducted, in two human skin cell lines, HaCaT (keratinocytes) and HFF-1 (fibroblasts). The results, depicted in Figure 6, showed significant differences between concentrations within the same formulation (statistical significance matrix on Table 3), and also when comparing the same concentration for different formulations (Table 4).

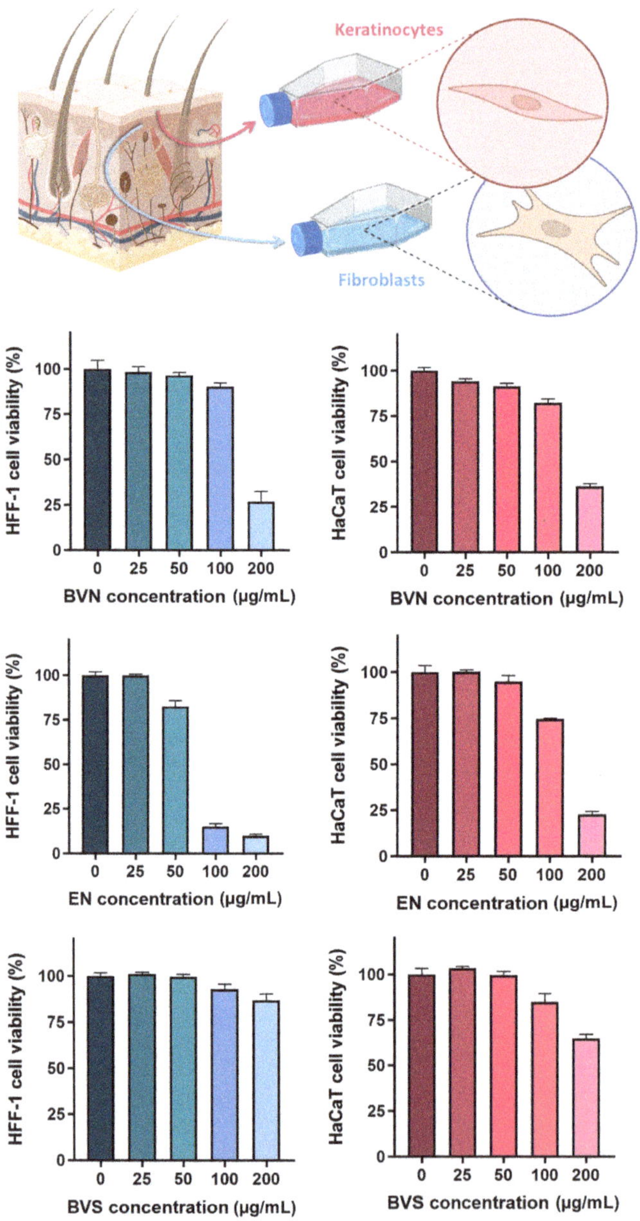

Figure 6. Cell viability percentage (%) variation with increasing applied formulation concentrations (µg/mL), on HFF-1 cell line (left bar graphs, in blue), and HaCaT cell line (right bar graphs, in pink), including the developed bee venom loaded niosomes (BVN), formulation vehicle (empty niosomes, EN), and compound solution (bee venom solution, BVS); data is represented as mean ± standard deviation; HaCaT—skin keratinocytes cell line; HFF-1—skin fibroblasts cell line.

Table 3. Significance matrix of the HaCaT and HFF-1 cell viability assay results (depicted in Figure 6), comparing the viability percentage variation with concentration variation within each studied formulation, for each cell type. The presented values correspond to p values, after the application of one-way ANOVA with Tukey's multiple comparisons' test.

HFF-1 Cells						**HaCaT Cells**					
Bee Venom-Loaded Niosomes						**Bee Venom-Loaded Niosomes**					
Concentration (μg/mL)	0	25	50	100	200	Concentration (μg/mL)	0	25	50	100	200
Overall			<0.0001			Overall			<0.0001		
0	-	NS	NS	0.0352	<0.0001	0	-	0.0025	<0.0001	<0.0001	<0.0001
25	-	-	NS	NS	<0.0001	25	-	-	NS	<0.0001	<0.0001
50	-	-	-	NS	<0.0001	50	-	-	-	0.0002	<0.0001
100	-	-	-	-	<0.0001	100	-	-	-	-	<0.0001
200	-	-	-	-	-	200	-	-	-	-	-
Empty niosomes						Empty niosomes					
Concentration (μg/mL)	0	25	50	100	200	Concentration (μg/mL)	0	25	50	100	200
Overall			<0.0001			Overall			<0.0001		
0	-	NS	<0.0001	<0.0001	<0.0001	0	-	NS	NS	<0.0001	<0.0001
25	-	-	<0.0001	<0.0001	<0.0001	25	-	-	NS	<0.0001	<0.0001
50	-	-	-	<0.0001	<0.0001	50	-	-	-	<0.0001	<0.0001
100	-	-	-	-	0.0392	100	-	-	-	-	<0.0001
200	-	-	-	-	-	200	-	-	-	-	-
Bee venom solution						Bee venom solution					
Concentration (μg/mL)	0	25	50	100	200	Concentration (μg/mL)	0	25	50	100	200
Overall			<0.0001			Overall			<0.0001		
0	-	NS	NS	0.0003	<0.0001	0	-	NS	NS	<0.0001	<0.0001
25	-	-	NS	0.0002	<0.0001	25	-	-	NS	<0.0001	<0.0001
50	-	-	-	0.0021	<0.0001	50	-	-	-	<0.0001	<0.0001
100	-	-	-	-	0.0087	100	-	-	-	-	<0.0001
200	-	-	-	-	-	200	-	-	-	-	-

NS—not significant (statistical significance); HaCaT—skin keratinocytes cell line; and HFF-1—skin fibroblasts cell line.

Overall, the results show that there is a concentration-dependent safety of the developed formulations ($p < 0.0001$, two-way ANOVA with Tukey's multiple comparisons' test), with the safest concentration in both HaCaT and HFF-1 cell lines appearing to reside between 50 and 100 μg/mL. Specifically for the bee venom solution, safety appears to be related to concentrations up to 200 μg/mL in the HFF-1 cell line, but only up to 100 μg/mL in the HaCaT cell line. These results are in accordance with the ones obtained by previous studies for the HaCaT cell line [99], where cell viability tended to reduce with increasing bee venom concentrations, and with safety existing up to 100 μg/mL, and appear to be more promising than the ones reported by previous studies for the HFF-1 cell line [100], where only concentrations equal or lower than 10 μg/mL were considered safe. Additionally, IC_{50} values (formulation concentrations causing 50% reduction of cell viability or proliferation, Table 5) were proven to be 165.7 ± 1.0 μg/mL and 161.0 ± 1.0 μg/mL for the bee venom-loaded niosomes, 138.2 ± 1.0 μg/mL and 69.8 ± 1.0 μg/mL for the formulation vehicle, and >200.0 μg/mL for the bee venom solution, in HaCaT and HFF-1 cells, respectively.

Table 4. Significance matrix of the HaCaT and HFF-1 cell viability assay results (depicted in Figure 6), comparing the viability percentage variation between studied formulations, for the same concentrations, for each cell type. The presented values correspond to p values, after application of two-way ANOVA with Tukey's multiple comparisons' test.

HFF-1 Cells						HaCaT Cells					
Bee Venom-Loaded Niosomes vs. Empty Niosomes						**Bee Venom-Loaded Niosomes vs. Empty Niosomes**					
Overall	0 μg/mL	25 μg/mL	50 μg/mL	100 μg/mL	200 μg/mL	Overall	0 μg/mL	25 μg/mL	50 μg/mL	100 μg/mL	200 μg/mL
<0.0001	0.0037	0.0104	0.0025	<0.0001	<0.0001	<0.0001	0.0058	<0.0001	0.0015	NS	<0.0001
Bee venom-loaded niosomes vs. bee venom solution						Bee venom-loaded niosomes vs. bee venom solution					
Overall	0 μg/mL	25 μg/mL	50 μg/mL	100 μg/mL	200 μg/mL	Overall	0 μg/mL	25 μg/mL	50 μg/mL	100 μg/mL	200 μg/mL
<0.0001	<0.0001	<0.0001	<0.0001	<0.0001	<0.0001	<0.0001	<0.0001	<0.0001	<0.0001	<0.0001	<0.0001
Empty niosomes vs. bee venom solution						Empty niosomes vs. bee venom solution					
Overall	0 μg/mL	25 μg/mL	50 μg/mL	100 μg/mL	200 g/mL	Overall	0 μg/mL	25 μg/mL	50 μg/mL	100 μg/mL	200 μg/mL
<0.0001	<0.0001	<0.0001	<0.0001	<0.0001	<0.0001	<0.0001	0.0004	0.0001	<0.0001	<0.0001	<0.0001

NS—not significant (statistical significance); HaCaT—skin keratinocytes cell line; and HFF-1—skin fibroblasts cell line.

Table 5. Cell viability of the developed bee venom-loaded niosomes, formulation vehicle (empty niosomes), and compound solution (bee venom solution), evaluated in HaCaT and HFF-1 cell lines, and represented by the calculated IC_{50} value.

	Cell Viability (IC_{50}, μg/mL)	
	HFF-1 Cells	**HaCaT Cells**
Bee venom-loaded niosomes	165.7 ± 1.0	161.0 ± 1.0
Empty niosomes	138.2 ± 1.0	69.8 ± 1.00
Bee venom solution	>200.0	>200.0

IC_{50} value corresponds to formulation concentrations causing 50% reduction of cell viability or proliferation; data is represented as mean ± standard deviation of tested formulations; HaCaT—skin keratinocytes cell line; and HFF-1—skin fibroblasts cell line.

Furthermore, the results showed that the developed niosomes without bee venom (formulation vehicle) appear to be less safe than the bee venom-loaded niosomes, in both cell lines ($p < 0.0001$, two-way ANOVA with Tukey's multiple comparisons' test). This seemingly unexpected cytotoxicity of the empty niosomes might be related to the quantities of the excipients used to formulate them. A previous study, on polysorbate 20 (Tween 20) formulations applied on HaCaT cells, showed that at elevated concentrations cytotoxicity could be detected, as well as after long periods of exposure [101]. Additionally, the lesser cytotoxicity of bee venom-loaded niosomes could be due to the absorption of the hydrophilic compound to the surface of the vesicles, thereby decreasing their toxicity due to decreasing the direct contact of the formulation compounds with the cells.

Hence, overall, the obtained results showed that the developed niosomes can only be administered on the skin up to certain concentrations, but since in vitro results have been reported to not always be directly related to what happens in vivo [102,103], and, even more, in a clinical context [104,105], further studies would have to be performed to assess the true safety of the developed nanocarriers. Therefore, safety was further assessed in the HET-CAM test (results shown in the following Section 2.5). It is also relevant to mention that given the known severe side effects related to the grand majority of anticancer therapies [106–108], a risk-benefit ratio would always have to be assessed if the developed formulations are proven to be of great therapeutic potential as primary or adjuvant anticancer therapies.

2.5. Ex Vivo Safety Assessment—HET-CAM Test

The HET-CAM test has been used for many years as a useful model to predict the potential of developed formulations to cause eye irritation, hence making the preparations that are proven to be safe after application onto the hen's egg chorioallantoic membranes, also potentially safe for administration through most administration routes, given that the eye is one of the most sensitive organs in the human body [109–111]. Hence, to evaluate the irritation degree of the developed bee venom-loaded niosomes, a HET-CAM test was conducted, with the application of 0.3 mL of each formulation (non-diluted) onto each fertilized egg's chorioallantoic membrane. Then, during the first 5 min after application, the membrane was observed for vascular reactions in the blood vessels, according to the described method's protocol [112]. Results are shown in Table 6 and Figure 7.

Table 6. HET-CAM results after application of the developed bee venom-loaded niosomes or formulation vehicle (empty niosomes), with respective positive (0.1 N NaOH) and negative (0.9% NaCl) controls, on hen's egg chorioallantoic membranes, and represented by the calculated average irritation score (IS) ± standard deviation, and visible vascular reactions and overall irritation degree.

Formulation	Average IS	Standard Deviation	Vascular Reactions Following Treatment	Irritation Degree
Bee venom-loaded niosomes	7.7	0.47	No lysis	Slightly irritative
Empty niosomes	14	0	Hemorrhage	Strongly irritative
0.9% NaCl	0.00	-	None	Non-irritant
0.1 N NaOH	19.00	-	Lysis and hemorrhage	Strongly irritative

IS—irritation score; HET-CAM—hen's egg chorioallantoic membrane.

Results showed that, as expected, no irritability was observed when 0.9% NaCl (negative control) was applied, and strong irritability was observed when 0.1 N NaOH (positive control) was applied. Furthermore, and in accordance with the results obtained from the in vitro cytotoxicity assays (Section 2.2), the empty niosomes showed a strongly irritative degree, with an IS value of 14, and caused hemorrhage 5 min after formulation application (Figure 7b). Again, just like in the in vitro assays, the unexpectedly high irritation degree of the empty niosomes could be related to its constituents, as some data has been found regarding the irritability of Tween 20 and cholesterol [113,114]. Additionally, in a previous study [115], where two different Tween 20 concentrations were tested (30% and 1%), results showed that higher concentrations of this non-ionic surfactant caused a higher irritation score than lower concentrations. Nevertheless, the bee venom-loaded niosomes had a much smaller irritative potential, with an IS value of 7.7, being half of the obtained for the empty niosomes, which indicates only a slight irritative degree, with no associated lysis or hemorrhage. Previous studies [116] have reported that bee venom, and more specifically melittin, can cause irritation in a dose-dependent manner. Hence, it seems that the bee venom concentrations used in the developed nanocarrier's composition appear to be safe. Moreover, and once again, the much lower IS obtained with the bee venom-loaded niosomes, when compared to the empty niosomes, could be due to the adsorption of some of the compound onto the vesicles' outer membrane, making the direct contact between the chorioallantoic membrane and the niosomes more reduced, and hence lowering the potential for irritation.

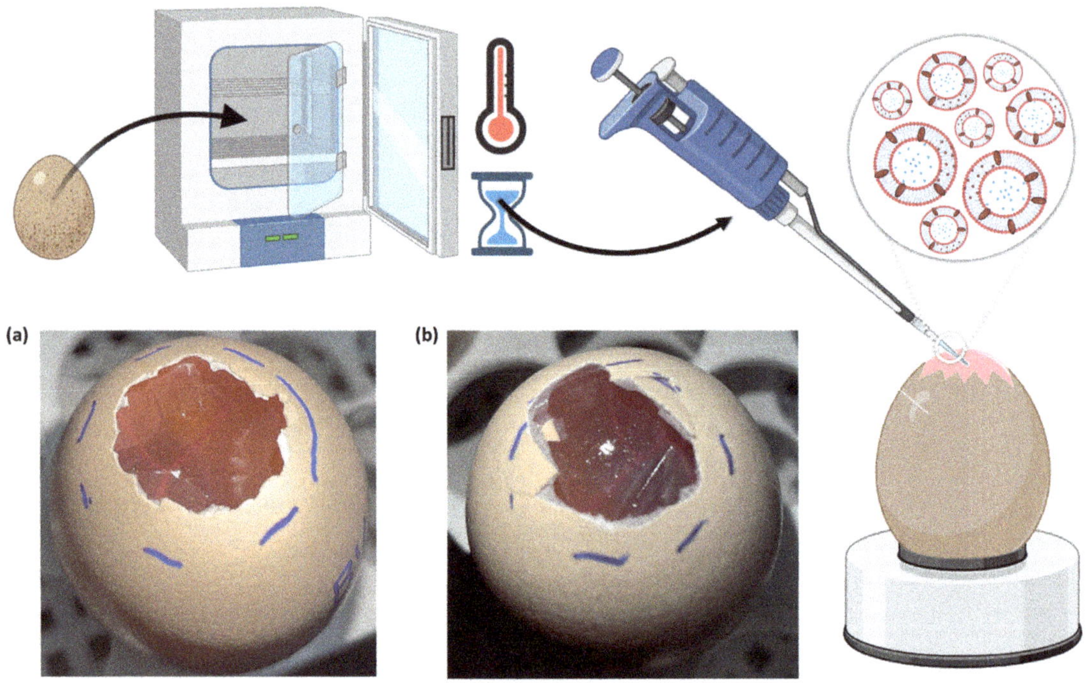

Figure 7. HET-CAM assay schematic representation, and photographs of the hen's egg chorioallantoic membranes after formulation application, either the developed bee venom-encapsulated niosomes (**a**), or the formulation vehicle (empty niosomes) (**b**); HET-CAM—hen's egg chorioallantoic membrane.

Therefore, since the bee venom-loaded niosomes showed hen's egg chorioallantoic membranes with normal blood vessels, with no lysis or other vascular reactions, and an overall low IS, the developed nanocarrier appears to have a reasonable safety profile. Nevertheless, again, additional tests are needed to confirm these results, to find the safest and, yet, most therapeutically effective concentrations of the developed formulation, with the assessment of a risk-benefit ratio being necessary to confirm the true value of the developed nanocarriers as primary or adjuvant anticancer therapies.

3. Materials and Methods

3.1. Materials and Reagents

Tween® 20, cholesterol, cetyl alcohol, chloroform, sulforhodamine B, lipopolysaccharide, trypan blue, dexamethasone, trichloroacetic acid, tris (hydroxymethyl)aminomethane buffer, cytochrome C from equine heart (purity $\geq$ 95%), melittin (purity $\geq$ 85%, HPLC grade) and phospholipase A2 (activity: 1775 units/mg solid) were purchased from Sigma-Aldrich (Saint Louis, MO, USA). Apamin (purity 98.3%) was purchased from CalBiochem (San Diego, CA, USA). Fetal bovine serum, penicillin, streptomycin, trypsin, L-glutamine, and Dulbecco's modified Eagle's medium (DMEM) were purchased from Gibco Invitrogen Life Technologies (Carlsbad, CA, USA). Formic acid (HPLC grade) and acetonitrile (HPLC grade) were obtained from Fisher Scientific (Loughborough, UK). The Griess reagent system kit was bought from Promega (Madison, WI, USA). Ultrapure water was obtained from adequate purification systems (Ellix Essential Millipore®, Darmstadt, Germany, and TGI Pure Water Systems, Brea, CA, USA).

3.2. Cell Lines

All human and animal cell lines used in this work are commercially available and were purchased from different authorized cell line resources, including the German Collection of Microorganisms and Cell Cultures (DSMZ) and the European Collection of Authenticated Cell Cultures (ECCAC). The human tumor cell lines used for the cytotoxicity assays included: MCF-7 (breast cancer), NCI-H460 (non-small-cell lung cancer), AGS (gastric adenocarcinoma), HeLa (cervical cancer) and Caco-2 (colorectal adenocarcinoma). All these cell lines were obtained from DSMZ, except the Caco-2 cell line, which was obtained from the ECACC. The non-tumoral macrophage derived cell line RAW 264.7, used for the anti-inflammatory in vitro studies, was purchased from the ECACC. Primary cell lines, obtained from porcine liver tissue (PLP2) and African green monkey kidney (Vero), were also used to study the cytotoxicity effect in non-tumoral cells. In order to maintain high scientific standards, all procedures were performed according to the best practices observed in the Guidance on Good Cell Culture Practice (GCCP).

3.3. Bee Venom Production and Harvesting

The bee venom used as the active compound to be encapsulated within the developed niosomes was collected between August and November of 2018 from *Apis mellifera intermissa* hives located in the northeast region of Morocco. To collect the bee venom, a double-face bee venom collector was used, especially developed for the purpose by the research team. The device was positioned in the hive at one of the outermost, diametrically opposed ends of the beehive, and produced mild electrical impulse shock waves on the beehive, which made the worker bees sting the glass, as a defense mechanism, leaving the bee venom deposited on it. Following the collection process, the venom was meticulously removed from the glass using a scraper and subsequently stored in pharmaceutical-grade vials. Samples were then freeze-dried, in a freeze dryer (Labconco FreeZone 4.5, Labconco Corporation, Kansas City, MO, USA), and kept at −20 °C until further analysis [78].

3.4. Ultra-High-Performance Liquid Chromatography Analysis

The ultra-high-performance liquid chromatography (UHPLC) analysis was executed utilizing a Dionex Ultimate 3000 UHPLC instrument (Thermo Scientific, Waltham, MA, USA), featuring a diode-array detector. The chromatographic system comprised a quaternary pump, an autosampler maintained at 5 °C, a degasser, a photodiode array detector, and an automatic thermostatic column compartment. Chromatographic separation was conducted on an XSelect CSH130 C18, 100 mm × 2.1 mm id, 2.5 μm XP column (Waters, Milford, MA, USA), with a constant temperature of 30 °C. The mobile phase consisted of 0.1% (v/v) formic acid in water and 0.1% (v/v) formic acid in acetonitrile, previously degassed and filtered. The used conditions were in accordance with previous studies [44]. Spectral data for all peaks were gathered within the range of 190–500 nm. Control and data acquisition were conducted using the Xcalibur® data system (Thermo Scientific, Waltham, MA, USA). Cytochrome C, employed as the internal standard, was prepared in deionized water at a concentration of 25 μg/mL. For analysis, the lyophilized bee venom (3 mg) was dissolved in 10 mL of internal standard. Each sample was filtered through a 0.2 μm polytetrafluoroethylene membrane. Bee venom peptide quantification was achieved using calibration curves for apamin (at a range of 2–60 μg/mL, $y = 0.040x + 0.055$, $R^2 = 0.999$), phospholipase A2 (at a range of 8–120 μg/mL, $y = 0.049x - 0.356$, $R^2 = 0.999$), and melittin (at a range of 15–250 μg/mL, $y = 0.062x + 0.029$, $R^2 = 0.997$).

3.5. Niosome Formulation Development and Characterization

For formulation preparation, the thin-film hydration method was applied (Figure 8), which is the most commonly used method for niosome production [38,117]. Firstly, the non-ionic surfactant and lipid fraction (3.5:2 molar ratio) were weighed into a round bottom flask and then dissolved in 6 mL of chloroform. The organic solvent was subsequently evaporated, in a rotary evaporator (Rotavapor R-210/215, BÜCHI, Meierseggstrasse, Flawil,

Switzerland), combined with a vacuum pump (V-700/710, BÜCHI, Switzerland), and a vacuum controller (V-850/855, BÜCHI, Switzerland), in a heating water bath (40 °C to 60 °C), with a rotation speed of 8 rpm, and under reduced pressure (120 mbar), for 60 min. After full organic solvent evaporation, a thin layer was formed on the interior of the flask, and this thin layer was then hydrated with either deionized water (6 mL) for the formulation vehicle (empty niosomes), or an aqueous compound solution (2 μg/mL) for the bee venom-loaded niosomes, under mild magnetic stirring, for 60 min. Although after thin-film hydration vesicles were already formed, to attain a nanometric and homogeneous particle size, the mixture was extruded (Avanti Mini-Extruder, Avanti Polar Lipids, Alabaster, AL, USA) through a synthetic polycarbonate membrane with a 200 nm pore size (Avanti Polar Lipids, USA). Various extrusion cycles were performed (11, 21, 31, 41, and 51), and the particle size and polydispersity index (PDI) for every performed cycle series were subsequently measured. Particle mean hydrodynamic size and PDI of the developed formulations were measured by dynamic light scattering, using a Zetasizer apparatus (ZetaSizer Nano ZS, Malvern Instruments, Malvern, UK). Samples were diluted 40-fold in deionized water and measured in disposable polymethyl methacrylate 12 mm square diameter cuvettes, at 25 °C. Zeta potential was also measured using the same apparatus, using a folded capillary cell (DTS1070), through electrophoretic light scattering. All the samples were measured in triplicate and the mean and standard deviation are reported. Formulations were stored in a refrigerator at 4 °C until further characterization.

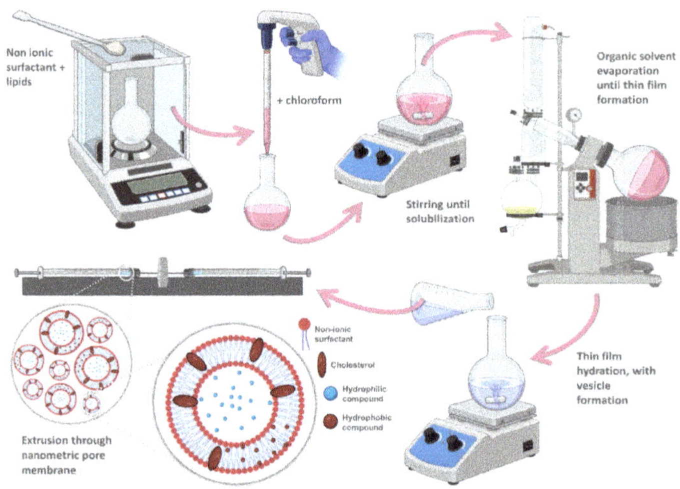

Figure 8. Schematic illustration of niosome composition and production, using the thin-film hydration method, followed by extrusion through a nanometric pore membrane (produced with Biorender).

3.6. *In Vitro Therapeutic Potential*

3.6.1. Cytotoxic Activity

The developed formulations' cytotoxic activity was tested in several different human cancer cell lines, namely: AGS (gastric adenocarcinoma), Caco-2 (colorectal adenocarcinoma), MCF-7 (breast adenocarcinoma), NCI-H460 (lung carcinoma), and HeLa (cervical carcinoma). For assessment of the potential toxicity of the developed formulations on non-cancerous tissues, non-tumor cell lines Vero (African green monkey kidney) and PLP2 (primary pig liver culture) were also tested. All cell lines were maintained in RPMI-1640 medium, supplemented with 10% fetal bovine serum, glutamine (2 mM), penicillin (100 U/mL), and streptomycin (100 mg/mL), except Vero cells, which were maintained in DMEM medium. The culture flasks were incubated at 37 °C, under a 5% CO_2 and high humidity atmosphere. Cells were used only upon reaching a 70 to 80% confluence.

Formulations were dissolved in water: dimethyl sulfoxide (DMSO) (1 mL; 1:1) to obtain stock solutions with a concentration of 1 μg/mL, from which successive dilutions were made, obtaining the samples at the concentrations to be tested (0.05–0.0008 μg/mL). Each sample (10 μL) was incubated with the cell suspension (190 μL) in 96-well microplates, for 72 h. The microplates were incubated at 37 °C, under a 5% CO_2 and high humidity atmosphere. All cell lines were tested at a concentration of 10,000 cells/well, except for Vero cells, in which a density of 19,000 cells/well was used. Subsequently to this incubation period, plates were incubated again, for 1 h, at 4 °C, after the addition of previously cooled trichloroacetic acid (10% *w*/*v*; 100 μL). The plates were then washed with water and, after drying, a sulforhodamine B solution (0.057% *w*/*v*, 100 μL) was added, and then left to stand at room temperature for 30 min. To remove non-adhered sulforhodamine B, the plates were washed three times with an acetic acid solution (1% *v*/*v*) and left to dry. Finally, the adhered sulforhodamine B was solubilized with Tris(hydroxymethyl)aminomethane (Tris) buffer (10 mM, 200 μL), and sample absorbance was measured at a wavelength of 540 nm, in a microplate reader (ELX800 Biotek microplate reader, Bio-Tek Instruments, Inc., Winooski, VT, USA). The results are expressed in terms of the sample concentration with the ability to inhibit cell growth by 50% (GI_{50}).

3.6.2. Anti-Inflammatory Activity

The anti-inflammatory activity of the developed formulations was also assessed. First, the formulations were diluted in water: DMSO solution to obtain a final concentration of 1 μg/mL, from which successive dilutions were carried out. Final concentrations ranged from 0.05 to 0.0008 mg/mL. A RAW 264.7 mouse macrophage cell line was used (Leibniz Institute DSMZ—German Collection of Microorganisms and Cell Cultures GmbH), and grown in DMEM medium, supplemented with heat-inactivated fetal serum (10%), glutamine and antibiotics, and kept in an incubator at 37 °C, with a 5% CO_2 and highly humid atmosphere. Cells were detached with a cell scraper, and an aliquot of macrophages cell suspension (300 μL), with a cell density of 5×10^5 cells/mL, and with a proportion of dead cells below 5% (according to the trypan blue exclusion test), was placed in each well. The microplate was incubated for 24 h, in an incubator, at the previously indicated conditions, to allow for adequate cell adherence and multiplication. After that period, the cells were treated with different concentrations of the developed formulations (15 μL) and incubated for one hour, with the range of tested concentrations being between 0.05 and 0.0008 μg/mL. Stimulation was performed with the addition of 30 μL of a liposaccharide (LPS) solution (1 mL/mL) and incubation for an additional 24 h. Dexamethasone (50 mM) was used as a positive control, and samples in the absence of LPS were used as a negative control. Quantification of nitric oxide was performed using a Griess reagent system kit (nitrophenamide, ethylenediamine, and nitrite solutions). The produced nitric oxide was determined by reading absorbances at 540 nm (ELX800 Biotek microplate reader, Bio-Tek Instruments, Inc., Winooski, VT, USA), on a 96-well microplate, and by comparison with a standard calibration curve. Results are depicted by a graphical representation of the percentage of inhibition of nitric oxide production versus sample concentration, and expressed in relation to the formulation concentration that causes the 50% inhibition of nitric oxide production (IC_{50}).

3.7. *Safety Assessment*

3.7.1. In Vitro Safety Assessment—Cytotoxicity Evaluation on HaCaT and HFF-1 Cell Lines

To assess the safety of the developed formulations in vitro, the colorimetric sulforhodamine B assay was conducted on two human cell lines: HFF-1 (human skin fibroblasts) and HaCaT (human immortalized keratinocytes). This assay measured cell survival after treatment with the developed formulations. The cell lines were cultured in DMEM medium, supplemented with fetal bovine serum (10%), glutamine, and antibiotics (penicillin and streptomycin 1%), in an incubator at 37 °C, with a 5% CO_2 atmosphere, and with saturated controlled humidity. Trypsin was used to disperse the cells from the inside of the flask where they were cultured, since these cells are adherent. The cell density for this assay was 10,000 cells per well. X-triton (1%), a detergent, served as a positive control due to its capacity to disrupt and destroy all cells. For the negative control group, only cells and medium were added (no formulation or other compound).

After the cells were dispersed by trypsin in the culture medium, centrifuged at 3000 rpm for 5 min, and resuspended in the medium, 10,000 cells per well were plated in a 96-well optical-bottom plate to adhere overnight. Afterwards, the bee venom-loaded niosomes and empty niosomes (formulation vehicle) samples were prepared by diluting them in water, for final concentrations equal to 0.1, 0.05, 0.025, and 0.0125 mg/mL, which were added to the plate. Samples at the exact same concentrations were also prepared for the bee venom compound solution, also by dilution with water. Each concentration level was tested in triplicate. The plates were then incubated for 48 h at 37 °C and in a 5% CO_2 atmosphere. After 48 h, the cells were fixated with trichloroacetic acid, for 1 h, at 4 °C. Afterwards, the liquid inside the plate was discarded, and the plate was washed 3 times with water, and left to dry. Once dried, 100 μL of sulforhodamine B was added to each well and left there for 30 min at room temperature. Acetic acid at 1% was used to remove the unbounded dye from the cells, and the bounded dye was dissolved with a 10 mM Tris buffer. The IC_{50} values were expressed as the concentration (μg/mL) of each formulation that caused 50% inhibition of cell growth. Samples were quantified by using UV-visible spectrophotometry in a microplate reader (ELX800 microplate reader, Bio-Tek Instruments, Winooski, VT, USA) at 540 nm, based on previously described methods [44,118].

3.7.2. Ex Vivo Safety Assessment—HET-CAM Test

The hen's egg chorioallantoic membrane (HET-CAM) test method was used to assess the irritation-inducing potential of the developed formulations, upon contact with a highly sensitive biological membrane, focusing on its ability to induce toxicity in the chorioallantoic membrane of a chicken egg. This type of membrane is known to resemble the human eye, and even if the product is not intended for ocular use, the test can still be quite useful since a formulation that is reasonably safe for eye application is probably also safe for contact with most other human organs [111].

The assay was done following the Interagency Coordinating Committee on the Validation of Alternative Methods (ICCVAM) recommended test method [119]. The experimental protocol consisted of the incubation of forty Leghorn fertilized chicken eggs, for 10 days, in an automatic rotating incubator, at 37 °C and 65% humidity. To confirm the presence of an embryo, a flashlight was used against each egg. If no embryo was detected that egg would be excluded from the experiment, and not used. For each tested formulation, a total of three eggs were used. After the 10-day incubation period, the top part of the eggshells was cut open to expose the chorioallantoic membrane, so that the formulation could then be applied. Nevertheless, before formulation application, all the membranes were hydrated using a 0.9% NaCl solution, for 30 min. Then, three formulation drops (approximately 0.1 mL per drop, for a total of 0.3 mL of formulation) were applied to the chorioallantoic membrane of each egg [119]. The negative control group was three eggs where a 0.9% NaCl solution was applied (no reaction intended), while for the positive control group, a 10% NaOH solution was applied on the membrane of three eggs (inflammatory reaction intended). The irritancy degree of each formulation was observed and monitored by the appearance of the following events: hemorrhage (bleeding of the vessels), lysis (disintegration of the vessels), and coagulation (intra and/or extra-vascular protein denaturation). The occurrence or non-occurrence of these events was observed at specific time points, namely 0.5, 2, and 5 min. A total score was then attributed, from 0 to 21, being the sum of the values attributed to each event and corresponding to a level of irritability (Table 7). Hence, after the 5 min time interval, formulations were given an irritation score (IS), with the following corresponding irritation levels: an IS score between 0 and 4.9 being slightly/non-irritative; an IS score between 5 and 8.9 being moderately irritative; and an IS score between 9 and 21 being strongly irritative [119,120].

Table 7. Numerical time-dependent scoring scheme for the HET-CAM test method.

Effect	Score		
	0.5 min	2 min	5 min
Lysis	5	3	1
Hemorrhage	7	5	3
Coagulation	9	7	5

HET-CAM—hen's egg chorioallantoic membrane.

3.8. Data Analysis

For a better understanding and interpretation of the results, whenever possible, statistical analysis was performed, using GraphPad Prism® (GraphPad, San Diego, CA, USA), version 8.0 software. More specifically, either a one-way ANOVA or a two-way ANOVA test was applied, with a Tukey's multiple comparisons post-test. A 95% confidence level was considered in all analysis, with a p value < 0.05 being considered statistically significant.

4. Conclusions

An innovative nanotechnological anticancer platform was successfully developed. The developed bee venom-loaded niosomes revealed small nanometric and homogeneous particle size, therapeutic efficacy in several in vitro cancer models, including breast, cervical, lung, gastric, and colorectal cell lines, and complementary anti-inflammatory potential, which has been proven to indirectly contribute to further synergistic anticancer effects. The developed formulations were shown to improve bee venom administration safety, in in vitro and ex vivo models. Although further studies will clarify the true potential of the developed bee venom-loaded niosomes, these findings are promising regarding both formulation safety and bioactivity, making them potentially promising alternatives for primary or adjuvant cancer treatment.

Author Contributions: Conceptualization, F.V., A.C.P.-S. and P.M.; methodology, P.C.P., A.C.P.-S., R.C.C., A.R.S., M.J.S. and S.I.F.; validation, P.C.P., F.V., A.C.P.-S., M.V.-B. and S.I.F.; formal analysis, M.B.P., P.C.P., F.V., A.C.P.-S., R.C.C., A.R.S. and M.J.S.; investigation, M.B.P., P.C.P. and P.M.; resources, F.V., A.C.P.-S., P.M. and S.I.F.; data curation, M.B.P., P.C.P., R.C.C., A.R.S., M.J.S. and S.I.F.; writing—original draft preparation, M.B.P., P.C.P. and A.C.P.-S.; writing—review and editing, P.C.P., F.V., A.C.P.-S., P.M., M.V.-B. and S.I.F.; supervision, P.C.P., F.V., A.C.P.-S. and S.I.F.; project administration, F.V., A.C.P.-S. and P.M.; funding acquisition, F.V. and A.C.P.-S. All authors have read and agreed to the published version of the manuscript.

Funding: The present study was supported by the Research and Development Project grant 2022.05270.PTDC, national funds FCT/MCTES (PIDDAC), CIMO funds (UIDB/00690/2020 and UIDP/00690/2020) and SusTEC funds (LA/P/0007/2021), supported by Fundação para a Ciência e a Tecnologia I.P. (FCT, Portugal). The authors are also grateful to Fundação para a Ciência e a Tecnologia I.P. (FCT, Portugal) for contracts' financial support through the institutional scientific employment program-contract for Soraia I. Falcão and Ricardo C. Calhelha.

Institutional Review Board Statement: Not applicable.

Informed Consent Statement: Not applicable.

Data Availability Statement: Data are contained within the article.

Acknowledgments: The authors thank Iouraouine El Mehdi for the bee venom sample collection.

Conflicts of Interest: The authors declare no conflicts of interest.

Abbreviations

COX-2—cyclooxygenase-2; DMEM—Dulbecco's modified Eagle's medium; DMSO—dimethyl sulfoxide; DSMZ—German Collection of Microorganisms and Cell Cultures; ECCAC—European Collection of Authenticated Cell Cultures; IC_{50}—formulation concentration that causes a 50% inhibition of nitric oxide production/cell growth; IS—internal standard; GCCP—Guidance on Good Cell Culture Practice; GI_{50}—sample concentration with the ability to inhibit cell growth by 50%; HET-CAM—hen's egg chorioallantoic membrane; ICCVAM—Interagency Coordinating Committee on the Validation of Alternative Methods; IFN—interferons; IgE—immunoglobulin E; IL—interleukins; IS—irritation score; LPS—liposaccharide; PDI—polydispersity index; TNF—tumor necrosis factor; Tris—Tris(hydroxymethyl)aminomethane; and UHPLC—ultra-high-performance liquid chromatography.

References

1. Siegel, R.L.; Miller, K.D.; Wagle, N.S.; Jemal, A. Cancer Statistics, 2023. *CA Cancer J. Clin.* **2023**, *73*, 17–48. [CrossRef] [PubMed]
2. Malvezzi, M.; Santucci, C.; Boffetta, P.; Collatuzzo, G.; Levi, F.; La Vecchia, C.; Negri, E. European Cancer Mortality Predictions for the Year 2023 with Focus on Lung Cancer. *Ann. Oncol.* **2023**, *34*, 410–419. [CrossRef] [PubMed]
3. Brown, J.S.; Amend, S.R.; Austin, R.H.; Gatenby, R.A.; Hammarlund, E.U.; Pienta, K.J. Updating the Definition of Cancer. *Mol. Cancer Res.* **2023**, *21*, 1142–1147. [CrossRef]
4. Iragorri, N.; de Oliveira, C.; Fitzgerald, N.; Essue, B. The Out-of-Pocket Cost Burden of Cancer Care—A Systematic Literature Review. *Curr. Oncol.* **2021**, *28*, 1216–1248. [CrossRef]
5. Chen, S.; Cao, Z.; Prettner, K.; Kuhn, M.; Yang, J.; Jiao, L.; Wang, Z.; Li, W.; Geldsetzer, P.; Bärnighausen, T.; et al. Estimates and Projections of the Global Economic Cost of 29 Cancers in 204 Countries and Territories from 2020 to 2050. *JAMA Oncol.* **2023**, *9*, 465–472. [CrossRef] [PubMed]
6. Mariotto, A.B.; Enewold, L.; Zhao, J.; Zeruto, C.A.; Yabroff, K.R. Medical Care Costs Associated with Cancer Survivorship in the United States. *Cancer Epidemiol. Biomark. Prev.* **2020**, *29*, 1304–1312. [CrossRef] [PubMed]
7. Berben, L.; Floris, G.; Wildiers, H.; Hatse, S. Cancer and Aging: Two Tightly Interconnected Biological Processes. *Cancers* **2021**, *13*, 1400. [CrossRef] [PubMed]
8. Li, D.; Ju, F.; Wang, H.; Fan, C.; Jacob, J.C.; Gul, S.; Zaliani, A.; Wartmann, T.; Polidori, M.C.; Bruns, C.J.; et al. Combination of the Biomarkers for Aging and Cancer?—Challenges and Current Status. *Transl. Oncol.* **2023**, *38*, 101783. [CrossRef] [PubMed]
9. Quinten, C.; Coens, C.; Ghislain, I.; Zikos, E.; Sprangers, M.A.G.; Ringash, J.; Martinelli, F.; Ediebah, D.E.; Maringwa, J.; Reeve, B.B.; et al. The Effects of Age on Health-Related Quality of Life in Cancer Populations: A Pooled Analysis of Randomized Controlled Trials Using the European Organisation for Research and Treatment of Cancer (EORTC) QLQ-C30 Involving 6024 Cancer Patients. *Eur. J. Cancer* **2015**, *51*, 2808–2819. [CrossRef]
10. Devlin, E.J.; Denson, L.A.; Whitford, H.S. Cancer Treatment Side Effects: A Meta-Analysis of the Relationship Between Response Expectancies and Experience. *J. Pain Symptom Manag.* **2017**, *54*, 245–258.e2. [CrossRef]
11. Mazzotti, E.; Antonini Cappellini, G.C.; Buconovo, S.; Morese, R.; Scoppola, A.; Sebastiani, C.; Marchetti, P. Treatment-Related Side Effects and Quality of Life in Cancer Patients. *Support. Care Cancer* **2012**, *20*, 2553–2557. [CrossRef] [PubMed]
12. Nurgali, K.; Jagoe, R.T.; Abalo, R. Adverse Effects of Cancer Chemotherapy: Anything New to Improve Tolerance and Reduce Sequelae? *Front. Pharmacol.* **2018**, *9*, 245. [CrossRef] [PubMed]
13. Gong, D.; Celi, N.; Zhang, D.; Cai, J. Magnetic Biohybrid Microrobot Multimers Based on Chlorella Cells for Enhanced Targeted Drug Delivery. *ACS Appl. Mater. Interfaces* **2022**, *14*, 6320–6330. [CrossRef] [PubMed]
14. Zhu, Y.; Jia, H.; Jiang, Y.; Guo, Y.; Duan, Q.; Xu, K.; Shan, B.; Liu, X.; Chen, X.; Wu, F. A Red Blood Cell-derived Bionic Microrobot Capable of Hierarchically Adapting to Five Critical Stages in Systemic Drug Delivery. *Exploration* **2024**, *4*, 20230105. [CrossRef]
15. Zhu, S.; Cheng, Y.; Wang, J.; Liu, G.; Luo, T.; Li, X.; Yang, S.; Yang, R. Biohybrid Magnetic Microrobots: An Intriguing and Promising Platform in Biomedicine. *Acta Biomater.* **2023**, *169*, 88–106. [CrossRef] [PubMed]
16. Paul, D.; Sanap, G.; Shenoy, S.; Kalyane, D.; Kalia, K.; Tekade, R.K. Artificial Intelligence in Drug Discovery and Development. *Drug Discov. Today* **2021**, *26*, 80–93. [CrossRef] [PubMed]
17. Vora, L.K.; Gholap, A.D.; Jetha, K.; Thakur, R.R.S.; Solanki, H.K.; Chavda, V.P. Artificial Intelligence in Pharmaceutical Technology and Drug Delivery Design. *Pharmaceutics* **2023**, *15*, 1916. [CrossRef]
18. El-Seedi, H.R.; Yosri, N.; Khalifa, S.A.M.; Guo, Z.; Musharraf, S.G.; Xiao, J.; Saeed, A.; Du, M.; Khatib, A.; Abdel-Daim, M.M.; et al. Exploring Natural Products-Based Cancer Therapeutics Derived from Egyptian Flora. *J. Ethnopharmacol.* **2021**, *269*, 113626. [CrossRef]
19. Giribaldi, J.; Smith, J.J.; Schroeder, C.I. Recent Developments in Animal Venom Peptide Nanotherapeutics with Improved Selectivity for Cancer Cells. *Biotechnol. Adv.* **2021**, *50*, 107769. [CrossRef]
20. Varghese, R.; Dalvi, Y.B. Natural Products as Anticancer Agents. *Curr. Drug Targets* **2021**, *22*, 1272–1287. [CrossRef]
21. Wehbe, R.; Frangieh, J.; Rima, M.; El Obeid, D.; Sabatier, J.-M.; Fajloun, Z. Bee Venom: Overview of Main Compounds and Bioactivities for Therapeutic Interests. *Molecules* **2019**, *24*, 2997. [CrossRef] [PubMed]
22. Pascoal, A.; Estevinho, M.M.; Choupina, A.B.; Sousa-Pimenta, M.; Estevinho, L.M. An Overview of the Bioactive Compounds, Therapeutic Properties and Toxic Effects of Apitoxin. *Food Chem. Toxicol.* **2019**, *134*, 110864. [CrossRef]
23. Carpena, M.; Nuñez-Estevez, B.; Soria-Lopez, A.; Simal-Gandara, J. Bee Venom: An Updating Review of Its Bioactive Molecules and Its Health Applications. *Nutrients* **2020**, *12*, 3360. [CrossRef] [PubMed]

24. El-Seedi, H.; El-Wahed, A.A.; Yosri, N.; Musharraf, S.G.; Chen, L.; Moustafa, M.; Zou, X.; Al-Mousawi, S.; Guo, Z.; Khatib, A.; et al. Antimicrobial Properties of Apis Mellifera's Bee Venom. *Toxins* **2020**, *12*, 451. [CrossRef] [PubMed]
25. Ahmed-Farid, O.A.; Taha, M.; Bakeer, R.M.; Radwan, O.K.; Hendawy, H.A.M.; Samaan, A.; Yousef, E. Effects of Bee Venom and Dopamine-Loaded Nanoparticles on Reserpine-Induced Parkinson's Disease Rat Model. *Sci. Rep.* **2021**, *11*, 21141. [CrossRef]
26. El-Didamony, S.E.; Kalaba, M.H.; El-Fakharany, E.M.; Sultan, M.H.; Sharaf, M.H. Antifungal and Antibiofilm Activities of Bee Venom Loaded on Chitosan Nanoparticles: A Novel Approach for Combating Fungal Human Pathogens. *World J. Microbiol. Biotechnol.* **2022**, *38*, 244. [CrossRef] [PubMed]
27. Garaj-Vrhovac, V.; Gajski, G. Evaluation of the Cytogenetic Status of Human Lymphocytes After Exposure to a High Concentration of Bee Venom In Vitro. *Arch. Ind. Hyg. Toxicol.* **2009**, *60*, 27–34. [CrossRef] [PubMed]
28. Gajski, G.; Garaj-Vrhovac, V. Genotoxic Potential of Bee Venom (Apis Mellifera) on Human Peripheral Blood Lymphocytes in Vitro Using Single Cell Gel Electrophoresis Assay. *J. Environ. Sci. Health* **2008**, *43*, 1279–1287. [CrossRef] [PubMed]
29. Gajski, G.; Garaj-Vrhovac, V. Bee Venom Induced Cytogenetic Damage and Decreased Cell Viability in Human White Blood Cells after Treatment in Vitro: A Multi-Biomarker Approach. *Environ. Toxicol. Pharmacol.* **2011**, *32*, 201–211. [CrossRef]
30. El-Wahed, A.A.A.; Khalifa, S.A.M.; Elashal, M.H.; Musharraf, S.G.; Saeed, A.; Khatib, A.; Tahir, H.E.; Zou, X.; Al Naggar, Y.; Mehmood, A.; et al. Cosmetic Applications of Bee Venom. *Toxins* **2021**, *13*, 810. [CrossRef]
31. Afzal, O.; Altamimi, A.S.A.; Nadeem, M.S.; Alzarea, S.I.; Almalki, W.H.; Tariq, A.; Mubeen, B.; Murtaza, B.N.; Iftikhar, S.; Riaz, N.; et al. Nanoparticles in Drug Delivery: From History to Therapeutic Applications. *Nanomaterials* **2022**, *12*, 4494. [CrossRef] [PubMed]
32. Abdel-Mageed, H.M.; AbuelEzz, N.Z.; Radwan, R.A.; Mohamed, S.A. Nanoparticles in Nanomedicine: A Comprehensive Updated Review on Current Status, Challenges and Emerging Opportunities. *J. Microencapsul.* **2021**, *38*, 414–436. [CrossRef] [PubMed]
33. Yusuf, A.; Almotairy, A.R.Z.; Henidi, H.; Alshehri, O.Y.; Aldughaim, M.S. Nanoparticles as Drug Delivery Systems: A Review of the Implication of Nanoparticles' Physicochemical Properties on Responses in Biological Systems. *Polymers* **2023**, *15*, 1596. [CrossRef] [PubMed]
34. Raghu, P.K.; Bansal, K.K.; Thakor, P.; Bhavana, V.; Madan, J.; Rosenholm, J.M.; Mehra, N.K. Evolution of Nanotechnology in Delivering Drugs to Eyes, Skin and Wounds via Topical Route. *Pharmaceuticals* **2020**, *13*, 167. [CrossRef] [PubMed]
35. Pires, P.C.; Paiva-Santos, A.C.; Veiga, F. Liposome-Derived Nanosystems for the Treatment of Behavioral and Neurodegenerative Diseases: The Promise of Niosomes, Transfersomes, and Ethosomes for Increased Brain Drug Bioavailability. *Pharmaceuticals* **2023**, *16*, 1424. [CrossRef] [PubMed]
36. Abd El-Alim, S.H.; Kassem, A.A.; Basha, M.; Salama, A. Comparative Study of Liposomes, Ethosomes and Transfersomes as Carriers for Enhancing the Transdermal Delivery of Diflunisal: In Vitro and in Vivo Evaluation. *Int. J. Pharm.* **2019**, *563*, 293–303. [CrossRef] [PubMed]
37. Moghtaderi, M.; Sedaghatnia, K.; Bourbour, M.; Fatemizadeh, M.; Salehi Moghaddam, Z.; Hejabi, F.; Heidari, F.; Quazi, S.; Farasati Far, B. Niosomes: A Novel Targeted Drug Delivery System for Cancer. *Med. Oncol.* **2022**, *39*, 240. [CrossRef]
38. Chen, S.; Hanning, S.; Falconer, J.; Locke, M.; Wen, J. Recent Advances in Non-Ionic Surfactant Vesicles (Niosomes): Fabrication, Characterization, Pharmaceutical and Cosmetic Applications. *Eur. J. Pharm. Biopharm.* **2019**, *144*, 18–39. [CrossRef] [PubMed]
39. Sharma, S.; Garg, A.; Agrawal, R.; Chopra, H.; Pathak, D. A Comprehensive Review on Niosomes as a Tool for Advanced Drug Delivery. *Pharm. Nanotechnol.* **2023**, *12*, 206–228. [CrossRef]
40. Yasamineh, S.; Yasamineh, P.; Ghafouri Kalajahi, H.; Gholizadeh, O.; Yekanipour, Z.; Afkhami, H.; Eslami, M.; Hossein Kheirkhah, A.; Taghizadeh, M.; Yazdani, Y.; et al. A State-of-the-Art Review on the Recent Advances of Niosomes as a Targeted Drug Delivery System. *Int. J. Pharm.* **2022**, *624*, 121878. [CrossRef]
41. Kuotsu, K.; Karim, K.; Mandal, A.; Biswas, N.; Guha, A.; Chatterjee, S.; Behera, M. Niosome: A Future of Targeted Drug Delivery Systems. *J. Adv. Pharm. Technol. Res.* **2010**, *1*, 374–380. [CrossRef]
42. Azeem, A.; Anwer, M.K.; Talegaonkar, S. Niosomes in Sustained and Targeted Drug Delivery: Some Recent Advances. *J. Drug Target.* **2009**, *17*, 671–689. [CrossRef]
43. Mawazi, S.M.; Ann, T.J.; Widodo, R.T. Application of Niosomes in Cosmetics: A Systematic Review. *Cosmetics* **2022**, *9*, 127. [CrossRef]
44. Sobral, F.; Sampaio, A.; Falcão, S.; Queiroz, M.J.R.P.; Calhelha, R.C.; Vilas-Boas, M.; Ferreira, I.C.F.R. Chemical Characterization, Antioxidant, Anti-Inflammatory and Cytotoxic Properties of Bee Venom Collected in Northeast Portugal. *Food Chem. Toxicol.* **2016**, *94*, 172–177. [CrossRef]
45. Kim, W. Bee Venom and Its Sub-Components: Characterization, Pharmacology, and Therapeutics. *Toxins* **2021**, *13*, 191. [CrossRef]
46. Manconi, M.; Vila, A.; Sinico, C.; Figueruelo, J.; Molina, F.; Fadd, A. Theoretical and Experimental Evaluation of Decypolyglucoside Vesicles as Potential Drug Delivery Systems. *J. Drug Deliv. Sci. Technol.* **2006**, *16*, 141–146. [CrossRef]
47. Abd-Elbary, A.; El-laithy, H.M.; Tadros, M.I. Sucrose Stearate-Based Proniosome-Derived Niosomes for the Nebulisable Delivery of Cromolyn Sodium. *Int. J. Pharm.* **2008**, *357*, 189–198. [CrossRef]
48. Vankayala, J.S.; Battula, S.N.; Kandasamy, R.; Mariya, G.A.; Franklin, M.E.E.; Pushpadass, H.A.; Naik, L.N. Surfactants and Fatty Alcohol Based Novel Nanovesicles for Resveratrol: Process Optimization, Characterization and Evaluation of Functional Properties in RAW 264.7 Macrophage Cells. *J. Mol. Liq.* **2018**, *261*, 387–396. [CrossRef]

49. Fersht, A.R. Denaturation (Proteins). In *Brenner's Encyclopedia of Genetics: Second Edition*; Elsevier Inc.: Amsterdam, The Netherlands, 2013; pp. 302–303. ISBN 9780080961569.
50. Zhang, S.; Wang, C. Effect of Stirring Speed on Particle Dispersion in Silica Synthesis. *Nano-Struct. Nano-Objects* **2023**, *35*, 100994. [CrossRef]
51. Danaei, M.; Dehghankhold, M.; Ataei, S.; Hasanzadeh Davarani, F.; Javanmard, R.; Dokhani, A.; Khorasani, S.; Mozafari, M. Impact of Particle Size and Polydispersity Index on the Clinical Applications of Lipidic Nanocarrier Systems. *Pharmaceutics* **2018**, *10*, 57. [CrossRef]
52. Aldayel, T.S.; Badran, M.M.; Alomrani, A.H.; AlFaris, N.A.; Altamimi, J.Z.; Alqahtani, A.S.; Nasr, F.A.; Ghaffar, S.; Orfali, R. Chitosan-Coated Solid Lipid Nanoparticles as an Efficient Avenue for Boosted Biological Activities of Aloe Perryi: Antioxidant, Antibacterial, and Anticancer Potential. *Molecules* **2023**, *28*, 3569. [CrossRef]
53. de Roodt, A.R.; Lanari, L.C.; Lago, N.R.; Bustillo, S.; Litwin, S.; Morón-Goñi, F.; Gould, E.G.; van Grootheest, J.H.; Dokmetjian, J.C.; Dolab, J.A.; et al. Toxicological Study of Bee Venom (Apis Mellifera Mellifera) from Different Regions of the Province of Buenos Aires, Argentina. *Toxicon* **2020**, *188*, 27–38. [CrossRef]
54. Yousefpoor, Y.; Amani, A.; Divsalar, A.; Mousavi, S.E.; Shakeri, A.; Sabzevari, J.T. Anti-Rheumatic Activity of Topical Nanoemulsion Containing Bee Venom in Rats. *Eur. J. Pharm. Biopharm.* **2022**, *172*, 168–176. [CrossRef]
55. Oršolić, N. Bee Venom in Cancer Therapy. *Cancer Metastasis Rev.* **2012**, *31*, 173–194. [CrossRef]
56. Duarte, D.; Falcão, S.I.; El Mehdi, I.; Vilas-Boas, M.; Vale, N. Honeybee Venom Synergistically Enhances the Cytotoxic Effect of CNS Drugs in HT-29 Colon and MCF-7 Breast Cancer Cell Lines. *Pharmaceutics* **2022**, *14*, 511. [CrossRef]
57. Premratanachai, P.; Chanchao, C. Review of the Anticancer Activities of Bee Products. *Asian Pac. J. Trop. Biomed.* **2014**, *4*, 337–344. [CrossRef]
58. Kwon, N.-Y.; Sung, S.-H.; Sung, H.-K.; Park, J.-K. Anticancer Activity of Bee Venom Components against Breast Cancer. *Toxins* **2022**, *14*, 460. [CrossRef]
59. Mahmoodzadeh, A.; Zarrinnahad, H.; Bagheri, K.P.; Moradia, A.; Shahbazzadeh, D. First Report on the Isolation of Melittin from Iranian Honey Bee Venom and Evaluation of Its Toxicity on Gastric Cancer AGS Cells. *J. Chin. Med. Assoc.* **2015**, *78*, 574–583. [CrossRef]
60. Alfaleh, M.A.; Fahmy, O.; Al-Rabia, M.W.; Abourehab, M.A.S.; Ahmed, O.A.A.; Fahmy, U.A.; Alsulimani, H.H.; Badr-Eldin, S.M.; Aldawsari, H.M.; Aldhabi, B.M.; et al. Hybrid Nanoparticulate System of Fluvastatin Loaded Phospholipid, Alpha Lipoic Acid and Melittin for the Management of Colon Cancer. *Sci. Rep.* **2022**, *12*, 19446. [CrossRef] [PubMed]
61. Lischer, K.; Sitorus, S.R.A.; Guslianto, B.W.; Avila, F.; Khayrani, A.C.; Sahlan, M. Anti-Breast Cancer Activity on MCF-7 Cells of Melittin from Indonesia's Apis Cerana: An In Vitro Study. *Asian Pac. J. Cancer Prev.* **2021**, *22*, 3913–3919. [CrossRef] [PubMed]
62. Choi, K.E.; Hwang, C.J.; Gu, S.M.; Park, M.H.; Kim, J.H.; Park, J.H.; Ahn, Y.J.; Kim, J.Y.; Song, M.J.; Song, H.S.; et al. Cancer Cell Growth Inhibitory Effect of Bee Venom via Increase of Death Receptor 3 Expression and Inactivation of NF-Kappa B in NSCLC Cells. *Toxins* **2014**, *6*, 2210–2228. [CrossRef]
63. Borojeni, S.K.; Zolfagharian, H.; Babaie, M.; Javadi, I. Cytotoxic Effect of Bee (A. Mellifera) Venom on Cancer Cell Lines. *J. Pharmacopunct.* **2021**, *23*, 212–219. [CrossRef] [PubMed]
64. Abd El-Gawad, A.; Kenawy, M.A.; El-Messery, T.M.; Hassan, M.E.; El-Nekeety, A.A.; Abdel-Wahhab, M.A. Fabrication and Characterization of Bee Venom-Loaded Nanoliposomes: Enhanced Anticancer Activity against Different Human Cancer Cell Lines via the Modulation of Apoptosis-Related Genes. *J. Drug Deliv. Sci. Technol.* **2023**, *84*, 104545. [CrossRef]
65. Liu, X.; Yin, L.; Shen, S.; Hou, Y. Inflammation and Cancer: Paradoxical Roles in Tumorigenesis and Implications in Immunotherapies. *Genes Dis.* **2023**, *10*, 151–164. [CrossRef]
66. Sohrab, S.S.; Raj, R.; Nagar, A.; Hawthorne, S.; Paiva-Santos, A.C.; Kamal, M.A.; El-Daly, M.M.; Azhar, E.I.; Sharma, A. Chronic Inflammation's Transformation to Cancer: A Nanotherapeutic Paradigm. *Molecules* **2023**, *28*, 4413. [CrossRef]
67. Afify, S.M.; Hassan, G.; Seno, A.; Seno, M. Cancer-Inducing Niche: The Force of Chronic Inflammation. *Br. J. Cancer* **2022**, *127*, 193–201. [CrossRef]
68. Zhao, H.; Wu, L.; Yan, G.; Chen, Y.; Zhou, M.; Wu, Y.; Li, Y. Inflammation and Tumor Progression: Signaling Pathways and Targeted Intervention. *Signal Transduct. Target. Ther.* **2021**, *6*, 263. [CrossRef] [PubMed]
69. Greten, F.R.; Grivennikov, S.I. Inflammation and Cancer: Triggers, Mechanisms, and Consequences. *Immunity* **2019**, *51*, 27–41. [CrossRef]
70. Coussens, L.M.; Werb, Z. Inflammation and Cancer. *Nature* **2002**, *420*, 860–867. [CrossRef]
71. Multhoff, G.; Molls, M.; Radons, J. Chronic Inflammation in Cancer Development. *Front Immunol* **2012**, *2*, 98. [CrossRef]
72. Murata, M. Inflammation and Cancer. *Environ. Health Prev. Med.* **2018**, *23*, 50. [CrossRef]
73. Grivennikov, S.I.; Greten, F.R.; Karin, M. Immunity, Inflammation, and Cancer. *Cell* **2010**, *140*, 883–899. [CrossRef]
74. Arfin, S.; Jha, N.K.; Jha, S.K.; Kesari, K.K.; Ruokolainen, J.; Roychoudhury, S.; Rathi, B.; Kumar, D. Oxidative Stress in Cancer Cell Metabolism. *Antioxidants* **2021**, *10*, 642. [CrossRef]
75. Zhang, Q.; Zhu, B.; Li, Y. Resolution of Cancer-Promoting Inflammation: A New Approach for Anticancer Therapy. *Front. Immunol.* **2017**, *8*, 71. [CrossRef]
76. Lai, H.; Liu, Y.; Wu, J.; Cai, J.; Jie, H.; Xu, Y.; Deng, S. Targeting Cancer-Related Inflammation with Non-Steroidal Anti-Inflammatory Drugs: Perspectives in Pharmacogenomics. *Front. Pharmacol.* **2022**, *13*, 1078766. [CrossRef]

77. Kolawole, O.R.; Kashfi, K. NSAIDs and Cancer Resolution: New Paradigms beyond Cyclooxygenase. *Int. J. Mol. Sci.* **2022**, *23*, 1432. [CrossRef]
78. El Mehdi, I.; Falcão, S.I.; Harandou, M.; Boujraf, S.; Calhelha, R.C.; Ferreira, I.C.F.R.; Anjos, O.; Campos, M.G.; Vilas-Boas, M. Chemical, Cytotoxic, and Anti-Inflammatory Assessment of Honey Bee Venom from Apis Mellifera Intermissa. *Antibiotics* **2021**, *10*, 1514. [CrossRef]
79. Jang, H.S.; Kim, S.K.; Han, J.B.; Ahn, H.J.; Bae, H.; Min, B. Il Effects of Bee Venom on the Pro-Inflammatory Responses in RAW264.7 Macrophage Cell Line. *J. Ethnopharmacol.* **2005**, *99*, 157–160. [CrossRef]
80. Moon, D.O.; Park, S.Y.; Lee, K.J.; Heo, M.S.; Kim, K.C.; Kim, M.O.; Lee, J.D.; Choi, Y.H.; Kim, G.Y. Bee Venom and Melittin Reduce Proinflammatory Mediators in Lipopolysaccharide-Stimulated BV2 Microglia. *Int. Immunopharmacol.* **2007**, *7*, 1092–1101. [CrossRef]
81. Khalil, A.; Elesawy, B.H.; Ali, T.M.; Ahmed, O.M. Bee Venom: From Venom to Drug. *Molecules* **2021**, *26*, 4941. [CrossRef]
82. Kocyigit, A.; Guler, E.M.; Kaleli, S. Anti-Inflammatory and Antioxidative Properties of Honey Bee Venom on Freund's Complete Adjuvant-Induced Arthritis Model in Rats. *Toxicon* **2019**, *161*, 4–11. [CrossRef]
83. An, H.; Kim, J.; Kim, W.; Gwon, M.; Gu, H.M.; Jeon, M.J.; Han, S.; Pak, S.C.; Lee, C.; Park, I.S.; et al. Therapeutic Effects of Bee Venom and Its Major Component, Melittin, on Atopic Dermatitis in Vivo and in Vitro. *Br. J. Pharmacol.* **2018**, *175*, 4310–4324. [CrossRef]
84. Shi, P.; Xie, S.; Yang, J.; Zhang, Y.; Han, S.; Su, S.; Yao, H. Pharmacological Effects and Mechanisms of Bee Venom and Its Main Components: Recent Progress and Perspective. *Front. Pharmacol.* **2022**, *13*, 1001553. [CrossRef]
85. Lee, Y.J.; Oh, M.J.; Lee, D.H.; Lee, Y.S.; Lee, J.; Kim, D.-H.; Choi, C.-H.; Song, M.J.; Song, H.S.; Hong, J.T. Anti-Inflammatory Effect of Bee Venom in Phthalic Anhydride-Induced Atopic Dermatitis Animal Model. *Inflammopharmacology* **2020**, *28*, 253–263. [CrossRef] [PubMed]
86. Kim, W.-H.; An, H.-J.; Kim, J.-Y.; Gwon, M.-G.; Gu, H.; Jeon, M.; Kim, M.-K.; Han, S.-M.; Park, K.-K. Anti-Inflammatory Effect of Melittin on Porphyromonas Gingivalis LPS-Stimulated Human Keratinocytes. *Molecules* **2018**, *23*, 332. [CrossRef]
87. Billingham, M.E.J.; Morley, J.; Hanson, J.M.; Shipolini, R.A.; Vernon, C.A. An Anti-Inflammatory Peptide from Bee Venom. *Nature* **1973**, *245*, 163–164. [CrossRef]
88. Jang, S.; Kim, K.H. Clinical Effectiveness and Adverse Events of Bee Venom Therapy: A Systematic Review of Randomized Controlled Trials. *Toxins* **2020**, *12*, 558. [CrossRef]
89. Aufschnaiter, A.; Kohler, V.; Khalifa, S.; Abd El-Wahed, A.; Du, M.; El-Seedi, H.; Büttner, S. Apitoxin and Its Components against Cancer, Neurodegeneration and Rheumatoid Arthritis: Limitations and Possibilities. *Toxins* **2020**, *12*, 66. [CrossRef] [PubMed]
90. You, D.; Kwon, Y. The Effect of Bee Venom Pharmacopuncture Therapy on the Condition of Different Concentration in Rheumatoid Arthritis Rat Model. *Int. J. Cardiol.* **2011**, *152*, S109–S110. [CrossRef]
91. Sharaf, S.E.; Alsanosi, S.; Alzahrani, A.R.; Al-Ghamdi, S.S.; Sharaf, S.E.; Ayoub, N. Knowledge, Attitude, and Practice of Bee Venom Acupuncture Therapy on Rheumatoid Arthritis Among Patients in Saudi Arabia. *Int. J. Gen. Med.* **2022**, *15*, 1171–1183. [CrossRef]
92. Lee, J.-D.; Park, H.-J.; Chae, Y.; Lim, S. An Overview of Bee Venom Acupuncture in the Treatment of Arthritis. *Evid.-Based Complement. Altern. Med.* **2005**, *2*, 79–84. [CrossRef] [PubMed]
93. Hamishehkar, H.; Rahimpour, Y.; Kouhsoltani, M. Niosomes as a Propitious Carrier for Topical Drug Delivery. *Expert Opin. Drug Deliv.* **2013**, *10*, 261–272. [CrossRef]
94. Rajera, R.; Nagpal, K.; Singh, S.K.; Mishra, D.N. Niosomes: A Controlled and Novel Drug Delivery System. *Biol. Pharm. Bull.* **2011**, *34*, 945–953. [CrossRef]
95. Teeranachaideekul, V.; Parichatikanond, W.; Junyaprasert, V.B.; Morakul, B. Pumpkin Seed Oil-Loaded Niosomes for Topical Application: 5α-Reductase Inhibitory, Anti-Inflammatory, and In Vivo Anti-Hair Loss Effects. *Pharmaceuticals* **2022**, *15*, 930. [CrossRef]
96. Planz, V.; Lehr, C.-M.; Windbergs, M. In Vitro Models for Evaluating Safety and Efficacy of Novel Technologies for Skin Drug Delivery. *J. Control. Release* **2016**, *242*, 89–104. [CrossRef]
97. Cruz, A.M.; Gonçalves, M.C.; Marques, M.S.; Veiga, F.; Paiva-Santos, A.C.; Pires, P.C. In Vitro Models for Anti-Aging Efficacy Assessment: A Critical Update in Dermocosmetic Research. *Cosmetics* **2023**, *10*, 66. [CrossRef]
98. Welss, T.; Basketter, D.A.; Schröder, K.R. In Vitro Skin Irritation: Facts and Future. State of the Art Review of Mechanisms and Models. *Toxicol. Vitr.* **2004**, *18*, 231–243. [CrossRef]
99. Kim, J.Y.; Lee, W.R.; Kim, K.H.; An, H.J.; Chang, Y.C.; Han, S.M.; Park, Y.Y.; Pak, S.C.; Park, K.K. Effects of Bee Venom against Propionibacterium Acnes-Induced Inflammation in Human Keratinocytes and Monocytes. *Int. J. Mol. Med.* **2015**, *35*, 1651–1656. [CrossRef]
100. Aburayan, W.S.; Alajmi, A.M.; Alfahad, A.J.; Alsharif, W.K.; Alshehri, A.A.; Booq, R.Y.; Alsudir, S.A.; Alsulaihem, F.M.; Bukhary, H.A.; Badr, M.Y.; et al. Melittin from Bee Venom Encapsulating Electrospun Fibers as a Potential Antimicrobial Wound Dressing Patches for Skin Infections. *Pharmaceutics* **2022**, *14*, 725. [CrossRef]
101. Rinaldi, F.; Del Favero, E.; Rondelli, V.; Pieretti, S.; Bogni, A.; Ponti, J.; Rossi, F.; Di Marzio, L.; Paolino, D.; Marianecci, C.; et al. Ph-Sensitive Niosomes: Effects on Cytotoxicity and on Inflammation and Pain in Murine Models. *J. Enzym. Inhib. Med. Chem.* **2017**, *32*, 538–546. [CrossRef]

102. Lu, Y.; Kim, S.; Park, K. In Vitro–in Vivo Correlation: Perspectives on Model Development. *Int. J. Pharm.* **2011**, *418*, 142–148. [CrossRef]
103. Qiu, Y.; Duan, J.Z. In Vitro/In Vivo Correlations. In *Developing Solid Oral Dosage Forms*; Elsevier: Amsterdam, The Netherlands, 2017; pp. 415–452.
104. Chain, A.S.Y.; Sturkenboom, M.C.J.M.; Danhof, M.; Pasqua, O.E. Della Establishing in Vitro to Clinical Correlations in the Evaluation of Cardiovascular Safety Pharmacology. *Drug Discov. Today Technol.* **2013**, *10*, e373–e383. [CrossRef]
105. Rath, S.; Kanfer, I. In Vitro–In Vivo Correlations (IVIVC) for Predicting the Clinical Performance of Metronidazole Topical Creams Intended for Local Action. *Pharmaceutics* **2023**, *15*, 268. [CrossRef] [PubMed]
106. Arunachalam, S.S.; Shetty, A.P.; Panniyadi, N.; Meena, C.; Kumari, J.; Rani, B.; Das, P.; Kumari, S. Study on Knowledge of Chemotherapy's Adverse Effects and Their Self-Care Ability to Manage—The Cancer Survivors Impact. *Clin. Epidemiol. Glob. Health* **2021**, *11*, 100765. [CrossRef]
107. Anand, U.; Dey, A.; Chandel, A.K.S.; Sanyal, R.; Mishra, A.; Pandey, D.K.; De Falco, V.; Upadhyay, A.; Kandimalla, R.; Chaudhary, A.; et al. Cancer Chemotherapy and beyond: Current Status, Drug Candidates, Associated Risks and Progress in Targeted Therapeutics. *Genes Dis.* **2023**, *10*, 1367–1401. [CrossRef]
108. Lustberg, M.B.; Kuderer, N.M.; Desai, A.; Bergerot, C.; Lyman, G.H. Mitigating Long-Term and Delayed Adverse Events Associated with Cancer Treatment: Implications for Survivorship. *Nat. Rev. Clin. Oncol.* **2023**, *20*, 527–542. [CrossRef]
109. Rivero, M.N.; Lenze, M.; Izaguirre, M.; Pérez Damonte, S.H.; Aguilar, A.; Wikinski, S.; Gutiérrez, M.L. Comparison between HET-CAM Protocols and a Product Use Clinical Study for Eye Irritation Evaluation of Personal Care Products Including Cosmetics According to Their Surfactant Composition. *Food Chem. Toxicol.* **2021**, *153*, 112229. [CrossRef] [PubMed]
110. Dahl, J.E. Potential of Dental Adhesives to Induce Mucosal Irritation Evaluated by the HET–CAM Method. *Acta Odontol. Scand.* **2007**, *65*, 275–283. [CrossRef]
111. Steiling, W.; Bracher, M.; Courtellemont, P.; de Silva, O. The HET–CAM, a Useful In Vitro Assay for Assessing the Eye Irritation Properties of Cosmetic Formulations and Ingredients. *Toxicol. Vitr.* **1999**, *13*, 375–384. [CrossRef]
112. Eiras, F.; Amaral, M.H.; Silva, R.; Martins, E.; Lobo, J.M.S.; Silva, A.C. Characterization and Biocompatibility Evaluation of Cutaneous Formulations Containing Lipid Nanoparticles. *Int. J. Pharm.* **2017**, *519*, 373–380. [CrossRef]
113. Mohammadi, M.; Elahimehr, Z.; Mahboobian, M.M. Acyclovir-Loaded Nanoemulsions: Preparation, Characterization and Irritancy Studies for Ophthalmic Delivery. *Curr. Eye Res.* **2021**, *46*, 1646–1652. [CrossRef]
114. Abdelkader, H.; Ismail, S.; Hussein, A.; Wu, Z.; Al-Kassas, R.; Alany, R.G. Conjunctival and Corneal Tolerability Assessment of Ocular Naltrexone Niosomes and Their Ingredients on the Hen's Egg Chorioallantoic Membrane and Excised Bovine Cornea Models. *Int. J. Pharm.* **2012**, *432*, 1–10. [CrossRef]
115. de Araujo Lowndes Viera, L.M.; Silva, R.S.; da Silva, C.C.; Presgrave, O.A.F.; Boas, M.H.S.V. Comparison of the Different Protocols of the Hen's Egg Test-Chorioallantoic Membrane (HET-CAM) by Evaluating the Eye Irritation Potential of Surfactants. *Toxicol. Vitr.* **2022**, *78*, 105255. [CrossRef]
116. Somwongin, S.; Chantawannakul, P.; Chaiyana, W. Antioxidant Activity and Irritation Property of Venoms from Apis Species. *Toxicon* **2018**, *145*, 32–39. [CrossRef]
117. Abdelkader, H.; Alani, A.W.G.; Alany, R.G. Recent Advances in Non-Ionic Surfactant Vesicles (Niosomes): Self-Assembly, Fabrication, Characterization, Drug Delivery Applications and Limitations. *Drug Deliv.* **2014**, *21*, 87–100. [CrossRef]
118. Vichai, V.; Kirtikara, K. Sulforhodamine B Colorimetric Assay for Cytotoxicity Screening. *Nat. Protoc.* **2006**, *1*, 1112–1116. [CrossRef]
119. *ICCVAM-Recommended Test Method Protocol: Hen's Egg Test-Chorioallantoic Membrane (HET-CAM) Test Method*; NIH: Bethesda, MD, USA, 2010.
120. Palmeira-de-Oliveira, R.; Monteiro Machado, R.; Martinez-de-Oliveira, J.; Palmeira-de-Oliveira, A. Testing Vaginal Irritation with the Hen's Egg Test-Chorioallantoic Membrane Assay. *ALTEX* **2018**, *35*, 495–503. [CrossRef]

pharmaceuticals

MDPI

Article

Contribution of Microbiota to Bioactivity Exerted by Bee Bread

Nikos Asoutis Didaras [1], Ioanna Karaiskou [1], Marios Nikolaidis [2], Christina Siaperopoulou [1], Irini Georgi [1], Christina Tsadila [1], Katerina Karatasou [3], Grigoris D. Amoutzias [2] and Dimitris Mossialos [1,*]

[1] Microbial Biotechnology-Molecular Bacteriology-Virology Laboratory, Department of Biochemistry & Biotechnology, University of Thessaly, 41500 Larissa, Greece; didasout@yahoo.gr (N.A.D.); ikaraiskou@uth.gr (I.K.); siaperopoulou@uth.gr (C.S.); egeorgi@uth.gr (I.G.); tsadila@uth.gr (C.T.)

[2] Bioinformatics Laboratory, Department of Biochemistry & Biotechnology, University of Thessaly, 41500 Larissa, Greece; marionik23@gmail.com (M.N.); amoutzias@uth.gr (G.D.A.)

[3] Apicultural Centre of Larissa, Federation of Greek Beekeepers Associations, 41222 Larissa, Greece; omse@otenet.gr

* Correspondence: mosial@uth.gr; Tel.: +30-2410565270

Abstract: Bee-collected pollen (BCP) and bee bread (BB) are honey bee products known for their beneficial biological properties. The main goal of this study was to investigate BB microbiota and its contribution to bioactivity exerted by BB. The microbiota of BB samples collected at different maturation stages was investigated via culture-independent (Next Generation Sequencing, NGS) and culture-dependent methods. Microbial communities dynamically fluctuate during BB maturation, ending in a stable microbial community structure in mature BB. Bee bread bacterial isolates were tested for phenotypes and genes implicated in the production and secretion of enzymes as well as antibacterial activity. Out of 309 bacterial isolates, 41 secreted hemicellulases, 13 cellulases, 39 amylases, 132 proteinases, 85 Coomassie brilliant blue G or R dye-degrading enzymes and 72 Malachite Green dye-degrading enzymes. Furthermore, out of 309 bacterial isolates, 42 exhibited antibacterial activity against *Staphylococcus aureus*, 34 against *Pseudomonas aeruginosa*, 47 against *Salmonella enterica* ser. Typhimurium and 43 against *Klebsiella pneumoniae*. Artificially fermented samples exerted higher antibacterial activity compared to fresh BCP, strongly indicating that BB microbiota contribute to BB antibacterial activity. Our findings suggest that BB microbiota is an underexplored source of novel antimicrobial agents and enzymes that could lead to new applications in medicine and the food industry.

Keywords: bee pollen; bee bread; microbiota; fermentation; bioactivity; antibacterial activity; enzyme production; pasteurization

1. Introduction

It has been suggested that honey bees evolved roughly 123 million years ago from carnivorous wasp species that replaced meat (as a food source) with pollen [1]. Bee-collected pollen (BCP), especially the fermented pollen designated bee bread (BB), is the main source of proteins, lipids, vitamins and minerals for honey bees. Furthermore, BB provides honey bees with valuable phytochemicals such as polyphenols [2,3].

The transition to a vegetarian diet was plausibly supported by the colonization of new microorganisms in the wasp gut, which facilitated pollen digestion [1]. A resilient outer layer consisting of a durable biopolymer called sporopollenin is present in pollen grains [4], which must be breached, to release essential nutrients bioavailable in the gut [5].

Highly nutritious pollen is not always abundant throughout the year [6]. Furthermore, pollen is a perishable food easily spoiled in the warm hive environment, due to its relatively high-water content and plethora of nutrients [7].

Bees have effectively dealt with all these issues by turning fresh pollen into BB, a fermented food that can be stored and preserved in the hive for a long time. Additionally,

BB is considered more nutritious and bioactive compared to BCP and is considered a functional food [8–10].

BB consists of pollen derived from the plants growing in the vicinity of the hive, honey bee glandular secretions containing symbiotic microorganisms, added nectar and honey containing a heterogeneous community of microorganisms of plant and environmental origin [11–14]. Although BB is an important honey bee product, BB bioactivity and especially BB microbiota, is so far poorly investigated. Recent studies regarding BB bioactivity with a special focus on antimicrobial properties have been published [15–17]; however, BB microbiota and its putative contribution to bioactivity are still elusive.

BB microbiota is important for honey bee nutrition and development [18,19]. It has been reported that BB microorganisms facilitate the enzymatic pre-digestion of pollen grains, thus increasing the digestibility and bioavailability of nutrients [20,21]. So far, the antimicrobial activity and biosynthetic potential of BB microbiota are largely unknown. Pelka et al., have shown that microorganisms isolated from BCP and BB produce antimicrobial compounds, as well as lipolytic, proteolytic, cellulolytic and esterolytic enzymes [22].

Furthermore, it has been demonstrated that BB exerted significantly higher antimicrobial activity than pollen [17]. Similarly, the antibacterial activity exerted by BB in water suspensions against clinically important pathogens was remarkable [16]. The application of chemical solvents (ethanol, methanol, ether), or the implementation of other processing techniques such as sonication, leads to breached pollen grains, thus increasing the availability of known antimicrobial phytochemicals such as polyphenols. The finding that virtually unprocessed BB demonstrated similarly high or even higher antimicrobial properties led us to hypothesize the presence of other than polyphenol antimicrobial agents, presumably produced by BB microbiota [16]. In a similar way, it has been recently reported that BB water suspensions exerted significant antiviral activity against Enterovirus D68 and Influenza A Virus (IVA) H1N1 [23,24].

BB microbiota consists of both plant and bee-derived microorganisms, but it seems that those of bee origin are relatively more abundant. It has been reported that changes in BCP microbiological and biochemical composition start as soon as pollen is collected [20]. Given that the nine bacterial phylotypes, which constitute the core gut microbiome of adult worker bees, are poorly represented in BB [18,25], it suggests that mainly microorganisms derived from honey bee stomach, including a variety of lactic acid bacteria, are present in BB microbiota [26,27].

Forager bees inoculate flower pollen with lactic acid bacteria (LABs) that are present in their honey stomach, an organ used to contain foraged nectar or water to be brought to the nest and for trophallaxis, the sharing of nectar among nest mates, which is part of honey production [11,28]. Indeed, forager bees regurgitate nectar and add it to collected pollen grains along with their secretions to form the pollen pellets they carry back to the hive. The pollen pellets end up in the comb cells where they are further processed by middle-aged bees by adding honey and glandular secretions. Finally, bees push the pollen pellets with their heads to pack them tightly into the cell, where BCP undergoes solid-state fermentation [29].

It has been suggested that BCP microorganisms are present inside the comb cell under aerobic, anaerobic and microaerophilic conditions [30], similar to microorganisms isolated from BB [31–35] that produce organic acids through both anaerobic and aerobic fermentation [36,37].

Researchers investigated the diversity of LABs previously isolated from the honey stomach of bees, in BCP samples, in two-week- and two-month-old BB samples. They identified twelve bacterial species belonging to *Lactobacillus* and *Bifidobacterium* genera. The majority of them remained viable in BCP and in two-week-old BB but not in older BB samples [11,38]. LABs might be considered as a starter culture of BCP fermentation [11,29] and they are known to produce antimicrobial compounds, thus contributing towards BB preservation in the hive [11,39]. Yeasts are also present in BB [29,31,32] and could similarly be implicated in BCP fermentation.

Recently, Dranca et al. [37] reported that lactic acid was not detected in BB but instead gluconic acid was the most abundant organic acid. They reported that mature BB contained 97.9 g/kg organic acids, with gluconic acid amounting to 79.2 g/kg, followed by acetic acid (10.4 g/kg) and formic acid (6.75 g/kg). Propionic acid (1.30 g/kg) and butyric acid (0.33 g/kg) were also detected [37]. Gluconic acid is produced from glucose either enzymatically by glucose oxidase, usually produced by fungi, or by glucose dehydrogenase produced by bacteria such as *Gluconobacter*, through aerobic fermentation [40].

Overall, BB contains microbial communities that flourish or perish during BB maturation. Gilliam [20] was the first to suggest that, during the transformation of BCP to BB, microbial succession takes place. Recent research has demonstrated that the diversity and community structure of BB microbiota indeed fluctuates during maturation [29,32,41,42].

The main goal of this study is to investigate how BB microbiota contributes towards BB bioactivity and identify the most relatively abundant microbial groups using both culture-independent (Next Generation Sequencing, NGS) and culture-dependent methods, starting from early fermentation to maturation. Moreover, it has been tested whether specific enzymes, such as amylases, proteinases, xylanases, cellulases and laccases, that presumably facilitate the digestion of pollen grains, could be produced by culturable microorganisms isolated from BB. Finally, the antimicrobial activity of BB isolates was assessed against important human pathogens, to elucidate the putative contribution of microbiota towards the high antimicrobial activity exerted by BB. Regarding this aspect, we fermented double pasteurized fresh BCP using BB isolates as a starter culture and then we tested the antimicrobial activity exerted by the fermented BCP.

2. Results

2.1. Metataxonomic Microbiota Analysis during BB Maturation

Metataxonomic analysis implementing Next Generation Sequencing (NGS) was performed to elucidate the microbiota dynamics during BB maturation. The basic statistics of each sample are shown in Supplementary Table S1. Rarefaction curves indicated that sequencing depth was sufficiently high regarding all samples (Supplementary Figures S1 and S2).

At the beginning of BB maturation, bacterial diversity fluctuated as depicted by Chao 1 index values: 46 (1-day-old BCP), 35 (11-day-old BB), 82 (27-day-old BB) and 42 (41-day-old BB) (see Supplementary Table S2). Regarding diversity and evenness, high fluctuation of Shannon index values was not observed, with a notable exception of samples S1 and S2 (Supplementary Table S2). Shannon index values were the following during maturation: 5.121 (1-day-old BCP), 4.778 (1-day-old BB), 5.714 (11-day-old BB), 5.603 (27-day-old BB) and 5.146 (41-day-old BB). Fungal diversity reduced gradually from day 1 to day 27, displaying Chao 1 index values of 26 (1-day-old BCP), dropping to 8 (27-day-old BB) and Shannon index values from 3.380 (1-day-old BCP) to 0.586 (27-day-old BB) (see Supplementary Table S3). These findings clearly indicate that during BB maturation, microbiota diversity dynamically fluctuates, ending up in a rather stable microbial community structure. Beta-diversity indices (Supplementary Tables S6–S13) showed no significant differences between samples. Figures 1 and 2 depict bacterial and fungal phyla as well as classes present in samples S1 to S9, while Supplementary Tables S4 and S5 summarize the most dominant (relative abundance >3%) families and genera of bacteria and fungi, respectively. Beta-diversity metric tables for bacteria are shown in Supplementary Tables S6–S9 and, for fungi, in Supplementary Tables S10–S13. Proteobacteria is the dominant phylum in BCP (S1), representing more than 60% of total operating taxonomic units (OTUs). Proteobacteria relative abundance increased rapidly within 24 h (S2), reaching almost 70% and gradually declined from day 11 to day 41, reaching approximately the initial relative abundance (S3–S5). Gammaproteobacteria were dominant (50% of total OTUs in S1) but dropped below 40% in S5. *Pseudomonas* genus abundance was significantly variable during BB maturation (S1: 4.62%, S2: 1.12%, S3: 6.1%, S4: 14.14%, S5 BB: 4.68%). The sharp decline from 4.62% to 1.12% within the first 24 h might be attributed to initial BB fermentation and honey inoculation. After that time, there is a progressive increase (days 11 to 27) and finally, a significant decrease from day 27 (S4) to day 41 (S5), possibly because BB was fully matured. From day 12 till day 41, the sampling frame was isolated within the hive so the honey bees could not add BCP or consume BB.

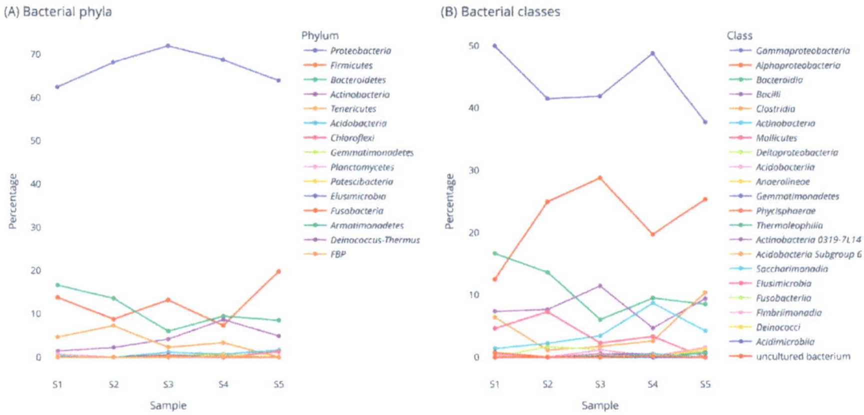

Figure 1. Bacterial phyla and classes detected via NGS in samples S1 to S5.

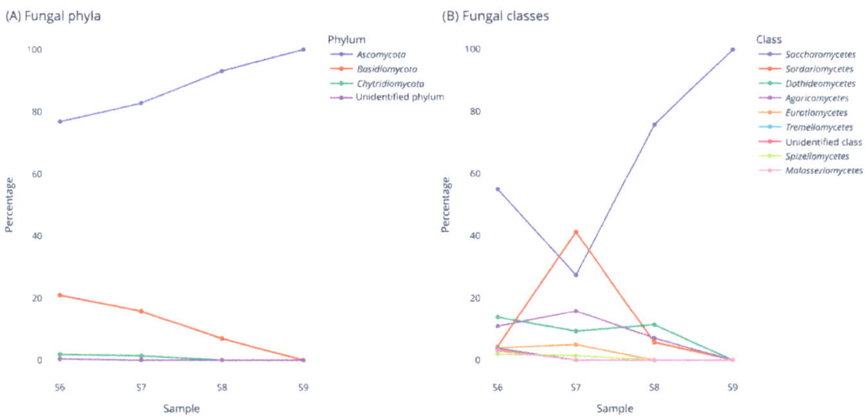

Figure 2. Fungal phyla and classes detected via NGS in samples S6 to S9.

Alphaproteobacteria constitute a significant class, amounting up to 30% in S3 but dropped to 25% in S5. *Sphingomonas* was a bacterial group that its abundance increased from 6.24% (S1) to 13.34% (S5).

Firmicutes relative abundance increased to 20% in S5. Bacilli and Clostridia are both dominant groups representing roughly 20%. Clostridia declined rapidly within the first 24 h and then progressively increased till day 41. On the contrary, *Lactobacillus* genus increased rapidly within the first 24 h, indicating the contribution of Lactobacilli in the fermentation process, especially at the very beginning. The fermentation process is crucial for BCP transformation to BB. Of note, *Lactobacillus* spp. are still present in 41-day-old BB, indicating their adaptability in this environment. Bacteroidetes is also an abundant phylum whose abundance gradually decreased.

In this study, NGS data demonstrated that *Sphingomonas, Pseudomonas, Acinetobacter* and *Lactobacillus* are important bacterial genera implicated in BB maturation as their relative abundance fluctuated at different maturation stages (Supplementary Table S4). These genera were present in S5 (41-day-old BB), each one representing more than 4% of total OTUs (Supplementary Table S4). *Enterobacter* spp. increased from 4.62% in one-day-old BCP (sample S1) to 7.08% in 1-day-old BB (sample S2). However, they were not detected in 11-day-old BB (sample S3). Furthermore, an unidentified genus of Enterobacteriaceae was detected in BB, ranging from 1.69% to 9.24% of OTUs, and remained present in 41-day-old BB (5.36%). *Massilia*, a bacterial genus detected in different environments but mostly related to plants, was the most abundant genus in the early BB fermentation stages (13.06% in 1-day-old BCP), dropping to 2.93% in 41-day-old BB (sample S5).

Regarding fungi, Ascomycota was the most abundant phylum, representing almost 100% of related OTUs in 27-day-old BB (Supplementary Table S5). The most dominant Ascomycota classes were *Saccharomycetes* and *Sordariomycetes*. Agaricomycetes relative abundance was almost 18% in sample S7 (1-day-old BB) and dropped to zero in sample S9 (27-day-old BB). Similarly, Dothideomycetes relative abundance was close to 15% in samples S6, S7 and S8, and dropped to zero in sample S9. *Zygosaccharomyces* was the most abundant genus, amounting to 99.58% of related OTUs in 27-day-old BB (S9 sample). Basidiomycota was the second most abundant fungal phylum, though its relative abundance decreased gradually from 20% in sample S6 (1-day-old BCP) to 0% in sample S9 (27-day-old BB).

2.2. Antimicrobial Activity and Biosynthetic Potential of Isolated BB Bacteria

Bacterial isolates (isolated from S10 and S11) were screened for antibacterial activity against four pathogens (*S. aureus*, *P. aeruginosa*, *S. enterica* ser. Typhimurium and *K. pneumoniae*), as well as for enzyme production, i.e., secretion of cellulases, hemicellulases, amylases, proteinases and oxidases, among them, laccases that are capable to degrade dyes. Isolates that exerted antibacterial activity at least against two pathogens and simultaneously produced diverse enzymes were selected for identification through 16S rRNA gene sequencing. Furthermore, we identified seven isolates that exerted antibacterial activity against one pathogen and three isolates that did not exert any antibacterial activity but still were able to produce various enzymes. The identified strains, the antibacterial activity and biosynthetic potential are presented in Tables 1 and 2. Overall, eleven strains were identified as *Apilactobacillus kunkeei*, one strain as *Fructobacillus fructosus*, one strain as *Pseudomonas aeruginosa*, one strain as *Staphylococcus hominis*, five strains as *Bacillus thuringiensis*, three strains as *Bacillus cereus*, three strains as *Bacillus siamensis*, two strains as *Bacillus licheniformis*, three strains as *Bacillus subtilis*, five strains as *Bacillus safensis*, one strain as *Bacillus halotolerans*, one strain as *Bacillus pumilus*, one strain as *Bacillus aerophilus* and 10 strains were identified at genus level as *Bacillus* spp.

Table 1. Antibacterial activity exerted by *Apilatobacillus* and *Fructobacillus* strains.

Accession Number (GenBank)	*K. pneumoniae* (cm ± [1]SD)	*S. enterica* ser. Typhimurium (cm ± [1]SD)	*P. aeruginosa* (cm ± [1]SD)	*S. aureus* (cm ± [1]SD)	% Identity	Identified Bacteria	16 S rRNA Gene Sequence (bp)	Strain
ON911239	3 ± 0.7	2.7 ± 0.9	3 ± 0.8	0.8 ± 0.1	99.79	*Apilactobacillus kunkeei*	1446	NADBB5
ON911241	3.1 ± 0.7	2.7 ± 0.9	3 ± 0.8	0.6 ± 0.1	100.00	*Apilactobacillus kunkeei*	1452	NADBB7
ON911243	3.2 ± 0.2	2.7 ± 0.4	3 ± 0.1	0	99.86	*Apilactobacillus kunkeei*	1424	NADBB9
ON911252	3.5 ± 0.5	3.4 ± 0.7	2.4 ± 1.4	0.7 ± 0.1	100.00	*Apilactobacillus kunkeei*	1447	NADBB20
ON911258	2.8 ± 1	3.4 ± 0.4	2.7 ± 1.2	0.9 ± 0	99.79	*Apilactobacillus kunkeei*	1412	NADBB27
ON911261	3 ± 0.9	2.8 ± 1	3 ± 0.8	0.7 ± 0.3	99.86	*Apilactobacillus kunkeei*	1433	NADBB30
ON911265	3 ± 1.3	3.3 ± 0.8	2.9 ± 1	0.9 ± 0.2	100.00	*Apilactobacillus kunkeei*	1413	NADBB34
ON911266	3.4 ± 0.8	3.2 ± 1.2	3.3 ± 0.8	1.6 ± 0.4	100.00	*Apilactobacillus kunkeei*	1208	NADBB35
ON911268	3.3 ± 0.9	3 ± 1.3	3.4 ± 0.9	1.1 ± 0.2	100.00	*Apilactobacillus kunkeei*	1446	NADBB37
ON911269	3.3 ± 0.9	3.1 ± 1.2	3.3 ± 1	1.1 ± 0.1	100.00	*Apilactobacillus kunkeei*	1443	NADBB38
ON911270	2.7 ± 0.6	1.8 ± 0.3	2.4 ± 0.4	0	99.43	*Fructobacillus fructosus*	1393	NADBB39
ON911279	3.3 ± 0.9	3 ± 1.2	3.3 ± 1	1.1 ± 0.4	100.00	*Apilactobacillus kunkeei*	1447	NADBB48

All tests have been performed at least in triplicates, [1]SD: standard deviation.

Table 2. Antibacterial activity and biosynthetic potential of bacteria isolated from BB.

Accession Number (GenBank)	Biosynthetic Potential	Antibacterial Activity	% Identity	Identified Bacteria	16S rRNA Gene Sequence (bp)	Strain
ON911235	A, P, R, G, L̲	1 *, 3 *	100.00	*Pseudomonas aeruginosa*	1400	NADBB1
ON911236	X, X̲, A, P, G, M	1 ***, 3 ***, 4 ***	100.00	*Bacillus* sp.	1395	NADBB2
ON911237	A, P, G, M, L̲	1 *, 3 *, 4 ***	99.93	*Bacillus thuringiensis*	1400	NADBB3
ON911238	A, P, R, G, L̲	1 ***, 2 ***, 3 ***	100.00	*Bacillus cereus*	1404	NADBB4
ON911240	C, X, A, P, GUA	1 **, 3 *, 4 *	100.00	*Bacillus siamensis*	1426	NADBB6
ON911242	X, A, G, M	1 **, 4 ***	100.00	*Bacillus* sp.	1416	NADBB8
ON911244	A, G, L̲	3 **, 4 *	99.86	*Bacillus thuringiensis*	1389	NADBB10
ON911245	X, X̲, **X**, A, P, G, M,	1 ***, 4 ***	99.93	*Bacillus* sp.	1417	NADBB11
ON911246	A, P, R, G, L̲	3 ***	99.93	*Bacillus thuringiensis*	1390	NADBB13
ON911247	C, X, X̲, P, R	1 **, 4 *	99.93	*Bacillus* sp.	1376	NADBB14
ON911248	C, A, P, G, M	1 **, 3 *, 4 ***	99.57	*Bacillus licheniformis*	1400	NADBB16
ON911249	C, X, A, P, M, L̲	1 **	100.00	*Bacillus subtilis*	1425	NADBB17
ON911250	A, P, G, M, L̲	1 **, 3 *, 4 *	99.86	*Bacillus* sp.	1419	NADBB18
ON911251	C, X, A, G, **L**, L̲		100.00	*Bacillus subtilis*	1423	NADBB19
ON911253	A, P, R, G, **L**, L̲	3 **	99.93	*Bacillus cereus*	1398	NADBB21
ON911254	X, X̲, P, G, M,	1 **	100.00	*Bacillus* sp.	1420	NADBB23
ON911255	C, X, **X**, X̲, P, G	1 **, 3 ***, 4 ***	100.00	*Bacillus* sp.	1414	NADBB24
ON911256	C, X, A, P, M	1 *	100.00	*Bacillus siamensis*	1410	NADBB25
ON911257	C, X, A, P, G, M	1 *, 3 *, 4 *	100.00	*Bacillus subtilis*	1392	NADBB26
ON911259	A, G, M, L̲		99.93	*Bacillus* sp.	1418	NADBB28
ON911260	A, P, G	1 **, 2 ***, 3 ***, 4 ***	100.00	*Bacillus cereus*	1402	NADBB29
ON911262	A, M, L̲		99.25	*Staphylococcus hominis*	1341	NADBB31
ON911263	C, X, X̲, P, G, M	1 ***, 3 ***, 4 ***	100.00	*Bacillus* sp.	1371	NADBB32
ON911264	C, X, A, P, M, G, L̲	1 ***, 3 ***	99.86	*Bacillus siamensis*	1417	NADBB33
ON911267	A, P, G, **L**, L̲	1 *, 3 *, 4 *	100.00	*Bacillus thuringiensis*	1313	NADBB36
ON911271	C, X, X̲, P, R, G, L̲	1 ***, 3 **, 4 ***	100.00	*Bacillus safensis*	1416	NADBB40
ON911272	C, X, X̲, P, G	1 ***, 4 ***	99.93	*Bacillus* sp.	1419	NADBB41
ON911273	C, X, A, P, G	1 **, 3 ***, 4 ***	99.71	*Bacillus halotolerans*	1393	NADBB42
ON911274	C, A, P, G, M	1 *, 4 **	99.86	*Bacillus licheniformis*	1395	NADBB43
ON911275	X, P, R, G	1 **, 4 **	100.00	*Bacillus safensis*	1383	NADBB44
ON911276	C, X, X̲, A, M;	1 *	100.00	*Bacillus pumilus*	1391	NADBB45
ON911277	C, X, P, R, G, M	1 **, 3 ***	100.00	*Bacillus aerophilus*	1412	NADBB46
ON911278	A, P, R, G, L̲	3 ***	100.00	*Bacillus thuringiensis*	1396	NADBB47
ON911280	X, **X**, X̲, P, G	1 *	99.85	*Bacillus safensis*	1323	NADBB49
ON911281	X, **X**, X̲, P, G	1 **, 3 **, 4 **	99.93	*Bacillus safensis*	1379	NADBB50

Antimicrobial activity against 1: *S aureus*, 2: *P. aeruginosa*, 3: *S. enterica* ser. Typhimurium, 4: *K. pneumoniae*. *: 3–7 mm, **: 7–11 mm, ***: >11 mm. **Biosynthetic potential:** C: cellulase positive phenotype, X: xylanase positive phenotype, **X**: endoxylanase gene confirmed via sequencing (336 bp fragment), X̲: endoxylanase gene PCR detection, A: amylase positive phenotype, P: proteinase positive phenotype, R: coomassie brilliant blue red degradation, G: coomassie brilliant blue green degradation, M: malachite green degradation, **L**: laccase gene confirmed via sequencing (142 bp fragment), L̲: laccase gene PCR detection.

2.3. Antibacterial Activity Exerted by BB Isolates

Out of 309 bacterial isolates, 42 exhibited antibacterial activity against *S. aureus* MRSA strain 1552, 34 against carbapenem-resistant *P. aeruginosa* strain 1773, 47 against *S. enterica* ser. Typhimurium and 43 against *K. pneumoniae*.

Apilactobacillus and *Fructobacillus* strains exerted higher antibacterial activity against Gram-negative pathogens (inhibition zone ranged from 1.8 cm to 3.5 cm, see Table 1). However, these strains exerted less antibacterial activity against Gram-positive *S. aureus*. *Bacillus* isolates demonstrated antibacterial activity against mainly *S. aureus*, though some exerted antibacterial activity against Gram-negative pathogens (Table 2).

2.4. Biosynthetic Potential of BB Isolated Bacteria

Out of 309 bacterial isolates, 41 secreted hemicellulases, 13 cellulases, 39 amylases, 132 proteinases, 85 Coomassie brilliant blue G or R dye-degrading enzymes and 72 Malachite Green dye-degrading enzymes. All identified strains were producing more than one of the above enzymes (Table 2).

Corresponding genes were partially amplified through PCR to investigate the bacterial gene content associated with laccase and hemicellulase production. The endoxylanase gene (336 bp fragment) was amplified from isolates, demonstrating a strong positive xylanase phenotype. Out of 35 tested isolates, 20 of them were positive, whereas 15 were negative, thus indicating the presence of various xylanolytic enzymes was probably exhibiting different modes of activity [43]. Furthermore, amplicons of ON911245 (*Bacillus* sp.), ON911255 (*Bacillus* sp.), ON911280 (*B. safensis*) and ON911281 (*B. safensis*) isolates were sequenced and indeed confirmed as endoxylanase gene fragments (Supplementary Table S14).

The lacasse gene (142 bp fragment) was amplified via PCR from isolates, demonstrating a strong dye degradation phenotype. Out of 55 tested isolates, 22 were positive, whereas 33 were negative. These findings indicate the presence of other dye-degrading enzymes such as lignin peroxidase, manganese peroxidase, versatile peroxidase and dye peroxidase [44]. Laccase activity has been detected on the guaiacol substrate. Positive colonies turned brown as expected and the surrounding substrate was turned light brown. Therefore, we assume that laccase-positive isolates may produce membrane-bound laccases. PCR amplicons of strains ON911251 (*B. subtilis*), ON911253 (*B. cereus*) and ON911267 (*B. thuringiensis*) were sequenced, thus confirming the presence of laccase gene in positive strains (Supplementary Table S14).

Cellulase and hemicellulase phenotypes were also directly detected in the protein fractions of BB, which further supports the hypothesis that BB microbiome facilitates the predigestion of pollen grains.

2.5. Antibacterial Activity Exerted by Double Pasteurized and Artificially Fermented BCP

The unpasteurized BCP (AF1) MIC has been determined at 12.5% *w*/*v* regarding pathogens *S. aureus* and *S. enterica* ser. Typhimurium, whereas MBC values were >12.5% *w*/*v* (Table 3). The MIC value of AF46D (non-inoculated, double pasteurized AF1) against *S. aureus* did not alter, thus implying that the antibacterial compounds inhibiting *S. aureus* growth were heat resistant. In contrast, AF46D MIC value was >12.5% *w*/*v* against *S. enterica* sub. Typhimurium, implying that the antimicrobial compounds inhibiting this pathogen were heat-labile. We assumed that due to fermentation, antimicrobial compounds contributing to exerted antibacterial activity might be produced. This hypothesis is further supported by the MIC and MBC values of AF42D, AF43D and AF 44D against *S. enterica* ser. Typhimurium. AF42D MIC value (6.25% *w*/*v*) is lower compared to AF46D and AF1 (MIC 12.5% *w*/*v*), thus demonstrating higher antibacterial activity. *A. kunkeei* strain NADBB37 was used as starter culture in AF42D. A different *A. kunkeei* strain (NADBB7) was used as a starter culture in AF43D. AF43D demonstrated the same MIC value compared to AF42D. However, AF43D (in contrast to AF42D) demonstrated bactericidal activity against *S. enterica* ser. Typhimurium (MBC 12.5% *w*/*v*). It is plausible that *A. kunkeei* NADBB7 produces different or at higher concentration antimicrobial compounds against *S. enterica* sub. Typhimurium compared to *A. kunkeei* NADBB37. A starter culture containing a mixture of two bacterial strains and a yeast (*A. kunkeei* NADBB37, *Fructobacillus fructosus* and *Zygosaccharomyces siamensis*) was implemented in fermentation of AF44D. It has been shown that AF44D did not exert bactericidal activity against *S. enterica* sub. Typhimurium (MBC > 12.5% *w*/*v*) but only bacteriostatic activity (MIC 12.5% *w*/*v*).

A starter culture consisted of *A. kunkeei* NADBB37 and prolonged fermentation time was applied to AF5U (29 days at 33 °C). AF5U MIC and MBC values were the lowest in this study against both tested pathogens (Table 3).

Our data have shown that the BCP lost its antibacterial activity against *Salmonella enterica* ser. Typhimurium after the double pasteurization process. Following fermentation, the artificially fermented BCP re-gained antibacterial activity against the tested pathogens, indicating that BB microbiota might contribute to antimicrobial activity either by antibacterial compound production or by releasing antibacterial compounds during the fermentation of BCP grains. Our data clearly indicate that the type of starter culture as well as fermentation conditions both affect the antibacterial activity of artificially fermented BCP (Table 3).

Table 3. MIC and MBC values of double pasteurized and artificially fermented BCP.

S. enterica ser. Typhimurium		*S. aureus*		Samples
MBC *w*/*v*	MIC *w*/*v*	MBC *w*/*v*	MIC *w*/*v*	
>12.5%	12.5%	>12.5%	12.5%	AF1
>12.5%	>12.5%	>12.5%	12.5%	AF46D
>12.5%	6.25%	>12.5%	12.5%	AF42D
12.5%	6.25%	>12.5%	12.5%	AF43D
>12.5%	12.5%	>12.5%	12.5%	AF44D
6.25%	6.25%	12.5%	6.25%	AF5

3. Discussion

Our findings indicate that during BB maturation, microbiota diversity dynamically fluctuates, ending up in a rather stable microbial community structure. Changes affecting microbial growth (production of metabolites, oxygen concentration, acidity, nutrients and water availability) might occur during BB maturation, thus forming a highly variable environment. Therefore, we assume that the observed variability regarding the diversity and abundance of specific microbial groups is due to antagonism or adaptation taking place during BB maturation.

Our data are in accordance with the study conducted by Ghosh et al. [30]. They compared BCP and BB bacterial diversity by implementing NGS (Illumina MiSeq) sequencing. Samples were collected from *Apis mellifera ligustica* colonies in Andong, Korea. The dominant phyla were Proteobacteria, followed by Firmicutes in BB [30]. However, Firmicutes were the most predominant phyla in BCP. Detected Firmicutes orders were Bacillales, Lactobacillales and Clostridiales. Lactobacillales were present only in BCP.

Similarly, Donkersley et al. [33] implemented NGS (Illumina MiSeq) sequencing to investigate the microbial diversity of North West England BB samples of unknown age collected from apiaries. They reported that Proteobacteria was the most dominant phylum, followed by Bacteroidetes and Firmicutes. *Pseudomonas* (32.4%), *Arsenophonus* (13.0%), *Lactobacillus* (8.2%), *Erwinia* (7.7%) and *Acinetobacter* (5.2%) were the most common genera. *Massilia* was identified in BB in relatively low abundance along with *Sphingomonas* [33].

Regarding fungi, our data showed that Ascomycota was the most abundant phylum, representing almost 100% of related OTUs in 27-day-old BB (Supplementary Table S5). The most dominant Ascomycota classes were *Saccharomycetes* and *Sordariomycetes*. *Zygosaccharomyces* was the most abundant genus, amounting to 99.58% of related OTUs in 27-day-old BB (S9 sample). Basidiomycota was the second most abundant fungal phylum, though its relative abundance decreased gradually from 20% in sample S6 (1-day-old BCP) to 0% in sample S9 (27-day-old BB). Our findings are in accordance with data reported in previous studies. Dimov et al. applied NGS-based metataxonomics (Illumina HiSec) to investigate the mycobiome of 2- to 4-day-old BB, collected from four locations in Bulgaria. All dominant genera belonged to the Ascomycota phylum (>99%) [45]. Sinpoo et al. combined PCR, DGGE and culture-dependent methods to identify fungal communities in BCP and 1-, 2-, 3-, 4- and 6-week-old BB in Thailand, whereas the bees foraged pollen mainly from *Mimosa pudica* L. Fungal populations and diversity decreased with storage. The dominant fungal species in BB were yeasts of the genus *Zygosaccharomyces* and filamentous fungi of *Cladosporium* and *Aspergillus* genera [41]. Similarly, Detry et al. isolated yeasts from 7-day-old and 20-day-old BB samples collected from apiaries in Belgium. Isolates were identified via PCR and analysis showed that most of the 252 identified isolates belonged to the genera *Starmerella*, *Metschnikowia* and *Zygosaccharomyces*. *Starmerella* (*Candida*) *apis* was the most dominant species in fresh BB, while *Zygosaccharomyces* spp. were more abundant in mature BB [42].

BB bacterial isolates were screened for antibacterial activity as well as for the production of diverse enzymes. Isolated bacteria demonstrated positive phenotypes regarding the secretion of cellulases, amylases and proteinases in accordance with a previous study [22]. Moreover, this is the first study reporting the secretion of hemicellulases, Coomassie Brilliant Blue G or R dye-degrading enzymes and Malachite Green dye-degrading enzymes by BB bacteria. The production of lignin-degrading enzymes (laccases or oxidases) by BB bacteria might promote exine (the outer layer of pollen grains) degradation. Moreover, the production of cellulases is essential for intine (the inner layer of pollen grains) degradation, which mainly consists of cellulose [46]. The ability of BB bacteria to breach pollen grain walls facilitates the release of nutrients and bioactive compounds contained in pollen grains. Recently, Damulienė et al. reported that enzymatic hydrolysis of BCP increased total phenolic content by 1.1 to 2.5 times, total flavonoid content by 1.1 to 3.0 times, radical scavenging activity by 1.1–3.5 times and antibacterial activity by 1.1 to 3.3 times [47]. Iorizzo et al. investigated LAB communities in BB as well as honey stomach and midgut of *Apis mellifera ligustica* in Italy. Three RAPD_isolates (Lpla.I, Lpla.II and Lpla.VI) present exclusively in BB, produced esterase, esterase lipase, α-glucosidase and β-glucosidase. RAPD_biotypes Lpla.I and Lpla.VI were also able to utilize raffinose, while the RAPD_isolate II metabolized melezitose [48]. Rokop et al. implemented culture -based methodology and molecular taxonomy to identify LAB communities present in different hive milieu. Both *Fructobacillus* spp. and *Lactobacillaceae* were isolated from brood cells, BB and nectar, and co-culture assays showed that these bacteria promote the growth of honey bee core bacterial species. Metabolic characterization of *Fructobacillus* spp. showed that these species could utilize simple sugars as well as the complex carbohydrate lignin [49]. Di Cagno et al. demonstrated that spontaneous fermentation of BB, after BCP inoculation with selected *L. kunkeei* strains and the yeast *Hanseniaspora uvarum* AN8Y27B, increased digestibility as well as bioavailability of nutrients and bioactive compounds naturally occurring in BCP. Artificially fermented BCP contained higher concentrations of peptides, free amino acids and free phytochemicals [29].

Investigation on biosynthetic potential (secondary metabolites and enzymes) of bacteria isolated from BB is underexplored. We have demonstrated that bee bread bacteria produce enzymes that could degrade pollen grains through the maturation process, thus releasing nutrients and bioactive compounds, leading to increased bioavailability. BB quality, nutritional value and potential health benefits for bees and humans depend indeed on the BB maturation process.

Further research could lead to biotechnological applications and a better understanding of BCP conversion to BB. Future research could explore the bioactive compounds produced by BB microbiota, and investigate the metabolic profile and the impact of environmental factors on BB composition in relationship with bee health and performance.

Apilactobacillus and *Fructobacillus* strains exerted high antibacterial activity against *Gram*-negative pathogens but exhibited lower antibacterial activity against *S. aureus*. On the other hand, *Bacillus* isolates demonstrated antibacterial activity against mainly *S. aureus*, though some exerted antibacterial activity against Gram-negative pathogens. It is plausible that BB antibacterial activity is the outcome of plant metabolites, such as polyphenols and antimicrobial compounds produced by BB microbiota [15]. LABs are known to produce antimicrobial compounds such as lactic acid, acetic acid, hydrogen peroxide, reuterin, diacetyl, reutericyclin, acetoin and more complex molecules like bacteriocins and antifungal peptides [39,50,51]. In a previous study, diverse Bacilli isolates were reported to exert antibacterial activity against *S. aureus* [22]. However, some of the isolates tested in this study exerted antibacterial activity against Gram-negative pathogens too. To our best knowledge, this is the first study demonstrating the antibacterial activity of *Apilactobacillus* and *Fructobacillus* strains isolated from BB.

In order to further investigate the contribution of BB microbiome to antibacterial activity, autochthonous microbial strains, isolated from BB samples, were implemented as a start culture in fermentation of double pasteurized BCP. It has been reported by several authors that BCP fermentation ameliorates BCP biological properties in terms of nutrient composition, bioactive components such as polyphenols and even flavor [7,8]. Potential health benefits include increased bioavailability of nutrients, prebiotic and probiotic potential and the possible degradation of allergenic compounds [29,52]. Kaškonienė et al. studied the impact of spontaneous and artificial solid-state lactic acid fermentation of natural and pasteurized BCP on its antibacterial, antifungal and antioxidant activities. *Lactococcus lactis* and *Lactobacillus rhamnosus* were used as starter cultures. It has been demonstrated that following BCP fermentation, total phenolic content, total flavonoid content and radical scavenging activity increased as well as antibacterial and antifungal activity against *Micrococcus luteus*, *Staphylococcus aureus*, *Escherichia coli* and *Penicillium roqueforti* respectively. Pasteurized BCP showed significantly lower antimicrobial and antioxidant activities after fermentation than unprocessed fermented BCP, indicating that BCP natural microbiota further contributes to antimicrobial and antioxidant properties exerted by artificially fermented BCP [21]. Urcan et al. showed that it is feasible to enhance the antioxidant and antimicrobial activity of BCP through solid-state fermentation [53]. Similarly, a recent study reported that microbiota enhanced BB antiviral activity against Influenza A virus, as shown by the higher antiviral potential of artificially fermented BCP compared to fresh unfermented BCP [23].

We implemented a double pasteurization protocol to eliminate most of the natural microbiota, thus demonstrating unequivocally the indigenous microbial contribution (starter culture) to antimicrobial activity exerted by BB. Our artificially fermented samples exhibited higher antibacterial activity compared to double pasteurized BCP as well as fresh BCP (unpasteurized) against *S. aureus* and *S.* Typhimurium, indicating that indigenous BB microbiota contributes towards BB bioactivity. To the best of our knowledge, this is the first study using double pasteurized BCP in solid-state fermentation.

4. Materials and Methods

4.1. Sampling

Out of 11 samples (Table 4), 10 were harvested in situ from bee colonies located in Mt Pelion, an area known for high plant diversity, attracting many beekeepers. Sample 11 was collected from a hive frame containing spring BB, provided by a beekeeper from Rethymno, Crete.

Sampling was performed after the placement of empty, marked honeycombs in the beehives. The surface of each honeycomb was divided into five segments. Sampling was performed (from each segment) during a different time point. Briefly, 1-day-old BB (S2 and S7) was collected on day one from one out of the five segments, 11-day-old BB (S3 and S8) was collected from another segment, and so on for BB 27-day-old (S4 and S9) and 41-day-old (S5 and S10). The honeycombs were filled with BCP in a few days, so it was plausible to figure out the age of the BB. BCP was collected using entrance traps after 24 h (BCP 1 day old, samples S1 and S10). Samples S1 and S6 originated by dividing the same initial sample, the same applies to samples S2 and S7, samples S3 and S8 and samples S4 and S9, respectively.

Table 4. Botanical origin, location and harvest month of BCP and BB samples.

Botanic Origin	Region	Month	Age of BB and BCP Samples	Samples
Multifloral	Pelion, Thessaly	May	1-day-old BCP	S1 and S6
Multifloral	Pelion, Thessaly	May	1-day-old BB	S2 and S7
Multifloral	Pelion, Thessaly	May	11-day-old BB	S3 and S8
Multifloral	Pelion, Thessaly	June	27-day-old BB	S4 and S9
Multifloral	Pelion, Thessaly	June	41-day-old BB	S5
Multifloral	Rethymno, Crete	May	Not determined	S11
Multifloral	Thessaly	May	BCP 24 h	AF1

Samples were collected aseptically in order to elucidate the diversity and relative abundance of microbial communities at different stages of BB maturation. From day 12 the BB comb used for sampling was isolated inside the hive environment (using a frame containing a metal net without touching the comb), so that the bees could not add BCP to stored BB or consume it (samples S4, S5, S9). Bacteria were isolated and cultured from samples S5 and S11. Although melissopalynological analysis was not performed, beekeepers provided information regarding the botanical origin of collected pollen. Regarding samples S1–S9, the most abundant plant families were Asteraceae, Lamiaceae, Cistaceae, Brassicaceae, Ranunculaceae and Papaveraceae, whereas regarding S11 sample, the most abundant plant families were Lamiaceae, Cistaceae, Brassicaceae, Ranunculaceae and Papaveraceae. Similarly, the AF1 sample, according to the beekeeper who provided it, contained mostly pollen derived from Brassicaceae, Ranunculaceae, Papaveraceae and Cistaceae.

4.2. Metataxonomic Analysis during BB Maturation

Total DNA was extracted from 0.2 g of S1–S10 samples using a Macherey Nagel NucleoSpin Food kit (Hoerdt, France) according to the manufacturer's instructions. Extracted DNA was used as a template to amplify the V3–V4 region of the 16S rRNA gene, using the primers 338F (5′-ACTCCTACGGGAGGCAGCA-3′) and 806R (5′-GGACTACHVGGGTWTCTAAT-3′). Similarly, the ITS1 region of fungi was amplified using the ITS1-1F-F (5′-CTTGGTCATTTAGAGGAAGTAA-3′) and ITS1-1F-R (5′-GCTGCGTTCTTCATCGATGC-3′) set of primers. Amplicon quality was assessed via agarose gel electrophoresis and Qubit assay. PCR products were used to construct an amplicon library. Subsequently, purified amplicons were paired-end sequenced on an Illumina MiSeq PE250 platform (Macrogen, Republic of Korea). Raw sequence reads were deposited into the NCBI Sequence Read Archive (SRA) database (Bioproject: PRJNA846146, BioSample Accession Numbers: SAMN28869225-SAMN28869233).

4.3. Bioinformatics Analysis

Bioinformatics analysis of raw sequencing data was performed with the QIIME2 platform [54]. Denoising, de-replication and chimera filtering were performed with the DADA2 plugin [55], whereas the bacterial sequences were trimmed (after manual inspection of the FASTQ scores) at 290 and 220 nucleotides long for forward and reverse reads, respectively. The fungal forward and reverse reads were trimmed at 240 and 180 nucleotides long, respectively. The chimera filtering was based on the default consensus method. Next mitochondrial, chloroplastic and non-assigned sequences were removed. Diversity analysis was performed with a sampling-depth cutoff of 530 for 16S and 890 for ITS. OTU clustering was based on a 97% sequence identity cutoff. Alpha- and beta-diversity metrics were calculated using the qiime diversity module. Faith, Shannon, observed OTUs, Chao1 and Evenness Alpha-diversity core metrics were calculated. Unweighted unifrac distance matrix, weighted unifrac distance matrix, Jaccard distance matrix, Bray–Curtis distance matrix and Beta-diversity metrics were also calculated. Alpha rarefaction was estimated with a maximum depth of 530 for 16S and 890 for ITS.

Taxonomic classification was based on the 16S Silva database version 132 (SILVA_132_97_16S.fna) [56] and UNITE ITS database version 8 (ver8_97_02.02.2019) [57] with the Vsearch algorithm, where the taxonomy cutoff was based on 97% nucleotide identity. In order to identify the core microbiota a filter was applied where the abundance of each genus should be at least 1% of the assigned sequences.

4.4. Isolation of BB Culturable Bacteria

Bacteria were isolated by spreading 100 μL of BB sterile saline dilutions (10^{-1}, 10^{-2} and 10^{-3}) on six agar plates of different culture media. Three out of six agar plates were incubated at 37 °C and the rest at 30 °C at least for 5 days. Culture media to isolate diverse bacterial groups were the following: Plate Count Agar (PCA) (Neogen, Heywood, UK), *Bacillus cereus* medium (LAB M, Bury, UK), containing 1.5% bacteriological agar and polymyxin B (LAB M, Bury, UK) were incubated aerobically. Man Rogosa and Sharpe (MRS) agar plates (NEOGEN, Heywood, UK) were incubated anaerobically in an AnaeroJar AG25 with the AnaeroGen Atmosphere Generation system (Oxoid, Basingstoke, UK) at 30 °C for approximately 5 days. In the case where several morphologically identical colonies were developed on a culture medium, at least three of them were picked up. Pure cultures were stored as glycerol stocks in Nutrient Broth (Biolab, Budapest, Hungary) supplemented with 0.5% *w*/*v* Yeast Extract (Neogen, Heywood, UK), 0.5% *w*/*v* glucose (SERVA, Heidelberg, Germany) and 20% *w*/*v* glycerol (SIGMA-ALDRICH, St. Louis, MO, USA) at −80 °C until further analysis.

4.5. Assessment of Antibacterial Activity Exerted by BB Bacterial Isolates

The method of cross streaking was performed to assess the antibacterial properties of isolated BB bacteria against human pathogens. BB isolates were inoculated on PCA plates in a line. After incubation long enough to allow growth (at least 5 mm wide) of the tested isolates, the pathogens were streaked perpendicularly, followed by incubation at 37 °C for 24 h. Broth cultures of pathogens, which were set up at OD 600 nm: 0.1, were further diluted 1/10 in Mueller–Hinton (NEOGEN, Heywood, UK) and implemented in cross streaking assay. The growth inhibition of pathogens in terms of distance from BB isolates was measured and recorded. The following pathogens were tested: methicillin-resistant *Staphylococcus aureus* 1552, carbapenem-resistant *Pseudomonas aeruginosa* 1773, *Salmonella enterica* serov. Typhimurium and *Klebsiella pneumoniae* [58].

4.6. BCP Double Pasteurization-Solid State BCP Fermentation

Multifloral bee-collected pollen (BCP) was collected in Thessaly, Greece in spring 2022, (sample AF1).

The double pasteurization process was performed as follows: AF1 BCP was pasteurized at 65 °C for 40 min in a water bath. In total, 11.5 gr of AF1 sample was mixed with 1 mL NB3 [NB3 is composed of Nutrient Broth containing 0.5% *w*/*v* yeast extract (Neogen, Heywood, UK) and 0.5% *w*/*v* glucose (SERVA, Heidelberg, Germany)] in a sterile 50 mL tube. After pasteurization, the tube was incubated at 33 °C for 48 h allowing bacteria that survived to grow. Then, a second pasteurization (65 °C for 40 min) took place.

- AF46D (negative control) sample: 1.3 mL NB3 broth mixed with 11.5 g of double pasteurized AF1 sample and incubated for 11 days at 33 °C.
- AF42D sample was fermented as follows: 11.5 g of double pasteurized AF1 sample inoculated with 10^8 CFUs of *A. kunkeei* strain NADBB37 was re-suspended in 1.3 mL NB3 broth. The sample was mixed and incubated for 11 days at 33 °C.
- AF43D sample was fermented as follows: 11.5 g of double pasteurized AF1 sample inoculated with 10^8 CFUs of *A. kunkeei* strain NADBB7 was re-suspended in 1.3 mL NB3 broth. The sample was mixed and incubated for 11 days at 33 °C.
- AF44D sample was fermented as follows: 11.5 g of double pasteurized AF1 sample inoculated with 10^8 CFUs of *A. kunkeei* strain NADBB37, 10^8 CFUs of *A. kunkeei* strain NADBB7, 10^8 CFUs *Fructobacillus fructosus* strain NADBB39 and 10^8 CFUs *Zygosaccharomyces siamensis* was resuspended in 1.3 mL NB3 broth. The sample was mixed and incubated for 11 days at 33 °C.
- AF5U sample was fermented as follows: 11.5 g of AF1 sample inoculated with 10^8 CFUs of *A. kunkeei* strain NADBB37 was re-suspended in 2.3 mL NB3 broth. The sample was mixed and incubated for 29 days at 33 °C.

4.7. Phenotypic Detection of Enzymes Produced by BB Isolates

In order to test whether BB isolates produce enzymes such as amylases, proteinases, hemicellulases cellulases and enzymes that degrade dyes such as copper oxidases (laccases), manganese oxidases and lignin oxidases [59], PCA plates containing appropriate substrates (see below) were used for qualitative screening. Bacteria were incubated for 1–7 days at 37 °C. Every day, the plates were checked for phenotype detection.

- Amylase activity: PCA + 1% starch. A clear halo was detected around the bacterial colony due to starch breakdown. To confirm amylase activity, the plate was covered with 1% iodine solution for 5–10 min, then washed with deionized water and the presence of light zones around the colony was observed under a light source [60].
- Protease activity: PCA + 2% skimmed milk powder. A clear halo was formed around the bacterial colony due to the breakdown of milk proteins [22].
- Hemicellulose activity (endo-1,4-b-Xylanase): PCA + 0.02% Megazyme AZCL-XYLAN (Megazyme, Bray, Ireland). A blue halo was detected around the bacterial colony due to the breakdown of the hemicellulose granules and the release of the bounded azo pigment [61].
- Cellulose activity (endo-Cellulase): PCA + 0.02% *w*/*v* Megazyme AZCL-HE-CELLULOSE (Megazyme, Bray, Ireland). In the case of cellulase secretion, a blue halo formed around the bacterial colony due to cellulose granule breakdown and the release of the azo pigment [62].
- Guaiacol assay and dye breakdown: PCA + 0.02% *w*/*v* Coomassie Brilliant Blue G (BIO-RAD, Richmond, CA, USA), PCA + 0.02% Coomassie Brilliant Blue R, PCA + 10% Malachite Green (oxalate solution 0.2% *w*/*v*, MERCK, Darmstadt, Germany), PCA + 0.5 mM guaiacol (Alfa Aecar, Kandel, Germany). The secretion of enzymes that break down dyes was detected as a clear halo formed around the bacterial colony. The appearance of brown color in the guaiacol assay indicated the positive phenotype [63].
- In order to determine whether cellulases and hemicellulases are produced and present in mature BB, the assays were carried out using the respective substrates mentioned above for the specific enzymes. Briefly, 6 mm diameter wells were opened in the plates and 100 μL of each protein fraction suspension of BB sample was placed in each of them.

4.8. Preparation of BB Protein Fractions

Protein fractions were prepared as follows: 500 mg of each BB sample was dissolved in sterile deionized water (dH_2O) to a final volume of 1.5 mL. Samples were incubated for 1 h at room temperature with occasional stirring and then centrifuged for 10 min at 10,000× *g*. The supernatant aqueous fraction was collected and solid ammonium sulfate $(NH_4)_2SO_4$ (AnalaR, BDH Chemicals Ltd., Poole, England) was then added stepwise to a final concentration of 60% *w*/*v*. Samples were mixed gently and left for 20 min at room temperature to equilibrate, then placed for 10 min at −20 °C and centrifuged for 30 min at 11,000× *g*. The supernatant was collected and used in the agar diffusion assays. The pellet was resuspended in 1 mL of sterile dH_2O.

4.9. Detection of Genes Encoding Enzymes in BB Isolates

Biosynthetic genes encoding laccases and hemicellulases produced by BB isolates were partially amplified via PCR. For the laccase gene, the primers Cu1AF and Cu2R [64,65] were used to amplify a 142 bp fragment. PCR reaction mix (50 μL total volume) comprised of 1 mM dNTPs (Invitrogen, Paisley, UK), 1 × Buffer B (Fastgene NIPPON Genetics, Tokyo, Japan), 0.5 mM $MgCl_2$ (Fastgene NIPPON Genetics, Tokyo, Japan), 25 pmol of each primer, 3 μL DNA template and 1 unit Taq Polymerase (Fastgene NIPPON Genetics, Tokyo, Japan). The thermal cycler Primus 25 (PEQLAB biotechnologie, Erlangen, Germany) conditions were as follows: 3 min at 95 °C for initial double-strand denaturation, followed by 30 cycles of DNA denaturation at 95 °C for 30 s, primer annealing at 50 °C for 30 s and elongation at 72 °C for 30 s, with a final 5 min extension at 72 °C. The PCR products were checked on a 1.5% (*w*/*v*) agarose gel, stained with ethidium bromide and the bands were visualized under UV light.

For endoxylanase genes, the degenerated primers GH11R and GH11F [66] were used to amplify a 336 bp fragment. Briefly, the DNA fragment was amplified in a 50 μL reaction mix, comprising 1 μM dNTPs (Invitrogen, Paisley, UK), 1 × Buffer A (Fastgene NIPPON Genetics, Tokyo, Japan), 0.5 mM $MgCl_2$ (Fastgene NIPPON Genetics, Tokyo, Japan), 25 pmol of each primer, 3 μL template and 1.5 unit Taq Polymerase (Fastgene NIPPON Genetics, Tokyo, Japan). The thermal cycler Primus 25 (PEQLAB biotechnologie, Erlangen, Germany) conditions for touch-down PCR were as follows: 3 min at 95 °C for initial double-strand denaturation, followed by 30 cycles of DNA denaturation at 95 °C for 30 s, primer annealing at 66 °C–0.5 °C/cyc for 30 s, followed by 25 cycles of DNA denaturation at 95 °C for 30 s, primer annealing at 50 °C for 30 s and elongation at 72 °C for 30 s, with a final 10 min extension at 72 °C. The PCR products were checked on a 1.5% (*w*/*v*) agarose gel, stained with ethidium bromide and the bands were visualized under UV light.

Amplicons of BB isolates exerting enzyme activity were purified using the NucleoSpin Gel and PCR clean-up kit (Macherey-Nagel, Düren, Germany) and directly sequenced via Sanger dideoxy termination method by Cemia (Larissa, Greece). Chromas version 2.6.6 software (Technelysium Pty Ltd., South Brisbane, Australia, www.technelysium.com.au (last accessed 5 June 2024)) was used to check the quality of the obtained sequencing data. Sequences were processed using Gene Runner version 6.5 software (www.generunner.net (last accessed 5 June 2024)) and subjected to a BlastN (Megablast) analysis (https://blast.ncbi.nlm.nih.gov/Blast.cgi (last accessed 5 June 2024)) to identify sequences with the highest similarity.

4.10. Determination of Minimum Inhibitory Concentration (MIC) and Minimum Bactericidal Concentration (MBC)

The determination of minimum inhibitory concentration (MIC) was carried out in sterile 96-well polystyrene microtiter plates (Kisker Biotech GmbH & Co. KG, Steinfurt, Germany) using a spectrophotometric bioassay as described by Didaras et al., 2021. Briefly, 0.5 g of BCP and artificially fermented BCP samples were suspended in sterile ddH_2O (2 mL final volume) for one hour at room temperature with occasional vortex and then centrifuged at 10,000× *g* for 7 min. The aqueous phase was filtered through a 0.22 μM filter and used for serial dilutions in Mueller–Hinton broth corresponding from 25 to 0.39% *v*/*v*. Overnight bacterial cultures grown in Mueller–Hinton broth were adjusted to a 0.5 McFarland turbidity standard (~1.5×10^8 CFU/mL). Ten μL Mueller–Hinton broth containing approximately 5×10^4 CFUs were added to 190 μL of tested 2-fold sample dilutions.

Mueller–Hinton broth inoculated only with pathogens in the absence of BCP serial dilutions was used as a positive control. Wells containing only Mueller–Hinton broth, not inoculated with bacteria, were monitored to test for contamination.

The optical density (OD) was determined at 600 nm using a PerkinElmer Multimode plate reader, (PerkinElmer, Inc., 940 Winter Street, Waltham, MA, USA) just prior to incubation (t = 0) and 24 h after incubation (t = 24) at 37 °C. The OD for each negative control replicate well at t = 24 was subtracted from the OD of the same replicate test well with bacteria at t = 24. The growth inhibition at each BCP dilution was determined using the formula % inhibition = [1 − (OD test well—OD of corresponding negative BB control well)] × 100. MIC was determined as the lowest bee bread concentration which results in 100% growth inhibition.

The MBC was determined by transferring a small quantity of sample contained in each replicate well of the microtiter plates to Mueller–Hinton agar plates by using a microplate replicator (BoekelScientific, Feasterville-Trevose, PA, USA). The plates were incubated at 37 °C for 24 h. The MBC was determined as the lowest concentration at which no colonies were observed [16].

4.11. Identification of Culturable Bacteria and Yeasts via 16S rRNA Gene and ITS SANGER Sequencing, Respectively

The identification of bacteria via 16S rRNA gene sequencing was performed as previously described [23]. Briefly, bacterial genomic DNA was extracted using the ExtractMe Genomic DNA Kit (Blirt, Gdansk, Poland). The 16S rRNA gene was amplified through PCR using the universal primers 27F (5′-AGAGTTTGATCMTGGCTCAG-3′) and 1492R (5′-GGTTACCTTGTTACGACTT-3′) (Eurofins Genomics, Ebersberg, Germany). PCR conditions: initial denaturation at 95 °C for 3 min, followed by 35 cycles of denaturation at 95 °C for 30 s, annealing at 50 °C for 30 s and elongation at 72 °C for 2 min. A final elongation step at 72 °C for 2 min was added (thermal cycler Primus 25, PEQLAB biotechnologie, Erlangen, Germany). For ITS amplification ITS1 (5′-TCCGTAGGTGAACCTGCGG-3′) and ITS4 (5′-TCCTCCGCTTATTGATATGC-3′) (Eurofins Genomics, Ebersberg, Germany) were used. The reaction mixture and PCR conditions were performed as described previously [23]. Amplicons were purified using the NucleoSpin Gel and PCR clean-up kit (Macherey-Nagel, Düren, Germany) and sequenced via the Sanger dideoxy termination method by Macrogen Europe (Amsterdam, The Netherlands). Yeast amplicons were sequenced via the Sanger dideoxy termination method by CeMIA SA (Larissa, Greece). Chromas version 2.6.6 software (Technelysium Pty Ltd., South Brisbane, Australia, www.technelysium.com.au (last accessed 5 June 2024)) was used to check the quality of the obtained sequencing data. Sequences were assembled into a single sequence via MEGA X version 10.1.6 software (Kumar et al., 2018 [67]) and Gene Runner version 6.5 software (www.generunner.net, accessed on 21 June 2022) and subjected to BlastN (Megablast) (https://blast.ncbi.nlm.nih.gov/Blast.cgi (last accessed 5 June 2024)) search in the 16S rRNA Database-GENEBANK to identify sequences with the highest similarity. Obtained sequences were deposited to GenBank under the following accession numbers ON911235-ON911282.

5. Conclusions

Most consumers are not familiar with bee bread, a honey bee product that should be considered a functional food due to its high content of nutrients (essential amino acids, sugars, fatty acids including ω-3, polyphenols, vitamins, macro and microelements) and exerted bioactivity (antioxidant, antimicrobial, anti-inflammatory). This study aims to investigate the microbiota during bee bread maturation and to elucidate the role of autochthonous microorganisms in the conversion of BCP to BB as well as exerted bioactivity. Our data demonstrated that during BB maturation microbial diversity dynamically fluctuated probably due to microbial competition and adaptation to highly volatile conditions, ending up rather stable in terms of relative abundance and microbial community structure. Implementing culture-dependent methods demonstrated that bacteria isolated from BB produce and secrete numerous enzymes, thus indicating a high biosynthetic potential. It is very plausible that the production of lignin-degrading enzymes (laccases or oxidases) and cellulases by BB bacteria breaches pollen grain walls. In that way, nutrients and bioactive compounds contained in pollen grains are further released, thus contributing to higher bioactivity exerted by BB compared to fresh BCP.

In this study, characterized bacteria isolated from BB have demonstrated antibacterial activity against human pathogens, thus indicating BB microbiota contribution to exerted bioactivity. Furthermore, it has been shown the antibacterial activity of *Apilactobacillus* and *Fructobacillus* strains isolated from BB for the first time. Secondary metabolites such as non-ribosomal peptides, polyketides and other antimicrobial compounds produced by BB microbiota during BCP fermentation and BB maturation could directly contribute to antimicrobial activity exerted by BB. This is further supported by our findings that artificial fermentation of BCP by indigenous microbial strains increased the MIC and MBC values against tested pathogens.

Overall, further studies on BB microorganisms regarding the antimicrobial activity as well as the biosynthetic and probiotic potential could lead to novel biotechnological applications in medicine (discovery of novel antimicrobial agents), in agriculture (production of novel functional food supplements for animals, or implementation of BB microbes for converting agriculture byproducts to added value products) as well as in human nutrition to discovery of novel enzymes implemented in paper industry for example. Furthermore, research may lead to a variety of products depending on BCP botanical origin and implemented microbial stains as a starter culture in artificial fermentation at an industrial scale.

Supplementary Materials: The following supporting information can be downloaded at https://www.mdpi.com/article/10.3390/ph17060761/s1, Figure S1: Rarefaction curve of 16S data for samples S1–S5; Figure S2: Rarefaction curve of ITS data for samples S6–S9; Table S1: Basic statistics of each sample; Table S2: Alpha diversity metrics for bacteria; Table S3: Alpha diversity metrics for fungi; Table S4: Relative abundance of bacterial families/genera in samples S1–S5; Table S5: Relative abundance of fungal families/genera in samples S6–S9; Table S6: Bray-Curtis beta-diversity matrix for bacteria (samples S1–S5); Table S7: Jaccard beta-diversity matrix for bacteria (samples S1–S5); Table S8: Weighted Unifrac beta-diversity matrix for bacteria (samples S1–S5); Table S9: Unweighted Unifrac beta-diversity matrix for bacteria (samples S1–S5); Table S10: Bray-Curtis beta-diversity matrix for fungi (samples S6–S9); Table S11: Jaccard beta-diversity matrix for fungi (samples S6–S9); Table S12: Weighted Unifrac beta-diversity matrix for fungi (samples S6–S9); Table S13: Unweighted Unifrac beta-diversity matrix for fungi (samples S6–S9); Table S14: Enzyme fragment amplicons sequences.

Author Contributions: Conceptualization, D.M. and N.A.D.; methodology, N.A.D., G.D.A. and D.M.; formal analysis, M.N. and G.D.A.; investigation, N.A.D., I.K., C.S., I.G. and C.T.; resources, N.A.D., K.K. and D.M.; data curation, M.N.; writing—original draft preparation, N.A.D., K.K., D.M. and G.D.A.; writing—review and editing, N.A.D., K.K., C.T., G.D.A. and D.M.; supervision, D.M. and G.D.A.; project administration, D.M.; funding acquisition, D.M. All authors have read and agreed to the published version of the manuscript.

Funding: This work was partly funded by the Postgraduate Programme "Biotechnology-Quality Assessment in Nutrition and the Environment" (Department of Biochemistry & Biotechnology, University of Thessaly), Grant No. 5838.

Institutional Review Board Statement: Not applicable.

Informed Consent Statement: Not applicable.

Data Availability Statement: All data regarding this study are available in the article and in its online Supplementary Materials.

Conflicts of Interest: The authors declare no conflicts of interest.

References

1. Cardinal, S.; Danforth, B.N. Bees Diversified in the Age of Eudicots. *Proc. R. Soc. B Biol. Sci.* **2013**, *280*, 20122686. [CrossRef]
2. Mărgăoan, R.; Stranţ, M.; Varadi, A.; Topal, E.; Yücel, B.; Cornea-Cipcigan, M.; Campos, M.G.; Vodnar, D.C. Bee Collected Pollen and Bee Bread: Bioactive Constituents and Health Benefits. *Antioxidants* **2019**, *8*, 568. [CrossRef]
3. Baky, M.H.; Abouelela, M.B.; Wang, K.; Farag, M.A. Bee Pollen and Bread as a Super-Food: A Comparative Review of Their Metabolome Composition and Quality Assessment in the Context of Best Recovery Conditions. *Molecules* **2023**, *28*, 715. [CrossRef]
4. Fan, T.-F.; Park, S.; Shi, Q.; Zhang, X.; Liu, Q.; Song, Y.; Chin, H.; Bin Ibrahim, M.S.; Mokrzecka, N.; Yang, Y.; et al. Transformation of Hard Pollen into Soft Matter. *Nat. Commun.* **2020**, *11*, 1449. [CrossRef] [PubMed]
5. Aylanc, V.; Falcão, S.I.; Ertosun, S.; Vilas-Boas, M. From the Hive to the Table: Nutrition Value, Digestibility and Bioavailability of the Dietary Phytochemicals Present in the Bee Pollen and Bee Bread. *Trends Food Sci. Technol.* **2021**, *109*, 464–481. [CrossRef]
6. Brodschneider, R.; Crailsheim, K. Nutrition and Health in Honey Bees. *Apidologie* **2010**, *41*, 278–294. [CrossRef]
7. Kostić, A.Ž.; Milinčić, D.D.; Barać, M.B.; Ali Shariati, M.; Tešić, Ž.L.; Pešić, M.B. The Application of Pollen as a Functional Food and Feed Ingredient—The Present and Perspectives. *Biomolecules* **2020**, *10*, 84. [CrossRef] [PubMed]
8. Kieliszek, M.; Piwowarek, K.; Kot, A.M.; Błażejak, S.; Chlebowska-Śmigiel, A.; Wolska, I. Pollen and Bee Bread as New Health-Oriented Products: A Review. *Trends Food Sci. Technol.* **2018**, *71*, 170–180. [CrossRef]
9. Bakour, M.; Fernandes, Â.; Barros, L.; Sokovic, M.; Ferreira, I.C.F.R. Badiaa lyoussi Bee Bread as a Functional Product: Chemical Composition and Bioactive Properties. *LWT* **2019**, *109*, 276–282. [CrossRef]
10. Ćirić, J.; Haneklaus, N.; Rajić, S.; Baltić, T.; Lazić, I.B.; Đorđević, V. Chemical Composition of Bee Bread (Perga), a Functional Food: A Review. *J. Trace Elem. Miner.* **2022**, *2*, 100038. [CrossRef]
11. Vásquez, A.; Olofsson, T.C. The Lactic Acid Bacteria Involved in the Production of Bee Pollen and Bee Bread. *J. Apic. Res.* **2009**, *48*, 189–195. [CrossRef]
12. Campos, M.G.R.; Frigerio, C.; Lopes, J.; Bogdanov, S. What Is the Future of Bee-Pollen? *J. ApiProduct ApiMedical Sci.* **2010**, *2*, 131–144. [CrossRef]
13. Anđelković, B.; Jevtić, G.; Mladenović, M.; Marković, J.; Petrović, M.; Nedić, N. Quality of pollen and honey bee bread collected in spring. *J. Hyg. Eng. Des.* **2012**, *1*, 275–277.
14. Bakour, M.; Laaroussi, H.; Ousaaid, D.; El Ghouizi, A.; Es-Safi, I.; Mechchate, H.; Lyoussi, B. Bee Bread as a Promising Source of Bioactive Molecules and Functional Properties: An Up-To-Date Review. *Antibiotics* **2022**, *11*, 203. [CrossRef] [PubMed]

15. Didaras, N.A.; Karatasou, K.; Dimitriou, T.G.; Amoutzias, G.D.; Mossialos, D. Antimicrobial Activity of Bee Collected Pollen and Bee bread: State of the Art and Future Perspectives. *Antibiotics* **2020**, *9*, 811. [CrossRef] [PubMed]
16. Didaras, N.A.; Kafantaris, I.; Dimitriou, T.G.; Mitsagga, C.; Karatasou, K.; Giavasis, I.; Stagos, D.; Amoutzias, G.D.; Hatjina, F.; Mossialos, D. Biological Properties of Bee Bread Collected from Apiaries Located across Greece. *Antibiotics* **2021**, *10*, 555. [CrossRef] [PubMed]
17. Pełka, K.; Otłowska, O.; Worobo, R.W.; Szweda, P. Bee Bread Exhibits Higher Antimicrobial Potential Compared to Bee Pollen. *Antibiotics* **2021**, *10*, 125. [CrossRef] [PubMed]
18. Saraiva, M.A.; Zemolin, A.P.P.; Franco, J.L.; Boldo, J.T.; Stefenon, V.M.; Triplett, E.W.; de Oliveira Camargo, F.A.; Roesch, L.F.W. Relationship between Honeybee Nutrition and Their Microbial Communities. *Antonie Van Leeuwenhoek* **2015**, *107*, 921–933. [CrossRef] [PubMed]
19. Dharampal, P.S.; Carlson, C.; Currie, C.R.; Steffan, S.A. Pollen-Borne Microbes Shape Bee Fitness. *Proc. R. Soc. B Biol. Sci.* **2019**, *286*, 20182894. [CrossRef]
20. Gilliam, M. Identification and Roles of Non-Pathogenic Microflora Associated with Honey Bees. *FEMS Microbiol. Lett.* **1997**, *155*, 1–10. [CrossRef]
21. Kaškonienė, V.; Adaškevičiūtė, V.; Kaškonas, P.; Mickienė, R.; Maruška, A. Antimicrobial and Antioxidant Activities of Natural and Fermented Bee Pollen. *Food Biosci.* **2020**, *34*, 100532. [CrossRef]
22. Pełka, K.; Worobo, R.W.; Walkusz, J.; Szweda, P. Bee Pollen and Bee Bread as a Source of Bacteria Producing Antimicrobials. *Antibiotics* **2021**, *10*, 713. [CrossRef] [PubMed]
23. Dimitriou, T.G.; Asoutis Didaras, N.; Barda, C.; Skopeliti, D.; Kontogianni, K.; Karatasou, K.; Skaltsa, H.; Mossialos, D. Antiviral Activity of Bee bread, Bee Collected Pollen and Artificially Fermented Pollen against Influenza A Virus. *Foods* **2023**, *12*, 1978. [CrossRef] [PubMed]
24. Asoutis Didaras, N.; Dimitriou, T.; Daskou, M.; Karatasou, K.; Mossialos, D. In vitro assessment of the antiviral activity of Greek Bee bread and bee collected pollen against Enterovirus D68. *J. Microbiol. Biotechnol. Food Sci.* **2022**, *11*, e4859. [CrossRef]
25. Martinson, V.G.; Moy, J.; Moran, N.A. Establishment of Characteristic Gut Bacteria during Development of the Honeybee Worker. *Appl. Environ. Microbiol.* **2012**, *78*, 2830–2840. [CrossRef] [PubMed]
26. Vásquez, A.; Forsgren, E.; Fries, I.; Paxton, R.J.; Flaberg, E.; Szekely, L.; Olofsson, T.C. Symbionts as Major Modulators of Insect Health: Lactic Acid Bacteria and Honeybees. *PLoS ONE* **2012**, *7*, e33188. [CrossRef] [PubMed]
27. Killer, J.; Dubná, S.; Sedláček, I.; Švec, P. *Lactobacillus apis* sp. Nov., from the Stomach of Honeybees (Apis Mellifera), Having an in Vitro Inhibitory Effect on the Causative Agents of American and European Foulbrood. *Int. J. Syst. Evol. Microbiol.* **2014**, *64*, 152–157. [CrossRef] [PubMed]
28. Tsadila, C.; Amoroso, C.; Mossialos, D. Microbial Diversity in Bee Species and Bee Products: Pseudomonads Contribution to Bee Well-Being and the Biological Activity Exerted by Honey Bee Products: A Narrative Review. *Diversity* **2023**, *15*, 1088. [CrossRef]
29. Di Cagno, R.; Filannino, P.; Cantatore, V.; Gobbetti, M. Novel Solid-State Fermentation of Bee Collected Pollen Emulating the Natural Fermentation Process of Bee Bread. *Food Microbiol.* **2019**, *82*, 218–230. [CrossRef]
30. Ghosh, S.; Namin, S.M.; Jung, C. Differential Bacterial Community of Bee Bread and Bee Pollen Revealed by 16s RRNA High-Throughput Sequencing. *Insects* **2022**, *13*, 863. [CrossRef]
31. Gilliam, M. Microbiology of pollen and bee bread: The yeasts. *Apidologie* **1979**, *10*, 43–53. [CrossRef]
32. Disayathanoowat, T.; Li, H.; Supapimon, N.; Suwannarach, N.; Lumyong, S.; Chantawannakul, P.; Guo, J. Different Dynamics of Bacterial and Fungal Communities in Hive-Stored Bee Bread and Their Possible Roles: A Case Study from Two Commercial Honey Bees in China. *Microorganisms* **2020**, *8*, 264. [CrossRef] [PubMed]
33. Donkersley, P.; Rhodes, G.; Pickup, R.W.; Jones, K.C.; Wilson, K. Bacterial Communities Associated with Honeybee Food Stores Are Correlated with Land Use. *Ecol. Evol.* **2018**, *8*, 4743–4756. [CrossRef] [PubMed]
34. Anderson, K.E.; Carroll, M.J.; Sheehan, T.; Mott, B.M.; Maes, P.; Corby-Harris, V. Hive-stored Pollen of Honey Bees: Many Lines of Evidence Are Consistent with Pollen Preservation, Not Nutrient Conversion. *Mol. Ecol.* **2014**, *23*, 5904–5917. [CrossRef] [PubMed]
35. Gilliam, M.; Hayden Bee, C. Microbiology of Pollen and Bee Bread: The Genus Bacillus. *Apidologie* **1979**, *10*, 269–274. [CrossRef]
36. Barene, I.; Daberte, I.; Siksna, S. Investigation of Bee bread and development of its dosage forms. *Med. Teor. Ir Prakt.* **2014**, *21*, 16–22. [CrossRef]
37. Dranca, F.; Ursachi, F.; Oroian, M. Bee Bread: Physicochemical Characterization and Phenolic Content Extraction Optimization. *Foods* **2020**, *9*, 1358. [CrossRef] [PubMed]
38. Olofsson, T.C.; Vásquez, A. Detection and Identification of a Novel Lactic Acid Bacterial Flora Within the Honey Stomach of the Honeybee Apis Mellifera. *Curr. Microbiol.* **2008**, *57*, 356–363. [CrossRef] [PubMed]
39. Reis, J.A.; Paula, A.T.; Casarotti, S.N.; Penna, A.L.B. Lactic Acid Bacteria Antimicrobial Compounds: Characteristics and Applications. *Food Eng. Rev.* **2012**, *4*, 124–140. [CrossRef]
40. Ramachandran, S.; Fontanille, P.; Pandey, A.; Larroche, C. Gluconic Acid: Properties, Applications and Microbial Production. *Food Technol. Biotechnol.* **2006**, *44*, 185–195.
41. Sinpoo, C.; Williams, G.R.; Chantawannakul, P. Dynamics of Fungal Communities in Corbicular Pollen and Bee Bread. *Chiang Mai J. Sci.* **2017**, *44*, 1244–1256.

42. Detry, R.; Simon-Delso, N.; Bruneau, E.; Daniel, H.M. Specialisation of Yeast Genera in Different Phases of Bee Bread Maturation. *Microorganisms* **2020**, *8*, 1789. [CrossRef] [PubMed]
43. Malgas, S.; Mafa, M.S.; Mkabayi, L.; Pletschke, B.I. A Mini Review of Xylanolytic Enzymes with Regards to Their Synergistic Interactions during Hetero-Xylan Degradation. *World J. Microbiol. Biotechnol.* **2019**, *35*, 187. [CrossRef]
44. Wang, X.; Yao, B.; Su, X. Linking Enzymatic Oxidative Degradation of Lignin to Organics Detoxification. *Int. J. Mol. Sci.* **2018**, *19*, 3373. [CrossRef] [PubMed]
45. Dimov, S.G.; Zagorchev, L.; Iliev, M.; Dekova, T.; Ilieva, R.; Kitanova, M.; Georgieva-Miteva, D.; Dimitrov, M.; Peykov, S. A Snapshot Picture of the Fungal Composition of Bee Bread in Four Locations in Bulgaria, Differing in Anthropogenic Influence. *J. Fungi* **2021**, *7*, 845. [CrossRef]
46. Iravani, S.; Varma, R.S. Plant Pollen Grains: A Move Towards Green Drug and Vaccine Delivery Systems. *Nano-Micro Lett.* **2021**, *13*, 128. [CrossRef] [PubMed]
47. Damulienė, V.; Kaškonienė, V.; Kaškonas, P.; Maruška, A. The Influence of Enzymatic Hydrolysis on Bee Pollen Antioxidant and Antibacterial Activities. *Foods* **2023**, *12*, 3582. [CrossRef]
48. Iorizzo, M.; Testa, B.; Lombardi, S.J.; Ganassi, S.; Ianiro, M.; Letizia, F.; Succi, M.; Tremonte, P.; Vergalito, F.; Cozzolino, A.; et al. Antimicrobial Activity against Paenibacillus Larvae and Functional Properties of Lactobacillus plantarum Strains: Potential Benefits for Honeybee Health. *Antibiotics* **2020**, *9*, 442. [CrossRef]
49. Rokop, Z.P.; Horton, M.A.; Newton, I.L.G. Interactions between Cooccurring Lactic Acid Bacteria in Honey Bee Hives. *Appl. Environ. Microbiol.* **2015**, *81*, 7261. [CrossRef]
50. Perez, R.H.; Zendo, T.; Sonomoto, K. Novel Bacteriocins from Lactic Acid Bacteria (LAB): Various Structures and Applications. *Microb. Cell Fact.* **2014**, *13*, S3. [CrossRef]
51. Ibrahim, S.A.; Ayivi, R.D.; Zimmerman, T.; Siddiqui, S.A.; Altemimi, A.B.; Fidan, H.; Esatbeyoglu, T.; Bakhshayesh, R.V. Lactic Acid Bacteria as Antimicrobial Agents: Food Safety and Microbial Food Spoilage Prevention. *Foods* **2021**, *10*, 3131. [CrossRef] [PubMed]
52. Cheng, Y.; Ang, B.; Xue, C.; Wang, Z.; Yin, L.; Wang, T.; Chen, Q.; Wang, Z.; Zeng, M.; Zhang, W.; et al. Insights into the Fermentation Potential of Pollen: Manufacturing, Composition, Health Benefits, and Applications in Food Production. *Trends Food Sci. Technol.* **2024**, *143*, 104245. [CrossRef]
53. Urcan, A.C.; Criste, A.D.; Dezmirean, D.S.; Bobiș, O.; Bonta, V.; Burtescu, R.F.; Olah, N.-K.; Cornea-Cipcigan, M.; Mărgăoan, R. Enhancing Antioxidant and Antimicrobial Activities in Bee Collected Pollen through Solid-State Fermentation: A Comparative Analysis of Bioactive Compounds. *Antioxidants* **2024**, *13*, 292. [CrossRef] [PubMed]
54. Bolyen, E.; Rideout, J.R.; Dillon, M.R.; Bokulich, N.A.; Abnet, C.C.; Al-Ghalith, G.A.; Alexander, H.; Alm, E.J.; Arumugam, M.; Asnicar, F.; et al. Reproducible, Interactive, Scalable and Extensible Microbiome Data Science Using QIIME 2. *Nat. Biotechnol.* **2019**, *37*, 852. [CrossRef] [PubMed]
55. Callahan, B.J.; McMurdie, P.J.; Rosen, M.J.; Han, A.W.; Johnson, A.J.A.; Holmes, S.P. DADA2: High-Resolution Sample Inference from Illumina Amplicon Data. *Nat. Methods* **2016**, *13*, 581–583. [CrossRef] [PubMed]
56. Quast, C.; Pruesse, E.; Yilmaz, P.; Gerken, J.; Schweer, T.; Yarza, P.; Peplies, J.; Glöckner, F.O. The SILVA Ribosomal RNA Gene Database Project: Improved Data Processing and Web-Based Tools. *Nucleic Acids Res.* **2012**, *41*, D590–D596. [CrossRef] [PubMed]
57. Kõljalg, U.; Larsson, K.H.; Abarenkov, K.; Nilsson, R.H.; Alexander, I.J.; Eberhardt, U.; Erland, S.; Høiland, K.; Kjøller, R.; Larsson, E.; et al. UNITE: A Database Providing Web-Based Methods for the Molecular Identification of Ectomycorrhizal Fungi. *New Phytol.* **2005**, *166*, 1063–1068. [CrossRef] [PubMed]
58. Tsavea, E.; Mossialos, D. Antibacterial Activity of Honeys Produced in Mount Olympus Area against Nosocomial and Foodborne Pathogens Is Mainly Attributed to Hydrogen Peroxide and Proteinaceous Compounds. *J. Apic. Res.* **2019**, *58*, 756–763. [CrossRef]
59. Pham, V.H.T.; Kim, J.; Chang, S.; Bang, D. Investigating Bio-Inspired Degradation of Toxic Dyes Using Potential Multi-Enzyme Producing Extremophiles. *Microorganisms* **2023**, *11*, 1273. [CrossRef]
60. Yassin, S.N.; Jiru, T.M.; Indracanti, M. Screening and Characterization of Thermostable Amylase-Producing Bacteria Isolated from Soil Samples of Afdera, Afar Region, and Molecular Detection of Amylase-Coding Gene. *Int. J. Microbiol.* **2021**, *2021*, 5592885. [CrossRef]
61. Maski, S.; Ngom, S.I.; Rached, B.; Chouati, T.; Benabdelkhalek, M.; El Fahime, E.; Amar, M.; Béra-Maillet, C. Hemicellulosic Biomass Conversion by Moroccan Hot Spring Bacillus Paralicheniformis CCMM B940 Evidenced by Glycoside Hydrolase Activities and Whole Genome Sequencing. *3 Biotech* **2021**, *11*, 379. [CrossRef] [PubMed]
62. Subramanian, V.; Farmer, S.J.; Heiland, K.L.; Moore, K.T.; Wall, T.A.V.; Sun, W.; Chaudhari, Y.B.; Himmel, M.E.; Decker, S.R. A Multi-Plex Protein Expression System for Production of Complex Enzyme Formulations in Trichoderma Reesei. *J. Ind. Microbiol. Biotechnol.* **2023**, *49*, 27. [CrossRef] [PubMed]
63. Sheikhi, F.; Roayaei Ardakani, M.; Enayatizamir, N.; Rodriguez-Couto, S. The Determination of Assay for Laccase of Bacillus Subtilis WPI with Two Classes of Chemical Compounds as Substrates. *Indian J. Microbiol.* **2012**, *52*, 701–707. [CrossRef] [PubMed]
64. Fernandes, T.A.R.; da Silveira, W.B.; Passos, F.M.L.; Zucchi, T.D. Oligonucleotide Primers for Specific Detection of Actinobacterial Laccases from Superfamilies I and K. *Antonie Van Leeuwenhoek* **2014**, *106*, 391–398. [CrossRef] [PubMed]
65. Ausec, L.; Berini, F.; Casciello, C.; Cretoiu, M.S.; van Elsas, J.D.; Marinelli, F.; Mandic-Mulec, I. The First Acidobacterial Laccase-like Multicopper Oxidase Revealed by Metagenomics Shows High Salt and Thermo-Tolerance. *Appl. Microbiol. Biotechnol.* **2017**, *101*, 6261–6276. [CrossRef] [PubMed]

66. Sheng, P.; Li, Y.; Marshall, S.; Zhang, H. High Genetic Diversity of Microbial Cellulase and Hemicellulase Genes in the Hindgut of Holotrichia Parallela Larvae. *Int. J. Mol. Sci.* **2015**, *16*, 16545–16559. [CrossRef]
67. Kumar, S.; Stecher, G.; Li, M.; Knyaz, C.; Tamura, K. MEGA X: Molecular Evolutionary Genetics Analysis across Computing Platforms. *Mol. Biol. Evol.* **2018**, *35*, 1547–1549. [CrossRef]

pharmaceuticals

MDPI

Article

The Influence of Geographical Origin on Poplar Propolis Composition and the Impact of Human Microbiota

Michał Miłek [1,*], Gabriela Franke [2], Monika Tomczyk [1], Miłosz Górecki [3], Olga Cwiková [2], Alžbeta Jarošová [2] and Małgorzata Dżugan [1]

[1] Department of Chemistry and Food Toxicology, Institute of Food Technology and Nutrition, University of Rzeszow, Ćwiklińskiej 1a St., 35-601 Rzeszow, Poland; mwesolowska@ur.edu.pl (M.T.); mdzugan@ur.edu.pl (M.D.)

[2] Department of Food Technology, Faculty of AgriSciences, Mendel University in Brno, Zemědělská 1 St., 613 00 Brno, Czech Republic; gabriela.franke@mendelu.cz (G.F.); olga.cwikova@mendelu.cz (O.C.); alzbeta.jarosova@mendelu.cz (A.J.)

[3] PROKIT—Miłosz Górecki, Świętokrzyska 25 St., Kazimierów, 05-074 Halinow, Poland; milosz.gorecki@prokit.pl

* Correspondence: mmilek@ur.edu.pl; Tel.: +48-178721730

Abstract: Ethanol extracts obtained from 13 poplar propolis samples originating from various European countries by traditional maceration were tested for total polyphenols, flavonoid content, and antioxidant activity. Moreover, the content of 18 polyphenolic compounds (from the group of phenolic acids and flavonoids) was determined using the HPLC method. The inhibitory effect of six selected extracts with the highest activity was assessed by well-diffusion method against five strains (*Bifidobacterium* spp., *L. rhamnosus*, *L. acidophilus*, *E. coli*, and *Bacteroides* spp.) of intestinal bacteria self-isolated from the faeces of obese probands with the use of selective media. It was found that the antioxidant activity of propolis varied depending on geographical origin and even among samples from the same region, which indicates that some other factors also influence propolis quality. The samples of different geographical origin varied mainly in the share of individual phenolic compounds, and it was not possible to find a characteristic marker of origin, excluding the galangin present in the Polish samples only. Assessing the inhibitory activity of propolis (in the range of 70 mg to 10 µg per mL) indicated that the concentration of 100 µg/mL was found as being safe for tested fecal bacteria (*Bifidobacterium* spp., *L. rhamnosus*, *L. acidophilus*, *E. coli*, and *Bacteroides* spp.). As no negative effect of low doses of propolis on the intestinal microflora was found, it can be suggested that its use in recommended doses brings only beneficial effects to the body.

Keywords: propolis; chemical composition; polyphenols; antibacterial activity; gut microbiota

1. Introduction

Propolis (or bee glue) is a resinous substance collected by honeybees (*Apis mellifera* L.) from plant buds, secretions, or resins found in the stems, branches, and leaves of various plants [1]. Considering that the main function of propolis is to support the sterility and health of the hive, the protective properties of the bioactive substances found in propolis may provide significant benefits to human health as well [2]. The mechanism by which propolis supports health seems to be related to its broad spectrum of action but is particularly based on its antioxidant, antimicrobial, anti-inflammatory, hepatoprotective, and immunomodulatory properties [3–6]. Therefore, propolis is widely used both in food and beverages, but also in cosmetics and pharmacology to improve human health and in the prevention of many diseases, among its other uses, such as inflammation, diabetes, heart disease, and even cancer [2,7–9]. Additionally, the literature describes the effect of propolis on various strains of viruses, such as the herpes simplex virus (HSV-1), the influenza virus (HIV-1), and even the SARS-CoV-2 virus [10–12]. Propolis also has the ability to inhibit the activity of various enzymes (acetylcholinesterase, lipoxygenase, α-glucosidase, xanthine oxidase, and hyaluronidase), which makes it a promising source of new active compounds used in the treatment of skin diseases, lifestyle diseases, and neurodegenerative diseases [13]. The beneficial properties of propolis are closely related to its rich chemical composition and the interaction of the individual components. According to actual literature, over 300 compounds have been described in propolis, including polyphenols, terpenoids, amino acids, sugars, steroids, minerals, and vitamins [1,4,14,15].

The composition of propolis is very variable and depends on various factors, such as the botanical and geographical origin (landforms), harvest time (month), season and climatic characteristics (weather), beekeeping practices (scraping from frames or propolis collector), and, finally, extraction method [8,16]. The basic composition of propolis is stable regardless of its origin and consists of about 50% resin, 30% wax, 5% pollen, 10% aromatic oils, and 5% other organic residues; however, the greatest variation is related to the presence or absence of selected polyphenolic compounds [6,17]. Flavonoids, such as galangin, apigenin, pinocembrin, pinostrobin, kaempferol, chrysin, and quercetin, as well as phenolic acids, including caffeic, ferulic, cinnamic, coumaric, and hydroxybenzoic, were determined in propolis samples from various geographic origins [10]. The most frequently identified compound in propolis from many countries, including Italy, Spain, Poland, and even India, is caffeic acid phenethyl ester (CAPE), characterized by its wide pharmacological effects, including anti-cancer activity [9,10]. Morphologically, there are three main types of propolis: temperate propolis, propolis from tropical regions, and propolis from the Pacific region [8]. In a temperate climate zone, bees collect propolis resin, mainly from the vegetative buds of poplars, primarily *Populus nigra* but also other *Populus* species including *P. tremula* (aspen), as well as from the leaf buds of *Betula* spp. and *Alnus* sp. (especially in Poland), which are also used by bees to produce propolis [8]. Poplar type propolis contains phenols typical of propolis from European poplar buds, i.e., flavonoids, phenolic acids, and their esters [18,19]. However, propolis is so botanically and geographically diversified and has such an extensive matrix that examining all the compounds is still a challenge for scientists.

The antibacterial effect of propolis is provided by polyphenolic substances, mainly flavonoids, which cause the inhibition of nucleic acid synthesis and DNA, cell wall, and membrane damage, as well as affecting the adhesion of bacteria to intestinal cells [20]. The bacteriostatic or bactericidal effect depends on the polyphenol structure and the particular strain of bacteria tested. It is estimated that only 5–10% of the total phenolic compounds are absorbed in the small intestine, while the remaining 90–95% are transported to the large intestine where they are biotransformed by the intestinal microflora. Studies by Ahn et al. [7] and Ozdal et al. [17] have demonstrated the degradation of propolis polyphenols at up to 80% and 87%, respectively. This claim is supported by many studies confirming the use of polyphenols as a substrate for colonic bacterial metabolism using enzymatic processes (deglycosylation, dehydroxylation, and demethylation). The resulting lower molecular weight metabolites (e.g., benzoic, phenylacetic, and phenylpropionic acids) have a bioactive effect on the organism and may exhibit anti-inflammatory activity [21–23]. Many studies confirm the metabolization of catechin and epicatechin by colonic bacteria; these are further absorbed by intestinal mucosal cells into the host bloodstream and subsequent metabolites are identified in blood plasma and urine [24–26].

While the antibacterial activity of propolis against pathogenic bacteria has been widely studied, the available literature completely lacks data on the impact of propolis on the microflora of the human gastrointestinal tract. Meanwhile, propolis is commonly used to treat infections and strengthen immunity by oral administration, which raises the question of whether such use does not strain the internal microflora. Thus, the main idea of this study was to evaluate the effect of poplar propolis extract on isolated human faecal bacteria during in vitro conditions. Considering the variability of the chemical composition of propolis, samples with extremely different levels of antioxidant activity and polyphenol profiles were selected at the preliminary stage from 13 propolis samples of distant geographical origin; thus, the comparative characterization of the chemical compositions of propolis from different parts of Europe was an additional result of the conducted research.

2. Results and Discussion

2.1. Variation in the Chemical Composition of Propolis Extract Resulted from Different Geographical Origin

Thirteen propolis extracts of different geographical origin were characterized in terms of the total content of polyphenols, flavonoids, and antioxidant activity, using three methods based on different mechanisms (Table 1). The study showed that the biological activity of propolis varied depending on its geographical origin. Moreover, the differences observed among samples from the same region indicate that the method of obtaining propolis influences its quality to a greater extent than its geographical origin does. The observed variability did not exceed 20%, except for the flavonoid content (39%), which seems to be unrelated to geographical origin. The samples with the highest antioxidant activity and polyphenol content included one from Ukraine (895), three from Poland (886, 887, 888), and one from Turkey (885). Among the tested samples of Polish propolis, three (75%) showed favorable values of the tested parameters, above the determined average. However, one sample (889) differed significantly from the others. Among the samples of different origins, those characterized by lower activity were the Bulgarian (890), Turkish (894, 897), and Ukrainian (896) samples.

Table 1. Total phenolic and flavonoid contents as well as antioxidant activity evaluation using different analytical methods for 13 samples of propolis differing in geographical origin.

Sample	TPC [mg GAE/g]	TFC [mg QE/g]	DPPH [μmol TE/g]	FRAP [μmol TE/g]	CUPRAC [μmol TE/g]
890 (BG)	80.51 ± 4.44 ^{a}	90.99 ± 4.78 ^{c}	171.63 ± 7.41 ^{ab}	284.49 ± 34.15 ^{ab}	1412.82 ± 138.91 ^{a}
891 (BG)	97.26 ± 5.65 ^{bde}	130.48 ± 5.66 ^{d}	207.48 ± 12.00 ^{bdef}	354.36 ± 6.45 ^{ce}	1874.36 ± 282.25 ^{af}
894 (TR)	67.38 ± 4.72 ^{a}	73.84 ± 2.88 ^{bc}	183.95 ± 23.54 ^{acdk}	330.16 ± 6.34 ^{bcd}	1667.95 ± 109.62 ^{acdi}
879 (TR)	78.97 ± 3.60 ^{a}	84.48 ± 3.64 ^{c}	201.38 ± 14.00 ^{ae}	306.83 ± 30.30 ^{ac}	1602.56 ± 193.59 ^{ab}
885 (TR)	109.74 ± 8.33 ^{b}	133.74 ± 5.03 ^{df}	287.25 ± 7.69 ^{l}	523.65 ± 26.99 ^{g}	2685.90 ± 276.99 ^{h}
892 (RO)	91.51 ± 7.75 ^{aef}	95.83 ± 4.82 ^{c}	236.47 ± 18.80 ^{e}	328.73 ± 29.89 ^{bcde}	1915.38 ± 362.21 ^{ag}
893 (RO)	98.15 ± 5.22 ^{bdf}	63.21 ± 2.54 ^{b}	209.47 ± 5.29 ^{bdeg}	364.21 ± 21.50 ^{cf}	2132.05 ± 311.05 ^{befgh}
895 (UA)	130.00 ± 5.45 ^{c}	160.46 ± 9.34 ^{e}	225.65 ± 11.79 ^{ejk}	390.49 ± 25.75 ^{ef}	2308.97 ± 99.88 ^{defgh}
896 (UA)	84.42 ± 6.69 ^{ad}	75.47 ± 2.95 ^{bc}	167.27 ± 8.44 ^{a}	278.03 ± 8.85 ^{ab}	1671.79 ± 207.70 ^{ae}
886 (PL)	121.48 ± 2.97 ^{bc}	151.60 ± 7.81 ^{e}	244.19 ± 12.96 ^{fghij}	358.96 ± 33.66 ^{ce}	2252.56 ± 180.99 ^{bcefgh}
887 (PL)	115.78 ± 3.75 ^{bc}	148.80 ± 10.69 ^{ef}	222.41 ± 11.20 ^{cei}	401.55 ± 24.78 ^{ef}	2271.79 ± 235.66 ^{efghi}
888 (PL)	117.52 ± 6.74 ^{bc}	143.31 ± 7.10 ^{de}	219.92 ± 11.79 ^{ceh}	386.77 ± 13.80 ^{def}	2021.79 ± 169.94 ^{ah}
889 (PL)	85.41 ± 4.17 ^{ad}	36.64 ± 1.59 ^{a}	163.17 ± 14.01 ^{a}	241.46 ± 0.57 ^{a}	1676.92 ± 182.48 ^{ae}
Min	61.98	34.81	148.98	241.13	1280.77
Max	136.30	167.02	293.10	545.34	2900.00
Mean	98.32	106.84	210.79	349.98	1961.14
SD	19.20	39.07	35.61	71.46	396.14
Variability [%]	19.53	36.57	16.89	20.42	20.20
F-value	35.42	135.74	21.26	28.17	7.67
p-value	0.000	0.000	0.000	0.000	0.000

BG—Bulgaria, TR—Turkey, RO—Romania, UA—Ukraine, PL—Poland; ^{a,b,c,d,e,f,g,h,i,j,k,l}—means marked with different letters are significantly different at $p < 0.05$. Data are presented as mean ± SD ($n = 3$).

The obtained results are in line with other studies where the high antioxidant activity of ethanolic extract of propolis was observed. For Polish propolis, in earlier studies, the polyphenol content ranged from 150.05 to 197.14 mg/g GAE, and total flavonoid content from 35.64 to 62.04 mg/g QE [19]. For Turkish propolis, the spread was even greater (TPC from 34.53 to 259.4 mg GAE/g and TFC from 21.28 to 152.56 mg CE/g) [1]. For propolis from various regions of Ukraine, the phenols content was 120.3 to 145.24 mg GAE/g, and the flavonoid fraction ranged from 53.9 to 82.71 mg QE/g [27]; similar values were reported for propolis from Romania [8]. Also, strong antioxidant activity, tested using various methods, is reflected in the available literature data for samples of similar geographical origin [8,27,28].

The results obtained using different methods were significantly correlated, as indicated by the values of Pearson correlation coefficients for DPPF-FRAP r = 0.89, DPPH-CUPRAC r = 0.88, and FRAP-CUPRAC r = 0.894. The total polyphenol content was significantly correlated with the flavonoid content TPC-TFC r = 0.832. A significant correlation was observed between antioxidant activity and polyphenol content, regardless of the research method used ($r > 0.63$), and between antioxidant activity and flavonoid content ($r > 0.657$), which indicates the pivotal role of these components in creating the antioxidant activity of the tested samples.

2.2. Variation in the Polyphenolic Profile of Propolis Extract According to Geographical Origin

The content of individual polyphenolic compounds in the extracts of the tested propolis was determined using the HPLC-DAD method (Table 2). Comparative analysis showed large differences in the content of individual polyphenolic ingredients depending on the origin of propolis. Based on the analysis of 13 samples, the average composition of the polyphenol fraction of propolis was established, and indicated that its active ingredients include phenolic acids (mainly caffeic, p-coumaric, and ferulic acid) and flavonoids (mainly chrysin, pinobanksin, and pinocembrin, as well as unidentified flavanones). This observation is in line with the literature data that indicate the presence of these compounds as typical for European poplar propolis [29–31].

The variability between samples of different geographical origin was mainly manifested in the different shares of individual compounds, and it was not possible to find characteristic marker compounds for samples from individual countries. For example, Polish propolis was characterized by the presence of an increased number of phenolic acids including, mainly, p-coumaric, caffeic, ferulic, and benzoic. However, the sample of Polish origin with the lowest activity contained mainly p-coumaric acid and a derivative of caffeic acid, while the content of other phenolic acids was lower than average. Among the flavonoids, Polish propolis was especially abundant in galangin, kaempferol, apigenin, and chrysin, while it contained less pinobanksin. Importantly, only in Polish propolis was galangin aglycone detected. This compound seems to be a promising origin marker. Two compounds from the flavanone group were also determined that could not be identified based on comparison with standards. These may include, for example, pinostrobin, the presence of which in European propolis is confirmed by the literature data [16,29].

The results of the total phenols and flavonoid content obtained using colorimetric and HPLC-DAD methods were compared. The distribution of the results is shown in Figure 1. A good correlation of the results was obtained, especially in the case of flavonoids (Pearson's coefficient r = 0.981), whereas polyphenols were less correlated (r = 0.889); however, it should be remembered that the Folin—Ciocalteu method is less specific for determining polyphenol compounds.

Based on the analysis of 13 samples, the average composition of the polyphenol fraction of propolis was established, and indicated that its active ingredients include phenolic acids (mainly caffeic, p-coumaric, and ferulic acid) and flavonoids (mainly chrysin, pinobanksin, and pinocembrin, as well as unidentified flavanones). This observation is in line with the literature data that indicate the presence of these compounds as typical for European poplar propolis [29–31].

Table 2. The individual polyphenolic compound content in tested propolis samples (mg/100 mg).

Propolis sample no. (country of origin)	Polyphenol Content [mg/100 g]																	
	Caffeic Acid	p-Coumaric Acid	Ferulic Acid	Isoferulic Acid	Caffeic Acid Derivative	Benzoic Acid	Vanillin	Quercetin	Kaempferol	Apigenin	Flavanone I	Pinobanksin	Chrysin	Pinocembrin	Galangin	Flavanone II	Galangin Derivative	Sum of polyphenols
890 (BG)	148.86 ± 11.22	181.47 ± 8.62	142.41 ± 18.53	82.13 ± 4.20	92.53 ± 7.08	72.80 ± 4.45	nd	240.80 ± 17.95	75.44 ± 22.95	188.87 ± 5.00	366.66 ± 31.11	688.68 ± 42.82	1873.22 ± 145.29	1155.22 ± 81.09	nd	1704.02 ± 136.13	nd	7013.11
891 (BG)	210.87 ± 12.05	135.56 ± 14.14	82.39 ± 3.73	132.68 ± 13.60	140.46 ± 12.11	92.58 ± 13.72	nd	423.88 ± 32.97	99.86 ± 38.84	268.00 ± 5.88	599.16 ± 24.41	815.14 ± 29.98	2694.24 ± 100.37	1699.43 ± 17.82	nd	2893.38 ± 123.84	nd	10,287.63
894 (TR)	127.81 ± 17.02	126.43 ± 34.37	58.71 ± 19.49	203.85 ± 27.46	127.35 ± 20.50	88.65 ± 28.87	12.45 ± 5.12	92.57 ± 7.59	64.44 ± 13.53	191.56 ± 11.05	298.86 ± 63.28	468.03 ± 42.33	2290.17 ± 208.16	739.58 ± 206.56	nd	1537.51 ± 352.02	nd	6427.97
879 (TR)	153.43 ± 4.12	159.28 ± 10.23	75.61 ± 5.08	168.92 ± 5.27	143.99 ± 9.99	179.63 ± 2.11	13.81 ± 0.66	85.30 ± 3.27	62.41 ± 4.92	191.90 ± 2.32	364.34 ± 35.14	492.12 ± 27.07	2432.83 ± 142.29	1065.96 ± 41.07	nd	1715.16 ± 71.17	96.15 ± 12.81	7400.84
885 (TR)	272.16 ± 6.54	302.83 ± 12.39	104.39 ± 10.69	433.07 ± 10.49	341.31 ± 9.76	458.91 ± 18.49	32.84 ± 1.95	nd	63.81 ± 4.09	144.26 ± 6.04	582.62 ± 25.43	675.30 ± 32.23	3728.38 ± 173.08	1697.07 ± 64.99	nd	2123.39 ± 20.86	141.93 ± 13.07	11,102.27
892 (RO)	156.98 ± 9.17	206.40 ± 19.80	142.43 ± 16.47	173.07 ± 9.85	184.61 ± 8.85	227.68 ± 13.72	48.54 ± 6.86	95.69 ± 6.82	54.91 ± 22.21	167.20 ± 22.24	500.10 ± 20.00	563.59 ± 28.81	2310.67 ± 85.51	1457.63 ± 63.02	nd	2056.45 ± 90.63	94.55 ± 3.77	8440.43
893 (RO)	112.47 ± 17.02	540.85 ± 51.52	482.88 ± 47.51	169.79 ± 28.36	175.53 ± 20.64	328.85 ± 33.85	113.71 ± 11.37	nd	nd	175.01 ± 11.37	270.26 ± 41.58	335.62 ± 51.79	1819.02 ± 561.25	781.53 ± 123.86	nd	1195.44 ± 173.84	nd	6500.96
895 (UA)	191.50 ± 13.89	950.12 ± 50.39	810.50 ± 37.69	180.15 ± 14.75	400.27 ± 23.10	569.85 ± 24.30	40.66 ± 1.95	159.04 ± 10.14	179.10 ± 19.98	540.27 ± 11.80	683.40 ± 39.44	862.48 ± 50.05	3723.49 ± 117.67	1906.02 ± 86.07	nd	3115.29 ± 167.31	380.85 ± 11.04	14,692.99
896 (UA)	122.90 ± 64.48	660.11 ± 273.44	429.33 ± 5.10	54.28 ± 7.02	nd	321.63 ± 6.40	139.57 ± 8.48	nd	108.51 ± 12.47	nd	190.22 ± 19.43	335.82 ± 38.95	2220.39 ± 348.32	350.84 ± 118.32	nd	837.42 ± 151.35	227.00 ± 21.54	5998.02
886 (PL)	300.24 ± 5.54	847.40 ± 96.13	492.66 ± 55.14	299.82 ± 8.20	130.60 ± 9.90	379.81 ± 67.42	50.03 ± 6.47	202.44 ± 5.57	164.31 ± 22.85	470.48 ± 23.75	757.57 ± 7.56	1068.69 ± 25.30	3140.17 ± 166.06	574.12 ± 26.69	2201.42 ± 2.29	3301.33 ± 113.70	234.24 ± 6.30	14,615.33
887 (PL)	251.81 ± 17.78	881.74 ± 21.56	515.37 ± 24.51	333.98 ± 27.94	148.32 ± 6.86	479.56 ± 21.30	77.81 ± 7.52	187.61 ± 16.85	163.82 ± 41.05	600.26 ± 31.72	674.49 ± 63.06	897.59 ± 100.91	3011.42 ± 213.99	497.22 ± 43.88	1933.68 ± 161.43	2883.25 ± 187.57	216.46 ± 15.16	13,754.39
888 (PL)	254.47 ± 25.51	738.65 ± 38.42	454.18 ± 48.15	306.31 ± 31.70	139.60 ± 18.84	341.33 ± 29.98	76.12 ± 8.49	198.94 ± 19.80	171.21 ± 34.64	507.80 ± 23.33	687.67 ± 44.90	1048.45 ± 82.87	2749.43 ± 324.41	456.49 ± 100.49	1673.06 ± 408.42	2370.49 ± 676.23	186.04 ± 109.80	12,360.24
889 (PL)	68.34 ± 7.85	1541.54 ± 198.10	717.36 ± 84.59	nd	nd	571.73 ± 59.60	61.74 ± 6.27	nd	nd	39.81 ± 6.27	nd	288.67 ± 40.08	nd	183.17 ± 67.96	nd	335.74 ± 95.02	nd	3808.1
Min	59.29	101.07	41.63	49.36	0.00	63.82	0.00	0.00	0.00	0.00	0.00	262.25	0.00	108.27	0.00	259.74	0.00	
Max	304.12	1739.98	839.53	439.35	421.47	638.47	146.71	460.84	187.68	700.08	765.78	1143.39	3856.90	1986.22	2202.94	3369.82	391.47	
Mean	182.45	559.26	346.79	195.23	316.39	155.74	51.33	129.71	92.91	268.11	459.64	656.94	2461.03	966.48	446.78	2005.30	121.32	
SD	71.77	425.86	254.38	118.76	172.67	109.42	41.75	121.35	60.73	192.82	226.22	264.33	954.23	563.96	839.08	903.22	122.06	
Variability [%]	38.98	76.15	73.35	60.83	54.57	70.26	81.35	93.55	65.37	71.92	49.22	40.24	38.77	58.35	187.81	45.04	100.61	
F-value	45,535	54.18	146.09	138.91	207.55	93.29	143.68	257.60	86.73	82.76	117.80	84.66	47.10	113.15	148.11	41.62	44.09	
p-value	0.000	0.000	0.000	0.000	0.000	0.000	0.000	0.000	0.000	0.000	0.000	0.000	0.000	0.000	0.000	0.000	0.000	

nd—not detected. Data are presented as mean ± SD (n = 3).

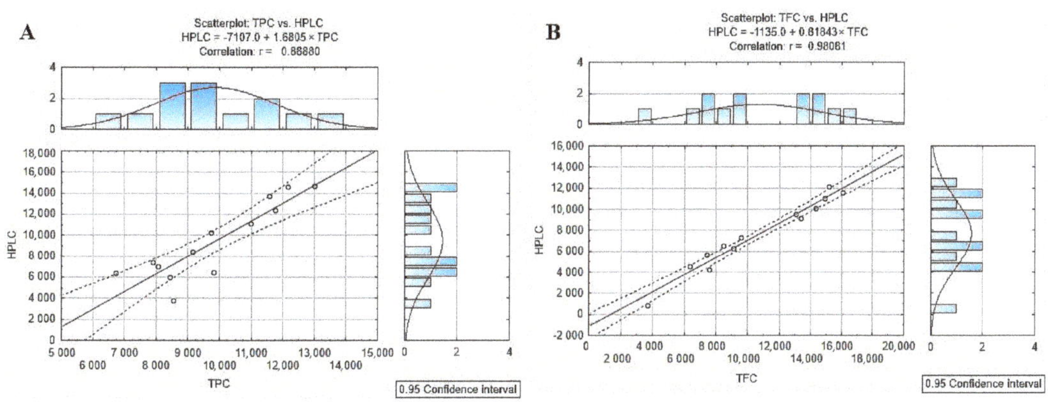

Figure 1. The correlation plots of total phenolic (**A**) and flavonoid (**B**) contents obtained by colorimetric and HPLC methods. Dashed lines indicate 0.95 confidence intervals.

The compositions of the tested propolis samples were varied and the resulting response of the bacteria to the presence of these substances is difficult to interpret. Some in-teractions can be inferred from the available studies, for example, the inhibitory effect of some flavonoids (chrysin and pinobanksin) on the growth of beneficial bacteria [32]. In our study, positive correlations were observed between the detected concentrations of flavanone I and II, chrysin, and pinobanksin and the inhibition effect on *L. rhamnosus* (r = 0.93, r = 0.89, r = 0.87, resp. r = 0.85; $p < 0.05$). The averaged polyphenol profiles for the samples from the analyzed countries compared to the overall average are shown in Figure 2. Generally, the polyphenol composition was similar, with some differences that are most evident in the content of phenolic acids (Poland and Ukraine) or flavonoids (Bulgaria and Turkey). For Bulgarian propolis, a characteristic predominance of quercetin content over kaempferol was observed, in contrast to the other samples.

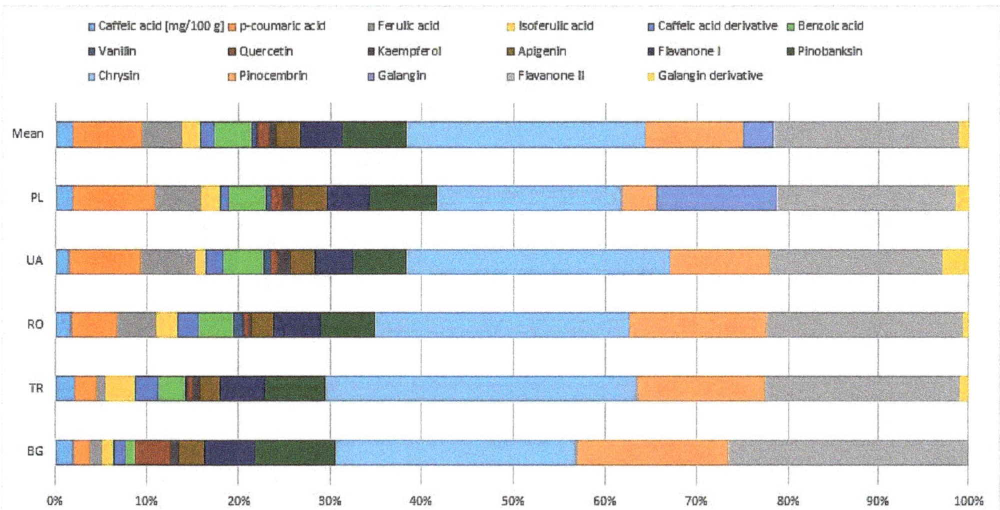

Figure 2. Average polyphenolic profiles for samples of different origins compared to the average profile of all tested samples. The shares of individual compounds are shown as percentages of the total sum of polyphenols determined by HPLC.

Based on differences in the obtained polyphenolic profiles, five samples were selected for the next step of analyzing the impact on the human microbiota (Figure 3). Samples with the highest content of polyphenols were selected from each country tested, and for comparison, the propolis sample with the lowest levels of these compounds (889, Poland) was applied. The specific feature of both Polish propolis samples was a lower pinocembrin content and the presence of galangin.

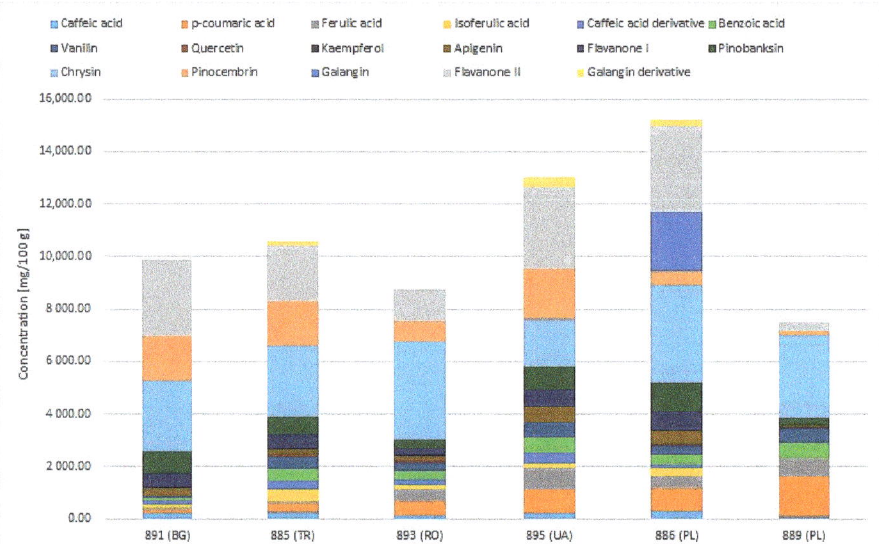

Figure 3. Polyphenolic profiles of propolis samples selected for in vitro microbiological study.

2.3. The Effect of Propolis on Fecal Bacteria In Vitro

Table 3 shows the antibacterial activity of the propolis extracts against bacteria obtained from the gut microbiome of probands. The concentration of the propolis samples tested at which they no longer showed an inhibitory effect against the micro-organisms tested was 100 μg/mL, except for sample 886, for which the inhibition of *L. rhamnosus* and *Bacteroides* spp. was observed at this concentration.

Table 3. Inhibition effect of EEP (diameter in mm) in tested concentrations on bacteria isolated from human faeces.

Sample	EEP Concentration	*Bifidobacterium* spp.	*L. rhamnosus*	*L. acidophilus*	*E. coli*	*Bacteroides* spp.
891 (BG)	70 mg/mL	16.3 ± 0.5^{c}	18.3 ± 05^{d}	28.3 ± 0.5^{e}	12.3 ± 0.5^{b}	8.3 ± 0.5^{a}
	40 mg/mL	13.7 ± 0.5^{c}	16.3 ± 0.5^{d}	23.7 ± 0.5^{e}	10.3 ± 0.5^{b}	8.3 ± 0.5^{a}
	10 mg/mL	11.7 ± 0.5^{b}	15.7 ± 0.5^{c}	20.3 ± 0.5^{d}	7.7 ± 0.5^{a}	7.3 ± 0.5^{a}
	1 mg/mL	8.7 ± 0.5^{bc}	7.7 ± 0.5^{b}	9.3 ± 0.5^{c}	nd	nd
	100 μg/mL	nd	nd	nd	nd	nd
	10 μg/mL	nd	nd	nd	nd	nd
885 (TR)	70 mg/mL	14.3 ± 0.5^{d}	18.3 ± 0.5^{a}	18.3 ± 0.5^{a}	12.3 ± 0.5^{c}	10.7 ± 0.5^{b}
	40 mg/mL	11.7 ± 0.5^{b}	15.7 ± 0.5^{c}	14.3 ± 0.5^{c}	10.3 ± 0.5^{ab}	9.7 ± 0.5^{a}
	10 mg/mL	9.7 ± 0.5^{b}	13.7 ± 0.5^{d}	11.7 ± 0.5^{c}	7.7 ± 0.5^{a}	7.7 ± 0.5^{a}
	1 mg/mL	8.3 ± 0.5^{a}	7.7 ± 0.5^{a}	7.7 ± 0.5^{a}	nd	7.3 ± 0.5^{a}
	100 μg/mL	nd	nd	nd	nd	nd
	10 μg/mL	nd	nd	nd	nd	nd

Table 3. *Cont.*

Sample	EEP Concentration	*Bifidobacterium* spp.	*L. rhamnosus*	*L. acidophilus*	*E. coli*	*Bacteroides* spp.
886 (PL)	70 mg/mL	14.3 ± 0.5 [c]	16.7 ± 0.5 [a]	12.3 ± 0.5 [b]	24.3 ± 0.5 [d]	16.3 ± 0.5 [a]
	40 mg/mL	13.7 ± 0.5 [a]	15.7 ± 0.5 [b]	12.3 ± 0.5 [a]	20.3 ± 0.5 [c]	12.3 ± 0.5 [a]
	10 mg/mL	11.7 ± 0.5 [a]	13.7 ± 0.5 [b]	10.3 ± 0.5 [a]	14.3 ± 0.5 [b]	10.3 ± 0.5 [a]
	1 mg/mL	8.3 ± 0.5 [a]	8.7 ± 0.5 [a]	nd	7.7 ± 0.5 [a]	7.7 ± 0.5 [a]
	100 µg/mL	nd	7.3 ± 0.5 [a]	nd	nd	7.3 ± 0.5 [a]
	10 µg/mL	nd	nd	nd	nd	nd
889 (PL)	70 mg/mL	18.3 ± 0.5 [a]	9.3 ± 0.5 [b]	18.3 ± 0.5 [a]	12.7 ± 0.5 [c]	16.3 ± 0.5 [d]
	40 mg/mL	14.7 ± 0.5 [a]	7.7 ± 0.5 [b]	14.3 ± 0.5 [a]	12.3 ± 0.5 [d]	10.3 ± 0.5 [c]
	10 mg/mL	13.7 ± 0.5 [c]	7.3 ± 0.5 [a]	11.7 ± 0.5 [b]	11.3 ± 0.5 [b]	8.3 ± 0.5 [a]
	1 mg/mL	7.3 ± 0.5 [b]	nd	7.3 ± 0.5 [b]	nd	nd
	100 µg/mL	nd	nd	nd	nd	nd
	10 µg/mL	nd	nd	nd	nd	nd
893 (RO)	70 mg/mL	10.7 ± 0.5 [a]	12.3 ± 0.5 [b]	16.3 ± 0.5 [c]	10.3 ± 0.5 [a]	12.7 ± 0.5 [b]
	40 mg/mL	9.7 ± 0.5 [b]	11.7 ± 0.5 [a]	12.3 ± 0.5 [a]	8.3 ± 0.5 [b]	11.7 ± 0.5 [a]
	10 mg/mL	9.7 ± 0.5 [a]	10.3 ± 0.5 [a]	9.7 ± 0.5 [a]	6.7 ± 0.5 [b]	9.7 ± 0.5 [a]
	1 mg/mL	7.7 ± 0.5 [b]	nd	nd	nd	nd
	100 µg/mL	nd	nd	nd	nd	nd
	10 µg/mL	nd	nd	nd	nd	nd
895 (UA)	70 mg/mL	14.3 ± 0.5 [c]	16.3 ± 0.5 [d]	10.3 ± 0.5 [a]	12.3 ± 0.5 [b]	10.3 ± 0.5 [a]
	40 mg/mL	13.7 ± 0.5 [d]	13.7 ± 0.5 [d]	8.3 ± 0.5 [a]	10.3 ± 0.5 [c]	9.7 ± 0.5 [ab]
	10 mg/mL	11.7 ± 0.5 [b]	11.7 ± 0.5 [b]	7.3 ± 0.5 [a]	8.3 ± 0.5 [a]	7.7 ± 0.5 [a]
	1 mg/mL	7.7 ± 0.5 [b]	8.3 ± 0.5 [b]	nd	nd	nd
	100 µg/mL	nd	nd	nd	nd	nd
	10 µg/mL	nd	nd	nd	nd	nd

[a,b,c,d,e]—significant differences ($p < 0.05$) between strains with the same concentration of EEP. nd—not determined. Data are presented as mean ± SD ($n = 3$).

The compositions of the tested propolis samples varied and the resulting response of the bacteria to the presence of these substances is difficult to interpret. Some interactions can be inferred from the available studies, for example, the inhibitory effect of some flavonoids (chrysin and pinobanksin) on the growth of beneficial bacteria [32]. In our study, positive correlations were observed between the detected concentrations of flavanone I and II, chrysin, and pinobanksin and the inhibition effect on *L. rhamnosus* (r = 0.93, r = 0.89, r = 0.87, resp. r = 0.85; $p < 0.05$) only.

The evaluation of the antibacterial effect of propolis regardless of its concentration (Figure 4) allowed for ranking the tested samples in terms of their impact on individual bacterial strains. The antioxidatively strongest propolis samples, 891 (BG) and 886 (PL), showed a tendency toward different effects: the first one strongly inhibited the growth of probiotic bacteria (*Bifidobacterium* spp., *L. rhamnosus*, and *L. acidophilus*), and the growth of *E. coli* and *Bacteroides* spp. less strongly, whereas the second one, on the contrary, tended to inhibit the growth of all bacteria except for *L. acidophilus*. This effect may be related to the different chemical profiles of the samples. Since a significant difference was found concerning the presence of galangin in Polish propolis as well as the high content of quercetin in Bulgarian propolis, it can be suspected that these flavonoids may play an important role in shaping the antibacterial properties of propolis. These results are confirmed by the study by Omidi et al. [33], who observed no antibacterial effect on *L. acidophilus* of the matrix with pure galangin.

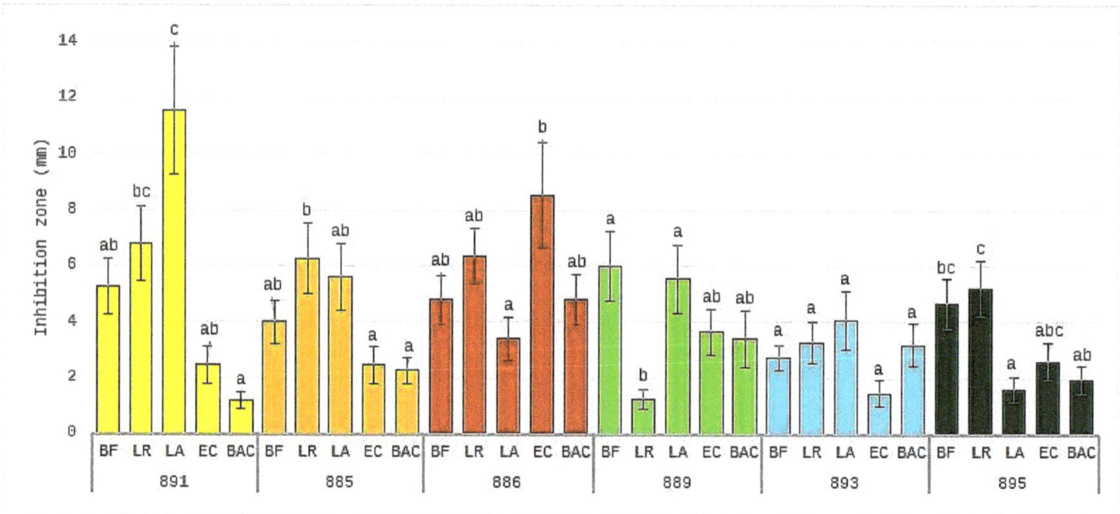

Figure 4. Diameter of inhibition zone (after subtraction diameter of well; in mm) of strains: *Bifidobacterium* spp. (BF), *Lactobacillus rhamnosus* (LR), *Lactobacillus acidophilus* (LA), *Escherichia coli* (EC), *Bacteroides* spp. (BAC) obtained after incubation with ethanolic extracts of propolis (EEP) regardless of the concentration. a–c letters mark significant differences ($p < 0.05$) between inhibition of strains by each sample of EEP.

In the case of *Bacteroides* spp., various inhibition effects among samples of propolis were detected. Recent genomic methods contributed to our understanding of the unique adaptive nature of the *Bacteroides* species. Bacteria of the *Bacteroides* genus are considered a reservoir of genes for antibiotic resistance [34].

However, taking into account the results from our previous work, where the MIC value determined for pathogenic bacteria (*E. coli* and *Staphylococcus* spp.) was 24–780 µg/mL [9], the applied concentrations of 100 µg/mL (0.01%) and 10 µg/mL (0.001%) seem to be safe for human microbiota. Assuming a daily intake of max. 30 drops of standard propolis extract, which corresponds to approximately 0.08 g of dry extract, and taking into account its dilution in the digestive content, the exposure of the microbiome in the intestine should not exceed the concentration of 0.01% tested in in vitro tests. It can be assumed that such therapy will be effective against pathogenic bacteria and, at the same time, safe against beneficial intestinal bacteria.

Many studies show an inhibitory effect of phenolics on pathogenic bacteria but a stimulatory effect on commensal bacteria of the digestive tract [35]. However, this area is still under-researched, and long-term in vivo research is needed to confirm the aforementioned hypothesis of a positive effect on beneficial intestinal bacteria. Some attempts were also made for single flavonoids, including quercetin and galangin, which were recognized as prebiotics [36,37].

In the study of Ferreira de Brito et al. [38], nine samples of Brazilian propolis extract were tested. An inhibition effect against *L. rhamnosus* was detected at concentrations of 500–1000 µg/mL and against *Staphylococcus aureus* and *Salmonella typhymurium* at 125–500 µg/mL and 250 µg/mL, respectively. Quercetin belongs to the important antibacterial substances of propolis and can be used for its effect in the prevention of bacterial diseases of the digestive tract of animals. The application of 0.4 g quercetin/kg to feed significantly increased ($p < 0.01$) the numbers of *Bifidobacterium* spp. and *Lactobacillus* spp. in the digestive tract of broilers, while the numbers of the pathogenic bacteria *P. aeruginosa*, *S. enterica*, and *S. aureus* decreased ($p < 0.05$, resp. $p < 0.01$) [39]. In the case of bifidobacteria, regression analysis confirmed the same effect, with a rising dose of quercetin increasing the number of bifidobacteria in the intestine ($p < 0.05$) [40]. The same effect was reported in a study of Kačániová et al. [41], who tested the addition of propolis extract to chicken feed. The numbers of lactobacilli in the digestive tract of chickens compared to the control group were increased in all experimental groups (100–800 mg of propolis/kg of feed).

A last study by Garzarella et al. [42] monitored the amount of polyphenols metabolized during a simulated digestive process. During the simulated digestion process and subsequent fermentation by the intestinal bacteria of healthy people, the polyphenol content was metabolized from the original 70.0 g of gallic acid equivalents/kg propolis to 2.5 ± 0.4 g of gallic acid equivalents/kg propolis after simulated digestion. However, the most significant decrease was observed in the case of the mixed bacterial microflora of obese people, where a value of up to 2.1 ± 0.2 g gallic acid equivalents/kg propolis was observed. In our study, bacterial strains from obese subjects were obtained (BMI > 25 kg/m^2); therefore, based on these results, it can be expected that the metabolism of phenolic compounds was at a higher level and, thus, the inhibitory effect was at a lower level than it would be in healthy individuals.

3. Materials and Methods

3.1. Chemicals

Chemicals (2,2-diphenyl-1-picrylhydrazyl, 2,2-azino-bis(3-ethylbenzothiazoline-6-sulfonic acid; 2,4,6-Tris(2-pyridyl)-s-triazine, neocuproine, copper(II) chloride, ammonium acetate, sodium carbonate, ferric chloride), reagents (Folin–Ciocalteu reagent), HPLC standards (gallic acid, caffeic acid, ferulic acid, benzoic acid, p-coumaric acid, vanillin, apigenin, quercetin, kaempferol, galangin, chrysin, pinobanksin, pinocembrin) were obtained from Sigma Aldrich (Saint Louis, MO, USA), and solvents (ethanol, acetonitrile, formic acid) were purchased from Avantor Performance Materials Poland SA (APM, Gliwice, Poland).

3.2. Media for Fecal Bacteria Isolation and Antibacterial Activity Testing

These included Bifidus selective medium agar with BSM Supplement (Sigma Aldrich, Saint Louis, MO, USA); MRS agar, *E. coli*/coliforms agar, Plate count agar (PCA), and Ringers solution tablets (¼ strength) (Neogen, Lansing, MI, USA); clindamycin hydrochloride, vancomycin, Bacteroides Bile esculin agar with Bacteroides Selective Supplement, and Nutrient Broth Peptone (Himedia, Mumbai, India); Mueller Hinton II agar and Gentamicin disk (30 µg) (Liofilchem, Roseto degli Abruzzi, Italy); and 70% ethanol (Lach-Ner, Neratovice, Czech Republic).

3.3. Propolis Samples and Extract Preparation

Thirteen samples of poplar propolis with various geographical origins were provided by the company PROKIT—MIŁOSZ GÓRECKI (Kazimierów, Poland), which specializes in purchasing raw propolis directly from beekeepers. The set included: 4 Polish (sample codes: 886, 887, 888, and 889), 3 Turkish (879, 885, and 894), 2 Romanian (892 and 893), 2 Ukrainian (895 and 896), and 2 Bulgarian (890 and 891) propolis samples. All samples showed organoleptic features (color, smell, texture) typical for poplar propolis.

For each propolis sample, an extract was prepared strictly by the same maceration procedure in duplicate. Specifically, 10 g of each propolis sample was poured with 100 mL of 70% ethanol in a glass bottle with a screw cap and shaken in the dark for 30 min at 400 rpm. After this time, propolis was macerated in dark at room temperature (20 ± 2 °C) within 5 days. Every day samples were manually shaken. Then, extract was filtered through a filter paper and subjected to the two-step condensation process, including ethanol evaporation (RVC 2–18 CDPlus, Martin Christ, Osterode am Harz, Germany) and freeze-drying (Alpha 1–2 LD plus, Martin Christ, Osterode am Harz, Germany). The obtained dry extract was dissolved in 70% ethanol (100 mg/mL concentration) and used for the determination of antioxidant activity, total polyphenols and flavonoid content, chromatographic analyzes, and antimicrobial effect in vitro study.

3.4. Antioxidant Activity Assays

DPPH radical scavenging activity was measured based on the procedure described by Miłek et al. [9]. Briefly, 0.02 mL of appropriate propolis extract was added to 0.18 mL of 0.1 mM DPPH solution in methanol and left in dark for 30 min. Then, the absorbance was measured at 517 nm using a UV–VIS Spectrometer (EPOCH 2 microplate spectrophotometer, BioTek, Winooski, VT, USA). The results obtained were expressed as μmol of Trolox equivalents (TE) per 1 g of the dry weight of the extract based on the prepared standard curve (25–300 nmol/mL of Trolox solution in methanol).

FRAP (Ferric Reducing Antioxidant Power) assay was also provided according to Miłek et al. [9]. Briefly, 0.02 mL of sample was mixed with 0.18 mL FRAP reagent consisted of 2.5 mL of a 10 mM 2,4,6-tripyridyltriazine (TPTZ) solution in 40 mM HCl, 2.5 mL of 20 mM $FeCl_3$ and 25 mL of 0.3 M acetate buffer (pH 3.6), and the absorbance of the mixture was measured spectrophotometrically (EPOCH 2 microplate spectrophotometer) at 593 nm after 10 min of incubation at 37 °C against blank. A calibration curve was prepared for Trolox ethanol solution in the range 25–300 nmol/mL, and the results were expressed as μmol of Trolox equivalents (TE) per 1 g of the dry extract.

CUPRAC (CUPric Reducing Antioxidant Capacity) assay was performed according to Dżugan et al. [43]. Briefly, 10 μL of diluted propolis dry extract was mixed with 40 μL of $CuCl_2$ (10 mM), 50 μL of neocuproine (7.5 mM), and 50 μL of ammonium acetate (1 M). The reaction mixture was then incubated at room temperature for 30 min and the absorbance was measured with a microplate reader (EPOCH2, BioTek, Winooski, VT, USA) at 450 nm. The results were expressed as Trolox equivalents per 1 g of dry extract based on a calibration curve (125–2000 nmol/mL).

3.5. Total Phenolic and Flavonoid Content Analysis

The total phenolic content (TPC) was also measured using the procedure described by Miłek et al. [9]. In summary, 0.02 mL of plant extract was mixed with 0.1 mL Folin–Ciocalteu reagent (10-fold diluted) and, next, 0.08 mL of 7.5% (*w*/*v*) Na_2CO_3 solution was added. After incubation at room temperature for 60 min, the absorbance was measured spectrophotometrically (EPOCH 2 microplate spectrophotometer) at 760 nm against the blank. TPC was calculated based on a calibration curve at the range 25–150 μg/mL prepared with gallic acid (GA). Results were expressed as mg of gallic acid equivalents (GAE) per 1 g of the extract.

The total flavonoid content (TFC) was assessed according to by Miłek et al. [9]. Briefly, 0.1 mL of the propolis solution was mixed with 0.1 mL 2% $AlCl_3$ (in methanol). The reaction mixture was incubated for 10 min at room temperature until the reaction was complete. The absorbance of the solution was then measured at 415 nm with a microplate reader EPOCH 2 against methanol blank. The total content of flavonoids in the extracts was expressed in mg of quercetin equivalent (QE) per g of dry extract (mg QE/g). The results were calculated based on a calibration curve prepared for quercetin in the range 0–125 μg/mL.

3.6. HPLC Analysis

The content of selected polyphenolic components of the propolis extracts have been quantified by HPLC-DAD method using Gilson HPLC System (Gilson Inc., Middleton, WI, USA). The analytical column (Poroshell 120, EC C-18, 4.6 × 150 mm, Agilent Technologies Inc., Santa Clara, CA, USA) has been applied. Before analysis, extracts were filtered through 0.22 μm syringe filters and diluted 5 times. A 10 μL injection was used, with a 1 mL/min flow gradient elution mode using 0.1% formic acid in distilled water (A) and acetonitrile (B). Gradient program with gradient: 0–1.5 min 10% B, 1.5–3 min 10–30% B, 3–9 min 30–50% B, 9–24 min 50% B, 24–29 min 50–100% B, 29–33 min 100% was applied and 10% B was used again to equilibrate the column. The components of the extracts were identified based on a comparison of UV-Vis spectra and retention times with standards. For quantitative analysis, the standard curve method was used for the following standards: caffeic acid, p-coumaric acid, ferulic acid, benzoic acid, vanillin, apigenine, quercetin, kaempferol, pinobanksin, pinocembrin, and galangin. For all compounds, calibration was linear, in the range of 12.5–250 μg/mL ($R^2 > 0.997$). The results were expressed as mg per 100 g of propolis.

3.7. *In Vitro Testing of the Propolis Effect on Fecal Bacteria*

3.7.1. Isolation of Intestinal Bacteria from Faeces

For isolation of five intestinal bacteria taxons: *Lactobacillus acidophilus, Lactobacillus rhamnosus, Bifidobacterium* spp., *Escherichia coli, Bacteroides* spp. the samples of human faeces from obese subjects were obtained (women, aged in the range of 18–52 years, BMI > 25 kg/m^2, without pharmacological treatment) were used. The method for isolation according Komprda et al. [44] with a little modification was applied. 0.5 g of faecal sample was homogenized with 4.5 mL of Nutrient Broth Peptone and pre-cultivated 4 h at 37 °C. After that, decimal dillutions were performed and following bacteria were isolated: *Bifidobacterium* spp. on Bifidus selective medium (BSM) agar at 37 °C after 72 h of anaerobic cultivation; *Lactobacillus acidophilus* and *Lactobacillus rhamnosus* on MRS medium adjusted with clindamycin hydrochloride 0.5 mg/mL, resp. vancomycin 2 mg/mL after 72 h of anaerobic cultivation at 37 °C; *Escherichia coli* on *E. coli*/coliforms agar after 48 h of aerobic cultivation at 37 °C; *Bacteroides* spp. on Bacteroides Bile esculin agar base adjusted with supplement after 72 h of anaerobical cultivation at 37 °C (colonies were harvested regardless esculin hydrolysis reaction).

After isolation on the selective media bacteria were purified on non-selective agar PCA and cultivated at the same conditions. The fresh purified cultures were used for isolation of DNA by NucleoSpin Tissue (Machery Nagel, Dueren, Germany) according to the producer instructions. The samples of purified bacterial DNA were identified by polymerase chain reaction (PCR) using primers selective for the following species, targeting marker DNA sequences deposited in the GenBank (GenBank, Bethesda, MD, USA): for *Bifidobacterium* spp., accession number AF261684; for *Lb. acidophilus*, U32971; for *Lb. rhamnosus*, U32966; and for *E. coli*, J01636. *Bacteroides* spp. were identified as typical colonies according the manufacturer's instructions for the selective medium.

3.7.2. Well-Diffusion Method

Antimicrobial activity of propolis ethanolic extracts by well-diffusion method was performed according to protocol CLSI M7 [45] and M11 [46]. Bacterial cultures were grown on PCA agar for 18 h at 37 °C aerobically, resp. anaerobically. The cell suspensions were prepared with sterile Ringer's solution to the 0.5 McFarland standard. Inoculation of Petri dishes with Mueller Hinton II agar were performed by sterile swabs immersion into cell suspensions. Using a cork borer (Fisher Scientific, Sunnyvale, CA, USA), the wells (in diameter 6 mm) were made and 30 μL of tested propolis solutions were pipetted into the wells. The antimicrobial effect of propolis solutions on bacterial cultures were evaluated after 24 h at 37 °C aerobically, resp. anaerobically. Gentamicin disk (30 μg) as a positive control and 70% ethanol (Lach-Ner, Czech Republic) as a negative control were used. The diameter of inhibition clear zones (in mm) was measured around the wells. All tests were carried out in triplicate.

3.8. *Statistical Analysis*

All analyses were performed in triplicates and the results are expressed as mean ± standard deviation. The results were subjected to one-way ANOVA and the significance of differences was determined based on Tukey's test ($p = 0.05$). Correlations between obtained results were calculated using r Pearson's coefficients. All calculations were made using the Statistica 13.3 software (StatSoft, Tulsa, OK, USA).

4. Conclusions

The study confirmed that the levels of antioxidant activity and the polyphenolic profiles of European poplar propolis show diversification depending on the geographical origin of the sample. The differences observed for samples from the same region suggest the great impact of other factors. Unfortunately, it was not possible to establish universal markers useful to determine the place of origin. The assessment of the impact of poplar propolis extracts (in the range of 70 mg to 10 µg per mL) on human microbiota indicates the concentration of 100 µg/mL as safe for all tested fecal bacteria. However, a significant correlation between phenolic compositions and an inhibitory effect was not found. It has been shown that appropriate dosing of propolis does not affect the intestinal microflora, which allows us to assume that there are only beneficial effects of the use of propolis extract in prevention and treatment. As such, research using propolis samples from various European countries was carried out for the first time, and, taking into account the complex and variable chemical compositions of propolis, further extensive research, including in vivo tests, is required.

Author Contributions: Conceptualization, M.M. and M.D.; methodology, M.M. and G.F.; software, M.M. and G.F.; validation, M.M. and G.F.; formal analysis, M.D. and A.J.; investigation, M.M., G.F., M.T. and O.C.; resources, M.G. and G.F.; data curation, M.M. and G.F.; writing—original draft preparation, M.M., G.F. and M.T.; writing—review and editing, M.D.; visualization, M.M.; supervision, A.J.; project administration, M.M.; funding acquisition, M.D. All authors have read and agreed to the published version of the manuscript.

Funding: This work was supported by the Polish Ministry of Science and Higher Education research project within the University of Rzeszów PB/ZCHTZ/2024.

Institutional Review Board Statement: Not applicable.

Informed Consent Statement: Not applicable.

Data Availability Statement: The data presented in this study are available in the article.

Conflicts of Interest: The authors declare no conflicts of interest.

References

1. Özkök, A.; Keskin, M.; Tanuğur Samancı, A.E.; Yorulmaz Önder, E.; Takma, Ç. Determination of antioxidant activity and phenolic compounds for basic standardization of Turkish propolis. *Appl. Biol. Chem.* **2021**, *64*, 37. [CrossRef] [PubMed]
2. Braakhuis, A. Evidence on the health benefits of supplemental propolis. *Nutrients* **2019**, *11*, 2705. [CrossRef] [PubMed]
3. Kocot, J.; Kiełczykowska, M.; Luchowska-Kocot, D.; Kurzepa, J.; Musik, I. Antioxidant potential of propolis, bee pollen, and royal jelly: Possible medical application. *Oxid. Med. Cell. Longev.* **2018**, *2018*, 7074209. [CrossRef]
4. Woźniak, M.; Mrówczyńska, L.; Waśkiewicz, A.; Rogoziński, T.; Ratajczak, I. Phenolic profile and antioxidant activity of propolis extracts from Poland. *Nat. Prod. Commun.* **2019**, *14*, 1–7. [CrossRef]
5. Rivera-Yañez, N.; Rivera-Yañez, C.R.; Pozo-Molina, G.; Méndez-Catalá, C.F.; Méndez-Cruz, A.R.; Nieto-Yañez, O. Biomedical properties of propolis on diverse chronic diseases and its potential applications and health benefits. *Nutrients* **2021**, *13*, 78. [CrossRef] [PubMed]
6. Akbar, A.; Gul, Z.; Aziz, S.; Sadiq, M.B.; Achakzai, J.K.; Saeed, S.; Chein, S.H.; Sher, H. Bio-Functional Potential and Biochemical Properties of Propolis Collected from Different Regions of Balochistan Province of Pakistan. *Oxid. Med. Cell. Longev.* **2022**, *2022*, 7585406. [CrossRef] [PubMed]
7. Ahn, M.R.; Kumazawa, S.; Hamasaka, T.; Bang, K.S.; Nakayama, T. Antioxidant activity and constituents of propolis collected in various areas of Korea. *J. Agric. Food Chem.* **2004**, *52*, 7286–7292. [CrossRef] [PubMed]
8. Kurek-Górecka, A.; Keskin, Ş.; Bobis, O.; Felitti, R.; Górecki, M.; Otręba, M.; Stojko, J.; Olczyk, P.; Kolayli, S.; Rzepecka-Stojko, A. Comparison of the Antioxidant Activity of Propolis Samples from Different Geographical Regions. *Plants* **2022**, *11*, 1203. [CrossRef] [PubMed]
9. Miłek, M.; Ciszkowicz, E.; Tomczyk, M.; Sidor, E.; Zaguła, G.; Lecka-zlachta, K.; Pasternakiewicz, A.; Dżugan, M. Poplar-Type Polish Propolis Considering Local Flora Diversity Breast Cancer Cells. *Molecules* **2022**, *27*, 725. [CrossRef]
10. Woźniak, M.; Sip, A.; Mrówczyńska, L.; Broniarczyk, J.; Waśkiewicz, A.; Ratajczak, I. Biological Activity and Chemical Composition of Propolis from Various Regions of Poland. *Molecules* **2023**, *28*, 141. [CrossRef] [PubMed]
11. Yosri, N.; El-Wahed, A.A.A.; Ghonaim, R.; Khattab, O.M.; Sabry, A.; Ibrahim, M.A.A.; Moustafa, M.F.; Guo, Z.; Zou, X.; Algethami, A.F.M.; et al. Anti-Viral and Immunomodulatory Properties of Propolis: Chemical Diversity, Pharmacological Properties, Preclinical and Clinical Applications, and In Silico Potential against SARS-CoV-2. *Foods* **2021**, *10*, 1776. [CrossRef]
12. Rocha, M.P.; Amorim, J.M.; Lima, W.G.; Brito, J.C.M.; da Cruz Nizer, W.S. Effect of honey and propolis, compared to acyclovir, against Herpes Simplex Virus (HSV)-induced lesions: A systematic review and meta-analysis. *J. Ethnopharmacol.* **2022**, *287*, 114939. [CrossRef] [PubMed]

13. Widelski, J.; Gaweł-Bęben, K.; Czech, K.; Paluch, E.; Bortkiewicz, O.; Kozachok, S.; Mroczek, T.; Okińczyc, P. Extracts from European Propolises as Potent Tyrosinase Inhibitors. *Molecules* **2023**, *28*, 55. [CrossRef] [PubMed]
14. Mihai, C.M.; Al Mărghitaş, L.; Dezmirean, D.S.; Bărnuţiu, L. Correlation between Polyphenolic Profile and Antioxidant Activity of Propolis from Transylvania. *Sci. Pap. Anim. Sci. Biotechnol.* **2011**, *44*, 100–103.
15. Osés, S.M.; Marcos, P.; Azofra, P.; de Pabl, A.; Fernández-Muíño, M.Á.; Sancho, M.T. Phenolic profile, antioxidant capacities and enzymatic inhibitory activities of propolis from different geographical areas: Needs for analytical harmonization. *Antioxidants* **2020**, *9*, 75. [CrossRef] [PubMed]
16. Pobiega, K.; Kot, A.M.; Przybył, J.L.; Synowiec, A.; Gniewosz, M. Comparison of the Chemical Composition and Antioxidant Properties of Propolis from Urban Apiaries. *Molecules* **2023**, *28*, 6744. [CrossRef]
17. Ozdal, T.; Ceylan, F.D.; Eroglu, N.; Kaplan, M.; Olgun, E.O.; Capanoglu, E. Investigation of antioxidant capacity, bioaccessibility and LC-MS/MS phenolic profile of Turkish propolis. *Food Res. Int.* **2019**, *122*, 528–536. [CrossRef] [PubMed]
18. Kurek-Górecka, A.; Rzepecka-Stojko, A.; Górecki, M.; Stojko, J.; Sosada, M.; Swierczek-Zieba, G. Structure and antioxidant activity of polyphenols derived from propolis. *Molecules* **2014**, *19*, 78–101. [CrossRef]
19. Socha, R.; Gałkowska, D.; Bugaj, M.; Juszczak, L. Phenolic composition and antioxidant activity of propolis from various regions of Poland. *Nat. Prod. Res.* **2015**, *29*, 416–422. [CrossRef]
20. Makarewicz, M.; Drożdż, I.; Tarko, T.; Duda-Chodak, A. The interactions between polyphenols and microorganisms, especially gut microbiota. *Antioxidants* **2021**, *10*, 188. [CrossRef]
21. Zheng, S.; Zhang, H.; Liu, R.; Huang, C.L.; Li, H.; Deng, Z.Y.; Tsao, R. Do short chain fatty acids and phenolic metabolites of the gut have synergistic anti-inflammatory effects?—New insights from a TNF-α-induced Caco-2 cell model. *Food Res. Int.* **2021**, *139*, 109833. [CrossRef] [PubMed]
22. Kemperman, R.A.; Bolca, S.; Roger, L.C.; Vaughan, E.E. Novel approaches for analysing gut microbes and dietary polyphenols: Challenges and opportunities. *Microbiology* **2010**, *156*, 3224–3231. [CrossRef] [PubMed]
23. Van Duynhoven, J.; Vaughan, E.E.; Jacobs, D.M.; Kemperman, R.A.; Van Velzen, E.J.J.; Gross, G.; Roger, L.C.; Possemiers, S.; Smilde, A.K.; Doré, J.; et al. Metabolic fate of polyphenols in the human superorganism. *Proc. Natl. Acad. Sci. USA* **2011**, *108*, 4531–4538. [CrossRef]
24. Wang, L.-Q.; Meselhy, M.R.; Li, Y.; Nakamura, N.; Min, B.-S.; Qin, G.-W.; Hattori, M. The Heterocyclic Ring Fission and Dehydroxylation of Catechins and Related Compounds by Eubacterium sp. Strain SDG-2, a Human Intestinal Bacterium. *Chem. Pharm. Bull.* **2001**, *49*, 1640–1643. [CrossRef] [PubMed]
25. Unno, T.; Tamemoto, K.; Yayabe, F.; Kakuda, T. Urinary Excretion of 5-(3′,4′-Dihydroxyphenyl)-γ-valerolactone, a Ring-Fission Metabolite of (−)-Epicatechin, in Rats and Its in Vitro. *J. Agric. Food Chem.* **2003**, *51*, 6893–6898. [CrossRef] [PubMed]
26. Wang, D.; Ho, L.; Faith, J.; Ono, K.; Janle, E.M.; Lachcik, P.J.; Cooper, B.R.; Jannasch, A.H.; D'Arcy, B.R.; Williams, B.A.; et al. Role of intestinal microbiota in the generation of polyphenol-derived phenolic acid mediated attenuation of Alzheimer's disease β-amyloid oligomerization. *Mol. Nutr. Food Res.* **2015**, *59*, 1025–1040. [CrossRef]
27. Okińczyc, P.; Widelski, J.; Szperlik, J.; Żuk, M.; Mroczek, T.; Skalicka-Woźniak, K.; Sakipova, Z.; Widelska, G.; Kuś, P.M. Impact of plant origin on eurasian propolis on phenolic profile and classical antioxidant activity. *Biomolecules* **2021**, *11*, 68. [CrossRef] [PubMed]
28. Tumbarski, Y.; Todorova, M.; Topuzova, M.; Gineva, G.; Yanakieva, V.; Ivanov, I.; Petkova, N. Comparative Study on Physico-chemical, Antioxidant and Antimicrobial Properties of Propolis Collected from Different Regions of Bulgaria. *J. Apic. Sci.* **2023**, *67*, 37–56. [CrossRef]
29. Ristivojević, P.; Trifković, J.; Andrić, F.; Milojković-Opsenica, D. Poplar-type propolis: Chemical composition, botanical origin and biological activity. *Nat. Prod. Commun.* **2015**, *10*, 1869–1876. [CrossRef]
30. Altuntaş, Ü.; Güzel, İ.; Özçelik, B. Phenolic Constituents, Antioxidant and Antimicrobial Activity and Clustering Analysis of Propolis Samples Based on PCA from Different Regions of Anatolia. *Molecules* **2023**, *28*, 1121. [CrossRef]
31. Zhu, L.; Zhang, J.; Yang, H.; Li, G.; Li, H.; Deng, Z.; Zhang, B. Propolis polyphenols: A review on the composition and anti-obesity mechanism of different types of propolis polyphenols. *Front. Nutr.* **2023**, *10*, 1066789. [CrossRef] [PubMed]
32. Pobiega, K.; Gniewosz, M.; Kraśniewska, K. Antimicrobial and antiviral properties of different types of propolis. *Zesz. Probl. Postępów Nauk Rol.* **2018**, *589*, 69–79. [CrossRef]
33. Omidi, B.; Sarveahrabi, Y.; Nejati Khoei, S. Comparison of the Effect of Fluoride 0.2% and a Combined Mouthwash (Flavonoid Compounds and Fluoride 0.2%) Against Streptococcus mutans and Lactobacillus acidophilus: In Silico and In Vitro Study. *Avicenna J. Dent. Res.* **2023**, *15*, 142–149. [CrossRef]
34. Wexler, H.M. Bacteroides: The good, the bad, and the nitty-gritty. *Clin. Microbiol. Rev.* **2007**, *20*, 593–621. [CrossRef] [PubMed]
35. Alkhaldy, A.; Edwards, C.A.; Combet, E. The urinary phenolic acid profile varies between younger and older adults after a polyphenol-rich meal despite limited differences in in vitro colonic catabolism. *Eur. J. Nutr.* **2019**, *58*, 1095–1111. [CrossRef] [PubMed]
36. Kawabata, K.; Sugiyama, Y.; Sakano, T.; Ohigashi, H. Flavonols enhanced production of anti-inflammatory substance(s) by bifidobacterium adolescentis: Prebiotic actions of galangin, quercetin, and fisetin. *BioFactors* **2013**, *39*, 422–429. [CrossRef] [PubMed]
37. Alves-Santos, A.M.; Sugizaki, C.S.A.; Lima, G.C.; Naves, M.M.V. Prebiotic effect of dietary polyphenols: A systematic review. *J. Funct. Foods* **2020**, *74*, 104169. [CrossRef]

38. Ferreira de Brito, L.; Bergara Pereira, F.; Lorenzon, M.C.; Castro, R.N.; Laureano Melo, R.; Guerra, A.F.; Luchese, R.H. What is the Effect of Propolis Extracts against Pathogenic Microorganisms and on Potentially Probiotic Strains of Lacticaseibacillus and Limosilactobacillus? *ACS Food Sci. Technol.* **2022**, *2*, 493–502. [CrossRef]
39. Wang, S.; Yao, J.; Zhou, B.; Yang, J.; Chaudry, M.T.; Wang, M.; Xiao, F.; Li, Y.; Yin, W. Bacteriostatic effect of quercetin as an antibiotic alternative in vivo and its antibacterial mechanism in vitro. *J. Food Prot.* **2018**, *81*, 68–78. [CrossRef]
40. Liu, H.N.; Liu, Y.; Hu, L.L.; Suo, Y.L.; Zhang, L.; Jin, F.; Feng, X.A.; Teng, N.; Li, Y. Effects of dietary supplementation of quercetin on performance, egg quality, cecal microflora populations, and antioxidant status in laying hens. *Poult. Sci.* **2014**, *93*, 347–353. [CrossRef]
41. Kačániová, M.; Rovná, K.; Arpášová, H.; Čuboň, J.; Hleba, L.; Pochop, J.; Kunová, S.; Haščík, P. In vitro and In vivo antimicrobial activity of propolis on the microbiota from gastrointestinal tract of chickens. *J. Environ. Sci. Health Part A Toxic/Hazardous Subst. Environ. Eng.* **2012**, *47*, 1665–1671. [CrossRef] [PubMed]
42. Garzarella, E.U.; Navajas-Porras, B.; Pérez-Burillo, S.; Ullah, H.; Esposito, C.; Santarcangelo, C.; Hinojosa-Nogueira, D.; Pastoriza, S.; Zaccaria, V.; Xiao, J.; et al. Evaluating the effects of a standardized polyphenol mixture extracted from poplar-type propolis on healthy and diseased human gut microbiota. *Biomed. Pharmacother.* **2022**, *148*, 112759. [CrossRef] [PubMed]
43. Dżugan, M.; Miłek, M.; Kielar, P.; Stępień, K.; Sidor, E.; Bocian, A. SDS-PAGE Protein and HPTLC Polyphenols Profiling as a Promising Tool for Authentication of Goldenrod Honey. *Foods* **2022**, *11*, 2390. [CrossRef] [PubMed]
44. Komprda, T.; Sládková, P.; Kolářová, M.; Zorníková, G.; Sládek, Z.; Rožnovská, D. Effect of probiotic and symbiotic yoghurt consumption on counts of human faecal bacteria and tyramine production. *J. Food Nutr. Res.* **2013**, *52*, 230–238.
45. Clinical and Laboratory Standards Institute. *Methods for Dilution Antimicrobial Susceptibility Tests for Bacteria That Grow Aerobically*, 11th ed.; CLSI standard M7; Clinical and Laboratory Standards Institute: Wayne, PA, USA, 2018.
46. Clinical and Laboratory Standards Institute. *Methods for Antimicrobial Susceptibility Testing of Anaerobic Bacteria*, 9th ed.; CLSI standard M11; Clinical and Laboratory Standards Institute: Wayne, PA, USA, 2018.

pharmaceuticals

MDPI

Article

The Effectiveness of a Dietary Supplement with Honey, Propolis, *Pelargonium sidoides* Extract, and Zinc in Children Affected by Acute Tonsillopharyngitis: An Open, Randomized, and Controlled Trial

Fabio Cardinale [1,*], Dionisio Franco Barattini [2], Valentina Martinucci [3], Maria Morariu Bordea [4], Luca Barattini [5] and Serban Rosu [6]

1 Complex Operating Unit Paediatrics, Giovanni XXIII Paediatric Hospital, University of Bari, 70124 Bari, Italy
2 Opera Contract Research Organization, Tigermed Company, 300209 Timisoara, Romania; barattini@operacro.com
3 Pediatrica S.r.l., 57121 Livorno, Italy; rd@pediatrica.it
4 Cabinet Medical Medicina de Familie Dr Morariu Bordea, 300425 Timisoara, Romania; cabinetmbmorariu@yahoo.com
5 Tigermed Italy S.r.l., 16129 Genova, Italy; personal@lucabarattini.com
6 Department of Oral and Cranio-Maxillo-Facial Surgery, University of Medicine and Pharmacy Victor Babes, 300041 Timisoara, Romania; serbanrosu@gmail.com
* Correspondence: fabiocardinale1961@gmail.com; Tel.: +39-080-5596732

Abstract: Physicians are currently finding products for pediatric respiratory diseases of viral etiology to reduce the inappropriate use of antibiotic therapy. This study evaluated PediaFlù (Pediatrica S.r.l.), a dietary supplement already on the market composed of honey, propolis, *Pelargonium sidoides* extract, and zinc (DSHPP), in children affected by acute tonsillopharyngitis (ATR). The open-label, randomized, and controlled study compared DSHPP + standard of care (SoC) versus SoC alone for six days. Children between 3 and 10 years with an ATR $\leq$ 48 h, a negative rapid test for beta-hemolytic *Streptococcus*, or a culture identification of nasal and/or pharyngeal exudates were included. A tonsillitis severity score (TSS) and the number of treatment failures (using ibuprofen or high-dose paracetamol as rescue medication) were the primary endpoints. DSHPP+ SoC showed better performance than SoC alone for TSS sub-scores: throat pain and erythema on day 6 ($p < 0.001$ and $p < 0.05$), swallowing ($p < 0.01$ on day 4), and TSS total score on days 4 and 6 ($p < 0.05$ and $p < 0.001$). Only one patient (SoC group) had treatment failure for ibuprofen administration. No adverse events were reported. DSHPP is an optimal adjuvant in the treatment of URTI and could potentially be useful in the daily clinical practice of paediatricians evaluating the correct antibiotic prescription.

Keywords: dietary supplements; tonsillitis; pharyngitis; nasopharyngitis; honey; propolis; zinc; *Pelargonium sidoides*; severity score

1. Introduction

Acute tonsillopharyngitis (ATR), which is typically caused by viruses, is a common reason for consultation with pediatricians and general practitioners (GPs). In contrast, bacterial etiology requires antibiotic therapy and is present in approximately 30% of all cases of ATR. Therefore, in the great majority of cases, ATR does not require antibiotic treatment [1]. Furthermore, guidelines [2] and a recent review [3] emphasize that antibiotics should not be applied in the pediatric population for apparent viral respiratory illnesses (sinusitis, pharyngitis, and bronchitis). Instead, they should be administered only to children with pharyngitis clearly caused by group A *Streptococcus*. Even when considering other bacterial infections that require antibiotic treatment, the discrepancy between the median incidence of *Streptococcal pharyngitis*, which is 1764 per 100,000 children [4], and the annual rate of antibiotic prescribing for childhood upper respiratory tract infections (URTI), which is 421 prescriptions per 100,000 population in the US [5], is evident. This explains the observation made by Fleming-Dutra KE that one-third of outpatient antibiotic prescriptions for pediatric URTI are inappropriate [6]. Consequently, research and clinical practice are currently exploring the potential benefits of products that can be used in pediatric respiratory diseases of viral etiology, with the aim of reducing the inappropriate use of antibiotic therapy.

In light of the aforementioned considerations, Pediatrica S.r.l. (Livorno, Italy) has developed a dietary supplement (DS) in an oral solution, PediaFlù® (DSHPP), designed for pediatric use as an adjuvant for respiratory tract health and well-being. The composition of this product is based on the synergistic action of honey and propolis, which have been demonstrated to have beneficial effects on the respiratory tract [7,8]. The DSHPP also contains *Pelargonium sidoides* extract (Pelagon P 70™) and zinc. Six clinical trials using honey in a total of nearly 900 children were analyzed in the Cochrane meta-analysis published on 2018 [9]. The analysis revealed that honey was associated with favorable outcomes in terms of cough frequency, patient quality of life, and the quality of sleep for both parents and children. The limitations of the evaluated studies included the small sample sizes, the heterogeneous administration of the tested product (different types of honey were used in different studies), and the short duration of treatment (often one night only). Nevertheless, the meta-analysis concluded that honey alleviated cough symptoms compared with no treatment or diphenhydramine but was not found to be more effective than dextromethorphan. The beneficial activity of honey has been linked to the reduction of free radicals produced at the site of inflammation and its capacity to reduce the use of antibiotics. Additionally, it has been demonstrated to enhance the immune system, promoting the proliferation of human peripheral blood B cells, neutrophils, and T lymphocytes [10,11]. A recent pragmatic randomized clinical trial (RCT) conducted in Spain evaluated the efficacy of honey in reducing cough symptoms in adult patients with acute bronchitis. Although the trial did not reach its original enrollment goal of 668 patients [12], it did demonstrate that the duration of severe-to-moderate cough in patients treated with 30 mg of honey for two weeks was comparable to that of patients in the other arms (dextromethorphan 15 mg t.i.d. and ipratropium bromide inhaler 20 μg 2 puffs t.i.d.). A systematic review demonstrated that propolis exerts a beneficial effect on glutathione, glutathione peroxidase (GPX), and total antioxidant capacity (TAC) levels and has been shown to be safe for use as a dietary supplement. Moreover, it can be employed as an adjuvant treatment in diseases where oxidative stress plays a crucial role in the pathogenesis [13]. A number of studies have demonstrated that the administration of propolis to patients diagnosed with respiratory disorders has resulted in improvements in symptoms. In an RCT with a double-blind design, propolis was found to produce a statistically significant reduction in the number of days required for symptom resolution in both bacterial and viral URTI [14]. The findings of this study are consistent with those of a prior case-control investigation conducted on children regarding the treatment of rhinopharyngitis [15]. Propolis has also demonstrated advantages in asthmatic patients, including increased forced vital capacity (FVC), pulmonary forced expiratory volume in the first second (FEV1), and peak expiratory flow rate (PEFR) [16]. A statistically significant reduction in the incidence of exacerbations and an improvement in symptoms and quality of life of patients affected by chronic obstructive pulmonary disease (COPD) was evidenced in RCTs using a combination of propolis and N-acetylcysteine (NAC) [17,18]. A systematic review [19] examined data from 8526 patients who received zinc supplementation, demonstrating a reduction in the duration of the common cold. As evidenced by the scientific literature, the extract of *Pelargonium sidoides* may be an effective treatment for disorders affecting the respiratory tract, particularly in pediatric populations with acute non-streptococcal tonsillopharyngitis [20,21]. These beneficial effects of *Pelargonium sidoides* are the result of reducing harmful inflammation [22] from one side and enhancing the immune response by increasing phagocytic activity, oxidative burst, intracellular killing of pathogens, release of nitric oxide (NO) in macrophages, and release of tumor necrosis factor (TNF)-α, and interleukin (IL)-1 and IL-12 [23].

The data provided above indicate the effectiveness of the honey, propolis, zinc, and *Pelargonium sidoides* extract components when administered separately. Published reviews and the daily clinical practice of thousands of pediatricians have also emphasized the safety of these components when used in combination with other products. Therefore, integrating the four components into a single DSHPP has the advantage of activating the synergic action of honey and propolis [7,8]. It also provides medical doctors with the opportunity of administering a single, effective, and safe product in conjunction with the traditional standard of care (SoC).

The present clinical trial was planned to confirm the results observed in clinical practice. The objective was to assess whether a six-day administration of the investigational DSHPP, in conjunction with SoC, could result in a more favorable ATR symptomatology compared to patients receiving SoC alone. The confirmation of this hypothesis would support the candidacy of DSHPP as an effective tool for pediatricians and general practitioners.

2. Results

2.1. Patient Disposition

The enrollment period began on 3 June 2021, and concluded on 6 August 2021. The study was terminated on 12 August 2021 (last patient and last visit). A total of 135 individuals were initially screened, and 130 of them were deemed eligible for participation in the trial. The children were randomly assigned to either the DSHPP + SoC group (n = 66) or the SoC alone group (n = 64). The intention-to-treat (ITT) population included all 130 subjects who were enrolled and completed the study. The per protocol (PP) population consisted of 129 patients, as one child from the DSHPP + SoC group was excluded from the analysis due to discontinuation of treatment and withdrawal from the study following the use of rescue medication (Figure 1).

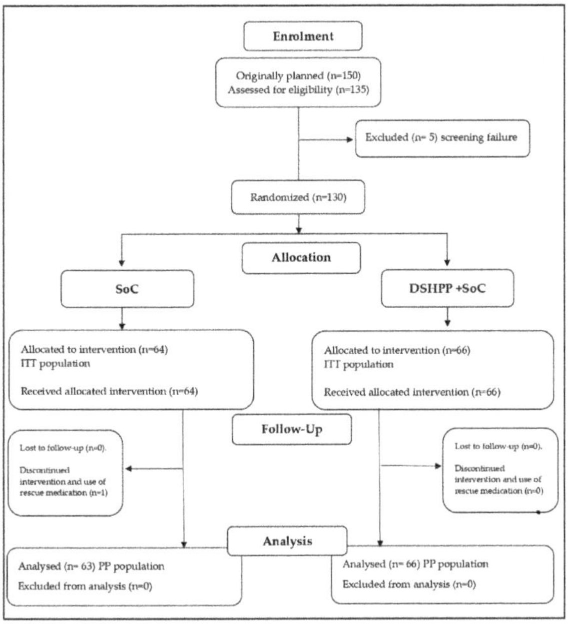

Figure 1. Flow diagram of the study. Standard of care (SoC); DSHPP dietary supplement PediaFlù® based on honey and propolis associated to zinc and *Pelargonium sidoides* extract.

The patient characteristics outlined in Table 1 showed no significant differences in baseline demographic and anthropometric variables between the DSHPP + SoC and SoC alone groups ($p > 0.05$, Mann–Whitney U test).

Table 1. Per protocol (PP) population: demographics of the patients at the baseline visit by assignment group. ns: non-significant.

Characteristics		All no. = 129	DSHPP + SoC no. = 66	SoC no. = 63	*p*-Value
Age (years)	Mean (SD)	5.52 (2.07)	5.8 (2.01)	5.22 (2.11)	ns
	Median	5	5.5	5	
	Range	3–10	3–10	3–10	
BMI (kg/m^2)	Mean (SD)	16.41 (3.06)	16.71 (3.0)	16.1 (3.11)	ns
	Median	15.54	15.97	15.42	
	Range	10.42–30.26	10.42–25.69	11.76–30.26	
Height (cm)	Mean (SD)	114.51 (14.95)	116.56 (15.36)	112.37 (14.31)	ns
	Median	114	116	108	
	Range	89–160	89–160	90–148	
Weight (kg)	Mean (SD)	22.1 (8.29)	23.32 (8.74)	20.83 (7.66)	ns
	Median	20	22	19	
	Range	11–60	12–60	11–54	

2.2. Administered Treatments and Compliance

All patients were fully compliant with the administration of DSHPP and SoC (low-dosage paracetamol and benzydamine hydrochloride). There were no significant differences in the number of doses and quantity of benzydamine hydrochloride administered between the groups. By contrast, there is a statistically significant difference ($p < 0.01$, Mann–Whitney U test) in the mean (SD) of administered doses of low-dosage paracetamol: 13.67 (4.34) and 15.92 (3.02) in DSHPP + SoC and SoC, respectively.

2.3. Efficacy

2.3.1. Primary Outcomes

Tonsillitis Severity Score

The primary efficacy outcome was the change in the tonsillitis severity score (TSS) from baseline to the final visit, analyzed separately for total score and for the five sub-scores: throat pain, difficulty in swallowing, salivation, erythema, and fever. The randomization between groups was executed properly (M diff. = +0.3, U = 1762, $p = 0.091$, CI95: 8.88–9.32). The balance between groups was maintained at the outset of medication and dietary supplement administration (M diff. = +0.3, U = 1763, $p = 0.114$, and CI95: 8.88–9.32).

TSS Total Score

The total score for TSS during the study period indicated that children treated with DSHPP + SoC exhibited a lower rating than children in the SoC alone group (Table 2). In particular, the difference between the two groups was statistically significant at days 4 and 6, with *p*-values of 0.034 and 0.002, respectively (Mann–Whitney U test).

Table 2. Tonsillitis severity score (TSS) total score mean ±SD ratings between administration groups, on day 0, day 4, and day 6 with Mann–Whitney U test. ** $p < 0.01$; * $p < 0.05$; ns: non-significant.

		DSHPP + SoC	SoC	*p*-Value
Start of administration	no.	66	63	
	Mean (SD)	9.2 (1.4)	8.9 (1.2)	ns
Day 4	no.	66	63	
	Mean (SD)	3.2 (1.4)	3.8 (1.7)	*
Day 6	no.	66	63	
	Mean (SD)	0.7 (0.7)	1.2 (1.0)	**

TSS Throat Pain Sub-Score

Two of the 66 subjects (3.03%) from the DSHPP + SoC group reported experiencing throat pain at the final visit. In contrast, 14 of the 63 subjects (23.33%) from the SoC alone group had throat pain on day 6. Consequently, a statistically significant lower number of subjects from the DSHPP + SoC group compared to the SoC alone group were experiencing throat pain at the final visit (chi-square test, $p < 0.001$). Figure 2 illustrates the change in TSS throat pain ratings from baseline to final visit. It shows a mean (SD) reduction in the DSHPP + SoC group from 2.2 (0.4) to 0.0 (0.2), while the SoC alone group exhibited a mean (SD) slight increase from 2.1 (0.3) to 0.2 (0.5). The statistical analysis revealed a significant difference between the two groups ($p < 0.001$, Mann–Whitney U test).

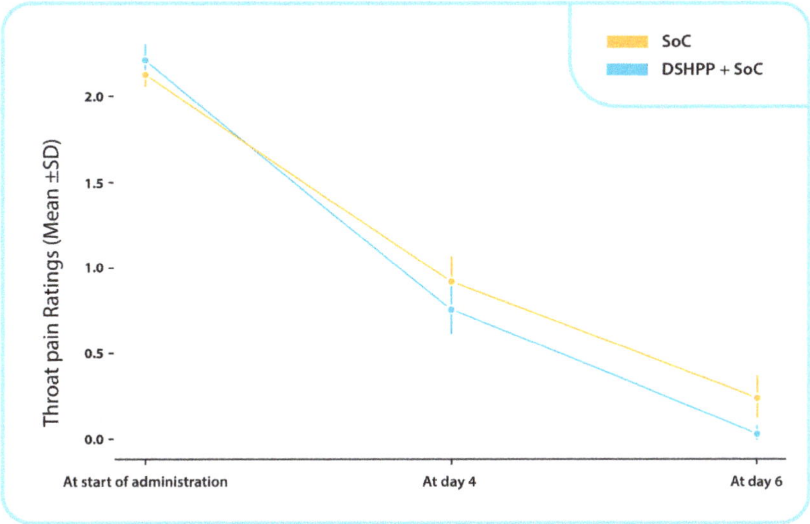

Figure 2. Change in TSS Throat pain; mean ± SD ratings from start of administration to final visit. On day 6 $p < 0.001$ (Mann–Whitney U test).

TSS Difficulty in Swallowing Sub-Score

At the final visit, none of the subjects in the DSHPP + SoC group exhibited any difficulty swallowing. In contrast, two of the sixty-three subjects in the SoC alone group (3.17%) reported difficulties swallowing at the final visit (day 6). The difference between the two groups was not statistically significant at the final visit, as determined by a chi-square test ($p = 0.146$). Figure 3 presents the comparison of the means (SD) between administration groups for difficulty in swallowing ratings from the beginning of administration to the final visit. A statistically significant difference was observed only on visit day 4 ($p < 0.01$, Mann–Whitney U test).

TSS Salivation and Fever Sub-Score

The statistical analysis of these two parameters during the course of the study showed no statistically significant difference between the group treated with DSHPP + SoC and the group treated with SoC alone.

TSS Erythema Sub-Score

The balance between groups was not altered at baseline or at the start of the administration, indicating that the randomization between groups was properly executed ($p = 0.065$, Mann–Whitney U test). At the final visit, 46 of 63 subjects (73.0%) from the SoC group and 36 of the 66 subjects (54.5%) in the DSHPP + SoC group reported erythema. Figure 4 demonstrated that the difference between the two groups was statistically significant ($p = 0.030$, chi-square test).

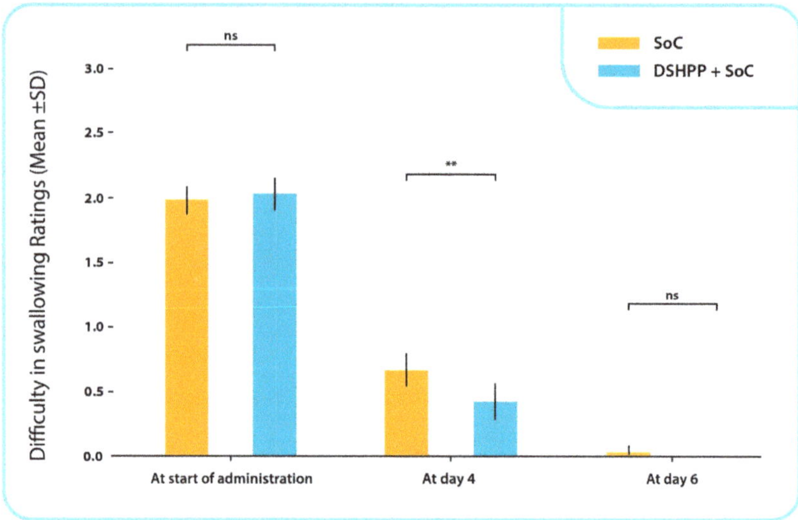

Figure 3. Difficulty in swallowing mean ± SD ratings with independent statistical tests between administration groups, from start of administration to final visit. ** $p < 0.01$; ns: non-significance.

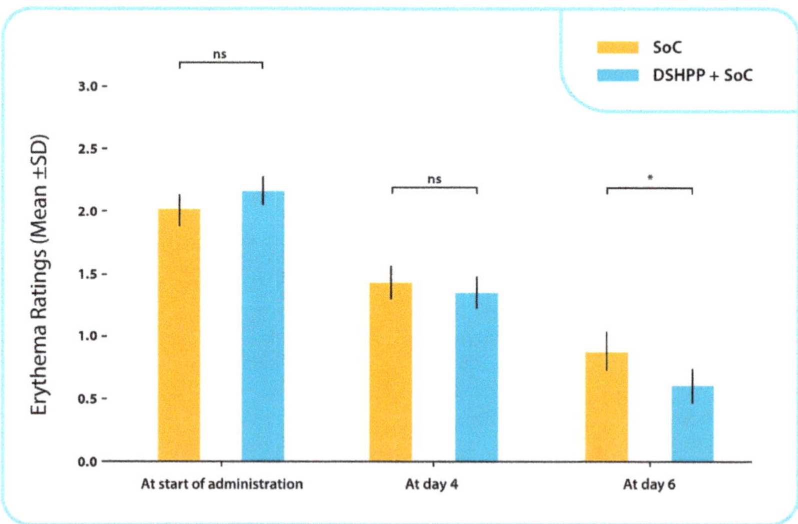

Figure 4. Erythema mean ± SD ratings from start of administration to final visit with chi-square test. * $p < 0.05$; ns: non-significance.

Use of Rescue Medications

The additional primary outcome was the use of rescue medications (ibuprofen and paracetamol above the limit as defined in the protocol of 30 mg/kg/dose) in the two groups and the resulting treatment failure. Only one patient in the SoC alone group received ibuprofen (1.6% of patients in the SoC alone group). The paracetamol doses administered to patients in both groups during the study were all below the threshold of 30 mg/kg/dose.

The mean (SD) paracetamol dose in the DSHPP + SoC group was 12.52 (2.83) mg/kg/dose, while the mean (SD) paracetamol dose in the SoC group was 12.79 (2.53) mg/kg/dose.

2.3.2. Secondary Outcomes

The secondary efficacy outcomes were the investigator global assessment (IGA) and the patient global assessment (PGA). A comparison was conducted for each of the parameters between the two groups at the final visit (Day 6).

IGA

Table 3 presents the IGA between groups on day 6. All subjects from the DSHPP + SoC group experienced high levels of treatment efficacy, with 83.3% rating it as very good and 16.7% rating it as good. Subjects from the SoC alone group rated the treatment as very good (58.7%), good (28.6%), and moderate (12.7%). The difference between the two groups was statistically significant (p = 0.04, chi-square test).

Table 3. Investigator global assessment (IGA) ratings in the two groups at final visit. p-values correspond to chi square tests.

IGA	Grade	DSHPP + SoC	SoC	p-Value
		66 (100.0%)	63 (100.0%)	
Subjects no. (%)	Very Good	55 (83.3%)	37 (58.7%)	0.040
	Good	11 (16.7%)	18 (28.6%)	
	Moderate	0 (0.0%)	8 (12.7%)	
	Poor	0 (0.0%)	0 (0.0%)	

PGA

The results of the PGA ratings indicate that none of the subjects in the DSHPP + SoC group reported poor treatment efficacy. In contrast, three (4.8%) subjects from the SoC alone group reported poor treatment efficacy. A statistically significant number of subjects (p = 0.013, chi square test) in the DSHPP + SoC group demonstrated superior treatment efficacy in comparison to those in the SoC alone group (Table 4).

Table 4. Patient global assessment (PGA) in the two groups at final visit. p-values correspond to chi square tests.

PGA	Grade	DSHPP + SoC	SoC	p-Value
		66 (100.0%)	63 (100.0%)	
Subjects no. (%)	Very Good	53 (80.3%)	35 (55.6%)	0.013
	Good	12 (18.2%)	19 (30.2%)	
	Moderate	1 (1.5%)	6 (9.5%)	
	Poor	0 (0.0%)	3 (4.8%)	

2.4. Safety

In both the DSHPP + SoC group and the SoC alone group, there were no adverse events (AEs) or serious adverse events (SAEs) reported by any children during the trial. Furthermore, a global evaluation of the safety of the treatment was conducted by the investigator at the conclusion of the study (Day 6). The ratings for the DSHPP + SoC group were 93.9% very good and 6.1% good, while the ratings for the SoC alone group were 55.6% very good and 30.2% good. The investigators did not record any concomitant medication.

3. Discussion

Our team has been trying for years to have a judicious antibiotic prescription for children with URTI [24]. In fact, we defined the child population in which we would avoid antibiotic prescriptions in our daily clinical practice as pediatricians, following international guidelines [24,25] that indicated stringent diagnostic criteria, weighing the benefits and harms of antibiotic therapy. The criteria we followed included as follows:

(1) ATR should be diagnosed early (possibly in the last 48 h) through clinical evaluation of symptoms, including sore throat and catarrhal angina.
(2) A negative result from a rapid test for group A beta-hemolytic *Streptococcus* (GABHS) or culture and the identification of nasal and/or pharyngeal exudate tests were mandatory.
(3) The severity of ATR should be clearly defined with the exclusion of cases with lacunar or follicular angina, indications for antibiotic therapy (i.e., abscess and septic tonsillitis), immunodeficiencies, and chronic illnesses.
(4) The exclusion of children under 3 years of age. This point was added because of the potential difficulty in justifying the exclusion of antibiotic therapy with the parents of infants of this age.

In general, the international guidelines [24,25] were characterized as follows:

- The target was the medical doctor visiting and treating children affected by URTI.
- The objective was to modify therapeutic strategies based on antibiotic prescription that have been proved to be not justified in the majority of cases
- The final result should be that thousands of medical doctors understand situations when antibiotics may not be indicated, and this should reduce the consumption of antibiotics inadequately administered to children.

Despite the efforts of scientific associations and institutions, incorrect antibiotic administration for URTI in children remains higher than the recommended benchmarks because of inappropriate prescribing habits [26]. In recent years, the medical literature has proposed a number of alternative strategies for achieving judicious antibiotic prescription in children with URTI. Some of these [27,28] involved Internet-based communication skills training in healthcare settings, which again were aimed solely at the prescribing physician. They obtained discrete success in reducing inappropriate antibiotic prescribing in adults, although they were not able to change the prescribing reality of antibiotic therapy in childhood URTIs. Other authors have based their work on the assumption that clinical uncertainty in primary care regarding the prognosis of children with respiratory tract infections contributes to the unnecessary use of antibiotics. Their aim was to reduce the misuse of antibiotic therapy in URTIs by improving the correct information aimed at the prescribing physician and focusing their task on equipping the physician with functional prognostic tools. An example of this approach was the RCT named CHICO, conducted with 294 GPs in the UK. The trial aimed to improve the early identification of children at low risk of future hospitalization to reduce clinical uncertainty [29]. The program utilized a web-based system with a prognostic algorithm to promptly identify children with acute cough and respiratory tract infections at low, average, or elevated risk of hospitalization in the next 30 days, accompanied by prescription guidance. The intervention was well received by GPs, but it did not alter prescribing habits, and antibiotic prescription rates remained largely unchanged. Kronman et al. [30] used a different approach, implementing the Dialogue Around Respiratory Illness Treatment (DART) quality improvement program. It was hypothesized that pairing Internet-based communication skills training with individualized antibiotic prescription audits and feedback would result in improved outcomes from 2015 to 2018 in 19 pediatric practices. The observed outcome (a 7% reduction in the probability of antibiotic prescription) is relatively modest, particularly when one considers the extensive resources deployed and the data regarding antibiotic prescription for *Streptococcal pharyngitis* (aRR 0.66; 95% CI, 0.50–0.87).

Finally, we believe that while communication, training, and information can be useful tools for improving the therapeutic strategies of physicians and increasing their prognostic ability, they are insufficient on their own. These approaches were designed to address the prescribing physicians alone. In our view, they should also engage the parents of children and even consider (in association with the traditional standard of care) the administration of new adjuvant tools that are accepted by both physicians and parents. Therefore, when the therapeutic strategy chosen by the clinician is not to use antibiotic therapy after performing a rapid test for GABHS, we believe that it is appropriate to flank the SoC already known to parents with other products that have been shown in clinical trials to have adjuvant action in total safety. The coordination carried out by the University of Timisoara (Romania) for the entire duration of the study and the supervision of Prof. Fabio Cardinale (Italy) were the fundamental key elements characterizing our research. The tested product (DSHPP) also has the advantage of being made up of ingredients such as honey and propolis, which are often used by parents themselves outside of prescription for their beneficial properties on the respiratory system. This can be an added advantage and ensure the maintenance of compliance, which is a prerequisite for the quick resolution of a child's disease.

4. Materials and Methods

4.1. Study Design

This multicenter, controlled, open-label, and randomized parallel-group superiority trial was conducted at three Romanian centers: Cabinet Medical Dr. Maria Morariu Bordea (Timișoara, Romania), Cabinet Medical Dr. Dorina Herteg (Timișoara), and Cabinet Medical Dr. Cristian Radu Matei (Otelu Rosu). The project team consisted of a scientific supervisor of the study, investigators, and was coordinated by the Academic Research Organization Department of Clinical Trials of the University of Medicine and Pharmacy Victor Babes. The contract research organization (CRO), Opera CRO, a Tigermed company based in Timișoara, Romania, was selected by the project team to manage the logistics and administration of the study. This included tasks such as protocol submission, project management, site monitoring, data management, and statistical analysis.

The project team created the study protocol following the methodology described by Fabio Cardinale et al., 2023 [31], and in accordance with the CONSORT-C Statement [32], which was specifically tailored for a trial involving a pediatric population. The study was registered at ClinicalTrials.gov (NCT04899401) and the overview of study methods (including ethics, design, randomization and allocation, setting, patient recruitment, inclusion and exclusion criteria, intervention and comparator, sample size calculation and statistical methods) was detailed in a recent publication [33].

Prior to the commencement of the trial, the protocol and related documents were submitted to the Romanian National Agency for Medicines and Medical Devices (ANSM) and were also approved by the local ethics committee (EC) of the involved centers (on 23 April and 27 April 2021).

The randomization procedure was executed through an internet-based platform provided by the CRO, accessible at all times. Patients were randomly assigned to either the control group, which received standard of care (SoC) alone, or the interventional group, which received DSHPP in addition to SoC. A non-involved staff member was responsible for carrying out the allocation process, without any input from the patients themselves. It should be noted that the patients' parents were not blinded to the randomization process.

4.2. Study Population

Only participants who were accompanied by their parents or caregivers to clinical sites from 6 June 2021 (start of enrollment) to 31 August 2021 (end of enrollment of 130 children) were eligible for the study. No additional recruitment efforts were made through the use of flyers, social media advertisements, or other promotional methods. The enrolled children must have been affected by ATR with a TSS score of at least 8 for no more than 48 h. They must also have had negative results on rapid tests for group A beta-haemolytic *Streptococcus* (GABHS) or negative culture and identification of nasal and/or pharyngeal exudates, and negative Severe Acute Respiratory Syndrome Coronavirus 2 (SARS-CoV-2) infection. Table 5 outlines the remaining inclusion and exclusion criteria.

Table 5. Study inclusion and exclusion criteria.

Inclusion Criteria	
1	Male and female (children aged 3 to 10 years).
2	Acute tonsillopharyngitis/rhinopharyngitis (ATR; sore throat, catarrhal angina), duration of symptoms $\leq$ 48 h.
3	Negative with rapid test for group A beta-hemolytic *Streptococcus* (GABHS) or culture and identification of nasal and/or pharyngeal exudates; negative for SARS-CoV-2 infection.
4	Tonsillitis symptom score (TSS) $\geq$ 8 points.
5	Both parents are willing to provide written informed consent prior to participation in the clinical trial.
6	Children older than 6 years must also have the ability and willingness to provide written informed consent.
Exclusion criteria	
1	Evidence of lacunar or follicular angina.
2	More than 2 past episodes of tonsillitis in the previous 12 months.
3	Mandatory indication for antibiotic therapy (e.g., abscess, septic tonsillitis, status postrheumatic fever, poststreptococcal glomerulonephritis, and minor Sydenham chorea).
4	Treatment with antibiotics within 4 months prior to study enrollment.
5	Hemorrhagic diathesis increases and chronic illnesses (e.g., severe heart, kidney, or liver disease, and primary or secondary immunodeficiencies).
6	Close contact history with individuals infected with SARS-CoV-2 within 10 days before showing symptoms.
7	Known or suspected allergic reactions to any study medication.
8	Concomitant therapy that may affect study results or have known interactions with study medications (such as coumarin derivatives).
9	Participation in another clinical trial within 3 months before enrollment.

Children who met all the study requirements were randomly assigned to either the DSHPP + SoC or SoC alone treatment arm and provided with the necessary products to complete the study. Parents were also instructed on how to follow the assigned treatment plan. Patients (by their parents or tutors) were permitted to withdraw from the trial at any time without providing a reason.

4.3. *Intervention Population*

4.3.1. Tested Product: DSHPP

The DSHPP tested is a dietary supplement already on the market in Italy as PediaFlù (Pediatrica Srl, Livorno, Italy). The formulation includes honey (5.5 g/100 mL), PropolNext Plus (equivalent to propolis, 7.7 mg/100 mL), Pelagon P-70 (equivalent to *Pelargonium sidoides*, 133.3 mg/100 mL), and zinc (13.3 mg/100 mL). DSHPP is supplied in the form of an oral solution. In the study DSHPP was administer it orally, at a dose of 5 mL, three times a day, for children under the age of 6 for a period of 6 days, while children over the age of 6 should take 10 mL, three times a day, for a period of 6 days. Due to concerns for patient safety, the investigator was authorized to discontinue the administration of DSHPP at any time and prescribe alternative treatments as needed for the patient's well-being.

4.3.2. Comparator: SoC

All patients included in the study were administered the SoC. This de facto included children assigned to the control group (who received SoC alone) and children assigned to the interventional group (who received SoC in addition to DSHPP).

The following products and treatments were administered as SoC:

- Nasopharyngeal lavage through the administration of hydrating fluids to facilitate the elimination of body fluids, along with the aspiration of secretions, saline solution for nasal irrigation and nasal sprays containing seawater.

- Paracetamol (acetaminophen) (120 mg/5 mL): as antipyretic (fever is defined as body temperature > 38.5 °C), as needed, 10 mg/kg/dose. The dosage was to be administered every 6 to 8 h, according to the leaflet. The maximum dosage was 30 mg/kg/day.
- Benzydamine hydrochloride was to be administered by throat sprays for 6 days in children under 6 years of age; the dosage was to be 1 spray per 4 kg of body weight, up to a maximum of 4 sprays at one time, 2 to 6 times daily. In children from 6 to 12 years, the benzydamine hydrochloride dosage was to be 4 sprays, administered two to six times daily. Each spray corresponds to 0.17 mL of solution.

4.3.3. Rescue Medication and Treatment Not Permitted

The administration of coumarin-based products and antibiotics was not permitted during the study.

Ibuprofen and paracetamol were the only permitted treatments in cases of necessity as rescue medications for the relief of severe symptoms of ATR. The following is a summary of the permitted treatments:

ibuprofen (100 mg/5 mL) orally;
high dose (>30 mg/kg/day) paracetamol (120 mg/5 mL) administered orally.

The use of rescue medication to a child was automatically classified as treatment failure.

4.4. Statistical Methods

4.4.1. Trial Hypothesis

We formulated a superiority hypothesis to assess whether symptoms in patients with ATR can be improved by a six-day course of DSHPP plus SoC compared with SoC alone. The primary hypothesis was that the minimal clinical difference between the test group (DSHPP + SoC) and the control group (SoC alone) should result in a two-point decrease in mean TSS after six days of treatment. The null hypothesis was that treatment with DSHPP + SoC would not result in a significant improvement in the symptoms of the treated patients compared to the control group (treated with SoC alone).

4.4.2. Sample Size Calculation

The sample size was determined based on the results of a prior study [21] that measured TSS as the primary outcome. The required sample size was calculated using the formula for comparing two means (two-sample) at a 5% significance level, 80% power, and a minimum clinically significant difference of 2 (SD 3.85 points). This indicated that 120 patients (130 with the estimated dropout) were required. To achieve this target, it was estimated that approximately 150 children should be screened.

4.4.3. Statistical Analyses

Categorical variables were described using frequencies and percentages, and comparative analyses were performed using the chi-squared test. Quantitative variables, if normally distributed, were described by means and standard deviations; non-normally distributed variables were described by medians and interquartile ranges. The Student's *t*-test and Mann–Whitney U test were used to perform comparative analyses according to the distribution of these variables. Factorial analysis of variance was employed to evaluate any interactions between quantitative variables and linear progression models, with the objective of identifying and addressing any potential confounding biases associated with the independent variables.

4.5. Evaluation Outcomes

4.5.1. Primary Outcomes

The primary efficacy outcomes were the change in TSS and the number of treatment failures between the two groups.

The TSS comprised five sub-scores: throat pain, difficulty in swallowing, salivation, pharyngeal erythema, and fever. The investigator evaluated and scored TSS at each visit as follows: throat pain, difficulty in swallowing, salivation, and pharyngeal erythema were rated on a scale of severe (3), moderate (2), mild (1), or absent (0), respectively. The investigator evaluated fever based on the following scale: The temperature scale is as follows: 37.5 °C to <38.5 °C = 1, 38.5 °C to <39.5 °C = 2, and ≥39.5 °C = 3. The results were compared in terms of the absolute change in the total score and for all sub-scores from baseline to the final visit.

The number of treatment failures was calculated by comparing the administration of rescue medications (ibuprofen and paracetamol > 30 mg/kg/dose) between the two groups.

4.5.2. Secondary Outcomes

The secondary efficacy outcomes were the investigator global assessment (IGA) and the patient global assessment (PGA). For both, the comparison was between groups at the end of the study period (Day 6). The investigator used a four-point scale, ranging from 1 (excellent) to 4 (poor), to assess the IGA. In contrast, the patient global assessment (PGA) was rated by patients on a 5-point scale, where 1 was defined as "very satisfied" and 5 as "very unsatisfied".

4.5.3. Safety

Any AE and SAE were recorded during the study to evaluate the incidence of AE/SAE. Furthermore, the investigators conducted a comprehensive assessment of the safety of the treatments using a four-point scale (1 = very good safety, 2 = good safety, 3 = moderate safety, and 4 = poor safety), with a comparison between groups at the conclusion of the trial.

4.5.4. Schedule of Examinations

Prior to initiating the study, the investigators informed each patient and their parent or legal guardian of the purpose and nature of the study, the potential risks and benefits, and requested consent by requiring them to sign an ICF. Furthermore, investigators provided the children with instructions on how to correctly respond to the tests, with a particular focus on the PGA. Finally, parents were requested to maintain a temperature log and report the usage of rescue medication in the patient diary during the study. Furthermore, it was emphasized that any unused medication be returned at the conclusion of the study and that the investigator be contacted in the event of an adverse event.

Table 6 outlines the schedule of examinations and procedures to be performed during the study period.

Table 6. Study schedule of examinations and procedures.

Time Point	Visit 1	Visit 2	Visit 3	Visit 4
	Day −2 to −1	Day 0	Day 4	Day 6
Informed consent	✓			
Inclusion criteria	✓			
Exclusion criteria	✓	✓	✓	✓
Demographics and medical history	✓			
Physical examination	✓	✓	✓	✓
Disease assessment	✓	✓	✓	✓
Rapid test for GABHS [a] or nasal and/or pharyngeal exudate culture plus SARS-CoV-2	✓			
Concomitant treatments	✓	✓	✓	✓
TSS [b]	✓	✓	✓	✓

Table 6. *Cont.*

Time Point	Visit 1	Visit 2	Visit 3	Visit 4
	Day −2 to −1	Day 0	Day 4	Day 6
Product delivery		✓		
Product return				✓
Subject diary delivery		✓		
Patient's diary verification			✓	
Subject diary return				✓
Products accountability				✓
IGA [c]				✓
PGA [d]				✓
Global assessment of the safety				✓
Adverse events	✓	✓	✓	✓

[a] GABHS: group A beta-hemolytic *Streptococcus*. [b] TSS: tonsillitis symptom score. [c] IGA: investigator global assessment. [d] PGA: patient global assessment.

5. Conclusions

The main limitation of this study is its open-label and controlled rather than double-blind design. This choice is motivated by logistical and economic reasons.

It is essential to highlight that our objective in this study was not merely to demonstrate that DSHPP associated with SoC will result in a clinical benefit. It was also crucial to prove that this administration was accompanied by optimal DSHPP compliance and safety, which are both essential requirements for a product to be administered to children. For this reason, our research hypothesis of associating the use of DSHPP with SoC may represent a potential alternative in the first-line treatment of acute respiratory tract infections, beyond the strict indication for antibiotic treatment, and can contribute to improving the judicious antibiotic prescription for children with URTI.

Author Contributions: F.C., D.F.B. and S.R. conceptualized the study. F.C., M.M.B., S.R. and D.F.B. were involved in the methodology. F.C., D.F.B. and S.R. were responsible for the formal analysis. The investigation during the study was performed by M.M.B.; F.C., S.R., D.F.B. and L.B. wrote the original draft, and F.C., S.R., D.F.B. and V.M. performed the review and editing of the manuscript. The visualization was created by L.B. and V.M. The project was supervised by F.C.; D.F.B. and V.M. were involved in the project's administration. All authors have read and agreed to the published version of the manuscript.

Funding: A grant support was received from Pediatrica S.r.l., Livorno, Italy (https://gruppopediatrica.it 3 June 2024). Pediatrica S.r.l. had no role in the study design, data collection and interpretation, or on the decision to submit the study results in abstract or paper for congress or publication.

Institutional Review Board Statement: The study was conducted in accordance with the Declaration of Helsinki and approved by the following ethics committees: Cabinet Medical Dr Cristian Radu Matei in Oțelu Roșu (Romania) on 23 April 2021 (OPPED/0120/FS); Cabinet Medical Medicina de Familie Dr. Morariu Bordea EC granted approval on 27 April 2021 (OPPED/0120/FS); Cabinet Medical Dr. Herteg Dorina EC approved on 27 April 2021 (OPPED/0120/FS).

Informed Consent Statement: Written informed consent was obtained from parents (or legal tutors) of all children involved in the study.

Data Availability Statement: The full protocol of the study has been deposited at Protocols.io [29]. The data sets analyzed for this study are available from the corresponding author upon request. The detailed description of the study protocol was recently published [31].

Acknowledgments: We thank Marius Ardelean for supporting us with the data management and statistical analysis.

Conflicts of Interest: D.F.B. is employed at Opera CRO, the contract research organization that managed the study. L.B. is employed at TIgermed Italy, the company that performed the data management of the study. V.M. is employed at Pediatrica S.r.l. F.C., S.R., and M.M.B. declare no conflicts of interest. The funder Pediatrica S.r.l., Livorno, Italy had no role in the design of the study; in the collection, analyses, or interpretation of data; in the writing of the manuscript; or in the decision to publish the results.

References

1. ESCMID Sore Throat Guideline Group; Pelucchi, C.; Grigoryan, L.; Galeone, C.; Esposito, S.; Huovinen, P.; Little, P.; Verheij, T. Guideline for the management of acute sore throat. *Clin. Microbiol. Infect.* **2012**, *18* (Suppl. S1), 1–28. [CrossRef]
2. Hersh, A.L.; Jackson, M.A.; Hicks, L.A.; American Academy of Pediatrics Committee on Infectious Diseases. Principles of judicious antibiotic prescribing for upper respiratory tract infections in pediatrics. *Pediatrics* **2013**, *132*, 1146–1154. [CrossRef]
3. Vicentini, C.; Vola, L.; Previti, C.; Brescia, V.; Dal Mas, F.; Zotti, C.M.; Bert, F. Antimicrobial Stewardship Strategies Including Point-of-Care Testing (POCT) for Pediatric Patients with Upper-Respiratory-Tract Infections in Primary Care: A Systematic Review of Economic Evaluations. *Antibiotics* **2022**, *11*, 1139. [CrossRef]
4. Yildiz, I.; Gonullu, E.; Soysal, A.; Oner, C.N.; Karabocuoglu, M. The Epidemiology of Influenza Virus Infection and Group A Streptococcal Pharyngitis in Children between 2011 and 2018 in an Outpatient Pediatric Clinic. *Cureus* **2023**, *15*, e33492. [CrossRef]
5. Hersh, A.L.; Shapiro, D.J.; Pavia, A.T.; Shah, S.S. Antibiotic prescribing in ambulatory pediatrics in the United States. *Pediatrics* **2011**, *128*, 1053–1061. [CrossRef]
6. Fleming-Dutra, K.E.; Hersh, A.L.; Shapiro, D.J.; Bartoces, M.; Enns, E.A.; File, T.M., Jr.; Finkelstein, J.A.; Gerber, J.S.; Hyun, D.Y.; Linder, J.A.; et al. Prevalence of inappropriate antibiotic prescriptions among US ambulatory care visits, 2010–2011. *JAMA* **2016**, *315*, 1864–1873. [CrossRef]
7. Al-Waili, N.; Al-Ghamdi, A.; Ansari, M.J.; Al-Attal, Y.; Salom, K. Synergistic effects of honey and propolis toward drug multi-resistant *Staphylococcus aureus*, *Escherichia coli* and *Candida albicans* isolates in single and polymicrobial cultures. *Int. J. Med. Sci.* **2012**, *9*, 793–800. [CrossRef]
8. Dimitriu, L.; Constantinescu-Aruxandei, D.; Preda, D.; Nichițean, A.-L.; Nicolae, C.-A.; Faraon, V.A.; Ghiurea, M.; Ganciarov, M.; Băbeanu, N.E.; Oancea, F. Honey and Its Biomimetic Deep Eutectic Solvent Modulate the Antioxidant Activity of Polyphenols. *Antioxidants* **2022**, *11*, 2194. [CrossRef]
9. Oduwole, O.; Udoh, E.E.; Oyo-Ita, A.; Meremikwu, M.M. Honey for acute cough in children. *Cochrane Database Syst. Rev.* **2018**, *4*, CD007094. [CrossRef]
10. Abuharfeil, N.; Al-Oran, R.; Abo-Shehada, M. The effect of bee honey on the proliferative activity of human B- and T lymphocytes and the activity of phagocytes. *Food Agric. Immunol.* **1999**, *11*, 169–177. [CrossRef]
11. Khan, R.U.; Naz, S.; Abudabos, A.M. Towards a better understanding of the therapeutic applications and corresponding mechanisms of action of honey. *Environ. Sci. Pollut. Res. Int.* **2017**, *24*, 27755–27766. [CrossRef]
12. Llor, C.; Moragas, A.; Ouchi, D.; Monfà, R.; Garcia-Sangenís, A.; Gómez-Lumbreras, A.; Pera, H.; Pujol, J.; Morros, R. Effectiveness of antitussives, anticholinergics, and honey versus usual care in adults with uncomplicated acute bronchitis: A multiarm randomized clinical trial. *Fam. Pr.* **2023**, *40*, 407–413. [CrossRef]
13. Nazari-Bonab, H.; Jamilian, P.; Radkhah, N.; Zarezadeh, M.; Ebrahimi-Mameghani, M. The effect of propolis supplementation in improving antioxidant status: A systematic review and meta-analysis of controlled clinical trials. *Phytother. Res.* **2023**, *37*, 3712–3723. [CrossRef]
14. Esposito, C.; Garzarella, E.U.; Bocchino, B.; D'Avino, M.; Caruso, G.; Buonomo, A.R.; Sacchi, R.; Galeotti, F.; Tenore, G.C.; Zaccaria, V.; et al. A standardized polyphenol mixture extracted from poplar-type propolis for remission of symptoms of uncomplicated upper respiratory tract infection (URTI): A monocentric, randomized, double-blind, placebo-controlled clinical trial. *Phytomedicine* **2021**, *80*, 153368. [CrossRef]
15. Crişan, I.; Zaharia, C.N.; Popovici, F.; Jucu, V.; Belu, O.; Dascălu, C.; Mutiu, A.; Petrescu, A. Natural propolis extract NIVCRISOL in the treatment of acute and chronic rhinopharyngitis in children. *Rom. J. Virol.* **1995**, *46*, 115–133.
16. Khayyal, M.T.; El-Ghazaly, M.A.; El-Khatib, A.S.; Hatem, A.M.; De Vries, P.J.F.; El-Shafei, S.; Khattab, M.M. A clinical pharmacological study of the potential beneficial effects of a propolis food product as an adjuvant in asthmatic patients. *Fundam. Clin. Pharmacol.* **2003**, *17*, 93–102. [CrossRef]
17. Buha, I.; Mirić, M.; Agić, A.; Simic, M.; Stjepanovic, M.; Milenkovic, B.; Nagorni-Obradovic, L.; Skodric-Trifunovic, V.; Ilic, B.; Popevic, S.; et al. A randomized, double-blind, placebo-controlled study evaluating the efficacy of propolis and N-acetylcysteine in exacerbations of chronic obstructive pulmonary disease. *Eur. Rev. Med. Pharmacol. Sci.* **2022**, *26*, 4809–4815. [CrossRef]
18. Kolarov, V.; Kotur Stevuljević, J.; Ilić, M.; Bogdan, M.; Tusek, B.; Agic, A.; Dugajlic, M.; Veres, K.T.; Stevic, S.K.; Zvezdin, B. Factorial analysis of N-acetylcysteine and propolis treatment effects on symptoms, life quality and exacerbations in patients with Chronic Obstructive Pulmonary Disease (COPD): A randomized, double-blind, placebo-controlled trial. *Eur. Rev. Med. Pharmacol. Sci.* **2022**, *26*, 3192–3199. [CrossRef]
19. Nault, D.; Machingo, T.A.; Shipper, A.G.; A Antiporta, D.; Hamel, C.; Nourouzpour, S.; Konstantinidis, M.; Phillips, E.; A Lipski, E.; Wieland, L.S. Zinc for prevention and treatment of the common cold. *Cochrane Database Syst. Rev.* **2024**, *5*, CD014914. [CrossRef]

20. Careddu, D.; Pettenazzo, A. *Pelargonium sidoides* extract EPs 7630: A review of its clinical efficacy and safety for treating acute respiratory tract infections in children. *Int. J. Gen. Med.* **2018**, *11*, 91–98. [CrossRef]
21. Bereznoy, V.V.; Riley, D.S.; Wassmer, G.; Heger, M. Efficacy of extract of *Pelargonium sidoides* in children with acute non-group A beta-hemolytic *Streptococcus* tonsillopharyngitis: A randomized, double-blind, placebo-controlled trial. *Altern. Ther. Health Med* **2003**, *9*, 68–79.
22. Nöldner, M.; Schötz, K. Inhibition of lipopolysaccharid-induced sickness behavior by a dry extract from the roots of *Pelargonium sidoides* (EPs 7630) in mice. *Phytomedicine* **2007**, *14* (Suppl. S6), 27–31. [CrossRef]
23. Kolodziej, H. Antimicrobial, Antiviral and Immunomodulatory Activity Studies of *Pelargonium sidoides* (EPs® 7630) in the Context of Health Promotion. *Pharmaceuticals* **2011**, *4*, 1295–1314. [CrossRef]
24. Shulman, S.T.; Bisno, A.L.; Clegg, H.W.; Gerber, M.A.; Kaplan, E.L.; Lee, G.; Martin, J.M.; Van Beneden, C. Infectious Diseases Society of America. Clinical practice guideline for the diagnosis and management of group A streptococcal pharyngitis: 2012 update by the Infectious Diseases Society of America. *Clin. Infect. Dis.* **2012**, *55*, e86–e102, Erratum in *Clin. Infect. Dis.* **2014**, *58*, 1496. [CrossRef]
25. Sauve, L.; Forrester, A.M.; Top, K.A. Group A streptococcal pharyngitis: A practical guide to diagnosis and treatment. *Paediatr. Child Health* **2021**, *26*, 319–320. [CrossRef]
26. Baillie, E.J.; Merlo, G.; Magin, P.; Tapley, A.; Mulquiney, K.J.; Davis, J.S.; Fielding, A.; Davey, A.; Holliday, E.; Ball, J.; et al. Antibiotic prescribing for upper respiratory tract infections and acute bronchitis: A longitudinal analysis of general practitioner trainees. *Fam. Pract.* **2022**, *39*, 1063–1069. [CrossRef]
27. Butler, C.C.; Simpson, S.A.; Dunstan, F.; Rollnick, S.; Cohen, D.; Gillespie, D.; Evans, M.R.; Alam, M.F.; Bekkers, M.J.; Evans, J.; et al. Effectiveness of multifaceted educational programme to reduce antibiotic dispensing in primary care: Practice based randomised controlled trial. *BMJ* **2012**, *344*, d8173. [CrossRef]
28. Little, P.; Stuart, B.; Francis, N.; Douglas, E.; Tonkin-Crine, S.; Anthierens, S.; Cals, J.W.; Melbye, H.; Santer, M.; Moore, M.; et al. Effects of internet-based training on antibiotic prescribing rates for acute respiratory-tract infections: A multinational, cluster, randomised, factorial, controlled trial. *Lancet* **2013**, *382*, 1175–1182. [CrossRef]
29. Blair, P.S.; Young, G.J.; Clement, C.; Dixon, P.; Seume, P.; Ingram, J.; Taylor, J.; Horwood, J.; Lucas, P.J.; Cabral, C.; et al. A multifaceted intervention to reduce antibiotic prescribing among CHIldren with acute COugh and respiratory tract infection: The CHICO cluster RCT. *Health Technol. Assess.* **2023**, *27*, 1–110. [CrossRef]
30. Kronman, M.P.; Gerber, J.S.; Grundmeier, R.W.; Zhou, C.; Robinson, J.D.; Heritage, J.; Stout, J.; Burges, D.; Hedrick, B.; Warren, L.; et al. Reducing Antibiotic Prescribing in Primary Care for Respiratory Illness. *Pediatrics* **2020**, *146*, e20200038. [CrossRef]
31. Cardinale, F.; Barattini, D.F.; Morariu Bordea, M.; Herteg, D.; Matei, C.R. A Randomized, Open, Controlled Study to Evaluate the Efficacy and Safety of Pediaflù® (Dietary Supplement) Along with Standard of Care in Children with Acute Tonsillopharyngitis/Rhinopharyngitis versus Standard of Care Only V.1. 2023. Available online: https://www.protocols.io/view/a-randomized-open-controlled-study-to-evaluate-the-kqdg398oqg25/v1 (accessed on 3 June 2024).
32. Saint-Raymond, A.; Hill, S.; Martines, J.; Bahl, R.; Fontaine, O.; Bero, L. CONSORT 2010. *Lancet* **2010**, *376*, 229–230. [CrossRef]
33. Cardinale, F.; Barattini, D.F.; Sbrocca, F.; Centi, A.; Giuntini, G.; Morariu Bordea, M.; Herteg, D.; Rosu, S.; Matei, C.R. The Effects of a Dietary Supplement (PediaFlu) Plus Standard of Care in Children with Acute Tonsillopharyngitis/Rhinopharyngitis: Protocol for a Randomized Controlled Trial. *JMIR Res. Protoc.* **2024**, *13*, e53703. [CrossRef]

pharmaceuticals

Article

Antitumor Effects and the Potential Mechanism of 10-HDA against SU-DHL-2 Cells

Yuanyuan Tian [1,2,†], Xiaoqing Liu [1,†], Jie Wang [1], Chuang Zhang [1] and Wenchao Yang [1,*]

1 College of Bee Science and Biomedicine, Fujian Agriculture and Forestry University, Fuzhou 350002, China; tianyuan4601@126.com (Y.T.); lxq7597@163.com (X.L.); wangjie01092023@163.com (J.W.); chuangzhang12@163.com (C.Z.)
2 College of JunCao Science and Ecology (College of Carbon Neutrality), Fujian Agriculture and Forestry University, Fuzhou 350002, China
* Correspondence: beesyang@gmail.com or 000q061005@fafu.edu.cn
† These authors contributed equally to this work.

Abstract: 10-hydroxy-2-decenoic acid (10-HDA), which is a unique bioactive fatty acid of royal jelly synthesized by nurse bees for larvae and adult queen bees, is recognized for its dual utility in medicinal and nutritional applications. Previous research has indicated that 10-HDA exerts antitumor effects on numerous tumor cell lines, including colon cancer cells, A549 human lung cancer cells, and human hepatoma cells. The present study extends this inquiry to lymphoma, specifically evaluating the impact of 10-HDA on the SU-DHL-2 cell line. Our findings revealed dose-dependent suppression of SU-DHL-2 cell survival, with an IC_{50} of 496.8 μg/mL at a density of 3×10^6 cells/well after 24 h. For normal liver LO2 cells and human fibroblasts (HSFs), the IC_{50} values were approximately 1000 μg/mL and over 1000 μg/mL, respectively. The results of label-free proteomics revealed 147 upregulated and 347 downregulated differentially expressed proteins that were significantly enriched in the complement and coagulation cascades pathway (adjusted p-value = 0.012), including the differentially expressed proteins prothrombin, plasminogen, plasminogen, carboxypeptidase B2, fibrinogen beta chain, fibrinogen gamma chain, and coagulation factor V. The top three hub proteins, ribosomal protein L5, tumor protein p53, and ribosomal protein L24, were identified via protein–protein interaction (PPI) analysis. This result showed that the complement and coagulation cascade pathways might play a key role in the antitumor process of 10-HDA, suggesting a potential therapeutic avenue for lymphoma treatment. However, the specificity of the effect of 10-HDA on SU-DHL-2 cells warrants further investigation.

Keywords: survival; 10-HDA; SU-DHL-2 cell; label-free proteomics; complement and coagulation cascades pathway

1. Introduction

Cancer remains a significant global health challenge, with an estimated 10 million fatalities in 2020, representing approximately one-sixth of all deaths, primarily due to prevalent malignancies such as breast, lung, colorectal, and prostate cancers [1]. Annually, diffuse large B-cell lymphoma (DLBCL) affects approximately 25,000 individuals worldwide, accounting for approximately 30% of non-Hodgkin lymphoma cases [2,3]. The etiology of DLBCL is multifactorial, with contributing factors ranging from genetic predispositions and viral infections (such as EBV) to environmental exposures such as agricultural pesticides and ionizing radiation, as well as physiological factors such as immunodeficiency and increased body mass index in young adults [4,5]. Over 60% of patients achieve remission through R-CHOP immunochemotherapy (including rituximab, cyclophosphamide, doxorubicin, vincristine, and prednisone), but other patients suffer from refractory or relapsed disease due to resistance to R-CHOP [4]. Consequently, extensive research efforts are dedicated to advancing DLBCL treatment modalities in clinical settings. The quest for safer therapeutics has propelled natural and dietary compounds to the forefront as promising substitutes for traditional chemotherapeutic agents. These endeavors include exploring the efficacy of chimeric antigen receptor (CAR) T cells, bispecific T-cell engagers, immunomodulatory drugs, checkpoint inhibitors, monoclonal antibodies, antibody–drug conjugates, targeted molecular pathway inhibitors, selective nuclear export inhibitors such as selinexor, and agents that modify epigenetic regulation [6,7].

Advances in the treatment of DLBCL have been marked by the exploration of novel therapeutic strategies and drug development. Recent studies have demonstrated that the combination of enzastaurin, a selective protein kinase C inhibitor, and ibrutinib, a Bruton's tyrosine kinase inhibitor, synergistically impedes DLBCL cell survival and proliferation. This synergy manifests as reduced cell proliferation, enhanced apoptosis, G1 phase arrest, and diminished cell invasion, migration, and downstream signaling of ERK, mTOR, and PLCγ2 phosphorylation [8]. In addition, the novel synthetic compound BR101801, a dual inhibitor targeting DNA-PK and PI3Kδ combined with rafoxanide, has exhibited antitumor effects on DLBCL cells both in vitro and in vivo [9,10]. Various agents, including curcumin, 25-hydroxyvitamin D, disulfide, the survivin suppressant YM155, miR-145-5p overexpression, and quinacrine, have been shown to exert antitumor effects on DLBCL cells through distinct mechanisms. Specifically, curcumin impedes the proliferation of DLBCL subtypes by inducing G2 phase arrest and modulating the PPARγ and Akt/mTOR pathways [11]. According to meta-analytical data, elevated levels of 25-hydroxyvitamin D correlate with reduced cancer incidence and mortality [12]. Disulfide promotes apoptosis and cell cycle arrest at the G0/G1 phase in various DLBCL cell lines by inhibiting the NF-κB signaling pathway [13]. YM155 effectively inhibits the growth of several DLBCL cell lines by inducing apoptosis [14]. The upregulation of miR-145-5p has been shown to antagonize tumor growth by affecting the S1PR1/STAT3/AKT pathway [15]. Finally, quinacrine induces G0/G1 cell cycle arrest and apoptosis through the MSI2-NUMB signaling pathway in a dose-dependent manner [16]. These findings underscore the heterogeneous nature of DLBCL and the potential for targeted therapies to exploit distinct molecular vulnerabilities.

Bee products, including honey, propolis, bee pollen, bee venom, royal jelly, bee bread, beeswax, queen bee larvae, and drone pupa, are considered important natural products and functional foods due to their nutritional value and remarkable biological activities. Compared with Tualang honey (made by *Apis dorsata*), manuka honey has been shown to exert an inhibitory effect on the progression of N-methyl-N-nitrosourea-induced breast cancer [17]. This inhibition encompasses a reduction in the grade, size, angiogenesis, and vascular endothelial growth factor levels in MCF-7 and MDA-MB-231 breast cancer cell lines induced by 7,12-dimethylbenz(a)anthracene [18,19]. Additionally, the antioxidants present in Iranian natural honey counteract croton oil-mediated skin carcinogenesis [20]. A spectrum of cancer cell lines, including human hepatocellular carcinoma (HepG2) [21], colon cancer HT-29 [22], prostate cancer (PC-3) [23], bladder cancer (RT4, T24, 253J, and murine MBT-2) [24], pancreatic cancer (MIA PaCa-2 and BxPC-3) [25], lung cancer (NCI-H460) [26], melanoma (human A375, B16-F1, and B16-F murine) [27,28], renal cell carcinoma (786-O and 769-P) [29], and both acute and chronic leukemia (K562 and MV4-11) [30], have been reported to respond to the anticancer effects of honey. However, certain types of honey have been shown to have dual impacts on the viability of MCF-7 cells [31], potentially attributable to variations in the concentration of phenolic compounds [32]. These findings suggest a complex interaction between honey constituents and cancer cell dynamics, warranting further investigation to elucidate the mechanisms involved and optimize the therapeutic potential of honey in oncology.

Propolis, which is synthesized by *Apis mellifera* from various plant exudates and subsequently enriched with salivary enzymes, stands out for its pronounced anticancer properties. Research has consistently demonstrated the efficacy of propolis and its bioactive constituents in inhibiting the proliferation of a diverse array of human cancer cell lines, including those from oral, gastric, cervical, and colon cancers, as well as leukemia, skin, breast, prostate, lung, colorectal, urological, and lymphoma origins [33–38]. Bee pollen, composed of plant pollen collected by worker bees, also exhibits significant antitumor activity. It has been shown to combat a spectrum of cancers, including those of the prostate, breast, lung, stomach, liver, cervix, and ovary [39,40]. Bee venom, which is secreted by the venom glands of worker bees, is another potent inhibitor of cancerous growth and is effective against a variety of cell lines, such as those from breast, liver, melanoma, ovarian, lung, glioblastoma, gastric, hepatocellular carcinoma, leukemia, prostate, pancreatic, and non-small cell lung cancers [41]. Royal jelly is distinguished by its content of 10-HDA, a fatty acid implicated in its pharmacological activity (Figure 1) [42]. The antitumor potential of 10-HDA has been extensively documented across several cancer types, including colon, lung, hepatoma, melanoma, skin, breast, leukemia, and various murine models, as well as in clinical observations of renal carcinoma patients [42–50]. Nevertheless, the specific antitumor mechanisms and effects of 10-HDA on SU-DHL-2 cells remain to be elucidated.

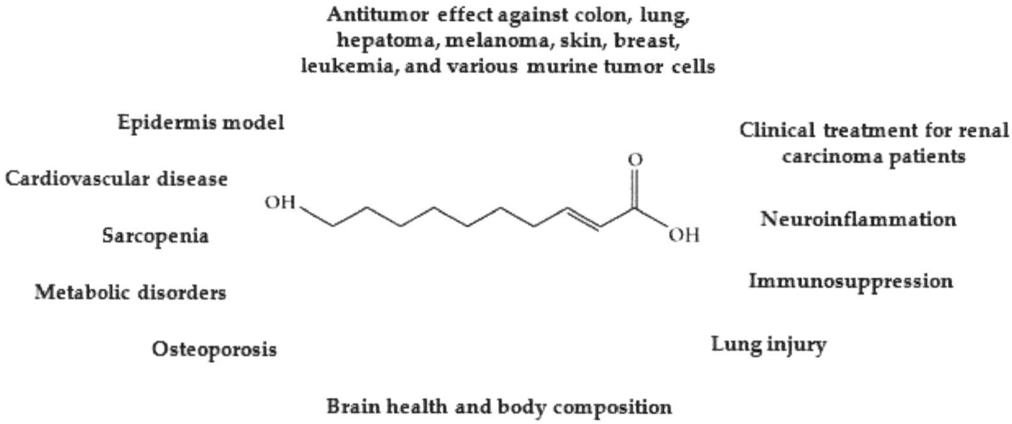

Figure 1. The structure and pharmacological properties of 10-hydroxy-2-decenoic acid (10-HDA).

To address this knowledge gap, we aimed to understand the link between the inhibitory effect of 10-HDA on SU-DHL-2 cells in vitro on cell survival, changes in protein expression determined using label-free proteomics, related gene expression trends, and conduction pathways.

2. Results

2.1. The Inhibitory Effects of 10-HDA on the Survival of SU-DHL-2 Cells

The control solvent (a complete culture medium with 0.02% ethanol, volume/volume) had no inhibitory effect on the survival of the SU-DHL-2 cells. However, significant inhibitory effects were observed in cells treated with 10-HDA at 250, 500, and 750 μg/mL ($p < 0.01$). Notably, there was no significant difference in cell death between the 750 μg/mL group and the 1000 μg/mL 10-HDA group. The data indicated that 10-HDA dose-dependently suppressed SU-DHL-2 cell survival (Figure 2A). The half-maximal inhibitory concentration (IC_{50}) for SU-DHL-2 cells was determined to be 496.8 μg/mL after a 24 h incubation period.

At concentrations up to 600 μg/mL, 10-HDA did not exhibit cytotoxic effects but promoted survival in the standard liver cell line LO2, with an IC_{50} value of approximately 1000 μg/mL (Figure 2B). Similarly, no cytotoxicity was observed at concentrations up to 800 μg/mL in normal human fibroblast HSFs (Figure 2C, $F_{(5, 12)} = 2.473$, $p = 0.0923$).

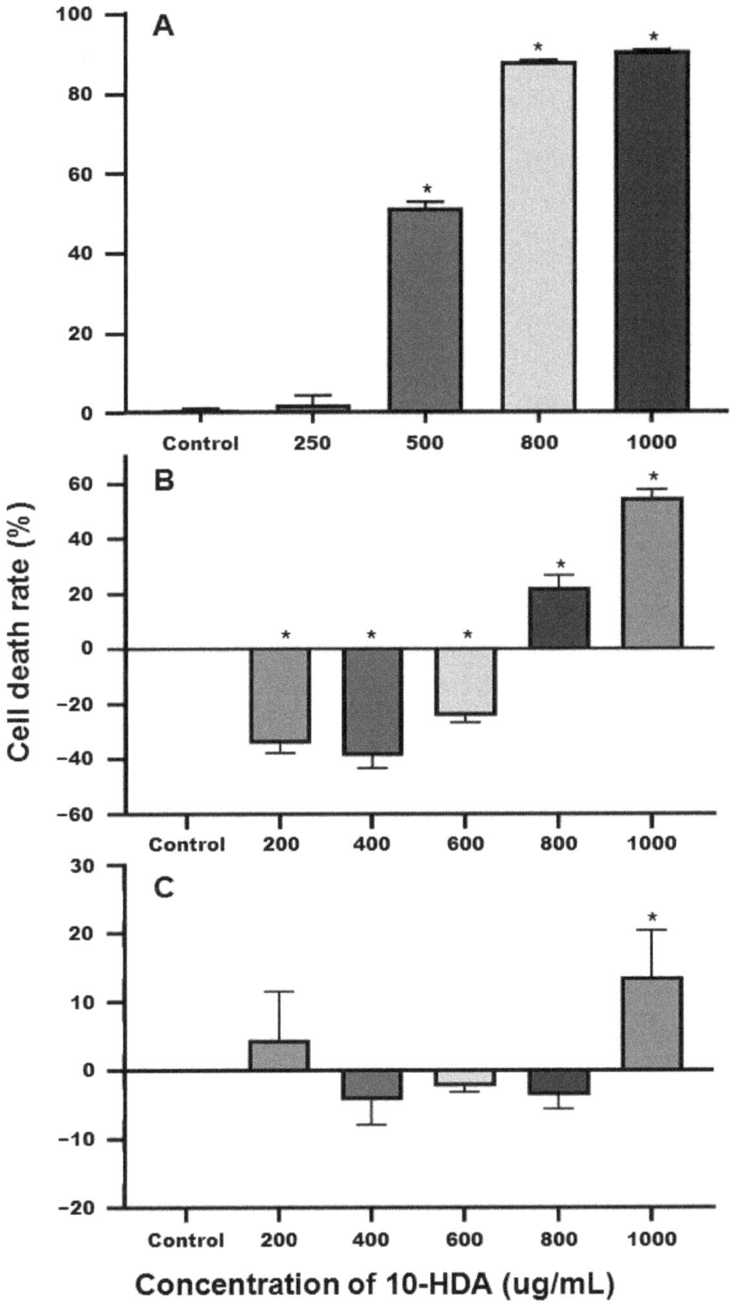

Figure 2. Cell death (%) of SU-DHL-2 cells (**A**), LO2 normal liver cells (**B**), and HSF normal human fibroblasts (**C**) treated with different concentrations of 10-HDA for 24 h. * indicates significant differences between the cell death rates of the treatment and control groups.

2.2. Differentially Expressed Proteins in Treated Cells

The results of the label-free proteomic analysis of SU-DHL-2 cells treated with the solvent control and the IC_{50} of 10-HDA (496.8 μg/mL) are shown in Figure 3 as a volcano plot. This analysis revealed 147 proteins with significantly increased expression and 347 proteins with decreased expression. Additionally, 3405 proteins exhibited no significant change in their expression levels.

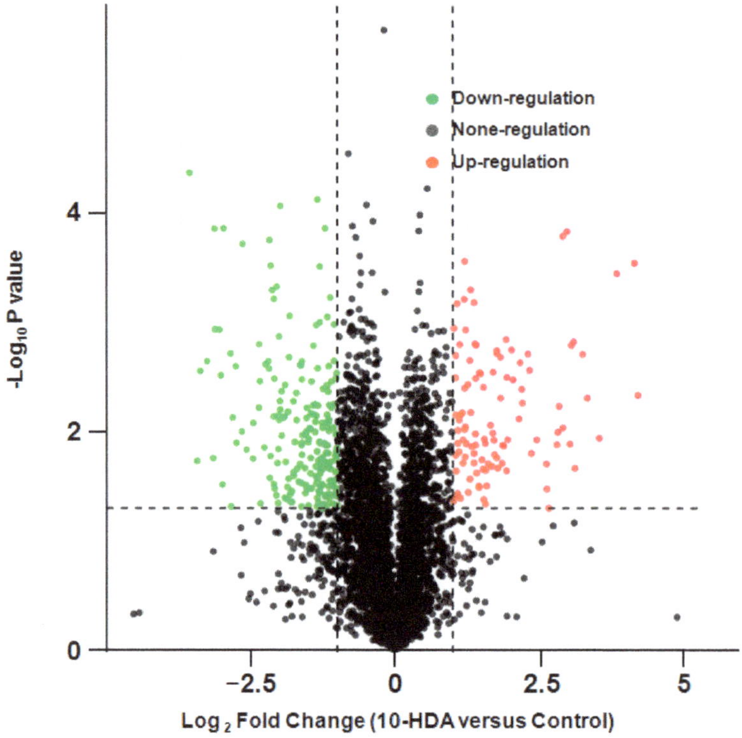

Figure 3. Volcano map of comparative protein expression determined using the label-free proteomic assay in SU-DHL-2 cells treated with 10-HDA (at the IC50 concentration) and untreated cells. Red dots represent significantly upregulated proteins, green dots represent significantly downregulated proteins, and black dots represent proteins whose expression did not significantly change.

DEPs were mainly located in the nucleus (41.85%), cytoplasm (14.77%), mitochondria (11.38%), plasma membrane (6.46%), endoplasmic reticulum (5.54%), Golgi apparatus (4.92%), cytoskeleton (4.92%), lysosome (3.69%), extracellular space (3.08%), endosome (1.23%), centrosome (0.92%), peroxisome (0.62%), synapse (0.31%), and microsome (0.31%).

Gene Ontology (GO) enrichment analysis revealed that 93 DEPs were enriched in biological process, 28 DEPs in cellular component, and 113 DEPs in molecular function, of which 22 biological terms were significantly enriched ($p < 0.05$), as illustrated in Figure 4. The 'response to stress' category encompassed the greatest number of DEPs, with eight downregulated proteins and two upregulated proteins, followed by the 'cell cycle' category, which included seven downregulated DEPs and one upregulated DEP, and the 'endoplasmic reticulum' category, which included five downregulated DEPs and two upregulated DEPs.

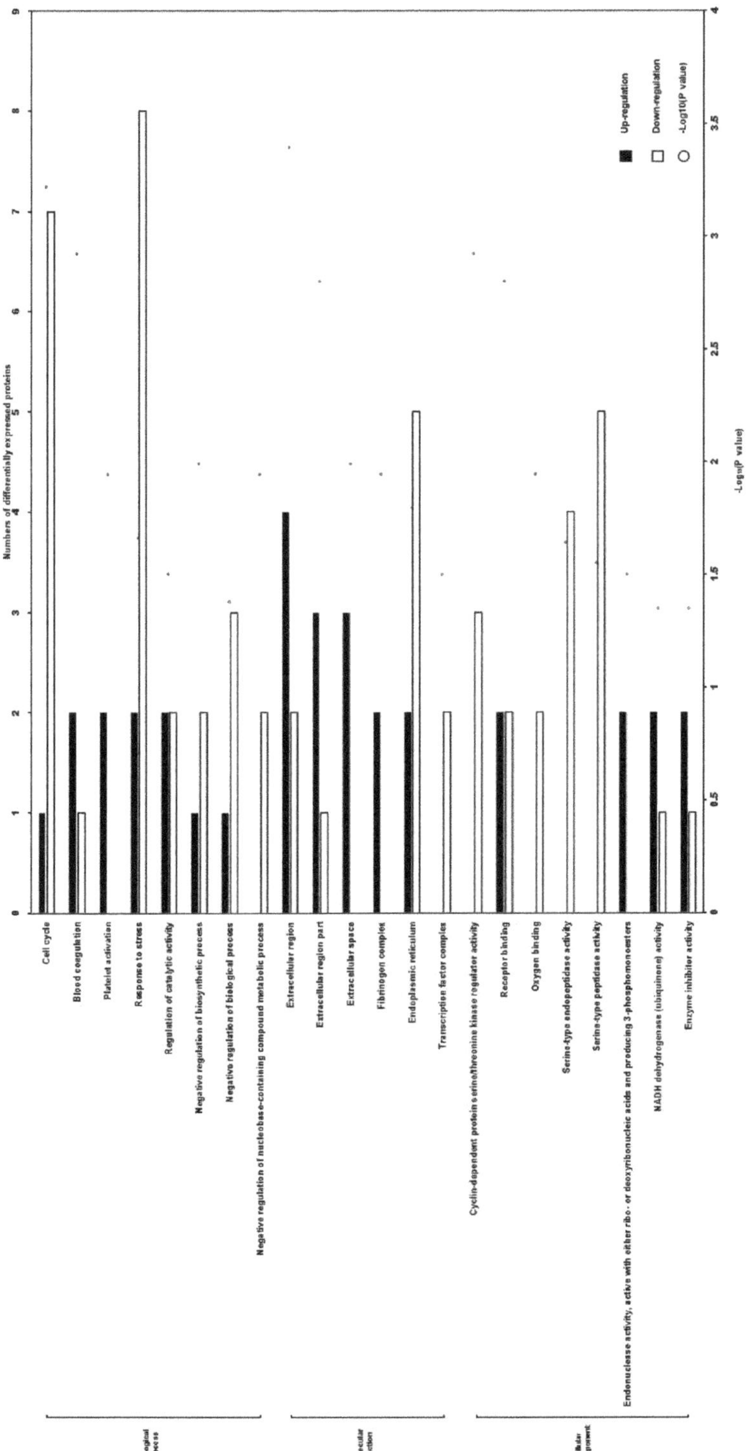

Figure 4. The GO enrichment terms of differentially expressed proteins ($p < 0.05$). The black and white bars indicate the number of upregulated or downregulated differentially expressed proteins in one term, respectively. The circles indicate the $-\log_{10}$ (p-value).

Kyoto Encyclopedia of Genes and Genomes (KEGG) pathway enrichment analysis revealed a significant difference in the DEPs in a distinct pathway, namely, the complement and coagulation cascades pathway (adjusted $p < 0.05$, Table 1); other pathways showed no significant difference (adjusted $p > 0.05$).

Table 1. The DEPs were enriched in significantly different pathways ($p < 0.05$).

Pathway	*p*-Value	Adjusted *p*-Value	Differentially Expressed Proteins	
			Upregulated	Downregulated
Complement and coagulation cascades	4.9×10^{-5}	0.0124	A0A0A0MRJ7, P02675, C9JC84	P00734, A0A0F7G8J1, B2R7F8, Q96IY4
Basal cell carcinoma	0.0013	0.1615	A0A3B3ITW1, Q92466, Q6TKP8	A0A0U1RQC9
Mineral absorption	0.0028	0.2324	B2R7U4, P02795, P04733, A0A140VJP7	A0A0U1RQC9
Neuroactive ligand–receptor interaction	0.0037	0.2360	-	P00734, A0A0F7G8J1, B2R7F8
Pathways in cancer	0.0131	0.5780	K7EP08, P15559, A0A3B3ITW1, B2R7U4, P02751, A0A024R728, Q92466, P63218, Q6TKP8, A0A2 × 0SFF5	B3KT21, A0A0U1RQC9, Q9HAV0, U6FVB0, X5D945, P11802, A8K725, P33552, A0A024R8H5, Q5T178, A0A024QYW7, B3KNJ3
Small-cell lung cancer	0.0147	0.5780	P02751, Q92466	A0A0U1RQC9, P11802, P33552, A0A024R8H5, Q5T178
Staphylococcus aureus infection	0.0161	0.5780	C9JC84	A0A0F7G8J1, B2R7F8
Pyrimidine metabolism	0.0210	0.6627	P36954	P23921, D6W4Z6, Q9BZX2, A0A024R8N6, O14802, A0A5F9ZHU7, P56282, Q3B726, Q9NR33, Q7Z3R8, A8K9A5
Melanoma	0.0285	0.7929	A0A024R728, Q92466	A0A0U1RQC9, X5D945, P11802
Thyroid cancer	0.0346	0.7929	Q92466	A0A0U1RQC9, U6FVB0, X5D945
Bladder cancer	0.0346	0.7929	-	A0A0U1RQC9, X5D945, P11802, B3KNJ3

The PPI network of the DEPs with interaction scores exceeding 0.9 is depicted in Figure 5. The most prominent nodes within this network were represented by ribosomal protein L5, which interacts with 13 other proteins. This interaction was closely followed by the interaction of the tumor protein p53 with 12 proteins and the ribosomal protein L24 with 9 proteins.

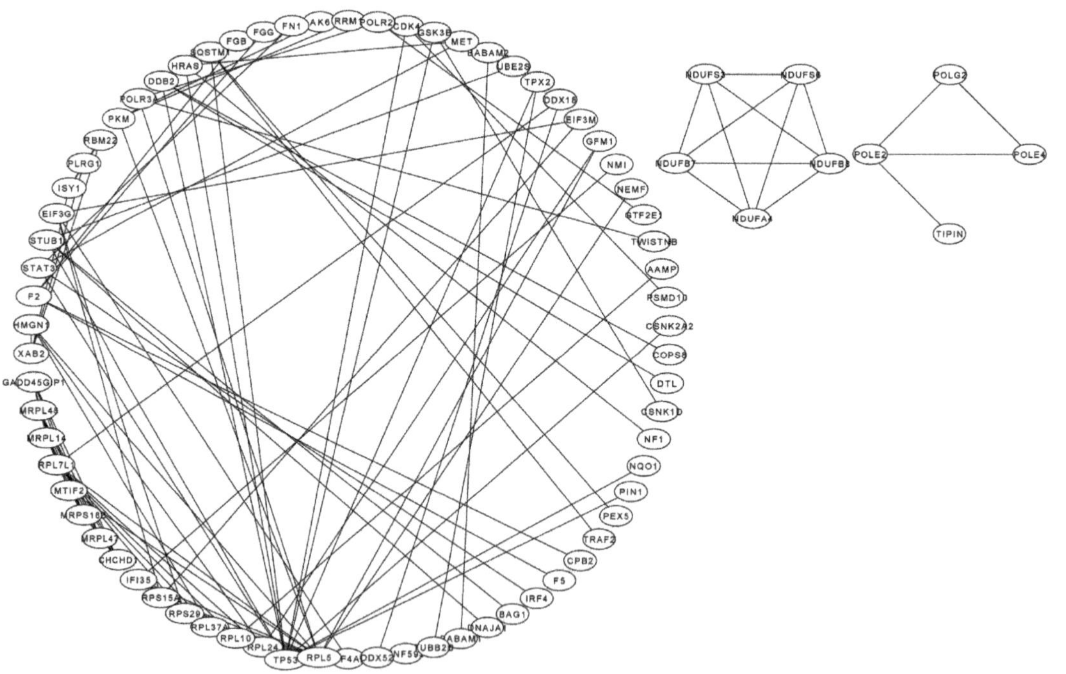

Figure 5. Protein–protein interactions of differentially expressed proteins (interaction score > 0.9). The characters indicate the gene names of differentially expressed proteins, and the lines between genes indicate that the differentially expressed proteins interact.

2.3. Relative Expression of Selected Genes

Figure 6 shows the relative expression levels of the selected genes. The genes *HO-1, NQO1, HSP70, P62, CD274, CDH1, FTH1*, and *GCLC* exhibited upregulated expression. In contrast, the genes *PLK1, BUB1B, FN1, P53, Cyclin B, Cyclin D*, and *Caspase 3* exhibited downregulated expression.

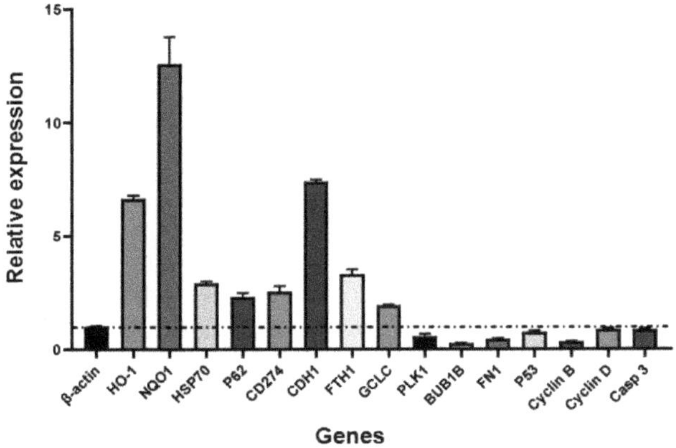

Figure 6. The relative expression of genes. Genes with a relative expression greater than 1 (dashed line) were upregulated, and those with a relative expression less than 1 were downregulated.

3. Discussion

The antitumor efficacy of 10-HDA has been documented across various cancer cell lines. The variability in IC_{50} values across different cancer cell lines and normal cell lines (Table 2) likely reflects the heterogeneity in cell density, determination methods, and differential sensitivity to 10-HDA [51,52]. A concentration of 200 μg/mL 10-HDA was found to be noncytotoxic to rat T cells from immunized animals (3×10^5 cells/well for 4 days) according to a 3H-thymidine incorporation assay [51]. In the present study, the IC_{50} values for 10-HDA in normal liver cells (LO2) and HSF were approximately 1000 μg/mL and over 1000 μg/mL, respectively, as displayed in Figure 2B,C. Further experiments on the cytotoxicity of 10-HDA against other normal cell lines should be performed.

Table 2. The IC_{50}s values of 10-HDA in different cell lines.

Cell Type	Cell Line	IC_{50} Value (μg/mL)	Method	References
Lung cancer cell	A549	4.22	CCK-8	[43]
Lung cancer cell	NCI-H460	8.20	CCK-8	[43]
Lung cancer cell	NCI-H23	8.34	CCK-8	[43]
Human hepatoma cell	HepG2	59.6	MTT	[44]
Human colorectal adenocarcinoma cell	CaCo-2	37.5	MTT	[50]
Breast cancer cell	MDA-MB231	651.88	-	[53]
Breast cancer cell	MDA-MB436	949.88	-	[53]
Breast cancer cell	HCC1937	979.68	-	[53]
Breast cancer cell	MCF-7	972.225	-	[53]
Human epithelial breast cell	MCF-10a	931.25	-	[53]
Human normal liver cell line	THLE-3	106.4	MTT	[44]
African green monkey kidney cell	Vero	3445.63	-	[53]
Fibroblast	NIH3T3 (Wt)	1862.5	-	[53]
Fibroblast	BRAF V600E mutation	1303.75	-	[53]
SIRC (Statens Seruminstitut Rabbit Cornea) cell	SIRC	2.38	MTT	[52]

The survival inhibition mechanisms of 10-HDA against cancer cell lines appear to be multifaceted and influenced by the diversity of cancer types and the respective cell lines. Proteomic technology, a critical tool in contemporary research, has been extensively utilized to identify differentially expressed proteins in response to various treatments [37,54–56]. In SU-DHL-2 cells treated with 10-HDA, 494 DEPs were identified, 147 of which were upregulated and 347 of which were downregulated. KEGG pathway enrichment analysis revealed a significant association of these DEPs with the complement and coagulation cascades pathway (adjusted $p < 0.05$), and nonsignificant differences in the other pathways are depicted in Table 2.

This particular pathway is integral to the survival inhibition of SU-DHL-2 cells, notably influencing the transport mechanisms of the protein corona associated with magnetic PEI/siRNA complexes [57]. Furthermore, comprehensive serum proteomic analyses have underscored the importance of this pathway in the pathophysiology of meningioma, as evidenced by studies across various grades of the disease using multiple quantitative proteomic and immunoassay-based methodologies [58]. Similarly, quantitative proteomic analysis has highlighted the complement and coagulation cascades pathway as a significant factor in epithelial ovarian cancer [59], malignant ascites in hepatocellular carcinoma [60], and other malignancies, including hepatocellular carcinoma [60–62], bladder cancer [63], and ovarian cancer [64], as determined through bioinformatics analyses.

Additionally, this pathway has been identified as a potential biomarker for predicting the response to immunotherapy in patients with metastatic urothelial cancer [65], further demonstrating its relevance in cancer treatment strategies. The breadth of evidence across various cancer types underscores the ubiquitous role of this pathway in tumor biology and its potential as a therapeutic target.

DEPs associated with the complement and coagulation cascades pathway include vital factors such as prothrombin, various plasminogen isoforms, carboxypeptidase B2, fibrinogen beta and gamma chains, and coagulation factor V. Prothrombin, a critical plasma glycoprotein, comprises a gamma-carboxyglutamic acid (Gla) domain, two kringle domains, and a serine protease domain and is essential for blood coagulation. Recombinant human prothrombin kringles 1, 2, and 1-2 (rk-1, -2, -1-2) have been shown to inhibit tumor growth and metastasis in Lewis lung carcinoma [66]. Genetic ablation of the prothrombin gene in mice is associated with embryonic and neonatal mortality, underscoring its physiological importance [67,68]. Thrombin, generated from prothrombin through proteolytic cleavage, catalyzes thrombus formation and regulates the coagulation cascade [69]. It has been implicated in promoting tumor progression via fibrin formation and the activation of protease-activated receptors and platelets; hence, thrombin inhibitors have shown efficacy in treating malignancies such as 4T1 mammary adenocarcinoma in murine models [70] and ovarian cancer [71]. In the present study, thrombin activity was attenuated by the downregulation of prothrombin expression, which induced apoptosis in SU-DHL-2 cells.

Plasminogen, another DEP, is a serine protease precursor converted to active plasmin. Plasmin, along with matrix metalloproteinases activated by plasminogen, plays a pivotal role in the degradation of the extracellular matrix. This degradation process is crucial for tumor-related inflammation, leukocyte infiltration, cancer cell invasion, and metastasis [72], influencing angiogenesis and cell migration [73]. In this study, the downregulation of plasminogen resulted in reduced plasmin levels, contributing to the inhibition of SU-DHL-2 cell survival.

Carboxypeptidase B2, a critical enzyme within the complement and coagulation cascades pathway, plays a significant role in modulating inflammation by inactivating substances that act as activators and attractants for neutrophils. It has been identified as a prognostic indicator for oral squamous cell carcinoma [74] and a colorectal cancer biomarker [75]. Moreover, carboxypeptidase B2 has been recognized as a central protein in the plasma of breast cancer patients [76], and its suppression by siRNA has been shown to impede the invasion and migration of breast cancer cells, suggesting its potential as a therapeutic target [77]. In this study, the downregulation of carboxypeptidase B2 was associated with inhibited survival of SU-DHL-2 cells.

Fibrinogen, a complex glycoprotein, comprises alpha, beta, and gamma chains and plays a multifaceted role in tumorigenesis and cancer progression. The therapeutic application of exogenous fibrinogen has been demonstrated in the entrapment of OK-432 within the tumor stroma, leading to the regression of colorectal carcinoma [78]. Furthermore, fibrinogen-like protein 2 has been proposed as an immunotherapeutic target for brain tumors [79]. In breast cancer, both fibrinogen beta and gamma chains have been implicated as key factors in tumor progression and metastasis [80]. Downregulation of the fibrinogen gamma chain has been associated with reduced resistance to anthracycline chemotherapy in breast cancer [81], and silencing of this chain has been shown to markedly increase apoptosis and reduce the proliferation, invasion, and migration of cancer cells [82]. The influence of fibrinogen on SU-DHL-2 cells is complex, impacting multiple aspects of cell behavior and response to treatment.

Coagulation factor V is essential for regulating blood coagulation and exhibits both procoagulant and anticoagulant effects. Its role extends beyond hemostasis, as it has been identified as a novel marker for immune cell infiltration in breast cancer. It has potential as an immunological biomarker with therapeutic implications for the nexus of cancer, inflammation, and thrombosis [83]. Elevated levels of coagulation factor V in estrogen receptor-positive breast tumors have been correlated with improved relapse-free survival in patients [84]. Furthermore, coagulation factor V has demonstrated antitumor activity against MDA-MB-231 cells, potentially by inhibiting tissue factor-induced activation of protease-activated receptor 2 [85]. This protein has also been recognized as a prognostic biomarker for gastric and prostate cancers, potentially affecting the immune microenvironment and patient survival by modulating transforming growth factor (TGF)-beta signaling [86–88]. In this study, increased expression of coagulation factor V was associated with decreased survival of SU-DHL-2 cells, potentially through immunological mechanisms.

PPI analysis revealed that DEPs were enriched across various pathways, interacting synergistically with other proteins. Notably, ribosomal protein L5, tumor protein p53, and ribosomal protein L24 were the top three interacting proteins (Figure 5). Ribosomal protein L5, which serves as a chaperone for 5S rRNA, was shown to regulate the MDM2/MDMX–p53 cascade, thereby inhibiting tumor cell proliferation [89]. It also interacts with MDM2 or MDMX, which are pivotal for tumor suppression by modulating the activity of p53 [90]. The tumor suppressor p53, encoded by the most frequently mutated gene in human cancers, is central to the cellular response to diverse stressors, including DNA damage, hypoxia, nutrient deprivation, and oncogene activation [91]. As a ferroptosis regulator, p53 controls cell death processes, highlighting its dual function in modulating this form of cell death [92]. Additionally, p53 modulates the expression of ribosomal protein L24, a translation factor implicated in tumorigenesis, further illustrating the intricate network of interactions that govern cellular fate and cancer progression [93]. These proteins play important roles in inhibiting the survival of SU-DHL-2 cells.

In the treated cells, the expression of genes encoding the hop proteins *P53*, *PLK1*, *BUB1B*, *FN1*, *Cyclin B*, *Cyclin D*, and *Caspase 3* decreased. Notably, the expression levels of these genes did not correspond with the abundance of their respective proteins. These data showed that the PPIs of the DEPs and differentially expressed genes (DEGs) were inconsistent. The expression of genes was less strongly correlated with the survival inhibition of SU-DHL-2 cells. This contradiction between mRNA and protein expression levels was consistent with findings in our previous study and other studies in the literature [38,94]. The correlation between protein and mRNA expression levels is generally moderate, with a reported coefficient of approximately 0.5 [95]. This correlation tends to be weaker for mRNAs and their structurally stable protein counterparts [94], suggesting that posttranscriptional and posttranslational mechanisms may play significant roles in determining protein abundance.

The limitations of this study are as follows: The xenograft tumor model in nude mice did not succeed many times, which may be caused by fewer cancer stem cells in the SU-DHL-2 cell samples injected in nude mice. The limitations of this study include the use of metabonomics, transcriptomics, cancer stem cells, molecular docking, or other advanced methods to accurately evaluate the antitumor mechanism of 10-HDA against SU-DHL-2 cells for new drug development. The positive control group was excluded because of the different antitumor mechanisms of 10-HDA and antitumor drugs against SU-DHL-2 cells, such as 5-fluorouracil, which has a higher IC_{50} than 10-HDA against A549, NIC-H460, and NCI-H23 cells [47]. This missing positive control was also found in other reports [96–98]. More in-depth research on the cell cycle of SU-DHL-2 cells inhibited by 10-HDA can be performed in the future.

10-HDA inhibits the survival of SU-DHL-2 cells by regulating proteins involved in the complement and coagulation cascade pathways, including the differentially expressed proteins prothrombin, plasminogen, plasminogen, carboxypeptidase B2, fibrinogen beta chain, fibrinogen gamma chain, and coagulation factor V. The combination of 10-HDA or royal jelly and R-CHOP or other potential antitumor drugs is a potential treatment strategy for the SU-DHL-2 cell line.

The IC_{50}s of 10-HDA against the normal liver cell line LO2 and normal human fibroblast line HSF were approximately 1000 μg/mL and greater than 1000 μg/mL, respectively. The lower specificity of 10-HDA against SU-DHL-2 cells should be considered. If we control the ADI of royal jelly according to the pharmacokinetics results or develop and apply a targeted sustained-release drug delivery system, then 10-HDA can be used for the practical treatment of cancer and enhance the proliferation of LO2 liver cells (B) and normal human fibroblasts (HSFs).

4. Materials and Methods

4.1. Determination of the IC50 of 10-HDA against SU-DHL-2 Cells

SU-DHL-2 cells (ATCC CRL-2956, purchased from Cellcook, Guangzhou, China) and LO2 normal liver cells were cultured in complete medium (composed of 89% modified RPMI-1640 basal medium (Wuhan Pricella Biotechnology Co., Ltd., Wuhan, China), 10% fetal bovine serum (Cellmax Bio Co., Ltd. Lanzhou, China), and a 1% penicillin and streptomycin mixture (HyClone Biochemical Products Co., Ltd. Shanghai, China)) in a 5% CO_2 humidified incubator at 37 °C (C150, Binder, Tuttlingen, German). Normal human HSF fibroblasts were cultured in complete medium (composed of 89% high-sugar DMEM purchased from Procell Life Technology Co., Ltd., Wuhan, China; 10% FBS; and a 1% penicillin and streptomycin mixture). The other chemicals and incubators used were the same as those described in our previous report [38].

Next, 50 milligrams of 10-HDA was dissolved in 100 μL of anhydrous ethanol. The 10-HDA solution was gradient diluted to 250, 500, 750, and 1000 μg/mL (the final concentration of 10-HDA in the complete medium) using complete culture medium until ready for use.

The concentration of SU-DHL-2 cells was adjusted to 3×10^6 cells/well in 96-well plates. Different concentrations of 10-HDA solution and a complete medium containing 0.02% ethanol (*v:v*, solvent control, equal to ethanol in 1000 μg/mL 10-HDA solution) were added after 24 h of incubation. After 24 h of further incubation, the cell suspensions were collected to determine cell viability with a CCK8 kit (purchased from Dojindo, Kumamoto, Japan) at 450 nm using a microplate reader (1510, Thermo Fisher, Waltham, MA, USA). The percentage of SU-DHL-2 cells that died due to 10-HDA treatment was calculated as the OD_{450} of the control group minus the OD_{450} of the treated group and then divided by the OD_{450} of the control group, which was multiplied by 100%. The IC_{50} of 10-HDA against SU-DHL-2 cells for 24 h was calculated using GraphPad Prism 8.4.3 for Windows (GraphPad Software, Inc., La Jolla, CA, USA). Similarly, LO2 normal liver cells and HSF normal human fibroblasts were treated with 10-HDA solution at 200, 400, 600, 800, and

1000 μg/mL (the final concentration of 10-HDA in complete medium) for determination of the IC_{50} values.

4.2. Proteomic Determination of Differentially Expressed Proteins in Cells Following Different Treatments

The SU-DHL-2 cells (3 × 10^6 cells/well in 96-well plates) were cultured with 10-HDA at the IC50 (496.8 μg/mL) or the solvent control (0.02% ethanol in complete medium) in a 5% CO_2 humidified incubator at 37 °C for 24 h of incubation. The cells were collected and subjected to the same procedures as those described in our previous report [38]. The concentration of the total proteins extracted from cells frozen in liquid nitrogen was determined using Coomassie brilliant blue staining (CBB-G250). Then, the spectra of proteins in SU-DHL-2 cells were determined by Novgene Biotech Co., Ltd., Beijing, China.

4.3. Detection of the Relative Expression of Genes

The relative expression of genes encoding hub proteins (top 10 proteins) involved in protein–protein interactions (PPIs), namely, *HO-1*, *NQO1*, *Hsp70*, *p62*, *CD274*, *CDH1*, *PLK1*, *BUB1B*, *p53*, *Cyclin B*, *Casp 3*, and *Cyclin D*, was determined via RT–PCR using a C1000 Touch Thermal Cycler (Bio-Rad). The RT–PCR procedure was performed as previously described [38]. Primers (Table 3) were designed via the NCBI free online primer design platform with β-actin as the internal reference gene.

Table 3. Primers utilized for the RT–PCR system.

Primer	Sequences (5′→3′)
β-actin-F	GATCATTGCTCCTCCTGAGC
β-actin-R	ACTCCTGCTTGCTGATCCAC
HO-1-F	TCTTGGCTGGCTTCCTTACC
HO-1-R	GGATGTGCTTTTCGTTGGGG
NQO1-F	TGAAAGGCTGGTTTGAGCGA
NQO1-R	TCCAGGCGTTTCTTCCATCC
GCL-F	AGGTCAAACCCAACCCAGT
GCL-R	TGTTAAGGTACTGAAGCGAGG
BUB1B-F	GGATGGGTCCTTCTGGAAACT
BUB1B-R	GTGGCCTCATCATTGGCATTC
FTH1-F	CAGAACTACCACCAGGACTCA
FTH1-R	TCAAAGCCACATCATCGCGG
HSP70-F	GTGTAACCCCATCATCAGCG
HSP70-R	GCTCCAAAACAAAAACAGCAATCT
p62-F	TACCAGGACAGCGAGAGGAAG
p62-R	ATCCTTTCTCAAGCCCCATGT
Cyclin B-F	GATACTGCCTCTCCAAGCC
Cyclin B-R	GCACACAATTATTCTCAAGTTGTC
Cyclin D-F	GCCGGGGACCGAAACT
Cyclin D-R	GCAGTGGCGAAGTGTTTACAAAG
CD274-F	TTTGCTGAACGCCCCATACA
CD274-R	TCCAGATGACTTCGGCCTTG
CDH1-F	GCTGGACCGAGAGAGTTTCC
CDH1-R	CAAAATCCAAGCCCGTGGTG
p53-F	ACACGCTTCCCTGGATTGG
p53-R	TCATCCATTGCTTGGGACGG
Casp 3-F	CTCTGGTTTTCGGTGGGTGT
Casp 3-R	CTTCCATGTATGATCTTTGGTTCC
FN1-F	CAAGCATGTCTCTCTGCCAAG
FN-R	CAGAACAGGCAATGTGCAGC
PLK1-F	CCTGCACCGAAACCGAGTTA
PLK1-R	ACCTCGAAACTGTGCCCTTT

4.4. Statistical Analysis

All experiments were performed in triplicate, and the results are expressed as the mean $\pm$ standard error. The cell death (%) was transformed to arcsin (degree) values (according to the formula: arc $\sin\sqrt{p}$) before ANOVA, which was performed using GraphPad Prism 8.4.3 for Windows (GraphPad Software, Inc., San Diego, CA, USA) to analyze the significance of differences ($p < 0.01$: highly statistically significant differences between the different treatment groups and $p < 0.05$: statistically significant differences).

All of the data obtained for differentially expressed proteins (DEPs) via a label-free technique were analyzed. The spectra obtained from LC–MS/MS were searched against the UniProt database using Proteome Discoverer 2.2 (Thermo) with credibility of more than 99% peptide spectrum matches. Proteins containing 1 or more unique peptides and with a probability of false discovery less than or equal to 1% were identified. The protein quantitation results were statistically analyzed with t-tests using GraphPad Prism 8.0.2 for Windows. DEPs were proteins with significantly different quantities between the treated group and the control group ($p \leq 0.05$ and fold change (FC) ≥ 2 or FC ≤ 0.5). All DEPs were sent to the Gene Ontology database (GO, http://www.geneontology.org/ (accessed on 5 January 2024)) to calculate the number of proteins in each term. A hypergeometric test was applied to find GO terms that were the most significantly enriched in DEPs compared with all protein backgrounds. Kyoto Encyclopedia of Genes and Genomes (KEGG) was used to analyze the enriched pathways (http://www.genome.ad.jp/kegg/ (accessed on 5 January 2024)). The PPIs of the DEPs were determined using the String-db server (http://string.embl.de/ (accessed on 5 January 2024)), in which the minimum required interaction score was >0.9. Then, the data exported from STRING-db were loaded into Cytoscape software (version 3.9.1; JAVA: 11.0.6 by AdoptOpenJDK) to construct the PPI network diagram.

The relative gene expression values are represented by the ratio of the expression of a gene in 10-HDA-treated cells to that in the solvent control group cells.

Author Contributions: Conceptualization, Y.T. and W.Y.; methodology, W.Y.; data curation, X.L., Y.T., J.W. and C.Z.; formal analysis, X.L. and J.W.; writing—original draft preparation, Y.T. and X.L.; writing—review and editing, W.Y.; supervision, W.Y. All authors have read and agreed to the published version of the manuscript.

Funding: This research received no external funding.

Institutional Review Board Statement: The animal study protocol was approved by the Ethics Committee of Fujian Agriculture and Forestry University (protocol code PZCASFAFU23074).

Informed Consent Statement: Not applicable.

Data Availability Statement: Data are contained within this article.

Conflicts of Interest: The authors declare no conflict of interest.

References

1. WHO. Cancer: Key Facts. Available online: https://www.who.int/news-room/fact-sheets/detail/cancer (accessed on 3 February 2024).
2. Sehn, L.H.; Salles, G. Diffuse large B-cell lymphoma. *N. Engl. J. Med.* **2021**, *384*, 842–858. [CrossRef]
3. Teras, L.R.; DeSantis, C.E.; Cerhan, J.R.; Morton, L.M.; Jemal, A.; Flowers, C.R. 2016 US lymphoid malignancy statistics by World Health Organization subtypes. *Ca-Cancer J. Clin.* **2016**, *66*, 443–459. [CrossRef]
4. Dickinson, M.J.; Carlo-Stella, C.; Morschhauser, F.; Bachy, E.; Corradini, P.; Iacoboni, G.; Khan, C.; Wróbel, T.; Offner, F.; Trněný, M.; et al. Glofitamab for relapsed or refractory diffuse large B-Cell lymphoma. *N. Engl. J. Med.* **2022**, *387*, 2220–2231. [CrossRef]
5. Alizadeh, A.A.; Eisen, M.B.; Davis, R.E.; Ma, C.; Lossos, I.S.; Rosenwald, A.; Boldrick, J.C.; Sabet, H.; Tran, T.; Yu, X. Distinct types of diffuse large B-cell lymphoma identified by gene expression profiling. *Nature* **2000**, *403*, 503–511. [CrossRef] [PubMed]
6. Wang, L.; Li, L.; Young, K. New agents and regimens for diffuse large B cell lymphoma. *J. Hematol. Oncol.* **2020**, *13*, 175. [CrossRef]
7. Susanibar-Adaniya, S.; Barta, S.K. 2021 Update on Diffuse large B cell lymphoma: A review of currentdata and potential applications on risk stratification andmanagement. *Am. J. Hematol.* **2021**, *96*, 617–629. [CrossRef]

8. He, Y.; Li, J.; Ding, N.; Wang, X.; Deng, L.; Xie, Y.; Ying, Z.; Liu, W.; Ping, L.; Zhang, C.; et al. Combination of Enzastaurin and Ibrutinib synergistically induces anti-tumor effects in diffuse large B cell lymphoma. *J. Exp. Clin. Cancer Res.* **2019**, *38*, 86. [CrossRef]
9. Jeon, B.; Lee, Y.J.; Shin, J.; Choi, M.J.; Lee, C.E.; Son, M.K.; Park, J.H.; Kim, B.; Kim, H.R.; Jung, K.H.; et al. A combination of BR101801 and venetoclax enhances antitumor effect in DLBCL cells via c-Myc/Bcl-2/Mcl-1 triple targeting. *Am. J. Cancer Res.* **2023**, *13*, 452. [PubMed] [PubMed Central]
10. He, W.; Xu, Z.; Song, D.; Zhang, H.; Li, B.; Gao, L.; Zhang, Y.; Feng, Q.; Yu, D.; Hu, L.; et al. Antitumor effects of ra-foxanide in Diffuse Large B Cell Lymphoma via the PTEN/PI3K/Akt and JNK/c-Jun Pathways. *Life Sci.* **2020**, *243*, 117249. [CrossRef] [PubMed]
11. Zhang, W.; Li, Q.; Yang, C.; Yang, H.; Rao, J.; Zhang, X. Curcumin exerts anti-tumor effects on diffuse large B cell lymphoma via regulating PPARγ expression. *Biochem. Biophys. Res. Commun.* **2020**, *524*, 70–76. [CrossRef]
12. Han, J.; Guo, X.; Yu, X.; Liu, S.; Cui, X.; Zhang, B.; Liang, H. 25-Hydroxyvitamin D and total cancer incidence and mortality: A meta-analysis of prospective cohort studies. *Nutrients* **2019**, *11*, 2295. [CrossRef]
13. Zhu, Y.; Lei, C.; Jiang, Q.; Yu, Q.; Qiu, L. DSF/Cu induces antitumor effect against diffuse large B-cell lymphoma through suppressing NF-κB/BCL6 pathways. *Cancer Cell Int.* **2022**, *22*, 236. [CrossRef]
14. Kita, A.; Nakahara, T.; Yamanaka, K.; Nakano, K.; Nakata, M.; Mori, M.; Kaneko, N.; Koutoku, H.; Izumisawa, N.; Sasamata, M. Antitumor effects of YM155, a novel survivin suppressant, against human aggressive non-Hodgkin lymphoma. *Leuk. Res.* **2011**, *35*, 787–792. [CrossRef] [PubMed]
15. Gao, Y.; Ding, X. miR-145-5p exerts anti-tumor effects in diffuse large B-cell lymphoma by regulating S1PR1/STAT3/AKT pathway. *Leuk. Lymphoma* **2021**, *62*, 1884–1891. [CrossRef]
16. Yang, S.; Sheng, L.; Xu, K.; Wang, Y.; Zhu, H.; Zhang, P.; Mu, Q.; Ouyang, G. Anticancer effect of quinacrine on diffuse large B-cell lymphoma via inhibition of MSI2-NUMB signaling pathway. *Mol. Med. Rep.* **2018**, *17*, 522–530. [CrossRef] [PubMed]
17. Othman, N.H.; Ahmed, S.; Sulaiman, S.A. Inhibitory effects of Malaysian *Tualang* honey and Australian/New Zealand Manuka honey in modulating experimental breast cancers induced by *N-methyl-N-nitrosourea* (mnu): A comparative study. *Pathology* **2016**, *48*, S148. [CrossRef]
18. Kadir, E.A.; Sulaiman, S.A.; Yahya, N.K.; Othman, N.H. Inhibitory effects of *Tualang* honey on experimental breast cancer in rats: A preliminary study. *Asian Pac. J. Cancer Prev.* **2013**, *14*, 2249–2254. [CrossRef]
19. Fauzi, A.N.; Norazmi, M.N.; Yaacob, N.S. *Tualang* honey induces apoptosis and disrupts the mitochondrial membrane potential of human breast and cervical cancer cell lines. *Food Chem. Toxicol.* **2011**, *49*, 871–878. [CrossRef]
20. Milani, S.M.; Najafi, M.; Alizadeh, P.; Rezazadeh, H. Inhibitory effect of honey on 7,12-dimethylbenz(a)anthracene- initiated and croton oil-promoted skin carcinogenesis. *Jundishapur J. Nat. Pharm. Prod.* **2018**, *13*, e57992. [CrossRef]
21. Hassan, M.I.; Mabrouk, G.M.; Shehata, H.H.; Aboelhussein, M.M. Antineoplastic effects of bee honey and Nigella sativa on hepatocellular carcinoma cells. *Integr. Cancer Ther.* **2012**, *11*, 354–363. [CrossRef]
22. Wen, C.T.P.; Hussein, S.Z.; Abdullah, S.; Karim, N.A.; Makpol, S.; Yusof, Y.A.M. Gelam and Nenas honeys inhibit proliferation of HT 29 colon cancer cells by inducing DNA damage and apoptosis while suppressing inflammation. *Asian Pac. J. Cancer Prev.* **2012**, *13*, 1605–1610. [CrossRef]
23. Aliyu, M.; Odunola, O.A.; Farooq, A.D.; Mesaik, A.M.; Choudhary, M.I.; Fatima, B.; Qureshi, T.A.; Erukainure, O.L. Acacia honey modulates cell cycle progression, pro-inflammatory cytokines and calcium ions secretion in PC-3 cell line. *J. Cancer Sci. Ther.* **2012**, *4*, 401–407. [CrossRef]
24. Swellam, T.; Miyanaga, N.; Onozawa, M.; Hattori, K.; Kawai, K.; Shimazui, T.; Akaza, H. Antineoplastic activity of honey in an experimental bladder cancer implantation model: In vivo and in vitro studies. *Int. J. Urol.* **2003**, *10*, 213–219. [CrossRef]
25. Angst, E.; Park, J.L.; Moro, A.; Lu, Q.Y.; Lu, X.; Li, G.; King, J.; Chen, M.; Reber, H.A.; Go, V.L.; et al. The flavonoid quercetin inhibits pancreatic cancer growth in vitro and in vivo. *Pancreas* **2013**, *42*, 223–229. [CrossRef] [PubMed]
26. Aliyu, M.; Odunola, O.A.; Farooq, A.D.; Rasheed, H.; Mesaik, A.M.; Choudhary, M.I.; Channa, I.S.; Khan, S.A.; Erukainure, O.L. Molecular mechanism of antiproliferation potential of Acacia honey on NCI-H460 cell line. *Nutr. Cancer* **2013**, *65*, 296–304. [CrossRef]
27. Pichichero, E.; Cicconi, R.; Mattei, M.; Muzi, M.G.; Canini, A. Acacia honey and chrysin reduce proliferation of melanoma cells through alterations in cell cycle progression. *Int. J. Oncol.* **2010**, *37*, 973–981. [CrossRef]
28. Fernandez-Cabezudo, M.J.; El-Kharrag, R.; Torab, F.; Bashir, G.; George, J.A.; El-Taji, H.; al-Ramadi, B.K. Intravenous administration of Manuka honey inhibits tumor growth and improves host survival when used in combination with chemotherapy in a melanoma mouse model. *PLoS ONE* **2013**, *8*, e5599. [CrossRef] [PubMed]
29. Song, W.; Dang, Q.; Xu, D.; Chen, Y.; Zhu, G.; Wu, K.; Zeng, J.; Long, Q.; Wang, X.; He, D.; et al. Kaempferol induces cell cycle arrest and apoptosis in renal cell carcinoma through EGFR/p38 signaling. *Oncol. Rep.* **2014**, *31*, 1350–1356. [CrossRef]
30. Man, N.M.K.N.; Hassan, R.; Ang, C.Y.; Abdullah, A.D.; Radzi, M.A.R.M.; Sulaiman, S.A. Antileukemic effect of *Tualang* honey on acute and chronic leukemia cell lines. *BioMed Res. Int.* **2015**, *2015*, 307094. [CrossRef]
31. Tsiapara, A.V.; Jaakkola, M.; Chinou, I.; Graikou, K.; Tolonen, T.; Virtanen, V.; Moutsatsou, P. Bioactivity of Greek honey extracts on breast cancer (MCF-7), prostate cancer (PC-3) and endometrial cancer (Ishikawa) cells: Profile analysis of extracts. *Food Chem.* **2009**, *116*, 702–708. [CrossRef]

32. Kyselova, Z. Toxicological aspects of the use of phenolic compounds in disease prevention. *Interdiscip. Toxicol.* **2011**, *4*, 173–183. [CrossRef] [PubMed]
33. Chiu, H.F.; Han, Y.C.; Shen, Y.C.; Golovinskaia, O.; Venkatakrishnan, K.; Wang, C.K. Chemopreventive and chemotherapeutic effect of propolis and its constituents: A mini-review. *J. Cancer Prev.* **2020**, *25*, 70–78. [CrossRef] [PubMed]
34. Ghazy, M.G.M.; Hanafy, N.A.N. Targeted therapies for breast and lung cancers by using propolis loaded albumin protein nanoparticles. *Int. J. Biol. Macromol.* **2024**, *260*, 129338. [CrossRef]
35. Kocyigit, A.; Guler, E.M.; Durmus, E.; Yenigun, V.B.; Kanimdan, E.; Ozman, Z.; Yasar, O.; Goren, A.C.; Hekimoglu, E.R.; Oruc, H.H.; et al. Propolis enhances 5-fluorouracil mediated antitumor efficacy and reduces side effects in colorectal cancer: An in vitro and in vivo study. *Chem. Biodivers.* **2023**, *20*, e202300591. [CrossRef]
36. Shen, M.; Liu, C.; Chang, K.; Lai, C.; Chang, S.; Huang, C. Propolis has an anticancer effect on early stage colorectal cancer by affecting epithelial differentiation and gut immunity in the tumor microenvironment. *Nutrients* **2023**, *15*, 4494. [CrossRef] [PubMed]
37. Salavatipour, M.S.; Kouhbananinejad, S.M.; Lashkari, M.; Bardsiri, M.S.; Moghadari, M.; Kashani, B.; Farsinejad, A.; Vahidi, R. Kermanian propolis induces apoptosis through upregulation of Bax/Bcl-2 ratio in acute myeloblastic leukemia cell line (NB4). *J. Cancer Res. Ther.* **2023**, *19*, 327–334. [CrossRef]
38. Liu, X.; Tian, Y.; Yang, A.; Zhang, C.; Miao, X.; Yang, W. Antitumor effects of poplar propolis on DLBCL SU-DHL-2 cells. *Foods* **2023**, *12*, 283. [CrossRef]
39. Aylanc, V.; Larbi, S.; Calhelha, R.; Barros, L.; Rezouga, F.; Rodríguez-Flores, M.S.; Seijo, M.C.; El Ghouizi, A.; Lyoussi, B.; Falcão, S.I.; et al. Evaluation of antioxidant and anticancer activity of mono- and polyfloral moroccan bee pollen by characterizing phenolic and volatile compounds. *Molecules* **2023**, *28*, 835. [CrossRef] [PubMed]
40. Rodríguez-Pólit, C.; Gonzalez-Pastor, R.; Heredia-Moya, J.; Carrera-Pacheco, S.E.; Castillo-Solis, F.; Vallejo-Imbaquingo, R.; Barba-Ostria, C.; Guamán, L.P. Chemical properties and biological activity of bee pollen. *Molecules* **2023**, *28*, 7768. [CrossRef] [PubMed]
41. Małek, A.; Strzemski, M.; Kurzepa, J.; Kurzepa, J. Can bee venom be used as anticancer agent in modern medicine? *Cancers* **2023**, *15*, 3714. [CrossRef]
42. Paredes-Barquero, M.; Niso-Santano, M.; Fuentes, J.M.; Martínez-Chacón, G. In vitro and in vivo models to study the biological and pharmacological properties of queen bee acid (QBA, 10-hydroxy-2-decenoic acid): A systematic review. *J. Funct. Foods* **2022**, *94*, 105143. [CrossRef]
43. Yang, Y.; Chou, W.; Widowati, D.; Lin, I.; Peng, C. 10-Hydroxy-2-decenoic acid of royal jelly exhibits bactericide and anti-inflammatory activity in human colon cancer cells. *BMC Complement. Altern. Med.* **2018**, *18*, 202. [CrossRef] [PubMed]
44. Lin, X.; Liu, S.; Luo, Y.; Xu, W.; Zhang, Y.; Zhang, T.; Xue, H.; Zuo, W.; Li, Y.; Lu, B.; et al. 10-HDA induces ROS-Mediated apoptosis in A549 human lung cancer cells by regulating the MAPK, STAT3, NF-κB, and TGF-β1 signaling pathways. *Biomed Res. Int.* **2020**, *2020*, 3042636. [CrossRef]
45. Saad Al Shehri, Z.; Alanazi, A.D.; Alnomasy, S.F. Anti-cancer effects of queen bee acid (10-Hydroxy-2-decenoic acid) and its cellular mechanisms against human hepatoma cells. *Molecules* **2023**, *28*, 1972. [CrossRef]
46. Peng, C.; Sun, H.; Lin, I.; Kuo, P.; Li, J. The functional property of royal jelly 10-Hydroxy-2-decenoic acid as a melanogenesis inhibitor. *BMC Complement. Altern. Med.* **2017**, *17*, 392. [CrossRef] [PubMed]
47. Atef, B.; Ishak, R.A.H.; Badawy, S.S.; Osman, R. 10-Hydroxy decanoic acid-based vesicles as a novel topical delivery system: Would it be a better platform than conventional oleic acid ufasomes for skin cancer treatment? *Pharmaceutics* **2023**, *15*, 1461. [CrossRef]
48. Pengpanich, S.; Srisupabh, D.; Tanechpongtamb, W.U. Potential role of royal jelly and 10-Hydroxy-2-decenoic acid as metastasis inhibitors in triple-negative breast cancer cells. *J. Med. Assoc. Thail.* **2019**, *102*, 17.
49. Miyata, Y.; Sakai, H. Anti-cancer and protective effects of royal jelly for therapy-induced toxicities in malignancies. *Int. J. Mol. Sci.* **2018**, *19*, 3270. [CrossRef]
50. Albalawi, A.E.; Althobaiti, N.A.; Alrdahe, S.S.; Alhasani, R.H.; Alaryani, F.S.; BinMowyna, M.N. Anti-tumor effects of queen bee acid (10-Hydroxy-2-decenoic acid) alone and in combination with cyclophosphamide and its cellular mechanisms against ehrlich solid tumor in mice. *Molecules* **2021**, *26*, 7021. [CrossRef] [PubMed]
51. Pengpanich, S.; Tanechpongtamb, W. The Inhibitory Effect of 10-Hydroxy-2decenoic acid (10-HDA) on Breast Cancer Cell Proliferation and Metastasis. Doctoral Dissertation, Srinakharinwirot University, Bangkok, Thailand, 2018. Available online: http://ir-ithesis.swu.ac.th/dspace/handle/123456789/129 (accessed on 4 May 2024).
52. Vucevic, D.; Melliou, E.; Vasilijic, S.; Gasic, S.; Ivanovski, P.; Chinou, I.; Colic, M. Fatty acids isolated from royal jelly modulate dendritic cell-mediated immune response in vitro. *Int. Immunopharmacol.* **2007**, *7*, 1211–1220. [CrossRef] [PubMed]
53. Perminaite, K.; Marksa, M.; Stančiauskaitė, M.; Juknius, T.; Grigonis, A.; Ramanauskiene, K. Formulation of Ocular In Situ Gels with Lithuanian Royal Jelly and Their Biopharmaceutical Evaluation In Vitro. *Molecules* **2021**, *26*, 3552. [CrossRef] [PubMed]
54. Verma, M.; Kagan, J.; Sidransky, D.; Srivastava, S. Proteomic analysis of cancer-cell mitochondria. *Nat. Rev. Cancer* **2003**, *3*, 789–795. [CrossRef] [PubMed]
55. Cohen, A.A.; Geva-Zatorsky, N.; Eden, E.; Frenkel-Morgenstern, M.; Issaeva, I.; Sigal, A.; Milo, R.; Cohen-Saidon, C.; Liron, Y.; Kam, Z.; et al. Dynamic proteomics of individual cancer cells in response to a drug. *Science* **2008**, *322*, 1511–1516. [CrossRef]

56. Nusinow, D.P.; Szpyt, J.; Ghandi, M.; Rose, C.M.; McDonald, E.R.; Kalocsay, M.; Jané-Valbuena, J.; Gelfand, E.; Schweppe, D.K.; Jedrychowski, M.; et al. Quantitative proteomics of the cancer cell line encyclopedia. *Cell* **2020**, *180*, 387–402.e16. [CrossRef] [PubMed]
57. Jiang, P.; Zhu, Y.; Kang, K.; Luo, B.; He, J.; Wu, Y. Protein corona of magnetic PEI/siRNA complex under the influence of a magnetic field improves transfection efficiency via complement and coagulation cascades. *J. Mater. Chem. B* **2019**, *7*, 4207–4216. [CrossRef]
58. Sharma, S.; Ray, S.; Moiyadi, A.; Sridhar, E.; Srivastava, S. Quantitative proteomic analysis of meningiomas for the identification of surrogate protein markers. *Sci. Rep.* **2014**, *4*, 7140. [CrossRef]
59. Zhang, W.; Peng, P.; Ou, X.; Shen, K.; Wu, X. Ovarian cancer circulating extracelluar vesicles promote coagulation and have a potential in diagnosis: An iTRAQ based proteomic analysis. *BMC Cancer* **2019**, *19*, 1095. [CrossRef]
60. Zhang, C.; Peng, L.; Zhang, Y.; Liu, Z.; Li, W.; Chen, S.; Li, G. The identification of key genes and pathways in hepatocellular carcinoma by bioinformatics analysis of high-throughput data. *Med. Oncol.* **2017**, *34*, 101. [CrossRef]
61. Gao, X.; Wang, X.; Zhang, S. Bioinformatics identification of crucial genes and pathways associated with hepatocellular carcinoma. *Biosci. Rep.* **2018**, *38*, BSR20181441. [CrossRef]
62. Zhang, Y.; Chen, X.; Cao, Y.; Yang, Z. C8B in complement and coagulation cascades signaling pathway is a predictor for survival in HBV-related hepatocellular carcinoma patients. *Cancer Manag. Res.* **2021**, *13*, 3503–3515. [CrossRef]
63. Gao, X.; Chen, Y.; Chen, M.; Wang, S.; Wen, X.; Zhang, S. Identification of key candidate genes and biological pathways in bladder cancer. *PeerJ* **2018**, *6*, e6036. [CrossRef] [PubMed]
64. Rahman, M.R.; Islam, T.; Al-Mamun, M.A.; Zaman, T.; Karim, M.R.; Moni, M.A. The influence of depression on ovarian cancer: Discovering molecular pathways that identify novel biomarkers and therapeutic targets. *Inform. Med. Unlocked* **2019**, *16*, 100207. [CrossRef]
65. Gong, Z.; He, Y.; Mi, X.; Li, C.; Sun, X.; Wang, G.; Li, L.; Han, Y.; Xu, C.; Xu, C.; et al. Complement and coagulation cascades pathway-related signature as a predictor of immunotherapy in metastatic urothelial cancer. *Aging* **2023**, *15*, 9479. [CrossRef]
66. Kim, T.H.; Kim, E.; Yoon, D.; Kim, J.; Rhim, T.Y.; Kim, S.S. Recombinant human prothrombin kringles have potent anti-angiogenic activities and inhibit Lewis lung carcinoma tumor growth and metastases. *Angiogenesis* **2002**, *5*, 191–201. [CrossRef]
67. Sun, W.Y.; Witte, D.P.; Degen, J.L.; Colbert, M.C.; Burkart, M.C.; Holmbäck, K.; Xiao, Q.; Bugge, T.H.; Degen, S.J. Prothrombin deficiency results in embryonic and neonatal lethality in mice. *Proc. Natl. Acad. Sci. USA* **1998**, *95*, 7597–7602. [CrossRef]
68. Xue, J.; Wu, Q.; Westfield, L.A.; Tuley, E.A.; Lu, D.; Zhang, Q.; Shim, K.; Zheng, X.; Sadler, J.E. Incomplete embryonic lethality and fatal neonatal hemorrhage caused by prothrombin deficiency in mice. *Proc. Natl. Acad. Sci. USA* **1998**, *95*, 7603–7607. [CrossRef] [PubMed]
69. Krishnaswamy, S. The transition of prothrombin to thrombin. *J. Thromb. Haemost.* **2013**, *11*, 265–276. [CrossRef]
70. Alexander, E.T.; Minton, A.R.; Hayes, C.S.; Goss, A.; Van Ryn, J.; Gilmour, S.K. Thrombin inhibition and cyclophosphamide synergistically block tumor progression and metastasis. *Cancer Biol. Ther.* **2015**, *16*, 1802–1811. [CrossRef]
71. Alexander, E.T.; Minton, A.R.; Peters, M.C.; van Ryn, J.; Gilmour, S.K. Thrombin inhibition and cisplatin block tumor progression in ovarian cancer by alleviating the immunosuppressive microenvironment. *Oncotarget* **2016**, *7*, 85291–85305. [CrossRef]
72. Bharadwaj, A.G.; Holloway, R.W.; Miller, V.A.; Waisman, D.M. Plasmin and plasminogen system in the tumor microenvironment: Implications for cancer diagnosis, prognosis, and therapy. *Cancers* **2021**, *13*, 1838. [CrossRef]
73. Kwaan, H.C.; McMahon, B. The role of plasminogen-plasmin system in cancer. *Cancer Treat. Res.* **2009**, *148*, 43–66. [CrossRef]
74. Vylliotis, A.; Yapijakis, C.; Nkenke, E.; Nisyrios, T.; Avgoustidis, D.; Adamopoulou, M.; Ragos, V.; Vassiliou, S.; Koronellos, N.; Vairakraris, E. Effect of thrombosis-related gene polymorphisms upon oral cancer: A regression analysis. *Anticancer. Res.* **2013**, *33*, 4033–4039.
75. Wu, Q.; Wang, X.; Wu, W.; Chen, Y.; Wang, J.; Zhang, X.; Qian, Y.; Du, S.; Sun, J.; Zeng, Z. Molecular mechanisms investigation for liver metastasis of colorectal cancer by combined bioinformatic gene expression profile analysis. *Cancer Treat. Res. Commun.* **2023**, *35*, 100694. [CrossRef]
76. An, R.; Yu, H.; Wang, Y.; Lu, J.; Gao, Y.; Xie, X.; Zhang, J. Integrative analysis of plasma metabolomics and proteomics reveals the metabolic landscape of breast cancer. *Cancer Metab.* **2022**, *10*, 13. [CrossRef] [PubMed]
77. Yu, C.; Luan, Y.; Wang, Z.; Zhao, J.; Xu, C. Suppression of TAFI by siRNA inhibits invasion and migration of breast cancer cells. *Mol. Med. Rep.* **2017**, *16*, 3469–3474. [CrossRef]
78. Monden, T.; Morimoto, H.; Shimano, T.; Yagyu, T.; Murotani, M.; Nagaoka, H.; Kawasaki, Y.; Kobayashi, T.; Mori, T. Use of fibrinogen to enhance the antitumor effect of OK-432. A new approach to immunotherapy for colorectal carcinoma. *Cancer* **1992**, *69*, 636–642. [CrossRef]
79. Zhang, S.; Rao, G.; Heimberger, A.; Li, S. Fibrinogen-like protein 2: Its biological function across cell types and the potential to serve as an immunotherapy target for brain tumors. *Cytokine Growth Factor Rev.* **2023**, *69*, 73–79. [CrossRef]
80. Patadia, H.; Priyadarshini, A.; Gangawane, A. Integrated proteomic, transcriptomic, and genomic analysis identifies fibrinogen beta and fibrinogen gamma as key modulators of breast cancer progression and metastasis. *Biomed. Biotechnol. Res. J.* **2022**, *6*, 266–277. [CrossRef]
81. Liu, Y.; Yan, Z.; Xia, Y.; Xie, X.; Zhou, K.; Xu, L.; Shi, Y.; Wang, Q.; Bi, J. Ligustrazine reverts anthracycline chemotherapy resistance of human breast cancer by inhibiting JAK2/STAT3 signaling and decreasing fibrinogen gamma chain (FGG) expression. *Am. J. Cancer Res.* **2020**, *10*, 939–952. [PubMed]

82. Peng, H.; Wang, J.; Xiao, L.; Yan, M.; Chen, S.; Wang, L.; Yang, K. Elevated serum fgg levels prognosticate and promote the disease progression in prostate cancer. *Front. Genet.* **2021**, *12*, 651647. [CrossRef] [PubMed]
83. Tinholt, M.; Stavik, B.; Tekpli, X.; Garred, Ø.; Borgen, E.; Kristensen, V.; Sahlberg, K.K.; Sandset, P.M.; Iversen, N. Coagulation factor V is a marker of tumor-infiltrating immune cells in breast cancer. *Oncoimmunology* **2020**, *9*, 1824644. [CrossRef]
84. Andresen, M.S.; Sletten, M.; Sandset, P.M.; Iversen, N.; Stavik, B.; Tinholt, M. Coagulation factor V (F5) is an estrogen-responsive gene in breast cancer cells. *Thromb. Haemost.* **2022**, *122*, 1288–1295. [CrossRef] [PubMed]
85. Lind, S.M. The Role of Coagulation Factor V in Breast Cancer: Effect on Treatment Response. Master's Thesis, Norwegian University of Life Sciences, Ås, Norway, 2021. Available online: https://hdl.handle.net/11250/2826527 (accessed on 6 February 2024).
86. Tong, Y.; Tan, Z.; Wang, P.; Gao, X. A machine learning method for predicting biomarkers associated with prostate cancer. *Front. Biosci.-Landmark* **2023**, *28*, 333. [CrossRef]
87. Liu, Y.; Liao, X.; Qin, Y.; Mo, X.; Luo, S. Identification of F5 as a prognostic biomarker in patients with gastric cancer. *BioMed Res. Int.* **2020**, *2020*, 9280841. [CrossRef] [PubMed]
88. Guan, Y.; Xu, B.; Sui, Y.; Chen, Z.; Luan, Y.; Jiang, Y.; Wei, L.; Long, W.; Zhao, S.; Han, L.; et al. Pan-cancer analysis and validation reveals that D-Dimer-Related genes are prognostic and downregulate CD8+ T cells via TGF-Beta signaling in gastric cancer. *Front. Mol. Biosci.* **2022**, *9*, 790706. [CrossRef] [PubMed]
89. Dai, M.; Lu, H. Inhibition of MDM2-mediated p53 ubiquitination and degradation by ribosomal protein L5. *J. Biol. Chem.* **2004**, *279*, 44475–44482. [CrossRef] [PubMed]
90. Zhou, X.; Liao, W.; Liao, J.; Liao, P.; Lu, H. Ribosomal proteins: Functions beyond the ribosome. *J. Mol. Cell Biol.* **2015**, *7*, 92–104. [CrossRef]
91. Kastenhuber, E.R.; Lowe, S.W. Putting p53 in context. *Cell* **2017**, *170*, 1062–1078. [CrossRef]
92. Jiang, X.; Stockwell, B.R.; Conrad, M. Ferroptosis: Mechanisms, biology and role in disease. *Nat. Rev. Mol. Cell. Biol.* **2021**, *22*, 266–282. [CrossRef]
93. Wilson-Edell, K.A.; Kehasse, A.; Scott, G.K.; Yau, C.; Rothschild, D.E.; Schilling, B.; Gabriel, B.S.; Yevtushenko, M.A.; Hanson, I.M.; Held, J.M.; et al. RPL24: A potential therapeutic target whose depletion or acetylation inhibits polysome assembly and cancer cell growth. *Oncotarget* **2014**, *5*, 5165–5176. [CrossRef]
94. Zhang, H.; Liu, T.; Zhang, Z.; Payne, S.H.; Zhang, B.; McDermott, J.E.; Zhou, J.; Petyuk, V.A.; Chen, L.; Ray, D.; et al. Integrated proteogenomic characterization of human high-grade serous ovarian cancer. *Cell* **2016**, *166*, 755–765. [CrossRef] [PubMed]
95. Akbani, R.; Ng, P.K.S.; Werner, H.M.; Shahmoradgoli, M.; Zhang, F.; Ju, Z.; Liu, W.; Yang, J.; Yoshihara, K.; Li, J.; et al. A pan-cancer proteomic perspective on the Cancer Genome Atlas. *Nat. Commun.* **2014**, *5*, 3887. [CrossRef] [PubMed]
96. Xiao, X.; Li, H.; Jin, H.; Jin, J.; Yu, M.; Ma, C.; Tong, Y.; Zhou, L.; Lei, H.; Xu, H.; et al. Identification of 11(13)-dehydroivaxillin as a potent therapeutic agent against non-Hodgkin's lymphoma. *Cell Death Dis.* **2017**, *8*, e3050. [CrossRef]
97. Jiang, L.; Sun, Y.; Wang, J.; He, Q.; Chen, X.; Lan, X.; Chen, J.; Dou, Q.P.; Shi, X.; Liu, J. Proteasomal cysteine deubiquitinase inhibitor b-AP15 suppresses migration and induces apoptosis in diffuse large B cell lymphoma. *J. Exp. Clin. Cancer Res.* **2019**, *38*, 453. [CrossRef]
98. Chauhan, D.; Catley, L.; Li, G.; Podar, K.; Hideshima, T.; Velankar, M.; Mitsiades, C.; Mitsiades, N.; Yasui, H.; Letai, A. A novel orally active proteasome inhibitor induces apoptosis in multiple myeloma cells with mechanisms distinct from Bortezomib. *Cancer Cell* **2005**, *8*, 407–419. [CrossRef] [PubMed]

pharmaceuticals

MDPI

Article

Comparative Assessment of Beeswax Alcohol and Coenzyme Q_{10} (CoQ_{10}) to Prevent Liver Aging, Organ Damage, and Oxidative Stress in Hyperlipidemic Zebrafish Exposed to D-Galactose: A 12-Week Dietary Intervention

Kyung-Hyun Cho *, Ashutosh Bahuguna, Ji-Eun Kim, Yunki Lee and Sang Hyuk Lee

Raydel Research Institute, Medical Innovation Complex, Daegu 41061, Republic of Korea
* Correspondence: chok@raydel.co.kr; Tel.: +82-53-964-1990; Fax: +82-53-965-1992

Abstract: The current study was designed to compare in vivo efficacy between beeswax alcohol (BWA) and coenzyme Q_{10} (CoQ_{10}) to treat fatty liver changes, oxidative stress, and damages in major organs of zebrafish by 12 weeks with high-cholesterol (HC) and galactose (Gal) supplementation. At week 12, the HC control and HC+Gal control groups showed 96% and 92% survivability, respectively, while co-supplementation of the 0.5% BWA and 1.0% BWA groups exhibited 96% and 100% survivability. However, co-supplementation of the 0.5% CoQ_{10} and 1.0% CoQ_{10} groups revealed the lowest survivability, around 92% and 89%, respectively. The 0.5% BWA and 1.0% BWA groups showed 21% ($p < 0.001$) and 41% ($p < 0.001$), respectively, lower total cholesterol (TC) than the HC+Gal control, while the 1.0% CoQ_{10} group showed only 15% lower TC than the control. Interestingly, the 0.5% BWA and 1.0% BWA groups showed 22% ($p < 0.001$) and 38% ($p < 0.001$), respectively, lower triglyceride (TG) than the HC+Gal control. However, both the 0.5% CoQ_{10} and 1.0% CoQ_{10} groups showed similar TG levels as the control, suggesting that CoQ_{10} supplementation had no effect on lowering serum TG. The 1.0% BWA group showed the highest plasma HDL-C and HDL-C/TC (%) up to 3.2-fold and 5.5-fold, respectively, higher than those of the HC+Gal control, while the 1.0% CoQ_{10} group showed 2.4-fold and 2.8-fold higher plasma HDL-C and HDL-C/TC (%), respectively, than the control. The plasma aspartate transaminase (AST) and alanine transaminase (ALT) levels were lowest in the 1.0% BWA group, 51% and 72%, respectively, lower than HC+Gal control, suggesting the lowest extent of hepatic damage. In hepatic tissue, neutrophil infiltration and interleukin (IL)-6 production were the lowest in the 1.0% BWA group, around 67% and 85%, respectively, lower than the HC+Gal control. Fatty liver change, cellular apoptosis, and cell senescence in hepatic tissue were remarkably lowered in the 1.0% BWA group, while the CoQ_{10} group showed much less effect than the BWA group. In kidney, ovary, and testis tissue, the 1.0% BWA group showed the lowest production of reactive oxygen species, the extent of cellular senescence, and cellular apoptosis with the healthiest cell morphology. In conclusion, supplementation of BWA remarkably protected the liver, kidney, ovary, and testis from oxidative damage by cholesterol and galactose consumption, with the least serum AST and ALT levels, inflammatory parameters, and senescence markers.

Keywords: beeswax alcohol (BWA); coenzyme Q_{10} (CoQ_{10}); cholesterol; galactose; aging; liver; inflammation; zebrafish

1. Introduction

Beeswax is a natural product produced by different species of honeybees [1,2]. The most commercially used beeswax is produced by the honeybee species *Apis mellifera* and *Apis cerana* [1]. Typically, beeswax is a complex mixture of more than 300 constituents that majorly comprises esters (67%), hydrocarbons of C27–C33 (12–16%), and free fatty acids (12%) [1,3]. The composition of beeswax may vary based on the families and breed of the honeybees [1]. Beeswax is processed by various methods to obtain the beeswax alcohol (BWA) [4], a typical mixture of long-chain aliphatic alcohols [1,3,5]. Nevertheless, the composition of the long-chain aliphatic alcohols (LCAAs) in BWA varies based on the beeswax source used for the BWA extraction.

BWA is well known for its antioxidant and anti-inflammatory activity [6–8]. BWA's potent antioxidant, hepatoprotective, and gastroprotective role in preventing oxidation of protein and lipids in the cell membrane has been described [9–11]. In addition, BWA's role in preventing LDL oxidation [12] and activity enhancement of HDL-associated PON-1 [12] and inhibition of HDL glycation has been recognized recently [13]. Despite the several beneficial effects, the most noteworthy effect of BWA was observed in protecting gastric health by improving gastric mucosa quality and quantity [11,14]. BWA oral supplementation in rats prevents gastric ulceration by augmenting antioxidant status, reducing neutrophil infiltration, and enhancing secretion and quality improvement of gastric mucosa [5]. Also, the BWA impact on preventing gastric ulcers by the inhibition of protein oxidation and generation of hydroxyl radicals along with the activity enhancement of catalase, superoxide dismutase (SOD), and glutathione peroxidase (GSH-PXs) has been depicted in the gastric mucosa strengthening its strong antioxidant property [5,11]. The antioxidant effect of BWA is not only limited to the mucosa, but it also reduces lipid peroxidation and protein oxidation and raises the activities of cellular antioxidants in the liver and brain [5,6]. In a clinical study, eight weeks of supplementation of BWA (100 mg/day) improved gastrointestinal health by reducing acidity, bloating, regurgitation, sucking, and flatulence scores [5]. A six-month BWA consumption study displayed substantial antioxidant and gastroprotective effects in middle-aged and elderly human subjects [15]. Besides the gastroprotective role, BWA also displayed a substantial effect on joint health by markedly reducing proinflammatory leukotriene B4 (LTB4) levels and the inhibition of cyclooxygenase (COX) and 5 lipoxygenase (5-LOX) activities [5]. Due to the notable advantages of BWA, it has recently been approved by the Korean Food and Drug Administration (KFDA) as a functional food ingredient to support gastric and joint health [16].

Among lipid-soluble antioxidants, coenzyme Q_{10} (CoQ_{10}) displayed substantial hepatoprotective effects and prevented nonalcoholic fatty liver diseases (NAFLDs) in experimental animals and humans [17,18]. However, a recent meta-analysis of randomized controlled trials revealed a statistically non-significant decrease in lipid profiles and liver enzymes of NAFLD patients after treatment with CoQ_{10} [17]. Under a cholesterol-rich diet, CoQ_{10} supplementation improved metabolic parameters and hepatic functions in rats in the presence of high doses of atorvastatin [19]. Also, CoQ_{10}, due to its antioxidant effect, prevents atorvastatin-induced myotoxicity in zebrafish embryos [20].

Aging in multi-organ systems, including the liver, kidney, and brain, is associated with functional loss and morphological changes, including a decrease in mitochondrial numbers and a reduction in hepatocyte telomere length due to the accumulation of oxidative stress and inflammation [21]. D-galactose is well known to accelerate aging via the accumulation of galactitol and H_2O_2, which are directly linked with the impairment of cell redox homeostasis and increased levels of inflammatory markers [22,23]. The galactose supplementation induced aging in the liver, kidney, brain, and reproductive systems with an elevation of malondialdehyde (MDA), reactive oxygen species (ROS), and proinflammatory cytokines, such as tumor necrosis factor (TNF)-alpha and interleukin (IL)-6 [24]. Moreover, D-galactose-induced aging is associated with fatty liver disease and dyslipidemia characterized by high serum cholesterol and triglyceride with low HDL-C levels [25]. Although D-galactose has been used to induce oxidative stress and to develop an aging process in rats and mice [26], there has been no study to induce artificial aging in adult zebrafish by galactose supplementation. Knowing this, in the present study, D-galactose was used as an inducer of aging in adult zebrafish, enabling the assessment of BWA and CoQ_{10} against D-galactose-induced adversity.

In our previous study, a substantial effect of BWA to prevent LDL oxidation [12], functionality improvement of HDL by augmenting PON-1 activity [12], and a protective effect against ethanol-induced toxicity in zebrafish were reported [27]. Additionally, BWA in reconstituted high-density lipoprotein (HDL) shields HDL from fructose-induced glycation and counteracts carboxymethyllysine (CML)-posed toxicity in zebrafish embryos and adults through its antioxidant and anti-inflammatory mechanisms which have been disclosed [13]. Although there is growing interest in the therapeutic potential of BWA, studies on the impact of BWA on conditions like dyslipidemia and liver toxicity, particularly induced by high cholesterol and galactose, are still scarce. To address this gap, the present study aims to evaluate the comparative effectiveness of BWA and CoQ_{10} following 12 weeks of supplementation in combating galactose-induced oxidative stress, inflammatory injuries, and dyslipidemia in hyperlipidemic zebrafish.

2. Results

2.1. Zebrafish Survivability and Body Weight

During 12 weeks of consumption, as shown in Figure 1A, HC+Gal groups showed 93% survivability, while the HC alone group showed 96% survivability, suggesting that co-supplementation of galactose caused more toxic and lethal effects to zebrafish. HC+Gal+0.5% BWA and HC+Gal+1.0% BWA groups showed 96% and 100% survivability, respectively, suggesting that co-consumption of BWA prevented the HC+Gal-induced premature death. However, HC+Gal+0.5% CoQ_{10} and HC+Gal+1.0% CoQ_{10} groups exhibited 93% and 89% survivability, respectively, suggesting that co-consumption of CoQ_{10} did not prevent premature death by hyperlipidemia and galactose toxicity.

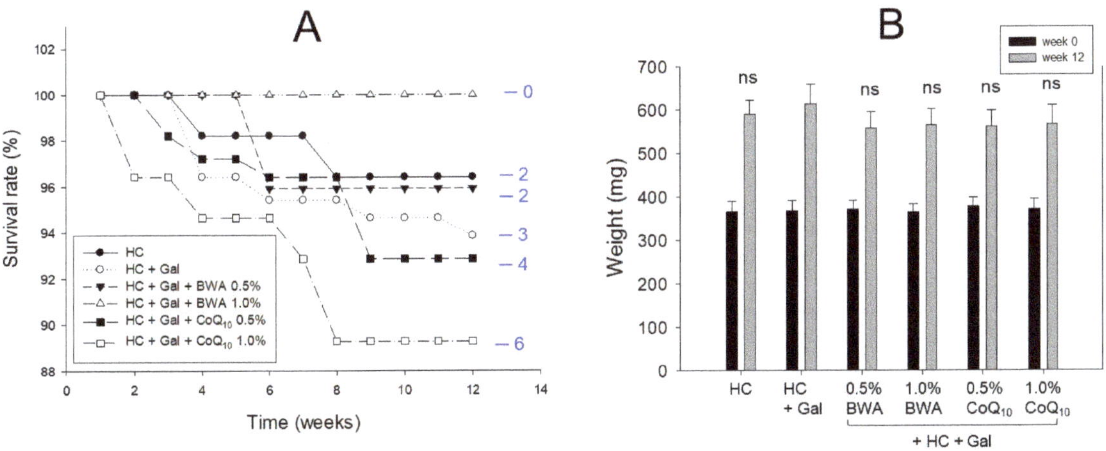

Figure 1. Comparative assessment of beeswax alcohol (BWA) and coenzyme Q_{10} (CoQ_{10}) under a high-cholesterol (HC, final 4%, *w/w*) and galactose (Gal, final 10%, *w/w*) diet on the survivability and body weight of zebrafish. (**A**) The survival rate of zebrafish across the different groups during 12 weeks of consumption of BWA or CoQ_{10}. The numerical values in the blue font represent the total number of dead zebrafish in the respective groups at 12 weeks. (**B**) Body weight of the zebrafish at the beginning (week 0) and after 12 weeks of consumption of BWA or CoQ_{10}. ns indicates a non-significant difference between the groups.

As shown in Figure 1B, during the 12 weeks, consumption of HC alone, HC+Gal, and HC+Gal with BWA or CoQ_{10} showed a nearly similar ~1.5-fold body weight enhancement with respect to the body weight observed on day 0. There is a non-significant difference in the net body weight attained at 12 weeks of consumption of different diets. The net body weight change during the 12 weeks of consumption across all the groups was in the range of 148–160% (Table 1).

Table 1. Survivability and body weight of zebrafish across the different groups at the beginning (week 0) and at 12 weeks of consumption of the respective diets.

Survivability and BW of Zebrafish	HC	HC+Gal	HC+Gal +0.5% BWA	HC+Gal +1.0% BWA	HC+Gal +0.5% CoQ_{10}	HC+Gal +1.0% CoQ_{10}
Week 0 (n)	56	56	56	56	56	56
Week 12 (n)	54	52	54	56	52	50
Survivability	96.4	92.9	96.4	100.0	92.9	89.3
BW at week 0	366.4 ± 24.5	368.3 ± 22.9	372.3 ± 20.1	365.1 ± 17.9	378 ± 21.5	372.3 ± 22.3
BW at week 12	590.9 ± 31.8	614.3 ± 45.3	558.7 ± 37.4	564.5 ± 36.8	561.7 ± 37.0	565.9 ± 45.0
Net increase in BW (mg)	224.5 ± 8.7	246.1 ± 25.4	180.1 ± 19.8	212.4 ± 20	175.5 ± 16.2	164.7 ± 27
Net increase in BW (%)	161.3 ± 2.3	166.8 ± 3.9	150.1 ± 3.9	154.6 ± 3.0	148.6 ± 2.1	152.0 ± 4.7

BW, body weight; BWA, beeswax alcohol; CoQ_{10}, coenzymeQ_{10}; Gal, galactose; HC, high cholesterol.

2.2. Change in Lipid Profiles

As shown in Figure 2A,B, the HC+Gal group showed a significant 9% ($p < 0.01$) and 10% ($p < 0.01$) higher TC and TG level than the HC alone group, suggesting that co-consumption of galactose augments the HC-induced blood TC and TG levels to exacerbate hyperlipidemia. However, the 1.0% BWA group showed the lowest plasma TC and TG levels, around 41% and 39%, lower than the HC+Gal control group, respectively, while the BWA 0.5% group showed 21% and 22% lower TC and TG levels than the HC+Gal control group. In contrast, both the 0.5% and 1.0% CoQ_{10} group showed around 14% lower TC level ($p < 0.01$) than the HC+Gal control. However, both the 0.5% and 1.0% CoQ_{10} groups showed similar TG levels (187–191 mg/dL) as observed in the HC+Gal control group (193.9 mg/dL), suggesting that consumption of CoQ_{10} was not effective in reducing blood TG level.

Compared to the CoQ_{10} group, a significantly 30% ($p < 0.05$) lower TC was observed in the 1.0% BWA group. Also, a significantly 20% ($p < 0.05$) and 36% ($p < 0.01$) lower TG was quantified in the 0.5% BWA and 1.0% BWA group compared to the 1.0% CoQ_{10} group, demonstrating the superior efficacy of BWA over CoQ_{10} in minimizing HC+Gal-induced TC and TG levels.

As shown in Figure 2C,D, the HC+Gal group showed 48% and 54% lower HDL-C and HDL-C/TC (%), respectively, than those of the HC alone group, suggesting that co-consumption of galactose caused a significant lowering of HDL-C and the percentage of HDL-C in TC. The 1.0% BWA group showed the highest HDL-C and HDL-C/TC (%), around 3.2-fold and 5.5-fold higher than the HC+Gal group, while the 0.5% BWA group showed 2.4-fold and 3.2-fold higher HDL-C and HDL-C/TC (%) than those of the HC+Gal group.

As shown in Figure 2E, the HC+Gal group showed the highest TG/HDL-C ratio, around 9.2, while the HC alone group showed 4.3, suggesting that co-consumption of galactose induced a 2.1-fold more atherogenic lipid profile. The co-supplementation of 1.0% BWA showed the lowest TG/HDL-C ratio, around 1.7, followed by the 0.5% BWA group (around 2.9), suggesting that 0.5% BWA and 1.0% BWA co-consumption resulted in a 69% and 82% reduction in the TG/HDL-C ratio compared with the HC+Gal control. The co-supplementation of 0.5% and 1.0% CoQ_{10} showed around 3.8 and 3.6 TG/HDL-C ratios, respectively, which is nearly similar to the TG/HDL-C ratio observed in the HC group. The ratio of LDL-C/HDL-C (L:H ratio) was highest in the HC+Gal group, around 5.1, while 0.5% BWA and 1.0% BWA groups showed the lowest level, around 1.0 and 0.2, respectively. In contrast, 0.5% CoQ_{10} and 1.0% CoQ_{10} groups showed a 1.2 and 1.0 L:H ratio. The combined outcomes of the plasma lipid profile indicate that BWA exhibits significantly greater efficacy than CoQ_{10} in mitigating HC+Gal-induced dyslipidemia.

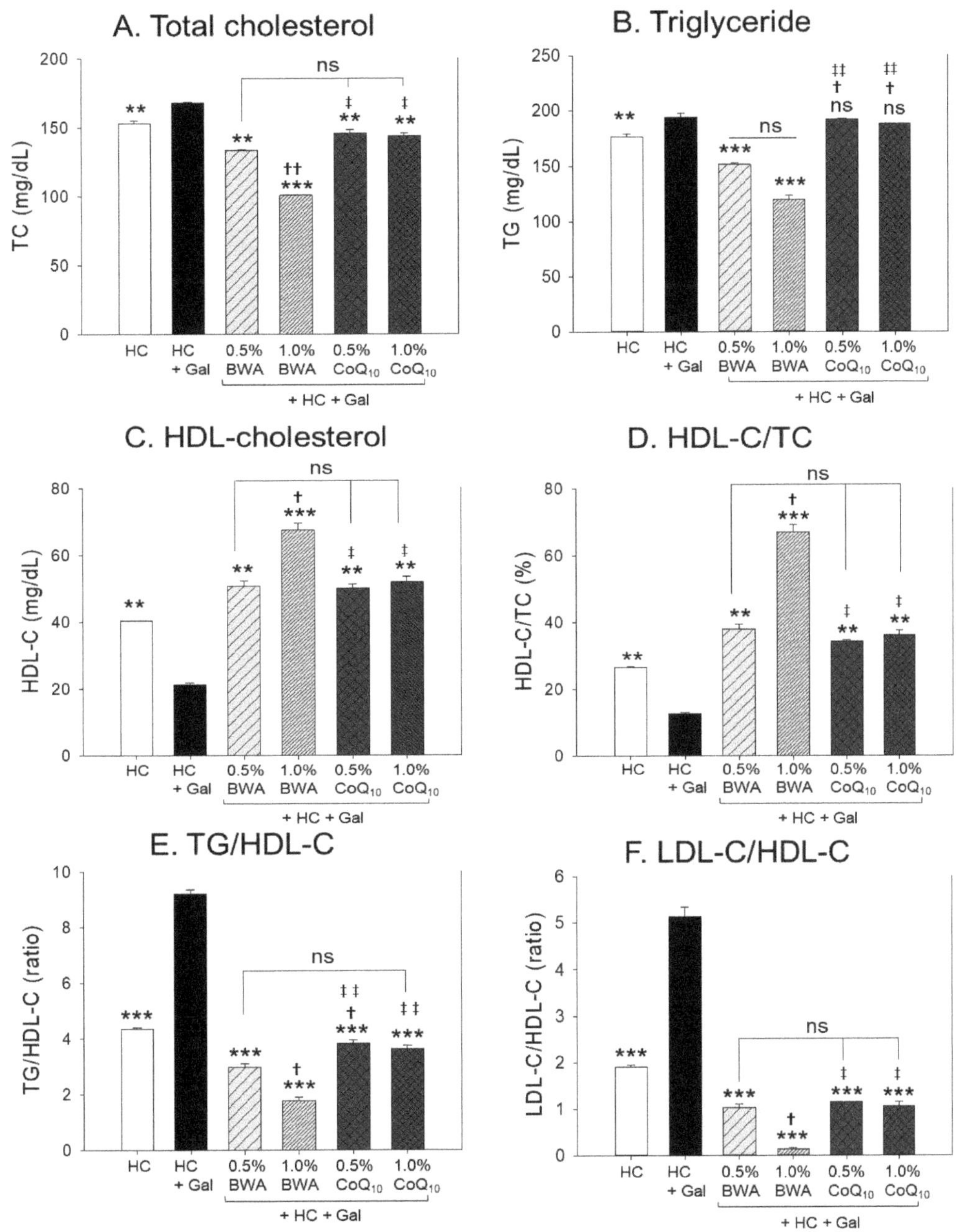

Figure 2. Change in plasma lipid profiles among beeswax alcohol (BWA) and coenzyme Q_{10} (CoQ_{10}) groups after 12 weeks of consumption under a high-cholesterol (HC, final 4%, *w/w*) and galactose (Gal, final 10%, *w/w*) diet. (**A**) Total cholesterol (TC); (**B**) triglyceride (TG); (**C**) high-density lipoprotein cholesterol (HDL-C); (**D**) percentage of HDL-C in total cholesterol (HDL-C/TC, %); (**E**) triglycerides (TG) and HDL-C ratio; (**F**) low-density lipoprotein cholesterol (LDL-C) and HDL-C ratio; Gal, galactose; high-cholesterol diet (HC); beeswax alcohol (BWA); and coenzyme Q_{10} (CoQ_{10}).

The statistical divergence between the groups was denoted by ** ($p < 0.01$) and *** ($p < 0.001$) for the HC+Gal group. † ($p < 0.05$) and †† ($p < 0.01$) displayed significant difference correspond to the HC+Gal+0.5% BWA group while ‡ ($p < 0.05$) and ‡‡ ($p < 0.01$) displayed significant difference correspond to the HC+Gal+1.0% BWA group; ns represents a non-significant difference between the groups.

2.3. Change in Hepatic Damage Parameters

As shown in Figure 3, the HC+Gal group showed the highest AST and ALT levels, i.e., 11% and 35% higher than the HC alone group, respectively, suggesting that co-supplementation of galactose caused more severe hepatic damage consequently increasing the AST and ALT levels. The 1.0% BWA group showed the lowest level of AST and ALT, i.e., 46% and 72%, lower than those of the HC+Gal control, respectively. The 0.5% BWA group showed the second lowest level of AST and ALT, i.e., 25% and 41%, lower than those of the HC+Gal control, respectively, suggesting the dose-dependent effect of BWA to protect HC+ Gal-induced hepatic damage. On the other hand, the 0.5% and 1.0% CoQ_{10} groups exhibited 22~25% lower ALT levels than those of the HC+Gal control; however, no significant changes in AST levels, regardless of the dosage of CoQ_{10}, were observed. These results suggest that co-consumption of BWA was more effective than CoQ_{10} in preventing the hepatic damage caused by intake of HC+Gal.

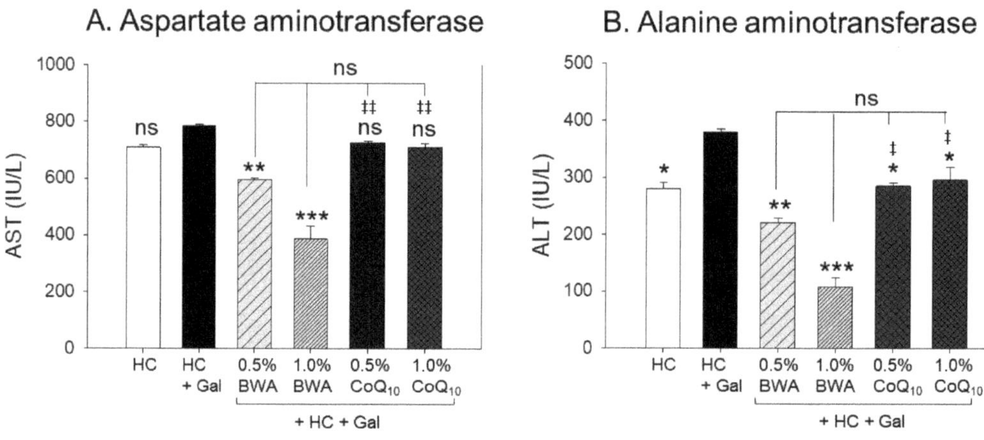

Figure 3. Change in plasma hepatic parameters, (**A**) aspartate aminotransferase (AST) and (**B**) alanine aminotransferase (ALT), among beeswax alcohol (BWA) and coenzyme Q_{10} (CoQ_{10}) groups after 12 weeks of consumption under high-cholesterol (HC, final 4%, *w/w*) and galactose (Gal, final 10%, *w/w*) supplementation. The statistical divergence between the groups was denoted by * ($p < 0.05$), ** ($p < 0.01$), and *** ($p < 0.001$) for the HC+Gal group, while ‡ ($p < 0.05$) and ‡‡ ($p < 0.01$) correspond to the HC+Gal+1.0% BWA group; ns represents a non-significant difference between the groups.

2.4. Histologic Analysis of Liver Tissue

As shown in Figure 4A, H&E staining with a microsection of hepatic tissue revealed that the HC+Gal group showed the highest H&E-stained area and number of infiltrated neutrophils (indicated by the red arrow), which is significantly1.9-fold and 2.5-fold more than the HC group. The consumption of 1.0% BWA showed the lowest H&E-stained area and neutrophil infiltration (red arrow), which was around 67% and 83% less than that of the HC+Gal control, respectively. Additionally, the least lipid droplets (indicated by the blue arrow) were observed in the 1.0% BWA group. The 0.5% BWA group showed the second lowest H&E-stained area and neutrophil infiltration, which was around 62% and 56%, lower than the HC+Gal control, respectively. Interestingly, the 0.5% and 1.0% CoQ_{10} groups exhibited weaker efficacy towards the HC+Gal-altered H&E-stained area and neutrophil infiltration as manifested by around 16~22% and 49~52% lesser H&E-stained area and neutrophil counts than the HC+Gal group.

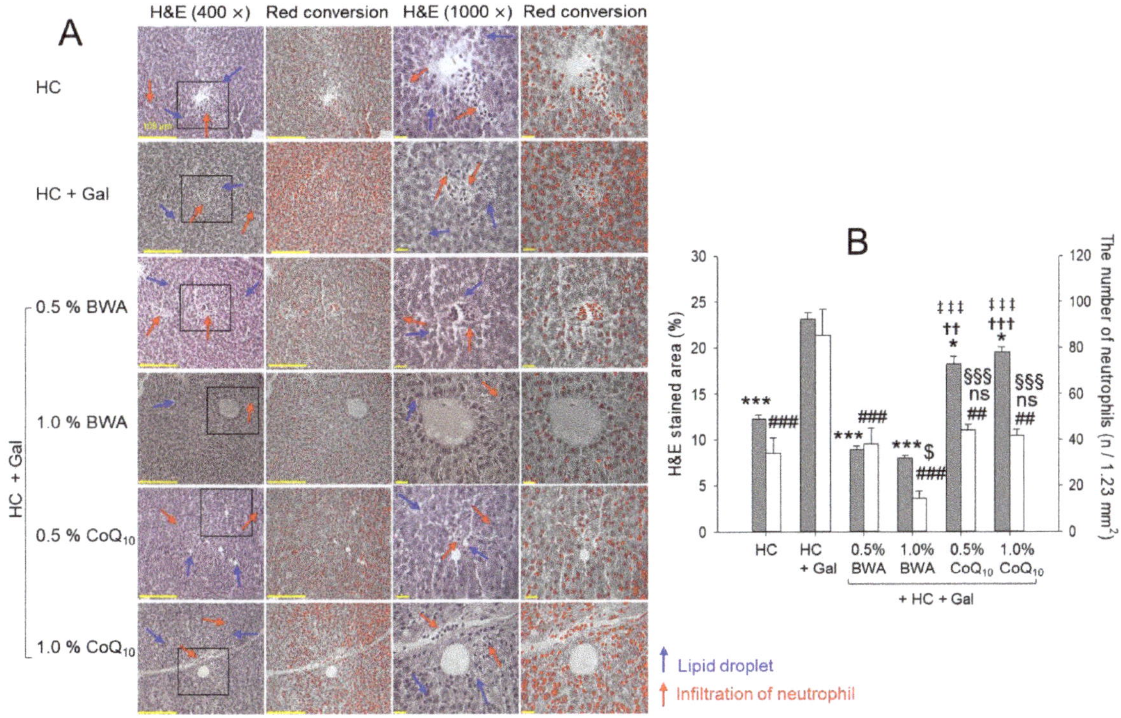

Figure 4. Liver histological analysis of zebrafish consuming a designated diet under high-cholesterol (HC, final 4%, *w/w*) and galactose (Gal, final 10%, *w/w*) supplementation. (**A**) Hematoxylin and eosin (H&E) staining visualized at 400× [scale bar = 100 μm] and 1000× [scale bar = 10 μm] magnification. The blue and red arrow indicates lipid droplets and infiltrated neutrophils. (**B**) Percentage of H&E-stained area and numbers of neutrophils in the H&E-stained area. A semiquantitative assessment of neutrophils (stained dark violet color) was carried out by microscopic examination of the designated area (1.23 mm^2) across three distinct sections and five different areas of each group. The statistical divergence between the groups was denoted by * ($p < 0.05$) and *** ($p < 0.001$) for the HC+Gal group, †† ($p < 0.01$) and ††† ($p < 0.001$) for the HC+Gal+5% BWA group, and ‡‡‡ ($p < 0.001$) for the HC+Gal+1.0% BWA group for the H&E-stained area. The statistical divergence for the number of neutrophils between the groups was denoted by ## ($p < 0.01$) and ### ($p < 0.001$) for the HC+Gal group, $ ($p < 0.05$) for the HC+Gal+0.5% BWA group, and §§§ ($p < 0.001$) for the HC+Gal+1.0% BWA group; ns denotes a non-significant difference between the groups.

2.5. Interleukin-6 Production in Liver

Immunohistochemical analysis revealed that the HC+Gal group showed the highest interleukin (IL)-6-stained area, around 39%, which was 2.5-fold higher than the HC alone group, suggesting that the co-consumption of galactose caused more hepatic inflammation (Figure 5A,B). The co-consumption of BWA remarkably decreased IL-6 production, which was around 66% and 91% lower, for the 0.5% BWA and 1.0% BWA groups, respectively, than that of the HC+Gal group. Contrary to this, the CoQ_{10} groups showed less effectiveness in minimizing the HC+Gal-induced IL-6 production. While compared to the 1.0% BWA group, a significantly ~6-fold ($p < 0.01$) higher IL-6 production was noticed in the 0.5% and

1.0% CoQ_{10}-consumed groups, suggesting the lower effectiveness of CoQ_{10} than the BWA to curtail the HC+Gal-induced inflammation measured in terms of IL-6 production.

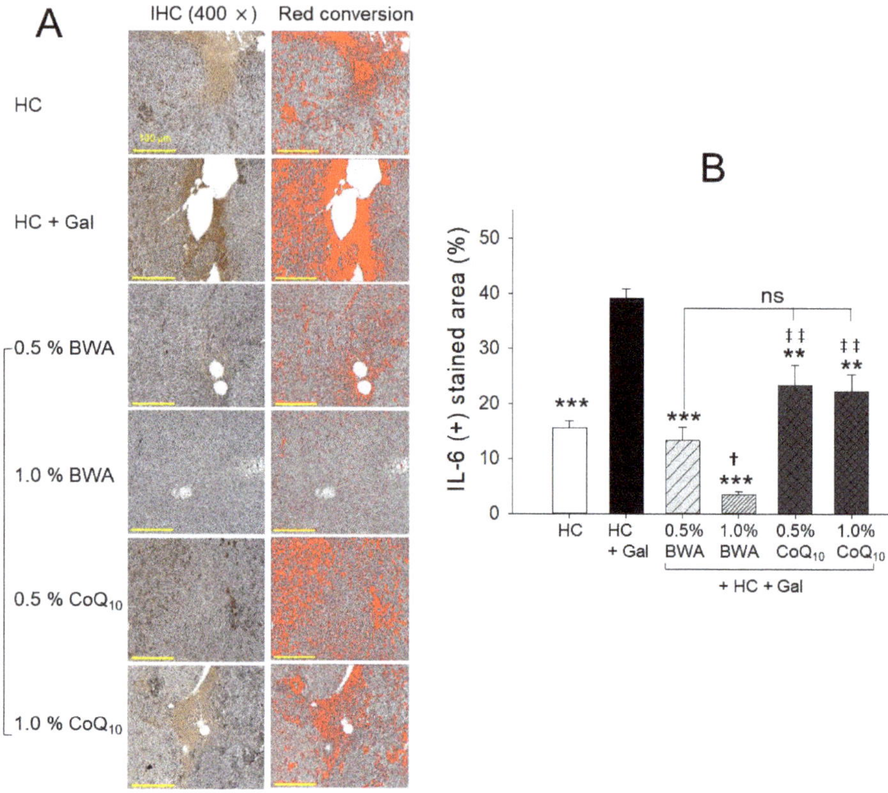

Figure 5. Interleukin (IL)-6 production in the liver section of zebrafish consuming a designated diet under high-cholesterol (HC, final 4%, *w/w*) and galactose (Gal, final 10%, *w/w*) supplementation. (**A**) Images of immunohistochemistry and red conversion images are IHC-stained areas (brown color) interchanged with red color [at a threshold value of (20–100)] using Image J software version 1.53r to enhance visualization. (**B**) Quantification of IL-6-stained area employing Image J software. The statistical divergence between the groups was denoted by ** ($p < 0.01$) and *** ($p < 0.001$) for the HC+Gal group and † ($p < 0.05$) for the HC+Gal+0.5% BWA group, while ‡‡ ($p < 0.01$) was for the HC+Gal+1% BWA group; ns represents a non-significant difference between the groups.

2.6. ROS Production, Apoptosis, Fatty Liver Change, and Cellular Senescence

As shown in Figure 6A,B, the HC+Gal group showed the highest extent of ROS production (DHE-stained red fluorescence) and apoptosis (AO-stained green fluorescence), around 1.5-fold and 1.4-fold, higher than the HC alone group, respectively. The consumption of BWA effectively prevented the HC+Gal-induced ROS production, as evidenced by significantly 3.0-fold- and 3.9-fold-reduced DHE fluorescent intensity in the 0.5% and 1.0% BWA-consumed groups against the HC+Gal control group. Contrary to this, CoQ_{10} at 0.5% was found ineffective in reducing the HC+Gal-provoked ROS production; however, CoQ_{10} at 1.0% consumption significantly reduced the ROS level evident by 1.6-fold ($p < 0.01$)-reduced DHE-stained areas than the DHE-stained area appeared in the HC+Gal group. Likewise, to the outcomes of DHE fluorescent staining, the AO staining represents the significant inhibition of HC+Gal-induced apoptosis in response to the consumption of BWA at both the consumed concentrations of 0.5% and 1.0%. Contrary to this, CoQ_{10} only at 1.0% consumption displayed the antiapoptotic effect. While compared to the 0.5% and 1.0% BWA, a ~2-fold higher AO fluorescent intensity was noticed in the 1.0% CoQ_{10}-consumed group, indicating higher efficacy of BWA to prevent HC+Gal-induced apoptosis in hepatic cells.

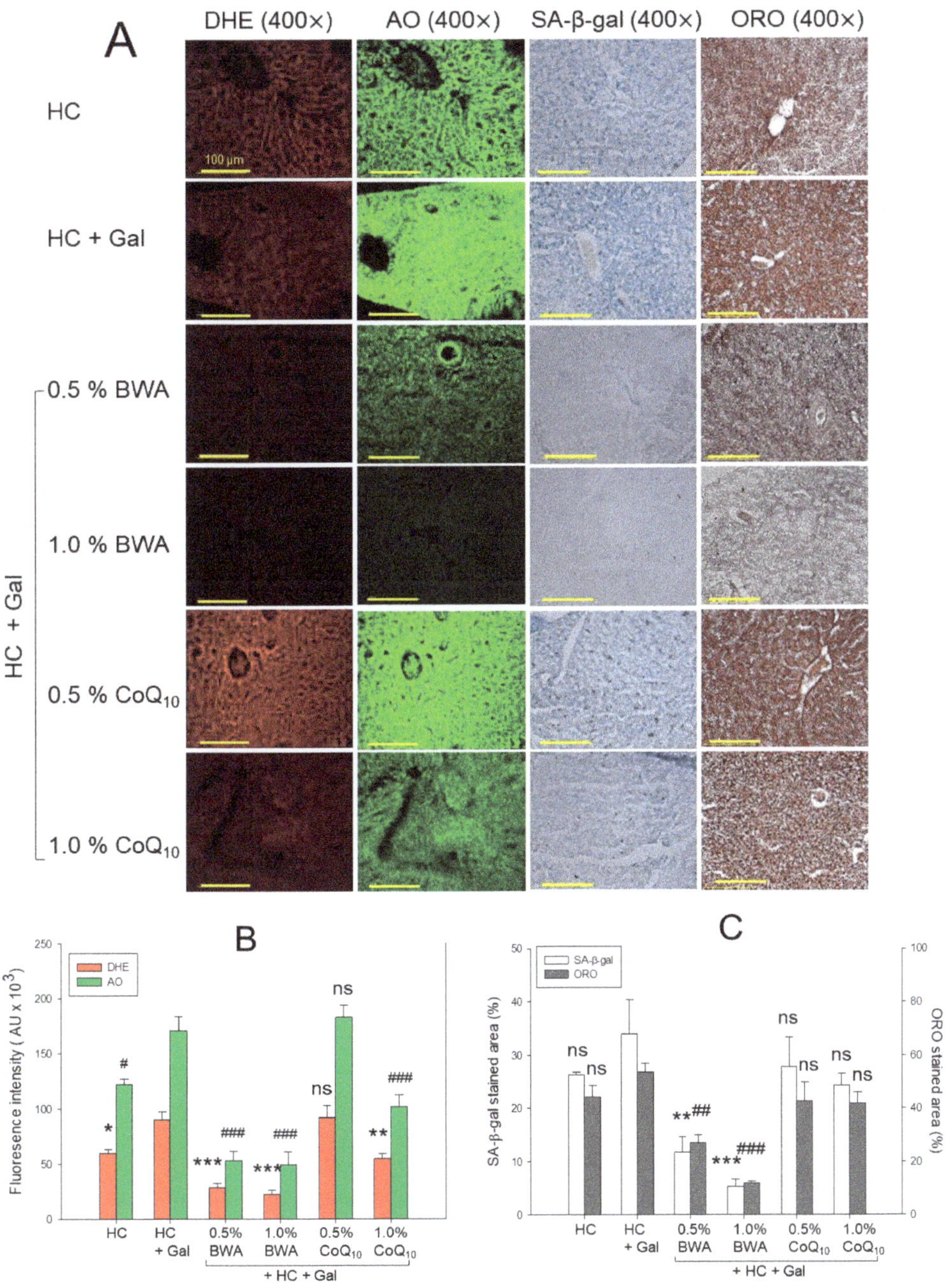

Figure 6. A comparative effect of beeswax alcohol (BWA) and coenzyme Q_{10} (CoQ_{10}) under a high-cholesterol (HC, final 4%, *w/w*) and galactose (Gal, final 10%, *w/w*) diet on hepatic reactive

oxygen species (ROS), apoptosis, senescence, and fatty liver. (**A**) Dihydroethidium (DHE) and acridine orange (AO) fluorescent staining align with reactive oxygen species (ROS) production and the extent of apoptosis, respectively. Oil red O (ORO) and senescent-associated βgalactosidase (SA-β-gal) staining. [100 μm, scale bar]. (**B**) Image J software (version 1.53r) based quantification of DHE and AO fluorescent intensity. (**C**) Quantification of ORO and SA-β-gal-stained area. The statistical divergence between the groups was denoted by * ($p < 0.05$), ** ($p < 0.01$), and *** ($p < 0.001$) for HC+Gal (for DHE and SA-β-gal) while # ($p < 0.05$), ## ($p < 0.01$), and ### ($p < 0.001$) were for HC+Gal (for AO and ORO); a non-significant difference between the groups is indicated by "ns".

The HC+Gal group showed the highest extent of cellular senescence and fatty liver change, up to 1.3-fold and 1.2-fold, higher than the HC alone group, respectively, implying that the addition of galactose causes more severe senescence and lipid accumulation in hepatic cells (Figure 6A,C). Consumption of BWA showed a dose-dependent effect in preventing HC+Gal-induced senescence and fatty liver changes. The 1.0% BWA group showed the least extent of cellular senescence and lipid accumulation, up to 85% and 78%, less than the HC+Gal group, respectively, while compared to the 0.5% BWA-consumed groups, a ~2-fold better inhibition of cellular senescence and lipid accumulation was detected in 1.0% BWA-consumed groups. In contrast to this, CoQ_{10}-consumed groups exhibited no detectable activity to improve cellular senescence and lipid accumulation (Figure 6A,C), indicating the ineffectiveness of CoQ_{10} in protecting against hepatic senescence and fatty liver damage imposed by the consumption of HC+Gal.

2.7. *Histological Analysis of Kidney*

The H&E staining of the kidney section highlighted the morphological changes in response to HC+Gal in the presence and absence of BWA and CoQ_{10} (Figure 7). A sparsely populated proximal and distal tubule with recurrent luminal debris in the tubular cast (indicated by a red arrow) was observed in the HC-consumed group. The consumption of Gal with HC aggravates the HC-induced kidney damage apparent by disorganized proximal tubules (PTs) and distal tubules (DTs) with frequent luminal debris and the presence of dark purple colored basophilic cluster indicating new nephron formation (highlighted by a green arrow), signifying the adverse effect of Gal in the presence of HC. The HC+Gal-induced kidney damage was considerably restored by the consumption of BWA at both the tested concentrations of 0.5% and 1.0%, evident by the well-differentiated and adequately organized proximal and distal tubules. However, the occasional luminal debris in the tubular cast was also noticed (indicated by a red arrow). Likewise, CoQ_{10} also displayed a protective effect against HC+Gal-induced kidney damage, though the efficacy is lower than the BWA. Notably, at 0.5% CoQ_{10}, luminal debris with the presence of a basophilic cluster corresponding to the new nephron generation was observed; on the contrary, at 1.0% CoQ_{10}, a substantial kidney preventive role was noticed.

The DHE and AO fluorescent staining documented the accentuated ROS generation and apoptosis in the HC+Gal group, which was significantly mitigated by consumption of BWA and CoQ_{10} at both the tested concentrations of 0.5% and 1.0%. A 4.1-fold- and 5.2-fold-reduced DHE fluorescent intensity was quantified in the 0.5% and 1.0% BWA-treated group that of the HC+Gal group (Figure 7A,B). Consistently, 3.2-fold- and 8.2-fold-diminished AO fluorescent intensity was noticed in 0.5% and 1.0% of the BWA-treated group compared to the HC+Gal group. Also, CoQ_{10} efficiently prevented the HC+Gal-induced ROS, as depicted by 1.6-fold- and 1.9-fold-reduced DHE fluorescent intensity in 0.5% and 1.0% CoQ_{10}-treated groups, respectively. Similarly, CoQ_{10} at 0.5% and 1.0% concentrations displayed a ~1.6-fold-diminished AO fluorescent intensity with respect to the HC+Gal group. However, compared to CoQ_{10}, BWA displayed a profound effect to reduce HC+Gal-induced ROS and apoptosis as quantified by 2.4-fold and 1.9-fold lower DHE fluorescent intensity and 2.6-fold- and 5.2-fold-diminished AO fluorescent intensity in the 0.5% and 1.0% BWA-consumed groups than that of the 0.5% and 1.0% CoQ_{10}-consumed group, respectively.

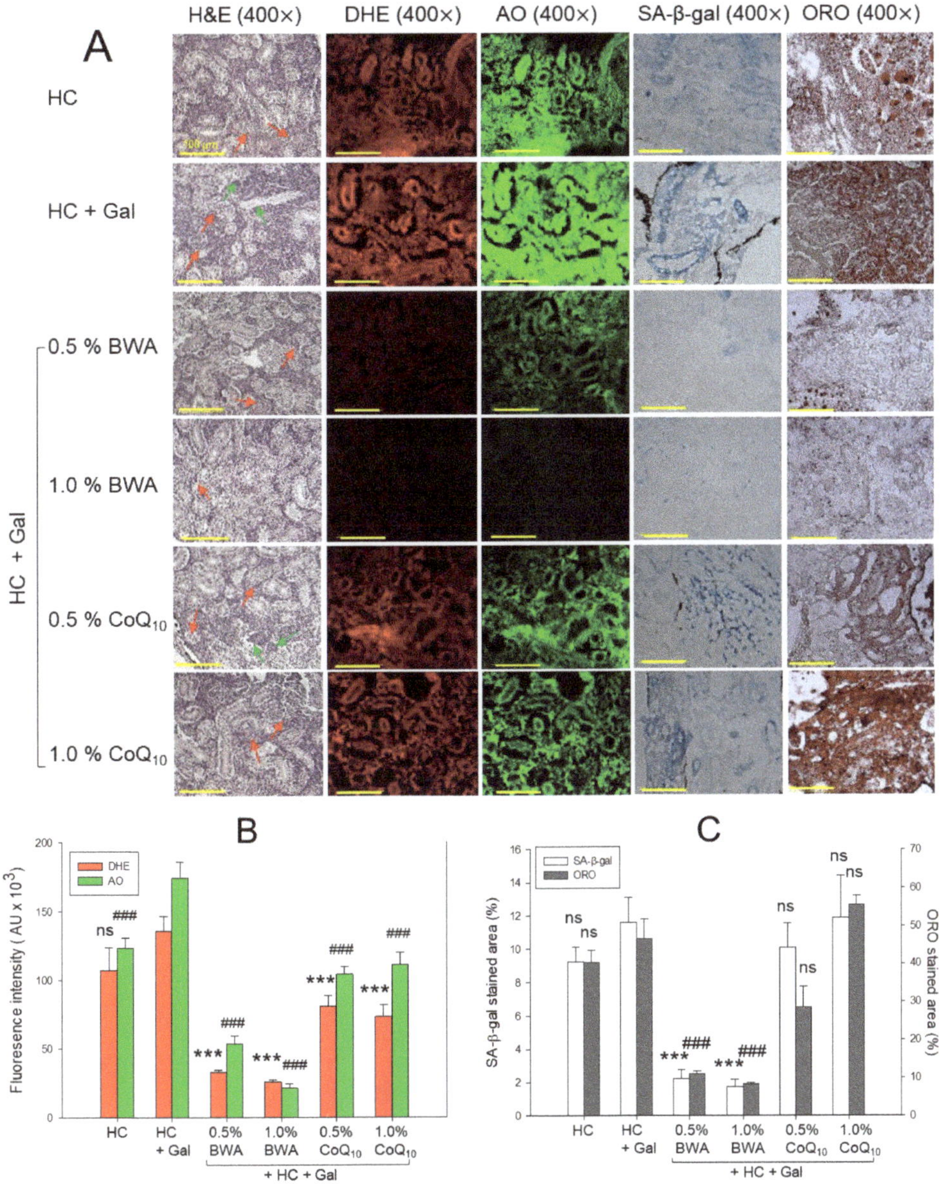

Figure 7. A comparative effect of beeswax alcohol (BWA) and coenzyme Q_{10} (CoQ_{10}) on the kidney of zebrafish fed with a high-cholesterol (HC, final 4%, *w/w*) and galactose (Gal, final 10%, *w/w*) diet. (**A**) Hematoxylin and eosin (H&E) staining; proximal and distal tubules are abbreviated as PT and DT; and the red arrow depicts luminal debris in the tubular cast, while the green arrow depicts the basophilic cluster complying with the new nephron. Dihydroethidium (DHE) and acridine orange (AO) fluorescent staining align with reactive oxygen species (ROS) production and the extent of apoptosis, respectively. Oil red O (ORO) and senescent-associated β-galactosidase (SA-β-gal) staining. [100 μm, scale bar]. (**B**) Image J-based quantification of DHE and AO fluorescent intensity.

(**C**) Quantification of ORO and SA-β-gal-stained area. The statistical divergence between the groups was denoted by *** ($p < 0.001$) for HC+Gal (for DHE and SA-β-gal) while ### ($p < 0.001$) was for HC+Gal (for AO and ORO); a non-significant difference between the groups is indicated by "ns".

ORO staining revealed the impact of HC+Gal on lipid accumulation in the kidney. The BWA at 0.5% and 1.0% concentrations effectively minimized HC+Gal augmented ORO-stained area by 4.2-fold and 5.6-fold compared to the HC+Gal groups (Figure 7A,C). Contrary to this, CoQ_{10} displayed no effect on preventing lipid accumulation stimulated by HC+Gal.

Similar to the ORO staining, higher cellular senescence was perceived in the HC+Gal group, which was significantly minimized by 5.2-fold and 6.7-fold by the treatment of 0.5% and 1.0% BWA, respectively (Figure 7A,C). Similar to the ORO staining, CoQ_{10} displayed no protective effect on cellular senescence actuated by the consumption of HC+Gal.

2.8. Examination of Ovarian Tissue

A significantly higher prevalence of previtellogenic oocytes was noticed in the HC+Gal group, which was 8.7% higher than in the HC group (Figure 8A,B). The BWA at 0.5% and 1.0% significantly, by 7.7% and 14.1%, diminished the previtellogenic oocyte counts affected by the consumption of HC+Gal. Similarly, the HC+Gal-affected early and mature vitellogenic oocyte counts were restored considerably by BWA consumption. Precisely, BWA at a 1.0% concentration displayed significantly 2.2-fold and 5.5-fold higher early and mature oocyte counts compared to the HC+Gal group, signifying the preventive effect of BWA against HC+Gal-induced ovary impairment. Contrary to the BWA, CoQ_{10} had no impact on the ovary morphology (concerning the restoration of pre-, early, and mature vitellogenic oocytes) altered by HC+Gal consumption.

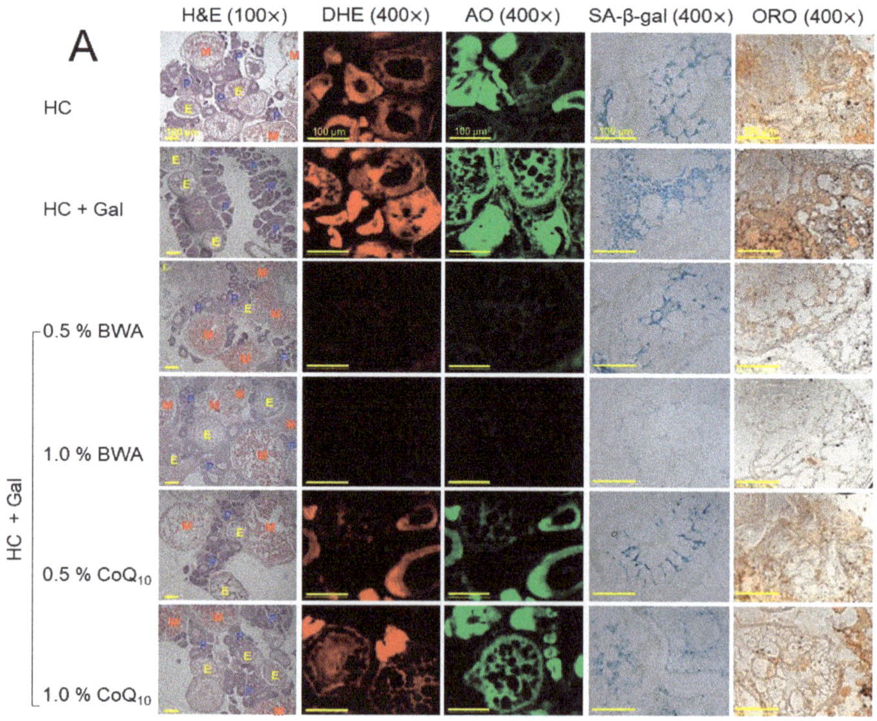

Figure 8. *Cont.*

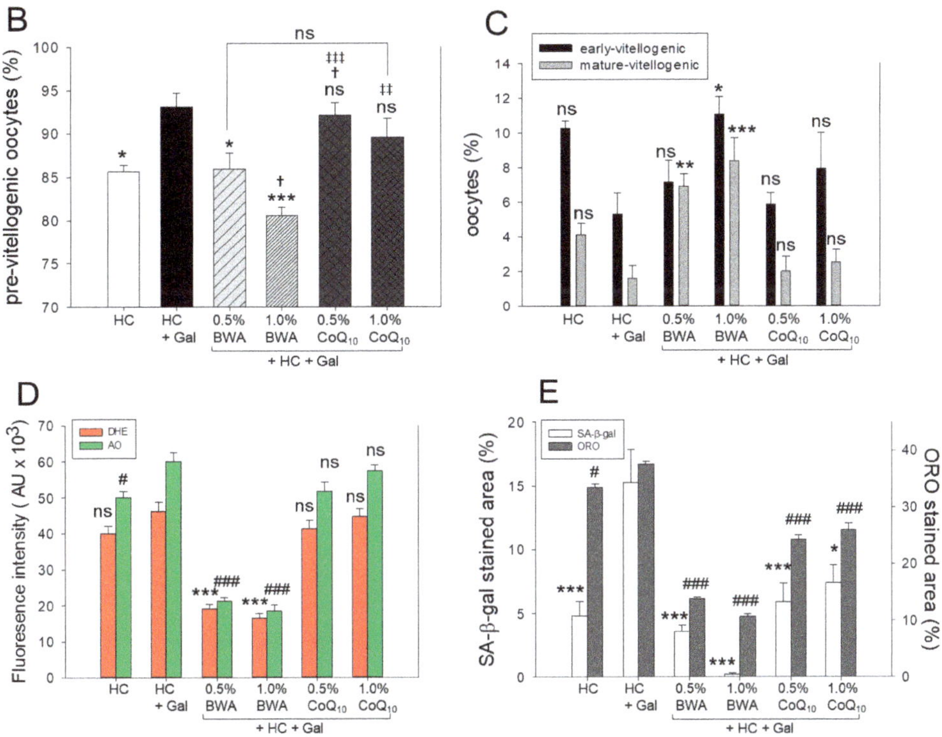

Figure 8. A comparative effect of beeswax alcohol (BWA) and coenzyme Q_{10} (CoQ_{10}) on the ovary of zebrafish fed with a high-cholesterol (HC, final 4%, *w/w*) and galactose (Gal, final 10%, *w/w*) diet. (**A**) Hematoxylin and eosin (H&E) staining; P, E, and M highlight the pre-, early, and mature oocytes, respectively. Dihydroethidium (DHE) and acridine orange (AO) decipher the generation of reactive oxygen species (ROS) and the degree of apoptosis, respectively. Oil red O (ORO) and senescent-associated β-galactosidase (SA-β-gal) staining [100 μm, scale bar]. (**B**) Pre-vitellogenic oocyte counts. (**C**) Early and mature vitellogenic oocyte counts. (**D**) DHE and AO fluorescence intensity quantification employing Image J software. (**E**) Presence of SA-β-gal and ORO-stained areas across the different groups. The statistical divergence between the groups was denoted by * ($p < 0.05$), ** ($p < 0.01$), and *** ($p < 0.001$) for HC+Gal (for DHE fluorescent intensity and SA-β-gal-stained area) while # ($p < 0.05$), ### ($p < 0.001$) were for HC+Gal (for AO fluorescent intensity and ORO-stained area). † ($p < 0.05$) was for the HC+Gal+0.5% BWA group while ‡‡ ($p < 0.01$) and ‡‡‡ ($p < 0.001$) were for the HC+Gal+1.0% BWA group; ns represents a non-significant difference between the groups.

DHE staining revealed a significant dose-dependent effect of BWA in preventing HC+Gal-induced ROS generation. In response to 0.5% and 1.0% BWA consumption, a 2.4-fold- and 2.8-fold-reduced DHE fluorescent intensity was quantified in the testis section compared to the HC+Gal group. Unlike BWA, a non-significant effect of CoQ_{10} (at 0.5% and 1.0% concentrations) was noticed on the HC+Gal-induced ROS level (Figure 8A,D).

The AO fluorescent staining revealed a significantly 2.8-fold- and 3.2-fold-reduced AO fluorescent intensity in the 0.5% and 1.0% BWA-consumed group, contrary to the HC+Gal group, documenting the antiapoptotic effect of BWA (Figure 8A,D). In contrast, C_OQ_{10} at a 0.5% concentration has a non-significant impact against HC+Gal-induced apoptosis.

A significantly 4.3-fold- and 69-fold-reduced cellular senescence was observed in the 0.5% and 1.0% BWA-consumed group compared to the HC+Gal group (Figure 8A,E). Like BWA, CoQ_{10} prevents the HC+Gal-induced cellular senescence, evidenced by ~2-fold lower SA-β-gal-positive cells in CoQ_{10} in the 0.5% and 1.0% consumption groups than that of the

HC+Gal group, while compared to 0.5% and 1.0% CoQ_{10}, significantly 1.6-fold and 32-fold lower SA-β gal-positive cells were detected in 0.5% and 1.0% BWA-consumed groups, signifying the functional superiority of BWA over CoQ_{10} to eliminate HC+Gal-induced cellular senescence.

The ORO staining revealed a significantly 12.2% higher lipid accumulation in the HC+BWA group than the HC group, suggesting the aggravative effect of Gal in the combination of HC towards the lipid accumulation in the ovary (Figure 8A,E). The HC+Gal-induced lipid accumulation is significantly alleviated by the consumption of BWA and CoQ_{10} as depicted by a significantly 2.7-fold-, 3.6-fold-,1.5-fold-, and 1.4-fold-reduced ORO-stained area in response to 0.5% and 1.0% BWA and CoQ_{10}, respectively, against the HC+Gal group.

2.9. Analysis of Testicular Tissue

The testis histology evaluated by H&E staining revealed a substantial adverse effect of HC on the testis that was further worsened in the presence of Gal. The HC+Gal group noticed a haphazard tubular structure with vague spermatocyte (ST) and spermatozoa (SZ) arrangement with dilatated interstitial space between the seminiferous tubules. The HC+Gal-induced testis damage was substantially prevented by the consumption of BWA and CoQ_{10}, as manifested by the significant 12%, 32%, 14%, and 19% reduction in the interstitial space between the seminiferous tubules in response to 0.5% and 1.0% BWA and 0.5% CoQ_{10} and 1.0% CoQ_{10}, respectively (Figure 9A,B).

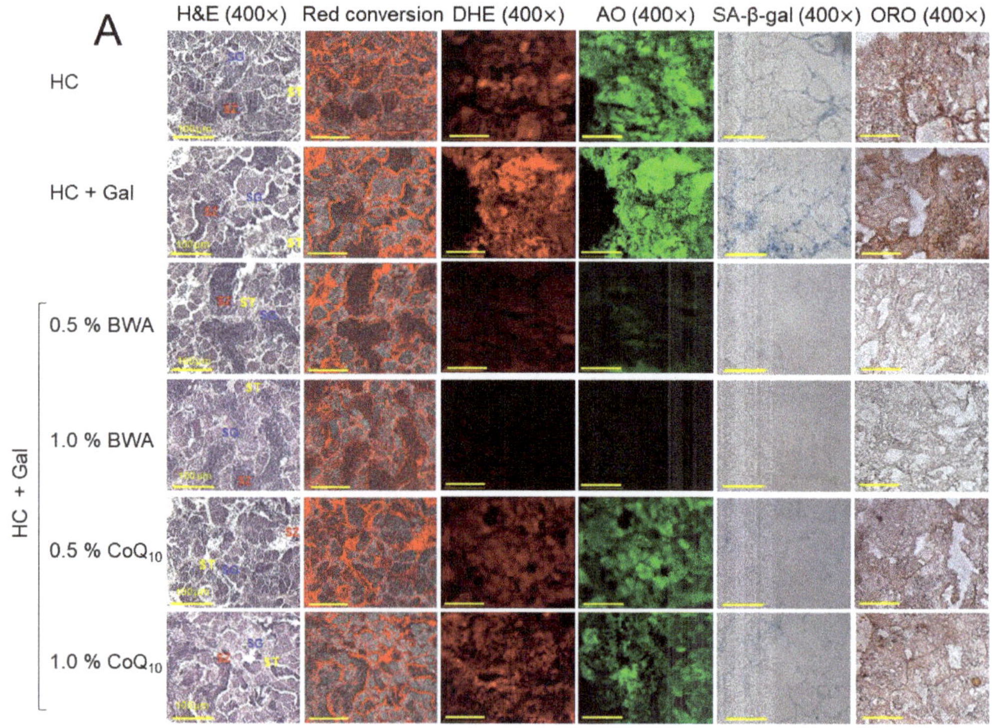

Figure 9. *Cont.*

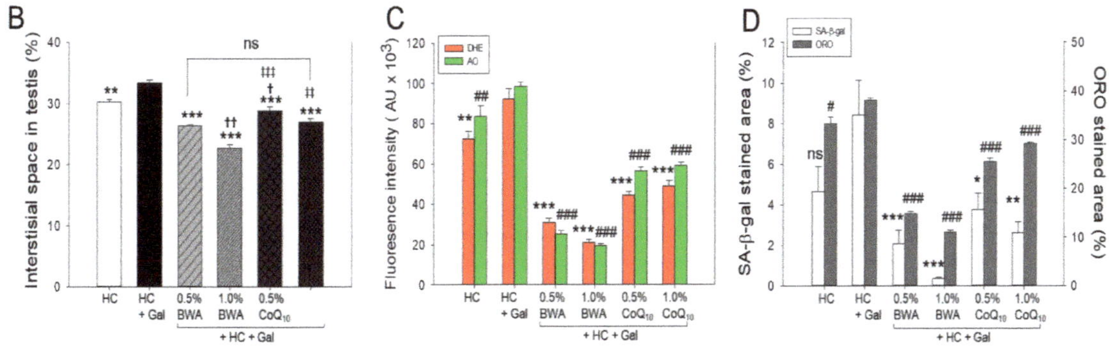

Figure 9. A comparative effect of beeswax alcohol (BWA) and coenzyme Q_{10} (CoQ_{10}) on the testicular tissue of zebrafish fed with a high-cholesterol (HC, final 4%, *w/w*) and galactose (Gal, final 10%, *w/w*) diet. (**A**) Hematoxylin and eosin (H&E) staining; Image J-based interchange of white color (depicting the interstitial space) to red color (red conversion) at the white color threshold value (20–120) to enhance the clarity; and SG, ST, and SZ abbreviated for spermatogonia, spermatocyte, and spermatozoa. Dihydroethidium (DHE) and acridine orange (AO) staining indicate the generation of reactive oxygen species (ROS) and apoptosis. Oil red O (ORO) and senescent-associated β-galactosidase (SA-β-gal) staining. [100 μm, scale bar]. (**B**) Quantification of interstitial space in the testis section. (**C**) DHE and AO fluorescence intensity quantification employing Image J software. (**D**) Estimation of SA-β-gal and ORO-stained areas across the different groups. The statistical divergence between the groups was denoted by * ($p < 0.05$), ** ($p < 0.01$), and *** ($p < 0.001$) for HC+Gal (for interstitial space, DHE fluorescent intensity, and SA-β-gal-stained area) while # ($p < 0.05$), ## ($p < 0.01$), and ### ($p < 0.001$) were for HC+Gal (for AO fluorescent intensity and ORO-stained area). † ($p < 0.05$) and †† ($p < 0.01$) were for the HC+Gal+0.5% BWA group while ‡‡ ($p < 0.01$) and ‡‡‡ ($p < 0.001$) were for the HC+Gal+1.0% BWA group; ns represents a non-significant difference between the groups.

The DHE and AO fluorescence imaging corresponding to ROS and apoptosis demonstrated the provocative effect of Gal to augment HC-induced ROS and apoptosis as documented by a significantly ~1.8-fold higher DHE and AO fluorescent intensity than the HC group (Figure 9A,C). The consumption of BWA at both 0.5% and 1.0% efficiently countered the HC+Gal-induced ROS production, as documented by a significantly 2.9-fold- and 4.3-fold-reduced DHE fluorescent intensity compared to the HC+Gal group. Likewise, a ~2-fold-reduced DHE-stained area was observed in both CoQ_{10} groups, 0.5% and 1.0%, compared to the HC+Gal group. The AO fluorescent staining revealed a substantial effect of BWA and CoQ_{10} in eliminating HC+Gal-induced apoptosis. However, when compared with CoQ_{10}, BWA at 0.5% and 1.0% was found to be more effective in preventing apoptosis, marked by 2.2-fold and 3.1-fold, respectively, reductions in AO fluorescent intensity compared to CoQ_{10} at the respective concentrations.

A higher accumulation of lipids in response to HC+Gal was noticed in the testis, which was significantly prevented by consuming BWA and CoQ_{10} (Figure 9A,D). However, compared to CoQ_{10}, BWA displayed much higher efficacy with 1.6-fold- and 2.6-fold-reduced ORO-stained areas in 0.5% and 1.0% BWA-consumed groups compared to CoQ_{10} at the respective concentrations. Similarly, both BWA and CoQ_{10} significantly altered the HC+Gal-induced cellular senescence; however, the higher efficacy of BWA compared to CoQ_{10} was noticed as depicted by significantly 1.8-fold- and 7.7-fold-reduced senescence-positive cells in response to 0.5% and 1.0% BWA than that of CoQ_{10} at 0.5% and 1.0%, respectively (Figure 9A,D).

3. Discussion

The composition of beeswax is substantially impacted by factors such as honeybee families and breed [1], the age of the wax, and varying climatic conditions [28], which also influence the quality of BWA. An earlier study documented the presence of fatty alcohols C33 and C35 in *A. mellifera* [29]. However, unlike this, we did not observe the presence of alcohols of C33 and C35 in used BWA, signifying that BWA composition substantially varied based on the honeybee types and source of beeswax. In contrast, the present findings are similar to the earlier study [28] documenting the presence of six distinct alcohols (C24, C26, C28, C30, C32, and C34) in the beeswax of *A. mellifera* L. with a high prevalence of C30 and C32 alcohols similar to the present study.

It is well known that a long-term HC diet, around 12~20 weeks, causes ruinous vascular lipid accumulation and damage to main organs, such as the liver, kidney, ovary, and testis with hypercholesterolemia and obesity in zebrafish [30,31]. Zebrafish were picked as a model organism in the present study owing to their significant genetic resemblance to humans [32], making them an excellent choice for preclinical research [33]. Of note, several key receptors and enzymes involved in lipid metabolism in zebrafish closely resemble those in humans [34], establishing them as a valuable model for investigating lipoprotein-related research.

In the current study, galactose (final 10%, *w/w*) combined with HC resulted in more rapid and severe damage in the major organs with rigorous inflammation, senescence, and atherogenic blood lipid profiles. After 12 weeks of consumption, the HC+Gal group showed the highest increase in body weight (Table 1), blood TC and TG, and blood AST/ALT (Figures 1–3). Interestingly, the HC+Gal group revealed the lowest blood HDL-C and the highest extent of cell senescence, fatty liver change, neutrophil infiltration, and IL-6 production in the liver (Figures 4–6). The HC+Gal group also exhibited the highest extent of ROS production, apoptosis, and senescence in the kidney, ovary, and testis (Figures 7–9). These results make a good agreement with previous reports that the administration of D-galactose accelerated aging and reduced fertility with exacerbation of cognitive dysfunction and neurodegeneration [35,36].

However, both the 0.5% and 1.0% BWA group showed higher survivability, 96% and 100%, respectively, than the HC+Gal group, around 92%, while the 0.5% and 1.0% CoQ_{10} group showed lower survivability, around 92% and 89%, respectively than the HC+Gal group (Table 1 and Figure 1). BWA groups exhibited higher efficacy than CoQ_{10} groups in ameliorating the lipid profile and organ injury, the least inflammation, cellular senescence, apoptosis, and ROS production in the liver, kidney, ovary, and testis. Among the BWA-supplemented groups, the 1.0% BWA group showed remarkably superior behaviors than the 0.5% BWA in improving blood lipid profiles by significantly lowering TC, TG, TG/HDL-C, and LDL-C:HDL-C with raising HDL-C and HDL-C/TC (%). However, CoQ_{10} groups did not show a difference between 0.5% and 1.0% in blood lipid profiles; they exhibited an atherogenic lipid profile without lowering TG and raising HDL-C. In blood profiles and histological analysis of the liver, there was no difference in neutrophil infiltration, IL-6 production, and cellular senescence between the 0.5% and 1.0% CoQ_{10} groups, suggesting that CoQ_{10} supplementation did not protect the zebrafish from galactose toxicity in both dosages.

Although CoQ_{10} is known to protect cellular membranes against oxidative stress in mitochondria and extra-mitochondria as a lipid-soluble antioxidant via removing ROS, there might be different efficacy depending on the dosage and supplementation period. A meta-analysis with a human study showed that 400–500 mg/day of CoQ_{10} supplementation decreased the TC and TG levels with an increase in HDL-C [37]; however, other clinical trials showed that consumption of 150 mg/day of CoQ_{10} in patients with diabetes for 12 weeks resulted in no change in TC, with TG and HDL-C being decreased [38]. While several research studies showed conflicting results, and there has been no established ideal dose of CoQ_{10}, it has been generally accepted that the recommended daily dose is 50 to 300 mg for adults to treat cardiovascular disease, dyslipidemia, and sarcopenia [39,40]. Recently, six-month supplementation with high-dose CoQ_{10}, 240 mg/day, has been shown to improve liver steatosis in patients with metabolic dysfunction associated with steatosis liver disease [41].

However, there was no beneficial effect on the decrease in blood TC and TG and increase in HDL-C levels in the CoQ_{10} group, except for a decrease in LDL-C [41]. The accumulating finding showed the disparity of the CoQ_{10} functionality [41]. In the present study, in the 1.0% CoQ_{10} group, an intake of 0.2 mg of CoQ_{10} per day is equivalent to the 616 mg and 456 mg per day humanized dose (assumption of 60 kg body weight) calculated based on the average body weight of zebrafish at 370 mg (week 0) and 580 mg (week 12), respectively, employing the equation suggested for conversion of the estimated human equivalent dose [42]. Despite the high dose, we have noticed no effect of CoQ_{10} to alleviate the TG level; though, a substantial effect was observed to restore HC+Gal-disturbed TC and HDL-C levels. However, the effect was substantially inferior compared to the effect exerted by BWA. The 1.0% CoQ_{10} supplemented group was found to be ineffective in diminishing HC+Gal-induced cellular senescence and fatty liver changes, suggesting that there is not much of an effect of CoQ_{10} in preventing hepatic damage. The outcome is supported by the elevated level of important hepatic function biomarker AST in response to CoQ_{10} consumption in the presence of HC+Gal.

It has been well known that high-cholesterol or galactose supplementation induces oxidative stress to cause proinflammatory and senescence signaling. However, no study has investigated the physiological effect of the co-supplementation with cholesterol and galactose. As far as the authors' knowledge, the current study is the first report to demonstrate that the co-supplementation of cholesterol and galactose induced more severe detrimental effects than the adverse effect posed by HC alone. Also, it is the first report deciphering a comparative effect of BWA and CoQ_{10} against high-cholesterol- and galactose-induced adversity.

The higher efficacy of BWA over CoQ_{10} to prevent HC+Gal-induced damage is probably due to the higher potency of BWA as an antioxidant, which efficiently manages the oxidative stress that has been recognized as the major culprit in inducing apoptosis [43,44] and cellular senescence [45,46]. This notion is supported by the earlier report signifying the higher antioxidant efficacy of BWA than CoQ_{10} [12] that leads to the protection of LDL oxidation and prevention of ROS generation against the CML-posed toxicity and consequently rescues the zebrafish embryos from the apoptotic cell death [12,13]. Also, the impact of BWA consumption on preventing lipid peroxidation oxidative damage of gastric mucosa of rats strengthens the present findings [5,11,47]. Even more, in the clinical study, BWA (100 mg/day) consumption improved the antioxidant status of middle-aged and older human subjects [12].

4. Materials and Methods

4.1. Materials

A block of beeswax from *Apis mellifera* (mainly mellifera linage) was used as a source material to extract beeswax alcohol (BWA). The BWA was extracted from beeswax using saponification and repeated organic solvent extraction at the National Center for Scientific Research (CNIC), Havana, Cuba. In brief, the beeswax was melted at shaking conditions in the presence of potassium hydroxide (KOH) for saponification. The saponified beeswax was processed for purification using organic solvents (acetone and hexane). Subsequently, the organic phase was evaporated, and the dried final product was processed for milling (stainless steel blade miller). The milled product was homogenized to obtain BWA. A schematic representation of the BWA extraction process is provided as Supplementary Figure S1. The CNIC-sourced BWA was examined for its purity and chemical composition of long-chain aliphatic alcohols (LCAAs) by Raydel® Australia Pty, Ltd. (Thornleigh, NSW, Australia). The quality analysis of BWA revealed $\geq$ 86% purity and the presence of six long-chain aliphatic alcohols (LCAAs) namely tetracosanol (6.1%), hexacosanol (10.7%), octacosanol (13.8%), triacontanol (30.5%), dotriacontanol (22.1%), and tetratriacontanol (2.9%). A certificate of analysis with the detailed chemical composition of the used BWA is provided in Supplementary Table S1. The CoQ_{10} was purchased from Sigma-Aldrich (>98% HPLC, Cat No. 303-98-0, St. Louis, MO, USA). All the other chemicals and reagents used in this study were of analytical grade and used as supplied. Supplementary Material S1 depicts the specifications of the used chemicals.

4.2. Zebrafish Aquaculture

An aerated tank with a constant water supply was used to maintain the zebrafish. The atmospheric conditions were maintained at 27 ± 1 °C with 14 h light and 10 h dark cycles. Zebrafish were fed with normal tetrabit (ND, Gmbh D49304, Melle, Germany) following the standard protocols adopted by the Animal Care Committee and the Use of Raydel Research Institute (approval code RRI-23-007; approval date 27 July 2023).

4.3. Preparation of High-Cholesterol Diet Infused with BWA or CoQ_{10}

The normal tetrabit (ND) was blended with cholesterol (final 4%, *w/w*) to make the high-cholesterol (HC) diet [48]. The HC diet was further mixed with galactose (Gal, final 10%, *w/w*) to make HC supplemented with galactose (HC+Gal). HC+Gal was further mixed with BWA at 0.5% or 1.0% (*w/w*) to make two distinct BWA-infused diets named HC+Gal with 0.5% BWA and HC+Gal with 1.0% BWA, respectively. Similarly, two distinct CoQ_{10}-supplemented diets were prepared by mixing HC+Gal with CoQ_{10} at 0.5% or 1.0% (*w/w*) and designated as HC+Gal with 0.5% CoQ_{10} and HC+Gal with 1.0% CoQ_{10}, respectively. Table 2 depicts the specific amount of ND, cholesterol, galactose, BWA, and CoQ_{10} to prepare different diets for zebrafish feeding. The specified diet, 10 mg/zebrafish (twice a day), was provided during the 12 weeks of the experimental period. The selection of BWA dosages (final 0.5% and 1.0%, *w/w*) was based on the preliminary experiments where we tested different dosages of BWA (final 0.1% and 10%, *w/w*) in hyperlipidemic zebrafish and observed their impact on blood lipid profile and hepatic function biomarkers (AST and ALT). The results indicated significant changes in plasma lipid profiles and AST and ALT levels at BWA concentrations between 0.5% (*w/w*) and 1.0% (*w/w*), while no significant difference was observed at concentrations exceeding 1.0% (*w/w*) up to 10% (*w/w*). Consequently, we chose 1.0% (*w/w*) BWA as the highest dose for the present study. For the comparative study (between BWA and CoQ_{10}), we used a similar dose of 1.0% (*w/w*) CoQ_{10}.

Table 2. Composition of the six different diets prepared by cholesterol, galactose, beeswax alcohol, and coenzyme Q_{10}.

Diet (10 mg)	HC	HC + Gal	HC+Gal + 0.5% BWA	HC+Gal + 1.0% BWA	HC+Gal + 0.5% CoQ_{10}	HC+Gal + 1.0% CoQ_{10}
Tetrabits	9.6	8.6	8.55	8.5	8.55	8.5
Galactose	0	1.0	1.0	1.0	1.0	1.0
Cholesterol	0.4	0.4	0.4	0.4	0.4	0.4
BWA	0	0	0.05	0.1	0	0
CoQ_{10}	0	0	0	0	0.05	0.1
Total (mg)	10.0	10.0	10.0	10.0	10.0	10.0

BW, body weight; BWA, beeswax alcohol; CoQ_{10}, coenzymeQ_{10}; Gal, galactose; HC, high cholesterol.

4.4. Zebrafish Fed with Different Diets

Adult zebrafish (n = 336) were fed with HC for 4 weeks prior to supplementation with different diets (Figure 10). The 4 weeks of supplementation of HC was performed to induce hyperlipidemia in zebrafish before introducing different dietary treatments [48]. The HC-supplemented zebrafish (4 weeks) were randomly allocated into six separate groups (n = 56 for each group) and fed with the specified diets for the 12 weeks. Zebrafish in groups I and II were fed with only HC and HC+Gal, respectively. Zebrafish in groups III and IV were maintained on the HC+Gal with 0.5% BWA and HC+Gal with 1.0% BWA diets, respectively. Likewise, the group V and VI zebrafish were nourished with HC+Gal with 0.5% CoQ_{10} and HC+Gal with 1.0% CoQ_{10}, respectively (Figure 10). During the 12 weeks of supplementation, the survivability and body weight of the zebrafish (Group I-VI) were monitored periodically.

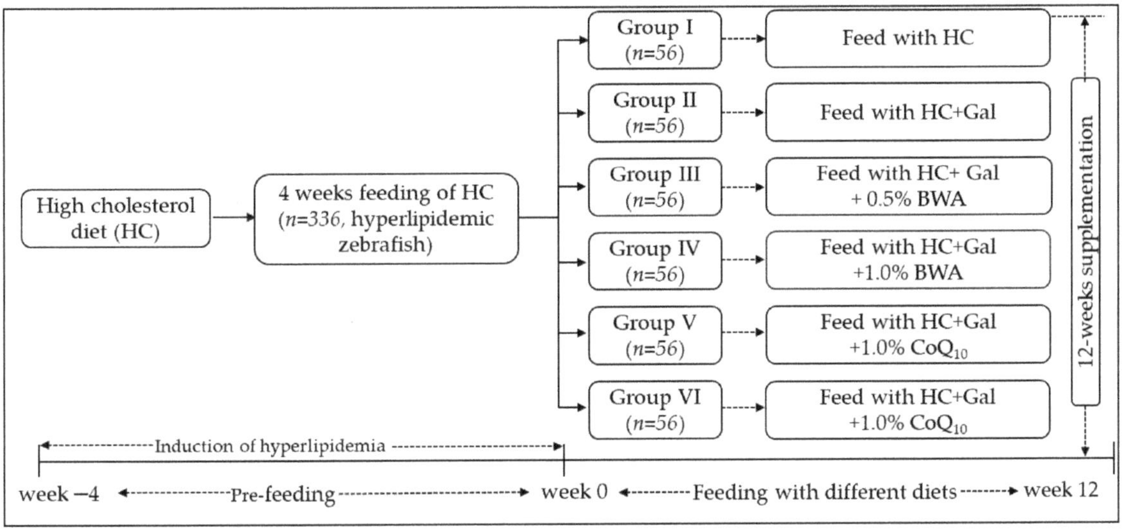

Figure 10. A schematic representation of the study plan. HC represents the high-cholesterol diet (final 4%, *w/w*) and Gal represents galactose (final 10%, *w/w*), while HC+Gal+BWA 0.5% and 1.0% represent HC+Gal supplemented with beeswax alcohol at 0.5% and 1.0% (final, *w/w*), and HC+Gal+CoQ_{10} 0.5% and 1.0% represent HC+Gal supplemented with coenzyme Q_{10} (CoQ_{10}) at 0.5% and 1.0% (final, *w/w*).

4.5. Blood and Tissue Collection

After 12 weeks, zebrafish in each group were sacrificed by hypothermal shock [48], and immediately, blood was collected from puncturing the heart. The blood was collected in tubes pre-washed with ethylenediaminetetraacetic acid (EDTA). The different organs (liver, kidney, testis, and ovaries) were surgically extracted and preserved in 10% formalin for further use.

4.6. Plasma Analysis

The collected blood was centrifuged to obtain plasma, which was processed for the quantification of total cholesterol (TC), triglycerides (TGs), high-density lipoprotein cholesterol (HDL-C), aspartate aminotransferase (AST), and alanine aminotransferase (ALT) using commercial kits following the manufacturers' suggested method. A detailed methodology of plasma analysis is described in Supplementary Material S2.

4.7. Histologic Analysis

The tissue (liver, kidney, testis, and ovary) was preserved and fixed in 10% formalin (Section 2.4), further dehydrated by treatment with a series of alcohols, and subsequently fixed in paraffin. A 7 μm section of the tissue embedded in the paraffin block was obtained using a microtome. The respective tissue sections were processed for Hematoxylin and eosin (H&E) staining to determine histological changes following the earlier described method [49].

The lipid accumulation in the tissue was examined by Oil red O (ORO) staining [48]. In brief, organ sections (5 μm) were pooled with ORO stain and subsequently incubated at 60 °C for 5 min. The excess ORO was rinsed, subsequently stained with hematoxylin for 30 s, and visualized under microscopy.

4.8. Immunohistochemical (IHC) Staining

The hepatic interleukin (IL)-6 level was examined by IHC analysis [50]. The tissue section was covered with IL-6-specified 200× diluted primary immunoglobulin (ab9324, Abcam, London, UK) followed by 16 hr incubation at 4 °C. The IL-6-complexed immunoglobulins were detected by applying 1000× diluted anti-IL-6 antibodies (enzyme-linked), and the section was developed using the chromogenic substrate utilizing the EnVison + system-HRP polymer kit (Dako, Glostrup, Denmark).

4.9. Dihydroethidium (DHE) and Acridine Orange (AO) Staining

The dihydroethidium (DHE) [51] and acridine orange (AO) [52] staining was performed by adding 200 μL of DHE (30 μM) and AO (5 μg/mL) solution to the tissue section. After 5 min incubation in the dark, the stained section was rinsed and analyzed under fluorescent microscopy operated at the 585 nm (excitation) and 615 nm (emission) wavelengths for DHE fluorescence and 505 nm (excitation) and 535 nm (emission) wavelengths for AO fluorescence.

4.10. Senescence Staining

Senescence was detected by a senescent-associated β-galactosidase (SA-β-gal) assay [53]. Briefly, the tissue section was treated with paraformaldehyde (4%) for 5 min, and subsequently, 0.1% of X-gal (5-bromo-4-chloro-3-indolyl-β-D-galactopyranoside) was added. After 14 hr, the section was washed with phosphate-buffered saline (PBS) and visualized under the microscope.

4.11. Statistical Analysis

Mean ± SEM of the triplicate values obtained from the experimental data was used to analyze the statistical divergence between the groups following One-Way Analysis of Variance (ANOVA)–Tukey's post hoc analysis using Statistical Package for the Social Sciences platform (SPSS, Inc., Chicago, IL, USA).

5. Conclusions

A comparable 12-week consumption study of BWA and CoQ_{10} disclosed the higher efficacy of BWA over CoQ_{10} in preventing adversity posed by the dietary consumption of HC+Gal. BWA, precisely at 1.0%, substantially prevents HC+Gal-provoked dyslipidemia by alleviating TC and TG levels and simultaneously increasing the HDL-C level. BWA also restricts HC+Gal-induced oxidative stress and inflammation, averts hepatic cellular senescence and fatty liver changes, and improves hepatic functionality. Consistently, BWA consumption was found effective in abolishing HC+Gal-invoked impairment of kidneys and reproductive organs. The findings underscore BWA's superior functionality over CoQ_{10} in mitigating HC+Gal-induced alterations, making BWA a viable nutraceutical for managing cholesterol- and galactose-related concerns.

Supplementary Materials: The following supporting information can be downloaded at https://www.mdpi.com/article/10.3390/ph17091250/s1: Supplementary Figure S1: Sequential steps for the extraction of beeswax alcohol (BWA) from the beeswax. Supplementary Table S1: Certificate of analysis and composition of beeswax alcohol (BWA). Supplementary Material S1: List of the used chemicals. Supplementary material S2: A detailed methodology for the quantification of plasma lipid profiles and hepatic function biomarkers.

Author Contributions: Conceptualization, K.-H.C.; methodology, A.B., J.-E.K., Y.L., and S.H.L.; data curation, writing—original draft preparation, K.-H.C.; writing—review and editing, K.-H.C., supervision, K.-H.C. All authors have read and agreed to the published version of the manuscript.

Funding: This research received no external funding.

Institutional Review Board Statement: The animal study protocol was approved by the Committee of Animal Care and Use of Raydel Research Institute (approval code RRI-23-001, approval date 27 July 2023).

Informed Consent Statement: Not applicable.

Data Availability Statement: Data is contained within the article and Supplementary Materials.

Conflicts of Interest: The authors declare no conflicts of interest.

References

1. Fratini, F.; Cilia, G.; Turchi, B.; Felicioli, A. Beeswax: A minireview of its antimicrobial activity and its application in medicine. *Asian Pacif. J. Tropic. Med.* **2016**, *9*, 839–843. [CrossRef]
2. Bradbear, N. *Bees and Their Role in Forest Livelihoods: A Guide to the Services Provided by Bees and the Sustainable Harvesting, Processing and Marketing of Their Products*; Food and Agriculture Organization of the United Nations: Rome, Italy, 2009.
3. Svečnjak, L.; Chesson, L.A.; Gallina, A.; Maia, M.; Martinello, M.; Mutinelli, F.; Muz, M.N.; Nunes, F.M.; Saucy, F.; Tipple, B.J.; et al. Standard methods for *Apis mellifera* beeswax research. *J. Apic. Res.* **2019**, *58*, 1–108. [CrossRef]
4. Srisaipet, A.; Phromchan, S.; Jaipaeng, T. Policosanol extraction from beeswax and improvement of the purity. *MATEC Web Conf.* **2017**, *111*, 02005. [CrossRef]
5. Molina, V.; Mas, R.; Carbajal, D. D-002 (beeswax alcohols): Concurrent joint health benefits and gastroprotection. *Indian J. Pharm. Sci.* **2015**, *77*, 127–134. [CrossRef]
6. Menéndez, R.; Amor, A.; González, R.; Jiménez, S.; Mas, R. Inhibition of rat microsomal lipid peroxidation by the oral administration of D002. *Braz. J. Med. Biol. Res.* **2000**, *33*, 85–90. [CrossRef] [PubMed]
7. Lopez, E.; Illnait, J.; Molina, V.; Oyarzabal, A.; Fernandez, L.; Perez, Y.; Mas, R.; Mesa, M.; Fernandez, J.; Mendoza, S. Effects of D-002 (beeswax alcohols) on lipid peroxidation in middle-aged and older subjects. *Lat. Am. J. Pharm.* **2008**, *27*, 695–703.
8. Rodriguez, I.; Illnait, J.; Molina, V.; Oyarzabal, A.; Fernandez, L.; Mesa, M.; Más, R.; Mendoza, S.; Gámez, R.; Jiménez, S. Comparison of the antioxidant effects of D-002 (beeswax alcohols) and grape seed extract (GSE) on plasma oxidative variables in healthy subjects. *Lat. Am. J. Pharm.* **2010**, *29*, 255–262.
9. Menéndez, R.; Más, R.; Illnait, J.; Pérez, J.; Amor, A.M.; Fernández, J.C.; González, R.M. Effects of D-002 on lipid peroxidation in older subjects. *J. Med. Food* **2001**, *4*, 71–77. [CrossRef]
10. Illnait, J.; Rodríguez, I.; Mendoza, S.; Fernández, Y.; Mas, R.; Miranda, M.; Piñera, J.; Fernández, J.C.; Mesa, M.; Fernández, L.; et al. Effects of D-002, a mixture of high molecular weight beeswax alcohols, on patients with nonalcoholic fatty liver disease. *Korean J. Intern. Med.* **2013**, *28*, 439. [CrossRef]
11. Pérez, Y.; Oyárzabal, A.; Mas, R.; Molina, V.; Jiménez, S. Protective effect of D-002, a mixture of beeswax alcohols, against indomethacin-induced gastric ulcers and mechanism of action. *J. Nat. Med.* **2013**, *67*, 182–189. [CrossRef]
12. Cho, K.-H.; Baek, S.-H.; Nam, H.-S.; Bahuguna, A.; López-González, L.E.; Rodríguez-Cortina, I.; Illnait-Ferrer, J.; Fernández-Travieso, J.C.; Molina-Cuevas, V.; Pérez-Guerra, Y.; et al. Beeswax alcohol prevents low-density lipoprotein oxidation and demonstrates antioxidant activities in zebrafish embryos and human subjects: A clinical study. *Curr. Issues Mol. Biol.* **2024**, *46*, 409–429. [CrossRef] [PubMed]
13. Cho, K.-H.; Baek, S.-H.; Nam, H.-S.; Bahuguna, A. Enhancement of antioxidant and anti-glycation properties of beeswax alcohol in reconstituted high-density lipoprotein: Safeguarding against carboxymethyllysine toxicity in zebrafish. *Antioxidants* **2023**, *12*, 2116. [CrossRef] [PubMed]
14. Puig, M.N.; Castaño, S.M.; Ferreiro, R.M.; Clara, M.V.; Hernansez, N.M. Effects of oral administration of D-002 (Beeswax alcohols) on histological and functional outcomes in a Rat model of antigen-induced arthritis: Preliminary Study. *Int. J. Pharmacol. Phytochem. Ethnomed.* **2016**, *5*, 60–68.
15. Illnait, J.; Rodriguez, I.; Molina, V.; Mendoza, S.; Mas, R.; Fernandez, L.; Oyarzabal, A.; Perez, Y.; Mesa, M.; Fernández, J. Effects of D-002 (beeswax alcohols) on gastrointestinal symptoms and oxidative markers in middle-aged and older subjects. *Lat. Am. J. Pharm.* **2013**, *32*, 166–174.
16. Korean Food and Drug Administration (KFDA). Available online: https://www.foodsafetykorea.go.kr/portal/healthyfoodlife/searchHomeHFDetail.do?prdlstReportLedgNo=2023021000330706 (accessed on 16 May 2023).
17. Ardekani, A.; Tabrizi, R.; Maleki, E.; Bagheri Lankarani, K.; Heydari, S.T.; Moradinazar, M.; Akbari, M. Effects of coenzyme Q_{10} supplementation on lipid profiles and liver enzymes of nonalcoholic fatty liver disease (NAFLD) patients: A systematic review and meta-analysis of randomized controlled trials. *Food Sci. Nutr.* **2023**, *11*, 2580–2588. [CrossRef]
18. Ashkani Esfahani, S.; Esmaeilzadeh, E.; Bagheri, F.; Emami, Y.; Farjam, M. The effect of co-enzyme q10 on acute liver damage in rats, a biochemical and pathological study. *Hepat. Mon.* **2013**, *13*, e13685. [CrossRef]
19. Jiménez-Santos, M.A.; Juárez-Rojop, I.E.; Tovilla-Zárate, C.A.; Espinosa-García, M.T.; Juárez-Oropeza, M.A.; Ramón-Frías, T.; Bermúdez-Ocaña, D.Y.; Díaz-Zagoya, J.C. Coenzyme Q10 supplementation improves metabolic parameters, liver function and mitochondrial respiration in rats with high doses of atorvastatin and a cholesterol-rich diet. *Lipids Health Dis.* **2014**, *13*, 22. [CrossRef] [PubMed]

20. Pasha, R.; Moon, T.W. Coenzyme Q_{10} protects against statin-induced myotoxicity in zebrafish larvae (*Danio rerio*). *Environ. Toxicol. Pharmacol.* **2017**, *52*, 150–160. [CrossRef] [PubMed]
21. Jaskelioff, M.; Muller, F.L.; Paik, J.-H.; Thomas, E.; Jiang, S.; Adams, A.C.; Sahin, E.; Kost-Alimova, M.; Protopopov, A.; Cadiñanos, J.; et al. Telomerase reactivation reverses tissue degeneration in aged telomerase-deficient mice. *Nature* **2011**, *469*, 102–106. [CrossRef]
22. Azman, K.F.; Zakaria, R. D-Galactose-induced accelerated aging model: An overview. *Biogerontology* **2019**, *20*, 763–782. [CrossRef]
23. Kumar, H.; Bhardwaj, K.; Valko, M.; Alomar, S.Y.; Alwasel, S.H.; Cruz-Martins, N.; Dhanjal, D.S.; Singh, R.; Kuča, K.; Verma, R.; et al. Antioxidative potential of *Lactobacillus* sp. in ameliorating D-galactose-induced aging. *Appl. Microbiol. Biotechnol.* **2022**, *106*, 4831–4843. [CrossRef] [PubMed]
24. Azman, K.F.; Safdar, A.; Zakaria, R. D-galactose-induced liver aging model: Its underlying mechanisms and potential therapeutic interventions. *Exp. Gerontol.* **2021**, *150*, 111372. [CrossRef]
25. Du, Z.; Yang, Y.; Hu, Y.; Sun, Y.; Zhang, S.; Peng, W.; Zhong, Y.; Huang, X.; Kong, W. A long-term high-fat diet increases oxidative stress, mitochondrial damage and apoptosis in the inner ear of D-galactose-induced aging rats. *Hear. Res.* **2012**, *287*, 15–24. [CrossRef]
26. Cui, X.; Zuo, P.; Zhang, Q.; Li, X.; Hu, Y.; Long, J.; Packer, L.; Liu, J. Chronic systemic D-galactose exposure induces memory loss, neurodegeneration, and oxidative damage in mice: Protective effects of R-α-lipoic acid. *J. Neurosci. Res.* **2006**, *84*, 647–654. [CrossRef]
27. Han, Y.; Zee, S.; Cho, K.-H. Beeswax alcohol and fermented black rice bran synergistically ameliorated hepatic injury and dyslipidemia to exert antioxidant and anti-inflammatory activity in ethanol-supplemented zebrafish. *Biomolecules* **2023**, *13*, 136. [CrossRef] [PubMed]
28. Bonvehí, J.S.; Bermejo, F.O. Detection of adulterated commercial Spanish beeswax. *Food Chem.* **2012**, *132*, 642–648. [CrossRef] [PubMed]
29. Aichholz, R.; Lorbeer, E. Investigation of combwax of honeybees with high-temperature gas chromatography and high-temperature gas chromatography–chemical ionization mass spectrometry: I. High-temperature gas chromatography. *J. Chromatogr. A* **1999**, *855*, 601–615. [CrossRef]
30. Cho, K.-H.; Kim, J.-E.; Nam, H.-S.; Baek, S.-H.; Bahuguna, A. Consumption of policosanol (Raydel®) improves hepatic, renal, and reproductive functions in zebrafish: In vivo comparison study among Cuban, Chinese, and American policosanol. *Pharmaceuticals* **2023**, *17*, 66. [CrossRef]
31. Yoon, Y.; Yoon, J.; Jang, M.Y.; Na, Y.; Ko, Y.; Choi, J.H.; Seok, S.H. High cholesterol diet induces IL-1beta expression in adult but not larval zebrafish. *PLoS ONE* **2013**, *8*, e66970. [CrossRef]
32. Patton, E.E.; Zon, L.I.; Langenau, D.M. Zebrafish disease models in drug discovery: From preclinical modelling to clinical trials. *Nat. Rev. Drug Discov.* **2021**, *20*, 611–628. [CrossRef]
33. Juan-García, A.; Bind, M.-A.; Engert, F. Larval zebrafish as an in vitro model for evaluating toxicological effects of mycotoxins. *Ecotoxicol. Environ. Saf.* **2020**, *202*, 110909. [CrossRef] [PubMed]
34. Fang, L.; Liu, C.; Miller, Y.I. Zebrafish models of dyslipidemia: Relevance to atherosclerosis and angiogenesis. *Transl. Res.* **2014**, *163*, 99–108. [CrossRef] [PubMed]
35. Shen, Y.X.; Xu, S.Y.; Wei, W.; Sun, X.X.; Yang, J.; Liu, L.H.; Dong, C. Melatonin reduces memory changes and neural oxidative damage in mice treated with D-galactose. *J. Pineal Res.* **2002**, *32*, 173–178. [CrossRef]
36. Liao, C.H.; Chen, B.H.; Chiang, H.S.; Chen, C.W.; Chen, M.F.; Ke, C.C.; Wang, Y.Y.; Lin, W.N.; Wang, C.C.; Lin, Y.H. Optimizing a male reproductive aging mouse model by D-galactose injection. *Int. J. Mol. Sci.* **2016**, *17*, 98. [CrossRef] [PubMed]
37. Liu, Z.; Tian, Z.; Zhao, D.; Liang, Y.; Dai, S.; Liu, M.; Hou, S.; Dong, X.; Zhaxinima; Yang, Y. Effects of coenzyme Q_{10} supplementation on lipid profiles in adults: A meta-analysis of randomized controlled trials. *J. Clin. Endocrinol. Metab.* **2023**, *108*, 232–249. [CrossRef] [PubMed]
38. Zahedi, H.; Eghtesadi, S.; Seifirad, S.; Rezaee, N.; Shidfar, F.; Heydari, I.; Golestan, B.; Jazayeri, S. Effects of CoQ_{10} supplementation on lipid profiles and glycemic control in patients with Type 2 diabetes: A randomized, double blind, placebo-controlled trial. *J. Diabetes Metab. Disord.* **2014**, *13*, 81. [CrossRef]
39. Bolt, J.; Sandhu, S.; Mohammadi, A. Effect of coenzyme Q_{10} supplementation on sarcopenia, frailty, and falls: A scoping review. *J. Nutr. Health Aging* **2023**, *27*, 586–592. [CrossRef]
40. Hou, S.; Tian, Z.; Zhao, D.; Liang, Y.; Dai, S.; Ji, Q.; Fan, Z.; Liu, Z.; Liu, M.; Yang, Y. Efficacy and optimal dose of coenzyme Q_{10} supplementation on inflammation-related biomarkers: AGRADE-assessed systematic review and updated meta-analysis of randomized controlled trials. *Mol. Nutr. Food Res.* **2023**, *67*, 220800. [CrossRef]
41. Soleimani Damaneh, M.; Fatahi, S.; Aryaeian, N.; Bavi Behbahani, H. The effect of coenzyme Q10 supplementation on liver enzymes: A systematic review and meta-analysis of randomized clinical trials. *Food Sci Nutr.* **2023**, *11*, 4912–4925. [CrossRef]
42. Nair, A.B.; Jacob, S. A simple practice guide for dose conversion between animals and human. *J. Basic Clin. Pharm.* **2016**, *7*, 27–31. [CrossRef]
43. Kannan, K.; Jain, S.K. Oxidative stress and apoptosis. *Pathophysiology* **2000**, *7*, 153–163. [CrossRef] [PubMed]
44. Lee, Y.-J.; Cho, H.-N.; Soh, J.-W.; Jhon, G.J.; Cho, C.-K.; Chung, H.-Y.; Bae, S.; Lee, S.-J.; Lee, Y.-S. Oxidative stress-induced apoptosis is mediated by ERK1/2 phosphorylation. *Exp. Cell Res.* **2003**, *291*, 251–266. [CrossRef] [PubMed]

45. Nousis, L.; Kanavaros, P.; Barbouti, A. Oxidative stress-induced cellular senescence: Is labile iron the connecting link? *Antioxidants* **2023**, *12*, 1250. [CrossRef]
46. Faraonio, R. Oxidative stress and cell senescence process. *Antioxidants* **2022**, *11*, 1718. [CrossRef] [PubMed]
47. Molina, V.; Valdés, S.; Carbajal, D.; Arruzazabala, L.; Menéndez, R.; Más, R. Antioxidant effect of D-002 on gastric mucosa of rats with experimentally induced injury. *J. Med. Food* **2001**, *4*, 79–83. [CrossRef]
48. Cho, K.-H.; Kim, J.-E.; Bahuguna, A.; Kang, D.-J. Long-term supplementation of ozonated sunflower oil improves dyslipidemia and hepatic inflammation in hyperlipidemic zebrafish: Suppression of oxidative stress and inflammation against carboxymethyllysine toxicity. *Antioxidants* **2023**, *12*, 1240. [CrossRef]
49. Fischer, A.H.; Jacobson, K.A.; Rose, J.; Zeller, R. Hematoxylin and eosin staining of tissue and cell sections. *Cold Spring Harb. Protoc.* **2008**, *2008*, prot4986. [CrossRef]
50. Al-Ghamdi, T.H.; Atta, I.S. Efficacy of interleukin-6 in the induction of liver cell proliferation after hemi-hepatectomy: Histopathologic and immunohistochemical study. *Int. J. Clin. Exp. Pathol.* **2020**, *13*, 1540–1549.
51. Owusu-Ansah, E.; Yavari, A.; Mandal, S.; Banerjee, U. Distinct mitochondrial retrograde signals control the G1-S cell cycle checkpoint. *Nat. Genet.* **2008**, *40*, 356–361. [CrossRef]
52. Umali, J.; Hawkey-Noble, A.; French, C.R. Loss of foxc1 in zebrafish reduces optic nerve size and cell number in the retinal ganglion cell layer. *Vis. Res.* **2019**, *156*, 66–72. [CrossRef]
53. Cho, K.-H.; Bahuguna, A.; Kang, D.-J.; Kim, J.-E. Prolonged supplementation of ozonated sunflower oil bestows an antiaging effect, improves blood lipid profile and spinal deformities, and protects vital organs of zebrafish (*Danio rerio*) against age-related degeneration: Two-years consumption study. *Antioxidants* **2024**, *13*, 123. [CrossRef] [PubMed]

pharmaceuticals

Article

Development of a Benzophenone-Free Red Propolis Extract and Evaluation of Its Efficacy against Colon Carcinogenesis

Iara Silva Squarisi [1], Victor Pena Ribeiro [1], Arthur Barcelos Ribeiro [1], Letícia Teixeira Marcos de Souza [1], Marcela de Melo Junqueira [1], Kátia Mara de Oliveira [1], Gaelle Hayot [2], Thomas Dickmeis [2], Jairo Kenupp Bastos [3], Rodrigo Cassio Sola Veneziani [1], Sérgio Ricardo Ambrósio [1,*] and Denise Crispim Tavares [1,*]

1 Research Group on Natural Products, Center for Research in Sciences and Technology, University of Franca, Franca 14404-600, SP, Brazil; iasquarisi79@outlook.com (I.S.S.); vpribeir@olemiss.edu (V.P.R.); arthur1_@hotmail.com (A.B.R.); leticiateixeiramds@gmail.com (L.T.M.d.S.); marcela.junqueira@cs.unifran.edu.br (M.d.M.J.); kmoliveiraq@gmail.com (K.M.d.O.); rodrigo.veneziani@unifran.edu.br (R.C.S.V.)

2 Institute of Biological and Chemical Systems—Biological Information Processing—Karlsruhe Institute of Technology, 76131 Karlsruhe, Germany; gaelle.hayot@kit.edu (G.H.)

3 School of Pharmaceutical Sciences of Ribeirão Preto, University of São Paulo, Ribeirão Preto 14040-903, SP, Brazil; jkbastos@fcfrp.usp.br

* Correspondence: sergio.ambrosio@unifran.edu.br (S.R.A.); denisecrispim2001@yahoo.com (D.C.T.)

Abstract: Background/Objectives: Brazilian red propolis has attracted attention for its pharmacological properties. However, signs of toxicity were recently observed in long-term studies using the hydroalcoholic extract of red propolis (RPHE), likely due to polyprenylated benzophenones. This study aimed to develop a benzophenone-free red propolis extract (BFRP) and validate an HPLC-PDA method to quantify its main constituents: isoliquiritigenin, vestitol, neovestitol, medicarpine, and 7-*O*-methylvestitol. Methods: BFRP's toxicity was assessed in zebrafish larvae through a vibrational startle response assay (VSRA) and morphological analysis. Genotoxicity was evaluated using the micronucleus test in rodents, and the extract's effects on chemically induced preneoplastic lesions in rat colon were studied. An HPLC-PDA method was used to quantify BFRP's main compounds. Results: BFRP primarily contained vestitol (128.24 ± 1.01 µg/mL) along with isoliquiritigenin, medicarpin, neovestitol, and 7-O-methylvestitol. Zebrafish larvae exposed to 40 µg/mL of BFRP exhibited toxicity, higher than the 10 µg/mL for RPHE, though no morphological differences were found. Fluorescent staining in the notochord, branchial arches, and mouth was observed in larvae treated with both BFRP and RPHE. No genotoxic or cytotoxic effects were observed up to 2000 mg/kg in rodents, with no impact on hepatotoxicity or nephrotoxicity markers. Chemoprevention studies showed a 41.6% reduction in preneoplastic lesions in rats treated with 6 mg/kg of BFRP. Conclusions: These findings indicate that BFRP is a safe, effective propolis-based extract with potential applications for human health, demonstrating reduced toxicity and chemopreventive properties.

Keywords: red propolis; benzophenone free; zebrafish; genotoxicity; colon cancer

1. Introduction

Propolis is a natural product of beekeeping widely used by humanity as a natural medicine, a supplement in the food industry, and an adjuvant in the cosmetic industry. Among the thirteen types of Brazilian propolis classified according to their physiochemical characteristics, the red propolis produced in the mangroves of northeast Brazil was the last identified [1] and is regarded as the second most significant type of Brazilian propolis, with increasing exports to various countries [2].

Since 2007, when red propolis was identified, studies have shown a variety of biological activities associated with this bee product [3], such as antioxidant [4], antibacterial [5–7], anti-periodontopathogenic bacteria, and anti-*Chikungunya* virus [8] activities; cutaneous wound healing [9]; and immunomodulatory, antiproliferative [10–12], anticarcinogenic [13], and gastroprotective [14,15] properties.

Chemically, red propolis is a rich source of phenolic compounds such as chalcones, flavonoids, isoflavones, isoflavans, and pterocarpans. These phenolic compounds originate from its botanical source *Dalbergia ecastaphyllum*, which is responsible for providing compounds such as liquiritigenin, isoliquiritigenin, formononetin, vestitol, neovestitol, medicarpine, and methylvestitol [16,17]. Moreover, phytochemical studies have also reported the presence of polyprenylated benzophenones, such as guttiferone E, xanthochymol, and oblongifolin B, whose source is *Symphonia globulifera* [18].

Although red propolis demonstrates promising biological activities, its potential advantages over conventional cancer therapies warrant further investigation. Chemotherapeutic agents are vital for cancer treatment but often come with significant side effects due to their non-specific targeting. These drugs can induce systemic toxicity by affecting normal cells, leading to problems such as anemia, hair loss, and gastrointestinal issues [19]. This highlights the urgent need for alternative therapeutic strategies.

Chemoprevention, which involves using agents like natural products to prevent cancer, plays a crucial role in reducing disease incidence. By focusing on prevention, these agents can minimize the necessity for aggressive treatments and lessen the overall cancer burden on patients [20]. Red propolis, with its bioactive compounds could offers a promising and less toxic alternative to conventional therapies, which are often associated with severe side effects.

Our research aims to develop a benzophenones-free red propolis extract (BFRP) to address the toxicity concerns related to the hydroalcoholic extract (RPHE) [21]. This new extract is intended to explore its potential in preventing colon carcinogenesis. By enhancing the safety and efficacy profile of red propolis, BFRP could become a valuable option for integrative oncology, appealing to patients who seek treatments with fewer side effects.

2. Results and Discussion

2.1. Obtaining the Standard Compounds and the Development and Validation of the RP-HPLC-PDA Method for the BFRP Analysis

As previously described, the compounds isoliquiritigenin, vestitol, neovestitol, medicarpine, and 7-*O*-methylvestitol were isolated from the BFRP, and their chemical structures were confirmed by the NMR data in comparison with the literature [18,22] (Figure 1). It is important to mention that during the isolation and analysis processes, the presence of polyprenylated benzophenones was not identified, thus denoting that the goal of obtaining a benzophenone-free red propolis extract was achieved. This fact can also be confirmed by analyzing the chemical profile displayed by the BFRP chromatogram obtained through the analysis performed according to the analytical method whose development is described herein (Figure 2). An analysis of the hydroalcoholic extract and the benzophenones-free red propolis extract was presented in supplementary materials (Figure S1).

Propolis is a complex natural product, abundant in flavonoids and other phenolic compounds. For phenolic compounds with strong chromophore groups, UV-based detectors provide excellent selectivity and sensitivity for the identification and quantification of bioactive compounds, making them an ideal choice for developing quality control methods. During the analytical method development, parameters such as temperature, flow rate, gradient, chromatographic conditions, including column and mobile phase, were optimized to achieve effective peak separation. The best peak resolution was obtained with a 30-min analysis (Figure 2). All parameters established during the method validation process comply with the relevant validation guidelines [23].

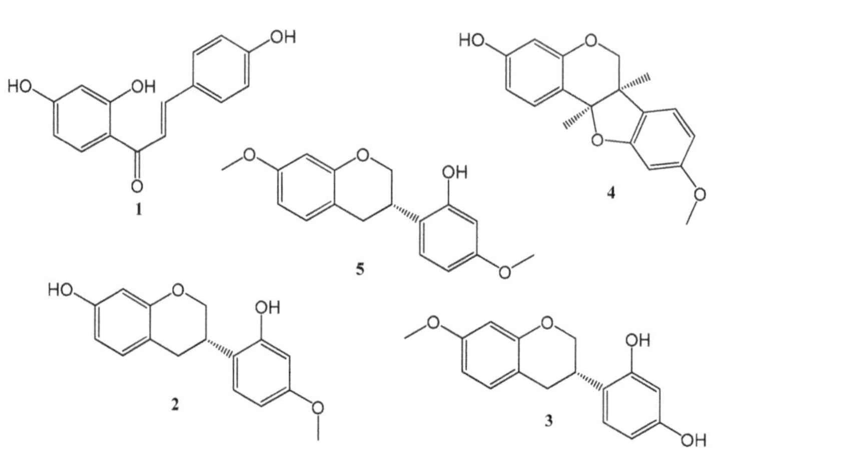

Figure 1. Chemical structures of isolated compounds from BFRP: 1—isoliquiritigenin; 2—vestitol; 3—neovestitol; 4—medicarpin; 5—7-O-methylvestitol.

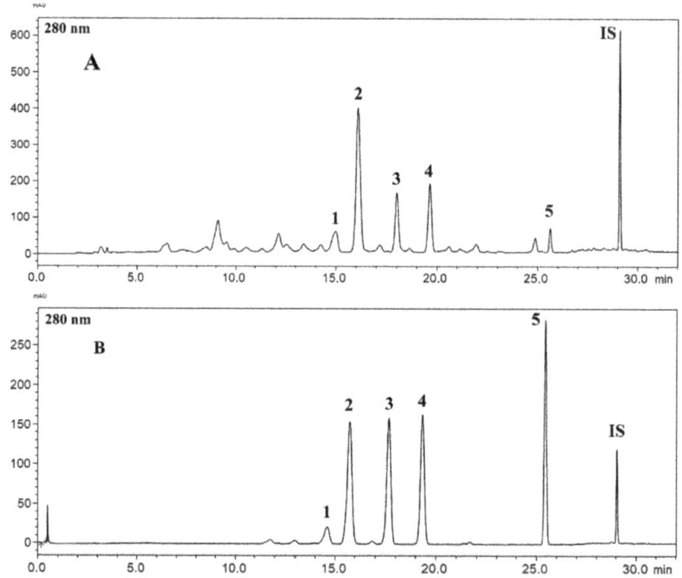

Figure 2. RP-HPLC-PDA chromatogram of the BFRP (A) in comparison with the respective standards (B): 1—isoliquiritigenin; 2—vestitol; 3—neovestitol; 4—medicarpin; 5—7-O-methylvestitol; and IS: benzophenone.

The UV spectra of each peak corresponded perfectly with their respective standards, confirming that each analytical signal aligns with its chromatographic counterpart. To assess linearity, standard solutions at eight different concentrations were analyzed using the HPLC-PDA method, yielding correlation coefficients (R) and determination coefficients (R^2) derived from the analytical curves, which were statistically analyzed using the least squares method. The R^2 values for all analytical curves exceeded 0.99, demonstrating linearity in accordance with validation guidelines. Furthermore, residual analyses were conducted, confirming the homoscedasticity of the data, as the analytical curves exhibited no lack of fit ($p > 0.05$). The intervals obtained for the limits of detection and quantification were also satisfactory, indicating that the chromatographic method can effectively detect and quantify the selected compounds at low concentrations (Table 1).

Table 1. Linearity, limits of detection, and quantification of the method.

Compound	Equation	R^2	R	LD	LQ	Minimum Observed Residual Value	Maximum Observed Residual Value	Lack of Fit *p* Value
(1)	y = 0.006x + 0.063	0.998	0.998	3.94	10.99	−3.31823	3.23520	0.61
(2)	y = 0.0356x + 0.3835	0.999	0.999	2.90	8.96	−2.2265	2.2288	0.79
(3)	y = 0.0313x + 0.4228	0.998	0.998	2.78	9.42	−2.26225	1.62954	0.74
(4)	y = 0.0293x + 0.4153	0.997	0.998	2.62	9.15	−2.26638	1.84199	0.81
(5)	y = 0.0292x + 0.4808	0.998	0.998	1.31	3.97	−1.59636	1.26722	0.93

R^2—determination coefficient; R—correlation coefficient; LD—limit of detection (µg/mL); LQ—limit of quantification (µg/mL); **1**—isoliquiritigenin; **2**—vestitol; **3**—neovestitol; **4**—medicarpin; and **5**—7-*O*-methylvestitol.

The accuracy of the method was evaluated for both repeatability (intraday accuracy) and intermediate accuracy (interday accuracy). Results demonstrated minimal variation between analyses, with both intraday and interday precisions exhibiting relative standard deviations (RSDs) below 2.99%. Accuracy results were approximately 100%, ranging from 96.05% to 113.93%, indicating that the analytical method yielded precise results with errors below 4.07% (Table 2). Consequently, the developed method is considered accurate and precise, adhering to ANVISA guidelines. For the recovery assessment, a Soxhlet appa-ratus was utilized for the exhaustive extraction of red propolis, yielding an extract yield of 52.6%. Recovery rates for all evaluated analytes were found to be between 96% and 108% at low, medium, and high concentrations. Thus, the optimized method can be deemed reliable for extracting chemically similar phenolic compounds. Additionally, the recovery of the internal standard was also high, ranging from 96% to 100%.

Table 2. Precision and accuracy of the method.

Compound	Level	Precision (RSD)		Accuracy (%)	E (%)	Recovery (%)
		Intraday	Interday			
(1)	High	0.08	2.13	100.89 ± 2.7	−0.89	104.02 ± 1.2
	Medium	0.79	1.38	113.93 ± 1.1	3.93	101.10 ± 2.8
	Low	0.66	2.97	97.93 ± 0.8	4.07	99.26 ± 1.9
(2)	High	0.35	1.65	98.49 ± 1.9	−1.51	107.02 ± 0.7
	Medium	0.65	2.99	107.7 ± 10.2	4.71	106.55 ± 1.1
	Low	0.46	1.15	104.04 ± 1.1	3.96	96.67 ± 0.9
(3)	High	0.57	0.72	99.50 ± 0.2	−0.50	108.69 ± 1.7
	Medium	0.61	0.44	110.92 ± 0.3	−2.92	105.01 ± 1.6
	Low	0.39	1.25	96.05 ± 0.9	3.59	99.50 ± 2.1
(4)	High	0.51	0.76	106.38 ± 1.2	2.38	97.52 ± 1.3
	Medium	0.56	0.43	108.05 ± 0.8	−1.35	100.94 ± 2.4
	Low	1.36	0.37	106.50 ± 1.2	2.65	102.86 ± 1.9
(5)	High	0.61	2.63	97.89 ± 2.5	2.11	99.65 ± 0.4
	Medium	0.44	0.43	101.94 ± 1.7	−1.94	96.90 ± 1.1
	Low	0.43	0.97	98.94 ± 2.3	−1.06	100.23 ± 2.2
I.S	High					100.98 ± 1.2
	Medium					96.71 ± 0.9
	Low					100.39 ± 1.6

RSD—relative standard deviation (%); E—error; **1**—isoliquiritigenin; **2**—vestitol; **3**—neovestitol; **4**—medicarpin; **5**—7-*O*-methylvestitol; and IS—internal standard, benzophenone.

The robustness was evaluated by the small variations in some parameters of the two-level method. The changes in these parameters led to a variation between 7 and 9% in the concentration of the compounds analyzed by the HPLC-PDA method. Staying within the limits established by the guides, therefore, the developed method proved to be robust.

Finally, it is possible to affirm that the developed method was successfully validated according to the guidelines of the Brazilian regulatory agency (ANVISA, Brasília, Brazil). Furthermore, the analyses performed using this method found that the phenolic compound content in the BFRP samples showed a predominant occurrence of vestitol (128.24 ± 1.01 μg/mL) in the extract, followed by isoliquiritigenin (87.94 ± 0.12 μg/mL), medicarpin (61.53 ± 0.42 μg/mL), neovestitol (53.36 ± 0.28 μg/mL), and 7-*O*-methylvestitol (29.69 ± 0.96 μg/mL). It is interesting to notice that vestitol was also identified as the major compound in the RPHE [17], although at a much lower concentration (65.06 ± 0.1796 μg/mL) than our findings in the BFRP. In fact, the concentration of the other main constituents of the BFRP that were previously quantified in the RPHE were also found at lower concentrations in the ethanolic extract (medicarpin: 48.72 ± 0.18 μg/mL; neovestitol: 33.03 ± 0.70 μg/mL; and 7-*O*-methylvestitol: 16.12 ± 0.29 μg/mL). These variations in the contents may be attributed to differences in the selectivity of the extraction process employed; however, other factors such as collection location and time of year, among others, could also be an influence.

2.2. *Toxicity Assessment*

2.2.1. Fish Toxicity Test

The toxicities of the BFRP and RPHE were initially evaluated in the zebrafish larvae using the VSRA assay. In this species, the startle response to a vibration stimulus starts at 5 dpf [24]. The larvae were exposed to the BFRP and RPHE at concentrations ranging from 2.5 to 160 μg/mL from 3 dpf to 5 dpf (48 h treatment), and their responses to a vibration stimulus are shown in Figure 3. Concentrations greater than or equal to 40 μg/mL of the BFRP (Figure 3A) and 10 μg/mL of the RPHE (Figure 3B) caused immobility in all the larvae, indicating toxicity at these concentrations ($p < 0.0001$). The larvae treated with BFRP and RPHE concentrations lower than or equal to 20 and 5 μg/mL, respectively, did not show significant immobilization when compared to the untreated larvae.

The lower toxicity of the BFRP when compared to the RPHE is related to the absence of polyprenylated benzophenones. In view of the known toxicity of these compounds [17,25,26], the BFRP was developed to remove the polyprenylated benzophenones with the aim of reducing the toxicity of the red propolis.

Previously, our research group reported the toxicity of RPHE to adult zebrafish at concentrations greater than or equal to 12.5 μg/mL after 96 h of exposure [17]. The data obtained in this present study revealed the greater sensitivity of zebrafish larvae to the effects of RPHE compared to adults, since its toxicity was observed in larvae at a lower concentration (10 μg/mL) and with a shorter exposure time (24 h).

The zebrafish larvae treated with 40 μg/mL of the BFRP, as well as those treated with the same concentration of the RPHE, exhibited an altered swimming behavior after 4 h of treatment. Specifically, the larvae were swimming upside down at the bottom of the plate. This behavior indicates that the central nervous system, the inner ear, or the swim bladder may have been altered by exposure to the extracts, compromising swimming ability and leading to the death of the individual.

In order to better understand the altered swimming behavior, morphological analyzes on these zebrafish larvae were conducted. The larvae treated with the BFRP and RPHE did not exhibit morphological abnormalities regarding the evaluated parameters when compared to those not treated (Figure 4B–H). Therefore, the altered swimming behavior induced by the extracts was not related to morphological changes in the inner ear or the swim bladder. It is noteworthy that the function of these organs may have been altered by the exposure of the larvae to the BFRP and RPHE, although no morphological changes were observed. Further studies should be carried out to clarify the abnormal swimming behavior of the larvae induced by the extracts.

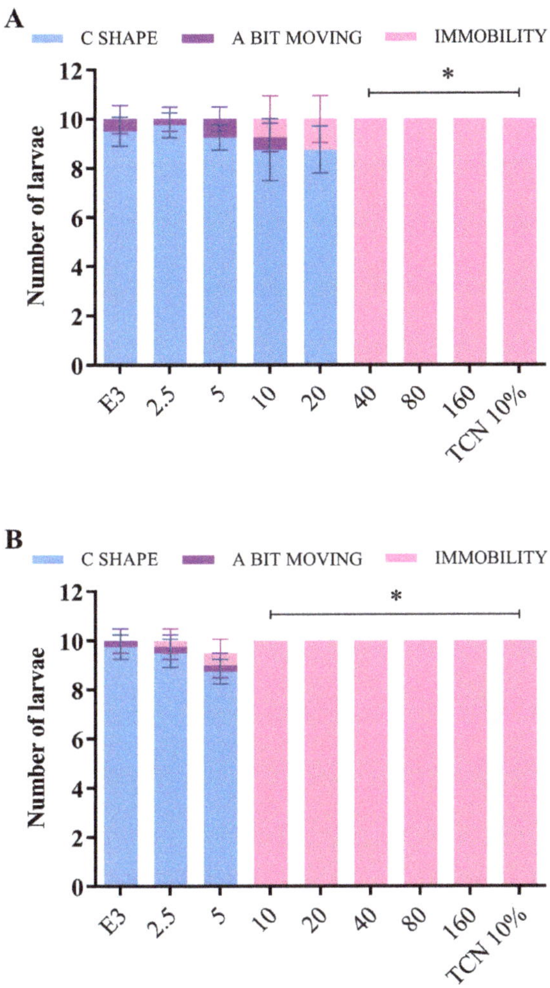

Figure 3. Effects of different concentrations of BFRP (**A**) and RPHE (**B**) on the startle response of zebrafish larvae (5 dpf) with VSRA assay. The count included the number of larvae that were immobile, a bit moving, and performing the C shape at the time of the stimulus. E3—E3 medium (negative control); BFRP—benzophenone-free red propolis extract; RPHE—red propolis hydroalcoholic extract; and TCN—tricaine 10% (positive control). The values are the mean ± SD ($n = 10$). The experiment was performed in triplicate. * significantly different from the negative control (E3) group ($p < 0.0001$).

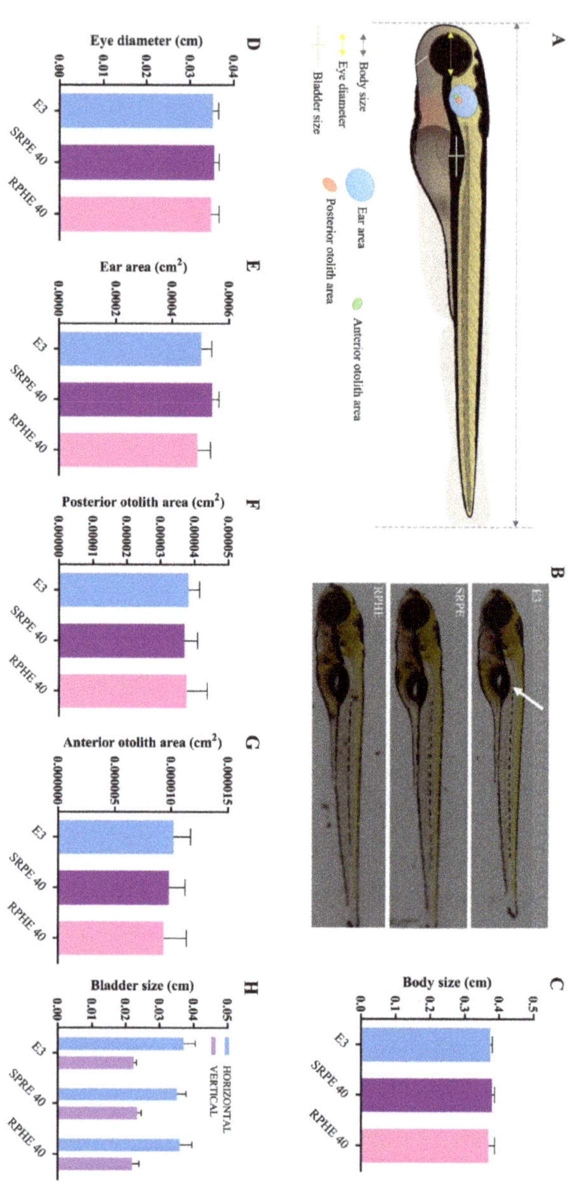

Figure 4. Effects of BFRP and RPHE on the morphology of zebrafish larvae at 5 dpf after 4 h of exposure. (**A**) Schematic representation of the different measurements of the larva (modified from Crouzier et al. [27]). (**B**) Lateral view of 5 dpf larvae. Swim bladder is indicated by a white arrow. (**C**) Measurement of body length, from the mouth to the end of the tail fin. (**D**) Measurement of the diameter of the eye. (**E–G**) Measurement of the ear. (**H**) Measurement of swim bladder size. BFRP—benzophenone-free red propolis extract (40 μg/mL); and RPHE—red propolis hydroalcoholic extract (40 μg/mL). No significant difference was observed between treated and untreated larvae ($p > 0.05$). The values are the mean ± SD (n = 10). Scale = 200 μm (75×) with a *brightfield microscope* Nikon SMZ18, with a camera Nikon Digital Sight 10.

Furthermore, a fluorescence microscopy analysis of these larvae was carried out. Interestingly, for the first time, it is being reported that the larvae treated with the BFRP or RPHE exhibited fluorescent staining in the notochord, branchial arches, and mouth, compared to the untreated larvae (Figure 5). The fluorescence displayed in these organs after the treatment with the extracts, especially of the notochord, may be involved in the altered swimming behavior.

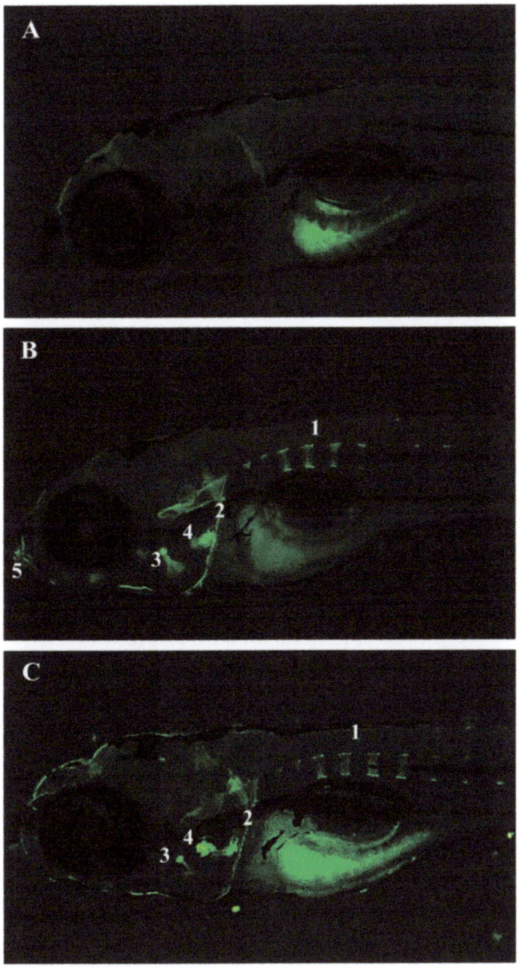

Figure 5. Effects of BFRP and RPHE on the development of zebrafish after 4 h of exposure. (**A**) Lateral view of 5 dpf zebrafish larvae treated with E3 medium (negative control). (**B**) Lateral view of 5 dpf zebrafish larvae treated with BFRP. (**C**) Lateral view of 5 dpf zebrafish larvae treated with RPHE. BFRP—benzophenone-free red propolis extract (40 µg/mL); RPHE—red propolis hydroalcoholic extract (40 µg/mL); 1—notochord; 2—branchial arch; 3 and 4—unrecognized structures; and 5—mouth. Fluorescence microscope (excitation wavelength 395 nm; emission wavelength 510 nm) Nikon SMZ18, with a camera Nikon Digital Sight 10. Scale = 200 µm (82×).

Additional studies are necessary to understand the relationship between the structures that exhibited fluorescence, and the toxicity observed in the larvae treated with the BFRP and RHPE. However, the mineralization of the notochord begins in the larval stage used in the experiments at 5 dpf [28]. Therefore, it can be speculated that the chemical constituents of the BFRP and RHPE have an affinity for calcium.

A segmented vertebral column is a distinctive feature of vertebrate species. In all vertebrates, somites are formed rhythmically and sequentially along the embryonic axis in a process regulated by a multicellular genetic oscillator known as the segmentation clock. This segmentation clock comprises a network of oscillating genes that exhibit variations among species [29]. It has been proposed that, in zebrafish [30] and salmon [31,32], the notochord rather than the sclerotome is the initial source of the bone matrix for cordacentra (vertebral body) formation, while in other species of teleost fish, the classic osteoblasts derived from the sclerotome have been suggested as the main drivers of the cordacentra formation [33,34]. The sclerotome occupies most of the somite, while skin and muscle are derived from the smaller dermatome. The cells within the sclerotome responsible for the production and mineralization of the organic aspect of bone (osteoid) are called osteoblasts. Cordacentra are first observed as they mineralize into rings around the notochord, forming sequentially along the axis in a process that begins several days after somitogenesis and muscle segmentation [28]. Thus, the beginning of the segmentation of the cordacentra can be observed through the fluorescence displayed by the BFRP and RPHE.

Among the flavonoids present in the BFRP and RPHE, isoliquiritigenin (ISL) is the only one reported in the literature to fluoresce [35]. The toxic effects of ISL have been reported on the development of zebrafish embryos (24 hpf) and larvae (96 hpf), especially on the heart, liver, and nervous system [36]. Nevertheless, the BFRP and RPHE are mixtures of substances. Therefore, studies with their substances isolated must be carried out, as well as molecular genetic analyses, to better understand the effects of the BFRP and RHPE on swimming behavior and the fluorescence displayed, especially by the notochord of zebrafish larvae.

2.2.2. Genetic Toxicology Test

The results obtained by the micronucleus assay in the Swiss mice's peripheral blood demonstrated that the frequencies of the MNPCEs of the animals treated with different doses of the BFRP (500, 1000, and 2000 mg/kg) did not differ significantly from the solvent group. In addition, the PCE/PCE + NCE (normochromatic erythrocyte) ratios were not significantly different between the treatment groups (Table 3). Therefore, the data revealed that the BFRP did not present genotoxicity and cytotoxicity, following the experimental recommendations of the OECD [37].

Table 3. Frequencies of micronucleated polychromatic erythrocytes (MNPCEs) in the peripheral blood of mice treated with different doses of BFRP.

Treatments (mg/kg)	MNPCEs	PCE/PCE + NCE
DMSO	6.0 ± 2.0	0.04 ± 0.02
500	5.0 ± 1.9	0.04 ± 0.01
1000	7.8 ± 2.6	0.04 ± 0.01
2000	9.2 ± 1.3	0.05 ± 0.00
PC	30.3 ± 3.2 *	0.03 ± 0.01

BFRP—benzophenone-free red propolis extract; PCEs—polychromatic erythrocytes; NCEs—normochromatic erythrocytes; DMSO—dimethyl sulfoxide (5%); and PC—positive control (doxorubicin, 10 mg/kg). The values are the mean ± SD ($n = 5$). * significantly different from the negative control group ($p < 0.05$).

The animals submitted to the different treatments presented serum levels of ALT (Figure 6A) and creatinine (Figure 6B) that did not differ from those observed in the negative control group, revealing the absence of hepatotoxicity and nephrotoxicity, respectively.

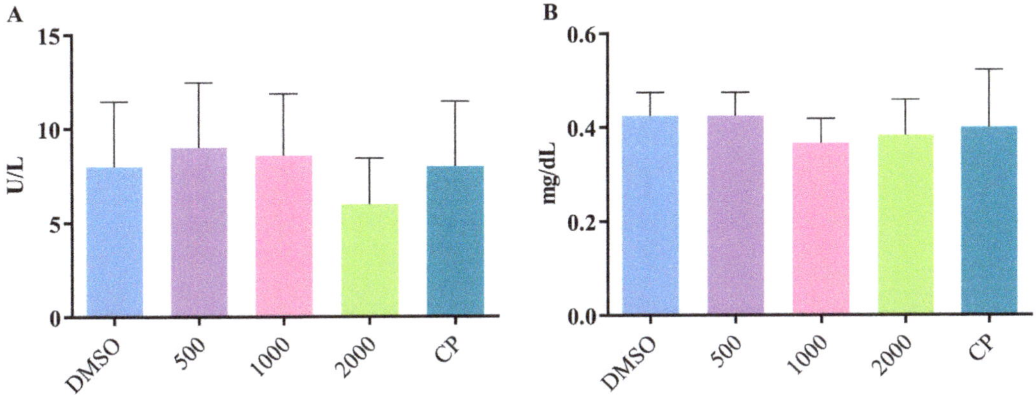

Figure 6. Serum levels of ALT (**A**) and creatinine (**B**) obtained in the peripheral blood of Swiss mice treated with different doses of BFRP (500, 1000, and 2000 mg/kg) and their respective controls. BFRP—benzophenone-free red propolis extract; ALT—alanine aminotransferase; DMSO—dimethyl sulfoxide (5%); and CP—positive control (doxorubicin, 10 mg/kg). The values are the mean ± SD ($n = 5$).

Genotoxicity tests are designed to identify the compounds capable of causing genetic damage through various mechanisms. These assessments facilitate the recognition of potential dangers related to DNA damage and its fixation. The fixation of DNA damage, such as genetic mutations; extensive chromosomal damage; or recombination is generally considered crucial in the intricate process of malignancy, where genetic alterations can play a contributory role. Numerical changes in the chromosomes have also been associated with tumorigenesis and may indicate susceptibility to aneuploidy in germ cells. The compounds that produce positive results in tests that detect these types of damage have the potential to act as human carcinogens and/or mutagens. Therefore, genotoxicity tests mainly serve to predict carcinogenicity [38].

The micronucleus test used in this present study is part of the standard genetic toxicology battery for the prediction of potential risks for pharmaceuticals intended for human use. Negative results, as obtained for the BFRP, are considered sufficient to demonstrate the absence of a significant genotoxic risk [39].

It is important to consider that, although BFRP did not show genotoxicity in acute exposure, the long-term use of propolis, particularly over extended periods, may still pose potential health risks [40]. Prolonged exposure to the bioactive compounds in propolis, whether through internal or external application, could lead to cumulative effects that might not be immediately apparent in short-term genotoxicity assays. For instance, the risk of allergic reactions, sensitization, and potential interactions with other med-ications may increase over time, especially in susceptible individuals [41]

Therefore, despite the absence of significant genotoxicity observed for BFRP, caution should be exercised with the long-term use of propolis, and further studies are recommended to thoroughly assess its safety profile under prolonged exposure.

2.3. Evaluation of the Effect of BFRP on Preneoplastic Colon Lesions

Preneoplastic lesions were observed only in the colons of animals that received DMH, whose results are presented in Figure 7. No significant differences were observed in the ACF/AC ratio between the treatment groups, which ranged from 1.1 to 2.0. The BFRP treatments led to reductions in the frequencies of the preneoplastic lesions induced by the carcinogen DMH. The differences were statistically significant for the group of animals treated with 6 mg/kg of the BFRP when compared to the group treated with DMH alone, corresponding to a 41.6% reduction in preneoplastic lesions.

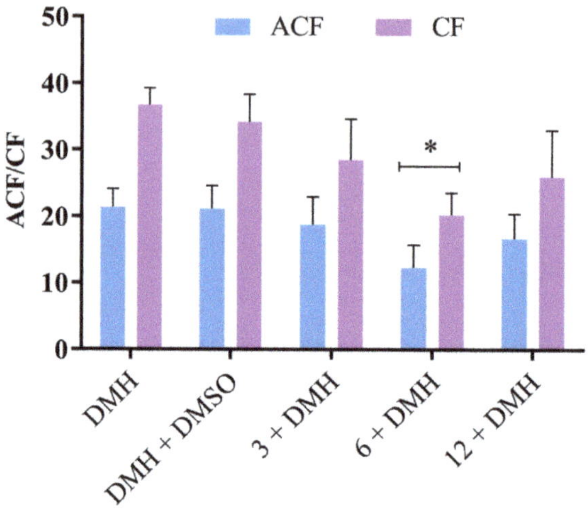

Figure 7. Effect of BFRP on DMH-induced carcinogenesis in the colon of Wistar Hannover rats. Rates of aberrant crypt foci (ACF) and aberrant crypts (AC) identified in the distal colon of rats administered BFRP and DMH. BFRP—benzophenone-free red propolis extract (3, 6, and 12 mg/kg); ACF—aberrant crypt foci; AC—aberrant crypt; DMH—1,2-dimethylhydrazine (40 mg/kg); and DMSO—dimethyl sulfoxide (5%). The values are the mean ± SD ($n = 5$). * significantly different from the DMH group ($p < 0.05$).

DMH is an alkylating procarcinogen that requires metabolic activation, involving various hepatic enzymes [42]. In the liver, it is metabolized into a diazonium ion, causing an imbalance in oxidative stress and DNA damage and contributing to carcinogenesis, including the development of ACF [43]. Processes related to inflammation have been demonstrated to play a role in the development of colon carcinogenesis, both in humans and in cases induced by DMH [44]. In this context, the reduction in preneoplastic lesions induced by DMH is related, at least in part, to the anti-inflammatory property of BFRP.

It is noteworthy that the literature has reported the anti-inflammatory activity of the RHPE, from which the BFRP was developed [11–13,15]. In addition, our previous study demonstrated that the animals treated with DMH showed a high expression of cyclooxygenase-2 (COX-2) in the colon tissue. RPHE significantly decreased the expression induced by DMH, indicating its anti-inflammatory properties [13]. COX-2 is an enzyme crucial in inducing inflammatory responses and is often associated with colorectal tumors. Under the same experimental conditions, we also observed the chemopreventive effect of the hydroalcoholic extract of *D. ecastaphyllum* stems, the botanical source of red propolis responsible for providing phenolic compounds. The treatments with this extract led to a reduction in DMH-induced preneoplastic lesions, which was accompanied by significantly lower levels of COX-2 expression [16]. Taken together, it is noted that the BFRP exhibited a protective effect against colon carcinogenesis at a dose lower (6 mg/kg) than that observed for the RPHE (12 mg/kg) and its botanical source (48 mg/kg).

Significant differences were observed in the weight gain of animals treated with DMH and DMSO plus DMH in relation to the control vehicle. In relation to water consumption, there were no statistically significant changes when compared to the vehicle control group (Table 4).

Table 4. Average initial body weight, final body weight, body weight gain, and water consumption of rats treated with varying doses of BFRP alongside DMH, along with their corresponding control groups, during the four-week experimental period.

Treatments (mg/kg)	Initial Weight (g)	Final Weight (g)	Weight Gain (g)	Water Consumption (mL/Animal/Day)
DMSO	225.8 ± 5.2	352.8 ± 2.7	128.0 ± 5.3	53.9 ± 18.1
24	229.3 ± 4.0	350.3 ± 5.5	121.0 ± 4.6	50.7 ± 12.1
DMH	227.0 ± 7.0	296.0 ± 9.5	89.8 ± 10.4 *	65.9 ± 22.2
DMSO + DMH	230.6 ± 7.0	295.7 ± 8.1	76.8 ± 14.0 *	49.0 ± 12.6
3 + DMH	219.8 ± 6.6	340.8 ± 6.2	122.2 ± 7.7	63.2 ± 12.5
6 + DMH	218.8 ± 5.5	341.7 ± 9.8	121.4 ± 6.9	52.2 ± 13.3
12 + DMH	225.8 ± 6.9	348.2 ± 7.2	122.4 ± 8.4	73.6 ± 23.3

BFRP—benzophenone-free red propolis extract; DMH—1,2-dimethylhydrazine (40 mg/kg); and DMSO—dimethyl sulfoxide (5%). The values are the mean ± SD (n = 5). * significantly different from the DMSO group ($p < 0.05$).

Previous studies have documented a notable reduction in body weight in rats treated with DMH when compared to the control group. This decline in body weight could be attributed to alterations in fat metabolism resulting from increased gluconeogenesis to meet the heightened energy demands of the hyperplastic cells [13,45]. Although there were no significant changes in food intake, the reduction in body weight observed after DMH treatment may be associated with the overall breakdown of lipids and proteins [46]. In contrast, the animals that received BFRP along with DMH did not exhibit significant decreases in body weight gain when compared to those that were not treated with DMH. These data indicate that the SPRE exhibited a protective effect against DMH-induced toxicity. Therefore, the BFRP was able to reduce not only the preneoplastic lesions induced by DMH but also its toxicity.

The complex chemical composition of an extract, containing various compounds, presents a notable challenge in understanding its mechanisms of action. These constituents can produce a range of biological effects, either working together or independently. Despite this complexity, an extract's biological activity is primarily tied to the synergistic effects of its constituents influencing various levels, targets, and pathways simultaneously. Thus, the extracts may demonstrate biological properties not observed in the isolated constituents [47,48].

Epidemiological studies show that flavonoid-rich foods prevent some diseases, including metabolic-related diseases and cancer. Further studies show that flavonoids have many properties, which include antioxidant, anti-inflammatory, anti-proliferative [49,50]. These results underscore the relevance of BFRP, an extract rich in flavonoids, as a potentially beneficial intervention in inflammatory bowel conditions [51].

3. Material and Methods

3.1. Obtaining the Hydroalcoholic Extract of Red Propolis (RPHE) and the Benzophenone-Free Red Propolis Extract (BFRP)

The Brazilian red propolis sample was sourced in February 2020 from the Association of Beekeepers of Canavieiras (COAPER, Bahia, Brazil), a cooperative situated in the southern region of Bahia, northeastern Brazil. The preparation of RPHE followed the method described by Aldana-Mejía et al. [21].

To prepare the BFRP, 50 g of crude red propolis was frozen at −80 °C for 3 h, then ground using a mill. The ground material was subjected to dynamic maceration in 500 mL of n-hexane at 35 °C and 140 rpm. The solvent was replaced every 24 h, completing three maceration cycles. After that, the precipitate was submitted to another three-times extraction using 300 mL of cold methanol (10 °C) for 30 min to give 22.7 g, a 45.4% yield of BFRP after concentration in a Buchi® rotary evaporator apparatus.

3.2. Isolation and Identification of the Standard Compounds

Twelve grams of BFRP was subjected to silica gel column chromatography (120 × 5 cm) with hexane/ethyl acetate in a gradient mode from 100% of hexane to 50% of hexane. This fractionation resulted in 247 fractions of 8 mL each that were analyzed by Thin Layer Chromatography (TLC) (hexane/ethyl acetate, 70:30) and reunited to give 26 fractions (F 1-26). Fraction 4 was submitted to a preparative scale using a high-performance liquid chromatography (HPLC; Shimadzu, Kyoto, Japan) with water plus 0.1% acetic acid (solvent A) and acetonitrile (solvent B). The separation method was a gradient starting in 30% of solvent B to 100% of solvent B in 25 min, furnishing isoliquiritigenin (**1**) (41 mg). Fraction 8 formed a precipitate, identified as vestitol (**2**) (1388 mg). Fraction 12 (1.7 g) was submitted to Sephadex column chromatography (90 × 3 cm) with methanol/water to give neovestitol (**3**) (33 mg) and medicarpin (**4**) (18 mg). Fraction 17 (685 mg) was submitted to a preparative HPLC with water plus 0.1% glacial acetic acid (solvent A) and acetonitrile (solvent B). The separation method was a gradient starting in 45% of solvent B to 100% of solvent B in 30 min, furnishing 7-*O*-methylvestitol (**5**) (41 mg).

The isolated compounds were identified through a nuclear magnetic resonance (NMR) analysis for the structural elucidation. The NMR spectra were obtained on a Bruker Advance DRX400, operating at 400 and 100 mHz for ^{1}H and ^{13}C, respectively. Deuterated solvent from Sigma Aldrich® was used.

3.3. RP-HPLC-PDA Method for BFRP Analysis

The analytical method for BFRP was developed using a Shimadzu HPLC system, model LC-20AR Prominence, equipped with an SIL-10AF autosampler, CTO-20A column oven, CBM-20A communication bus module, DGU-20A3R in-line degasser, and an SPD-M20A photodiode array detector. All experiments were conducted in triplicate under controlled temperature conditions. The HPLC analysis employed a Shim-pack VP-ODS analytical column (250 × 4.6 mm i.d., 5 μm; Shimadzu), with acidified water (0.2% acetic acid) as solvent A and acetonitrile as solvent B, using the following parameters: 0.01−15.00 min, 30−48% of B; 15.00−20.00 min, 48−55% of B; 20.00−23.00 min, 55−73% of B; 23.00−24.00 min, 73−100% of B; 24.00−29.00 min, 100% of B; 29.00−30.00 min, 100−40% of B; and 30.00−32.00 min, 40% of B. The flow rate was set at 1 mL/min and the UV detection at 280 nm for the compounds. The temperature of the column was set at 40 °C, and the injected volume was 20 μL. The Lab solution® software was used to process the data.

3.4. Validation of the Method

The validation followed the guidelines set by the Brazilian National Health Surveillance Agency (ANVISA) [23]. Parameters such as selectivity, linearity, detection and quantification limits, accuracy, precision, recovery, and robustness were assessed. All validation experiments were conducted in triplicate.

3.4.1. Selectivity

Method selectivity was determined based on the separation efficiency of chromatographic peaks, evaluated by assessing the chromatographic resolution. The peaks were compared to authentic standards to confirm the selectivity of red propolis compounds, using parameters such as relative retention time, peak area, resolution, and UV spectra.

3.4.2. Linearity, Limit of Detection, and Limit of Quantification

The linearity was estimated by calibration curves. The linear dynamic range was performed for the concentrations of 600, 500, 400, 300, 200, 100, 75, 25, and 15 μg/mL from the analytes. 1,2,4,5- tetramethylbenzene (TMB) was used as the internal standard at a final concentration of 100 μg/mL. TMB was selected as the internal standard due to its chemical stability, and non-interference with their detection, ensuring reliable chromatographic performance. From the solutions, 20 μL were injected in triplicate for three consecutive days. The analytical curve was generated by plotting the ratio of each analyte standard to the internal standard areas. Linearity was assessed by calculating the correlation coefficient (R), determination coefficient (R^2), and performing the lack of fit test. The Statistic 8.0 software was used to determine the minimum and maximum observed residual values. Limits of detection (LD) and quantification (LQ) were calculated based on baseline noise, using the following equations: LD = (3.3 × SD) / IC and LQ = (10 × SD) / IC, where SD represents the standard deviation of the y-intercept when x equals zero from the calibration curves, and IC is the slope of the analytical curve [23].

3.4.3. Precision and Accuracy

Three concentrations were selected to evaluate the precision and accuracy of the method. The method's precision was evaluated by calculating the relative standard deviation (RSD) for repeatability at three concentration levels: high (400 μg/mL), medium (100 μg/mL), and low (25 μg/mL). Measurements were taken on the same day (intraday precision) and across three consecutive days (interday precision). Accuracy was determined by comparing the theoretical and actual values of the solutions at the same three concentrations.

3.4.4. Recovery

For the recovery assessment, 15 g of ground propolis matrix underwent exhaustive extraction in a Soxhlet apparatus for 8 h with 300 mL of 96% ethanol. The matrix was then dried in an air-circulating oven at 50 °C for 12 h, and the extract was concentrated under vacuum. A standard solution of the compounds was prepared at a final concentration of 100 μg/mL for each compound. Following this, 200 mg of propolis matrix was spiked with the standard solution at three concentration levels: 4 mL (400 μg/mL, high level), 1 mL (100 μg/mL, medium level), and 0.25 mL (25 μg/mL, low level), and dried at room temperature. For extraction, 70% ethanol was used, with TMB (100 μg/mL) as the internal standard, and benzophenone (100 μg/mL) as the secondary internal standard. The extraction process was carried out using a shaker incubator at 35 °C and 140 rpm for 120 min. The standard compounds were quantified using the developed HPLC method. All experiments were performed in triplicate, and recovery percentages were calculated by comparing the theoretical and actual concentration values.

3.4.5. Robustness

The robustness was determined with the Plackett–Burman design for seven factors and eight experiments that combined the higher (+1) and lower (−1) levels of each factor. The factors were the flow rate (0.9 and 1.1 mL/min), the oven temperature (35 and 45 °C), the percentage of organic solvent (+1 and −1%), the detection wavelength (271 and 281 nm), and the volume of injection (19 and 21 μL). These factors were slightly changed for the higher and lower levels. To calculate the effects, the following equation was used: $Ex = \frac{\Sigma y(+) - \Sigma y(-)}{n/2}$, where Ex is the estimated effect of the response; Σy(+) is the sum of the responses at the positive level; Σy(−) is the sum of the responses at the negative level; and n is the number of experiments of the experimental design. These were expressed as the variation coefficients in percentages. The concentrations used to evaluate the robustness were the low, medium, and high levels, which were the same as were used in the precision test.

3.5. Toxicity Assessment

3.5.1. Fish Toxicity Test

Zebrafish Husbandry

Adult zebrafish (*Danio rerio*, AB2O2 line, Karlsruhe Institute of Technology; Eggenstein-Leopoldshafen, Germany) were bred and reared according to the standard methods [52]. The adult fish were kept under a light-dark cycle of 14 h of light and 10 h of darkness at a temper-ature of 28 °C. Fertilized eggs were gathered within 2 h of being laid and placed in petri dishes (10 cm in diameter) filled with E3 medium (5 mM NaCl, 0.17 mM

KCl, 0.33 mM $CaCl_2$) for incubation at 28.5 °C. The eggs from different clutches were kept separately to carry out the experiments, and all the experiments were performed in triplicate. All zebrafish care and procedures were carried out in accordance with the animal welfare regulations in Germany and received approval from the Government of Baden-Württemberg, Regierungspräsidium Karlsruhe, Germany (reference number 35-9185.64/BH KIT/March 1, 2022).

Vibration Startle Response Assay

A vibration startle response (VSRA) assay was conducted on 5 days postfertilization (dpf) larvae, after exposure to seven concentrations of BFRP (2.5, 5, 10, 20, 40, 80, and 160 µg/mL) for 48 h. In parallel, assays were conducted with the red propolis hydroalcoholic extract (RPHE), under the same experimental conditions, aiming to compare the effects. Ten larvae 72 h postfertilization (hpf) per condition were distributed in 5 cm diameter Petri dishes. The E3 medium was completely removed and replaced with 9 mL of E3 and 1 mL of the BFRP or RPHE solution. The exposure concentrations, based on previous studies, ranged from 2.5 to 160 µg/mL [17]. A stock solution of the BFRP and RPHE at 50 mg/mL was prepared, diluted in a mixture composed of 50% dimethyl sulfoxide (DMSO; Sigma-Aldrich) and 50% E3 medium. The DMSO concentration in the plate at the highest evaluated concentration of the BFRP and RPHE (160 µg/mL) was equivalent to 0.1%. Negative (E3 medium) and positive (10% tricaine) controls were added to the experiment [53].

The VSRA assay was based on the automated delivery of vibrational stimuli. The larvae were subjected to vibration at 5 dpf using sound-based vibration equipment, which was developed by the Screening Center at the Karlsruhe Institute of Technology and the Institute of Toxicology and Genetics (Karlsruhe, BW, Germany). The videos recorded by the equipment were manually analyzed, and the number of larvae that exhibited a 'c-shape', as well as those with little movement and/or that were immobile, was assessed as described in Hayot et al. [53].

Morphological Analyses

The larvae at 4.5 dpf were treated with 40 µg/mL of the BFRP and RPHE for 4 h, and the larval behavior before death was assessed. The choice of the concentration and treatment time was based on the results of the VSRA test. In this assay, the BFRP exhibited toxicity starting at 40 µg/mL. The RPHE was treated at the same concentration for comparison. The larvae were imaged using a *brightfield and* fluorescence microscope (with an excitation wavelength of 395 nm and an emission wavelength of 510 nm) Nikon SMZ18, with a camera Nikon Digital Sight 10, on a lateral view. The body thickness was measured as a toxicity parameter, as well as the swim bladder and otic vesicle area. Three replicates of ten larvae were analyzed. The parameters were measured using ImageJ, and the averages of the obtained values were calculated.

3.5.2. Genetic Toxicology Test

The peripheral blood micronucleus assay was utilized to evaluate the genotoxicity of BFRP and was carried out in accordance with the guidelines outlined in OECD 474 [37] recommendations. Male Swiss mice (*Mus musculus*), each weighing around 30 g, were sourced from the Faculty of Pharmaceutical Sciences at the University of São Paulo (Ribeirão Preto, SP, Brazil). The study protocols received approval from the Animal Use Ethics Committee of the University of Franca (process number 9907081122).

Following a one-week acclimatization period, the rodents were assigned into groups of five. Three distinct doses of BFRP were tested: 500, 1000, and 2000 mg/kg. The extract was administered to the animals via gavage over two consecutive days, once per day. Control groups included a solvent (DMSO, 1%) and a positive control group (doxorubicin; Bergamo, Taboão da Serra, SP, Brazil; 10 mg/kg). Peripheral blood samples were collected from the tail vein 48 h after the final treatment. Euthanasia of the rodents was performed through the intraperitoneal injection of thiopental sodium (840 mg/kg, Cristália, Itapira, SP, Brazil).

Blood samples were obtained through cardiac puncture under anesthesia (sodium pentobarbital, 45 mg/kg, intraperitoneal, 0.3 mL) for biochemical toxicity analysis. Serum levels of alanine aminotransferase (ALT) and creatinine were measured to assess hepatotoxicity and nephrotoxicity, respectively. For this, 0.3 mL serum samples were prepared using biochemical reagent kits Creatinine K (ref. 96) and ALT Liquiform (ref. 108) from Labtest Diagnóstico (Lagoa Santa, MG, Brazil), following the manufacturer's instructions. Measurements were conducted using a microprocessor-controlled random access biochemical analyzer (Bioplus, Barueri, SP, Brazil).

The frequency of micronucleated polychromatic erythrocytes (MNPCEs) was evaluated by examining 5000 polychromatic erythrocytes (PCEs) per mouse using a bright-field microscope (immersion objective, ×1000). Cytotoxicity resulting from the treatments was determined by calculating the ratio of PCE to the total erythrocyte count (PCE + normochromatic erythrocytes), analyzing 2000 erythrocytes per mouse.

3.6. Evaluation of the Effect of BFRP on Preneoplastic Colon Lesions

The aberrant crypt foci (ACF) assay was conducted following the methodology established by Bird [54] to assess the anticarcinogenic potential of BFRP. Male Wistar Hannover rats (Rattus norvegicus), each weighing approximately 120 g, were supplied by the Faculty of Pharmaceutical Sciences at the University of São Paulo (Ribeirão Preto, SP, Brazil) for the experiments. The animals (five animals/group) were housed in plastic cages in an experimental facility with controlled temperature (23 ± 2 °C) and humidity (50 ± 10%) under a 12-h light/dark cycle, with unrestricted access to food and water. The treatment protocols received approval from the Ethics Committee on Animal Use of the University of Franca (process number 9907081122).

The doses of the extract evaluated (6, 12, 24, and 48 mg/kg) were established based on a previous study involving red propolis hydroalcoholic extract [13]. The carcinogen 1,2-dimethylhydrazine (DMH; Sigma-Aldrich; 40 mg/kg) was utilized to induce preneoplastic lesions, specifically ACF, in the colon of the rats. This carcinogen was dissolved immediately prior to administration in 1 mM ethylenediaminetet-raacetic acid (EDTA; Labsynth, Diadema, SP, Brazil).

Following a week of acclimatization, various doses of BFRP were administered daily, once per day, for two weeks (during the second and third weeks) via gavage (1.0 mL/animal). Concurrently, DMH was administered subcutaneously twice a week (on the second and fifth days) for two weeks, totaling four administrations. Control groups included solvent (DMSO, 1%), DMH (40 mg/kg), and a combination of solvent and DMH. For the subsequent two weeks, the animals received no treatment. Body weight and water intake were recorded three times a week throughout the experimental period. The procedures for colon removal, slide preparation, and analysis were performed in accordance with Furtado et al. [55]. The frequencies of ACF and aberrant crypts (AC) were assessed by examining 15 sequential fields per colon segment.

3.7. Statistical Analysis

The data obtained in animals, zebrafish and rodents, were analyzed using analysis of variance (ANOVA) for fully randomized experiments, where F statistics and corresponding p-values were calculated. For results where $p < 0.05$, treatment means were compared using Tukey's test, and the minimum significant difference was determined for $\alpha = 0.05$. The statistical analysis was performed using Graph Pad Prism program 6. The percentage reduction in preneoplastic lesions was calculated according to Furtado et al. [55].

4. Conclusions

A benzophenones-free red propolis extract was obtained by a high-performance liquid chromatography with photodiode array detection method that is in accordance with the validation guidelines of the Brazilian regulatory agency. Toxicological evaluation assays revealed that benzophenones-free red propolis extract was significantly less toxic than hydroalcoholic extract of red propolis in zebrafish larvae and showed no genotoxicity in rodents. Therefore, it is confirmed that the removal of polyprenylated benzophenones from Brazilian red propolis leads to a reduction in the toxicity of this beekeeping product. Furthermore, benzophenones-free red propolis extract has promising effect on preventing colon cancer. How-ever, future research should focus on investigating the long-term effects of this extract in larger animal models and human clinical trials to further validate its safety and efficacy. Additionally, exploring the underlying mechanisms by which the extract exerts its chemopreventive effects is essential for fully understanding its therapeutic potential.

Supplementary Materials: The following supporting information can be downloaded at: https://www.mdpi.com/article/10.3390/ph17101340/s1, Figure S1: HPL-DAD chromatogram of (A) hydroalcoholic extract of red propolis and (B) benzophenones-free red propolis extract in a method developed by Aldana-Mejía et al. (2021).

Author Contributions: Conceptualization: I.S.S. and D.C.T.; Investigation: V.P.R., I.S.S., G.H., T.D., A.B.R., L.T.M.d.S., M.d.M.J., K.M.d.O.; Resources: J.K.B., R.C.S.V., S.R.A. and D.C.T.; Writing—Original Draft Preparation: I.S.S. and D.C.T.; Writing—Review & Editing: A.B.R. and D.C.T.; Data Curation: I.S.S., A.B.R. and D.C.T.; Project Administration: I.S.S. and D.C.T.; Supervision: D.C.T.; Funding Acquisition: D.C.T. and J.K.B. All authors approved the final manuscript. All authors have read and agreed to the published version of the manuscript.

Funding: This research was funded by São Paulo Research Foundation (FAPESP, Brazil; grants #2017/04138-8, #2018/05080-6, #2022/00659-1, and #2024/02434-2) for the financial support. I.S. Squarisi was the recipient of a doctorate fellowship from the Coordination for the Improvement of Higher Education Personnel (CAPES, Brazil; grant # 88887.505577/2020-00). The APC was funded by National Council for Scientific and Technological Development (CNPq, Brazil; grants #307379/2023-0, #307707/2021-0, #307778/2021-5, and #301440/2019-0).

Institutional Review Board Statement: The animal study protocol was approved by the Animal Use Ethics Committee of the University of Franca (approval number 9907081122, 13 March 2023).

Informed Consent Statement: Not applicable.

Data Availability Statement: Data is contained within the article.

Acknowledgments: The authors thank the São Paulo Research Foundation (FAPESP, Brazil; grants #2017/04138-8, #2018/05080-6, #2022/00659-1, and #2024/02434-2) for the financial support. I.S. Squarisi was the recipient of a doctoral fellowship from the Coordination for the Improvement of Higher Education Personnel (CAPES, Brazil). The authors are grateful to the National Council for Scientific and Technological Development (CNPq, Brazil) for the fellowships granted.

Conflicts of Interest: The authors declare that there are no conflicts of interest regarding the content of this paper.

References

1. Daugsch, A.; Moraes, C.S.; Fort, P.; Park, Y.K. Brazilian red propolis—Chemical composition and botanical origin. *Evid.-Based Complement. Altern. Med.* **2006**, *5*, 435–441. [CrossRef] [PubMed]
2. Salatino, A. Perspectives for uses of propolis in therapy against infectious diseases. *Molecules* **2022**, *27*, 4594. [CrossRef] [PubMed]
3. Rufatto, L.C.; Luchtenberg, P.; Garcia, C.; Thomassigny, C.; Bouttier, S.; Henriques, J.A.P.; Roesch-Ely, M.; Dumas, F.; Moura, S. Brazilian red propolis: Chemical composition and antibacterial activity determined using bioguided fractionation. *Microbiol. Res.* **2018**, *214*, 74–82. [CrossRef] [PubMed]
4. de Mendonça, I.C.G.; Porto, I.C.; do Nascimento, T.G.; de Souza, N.S.; Oliveira, J.M.; Arruda, R.E.; Mousinho, K.C.; dos Santos, A.F.; Basílio-Júnior, I.D.; Parolia, A.; et al. Brazilian red propolis: Phytochemical screening, antioxidant activity and effect against cancer cells. *BMC Complement. Altern. Med.* **2015**, *15*, 357. [CrossRef]
5. Souza Silva, T.; Silva, J.M.; Braun, G.H.; Mejia, J.A.; Ccapatinta, G.V.; Santos, M.F.C.; Tanimoto, M.H.; Bastos, J.K.; Parreira, R.L.T.; Orenha, R.P.; et al. Green and red brazilian propolis: Antimicrobial potential and anti-virulence against ATCC and clinically isolated multidrug-resistant bacteria. *Chem. Biodivers.* **2021**, *18*, e2100307. [CrossRef]

6. Oliveira Neto, N.F.; Bonvicini, J.F.S.; de Souza, G.L.; Santiago, M.B.; Veneziani, R.C.S.; Ambrósio, S.R.; Bastos, J.K.; Silva, M.J.B.; Martins, C.H.G.; Moura, C.C.G.; et al. Antibacterial activity of Brazilian red propolis and in vitro evaluation of free radical production. *Arch. Oral Biol.* **2022**, *143*, 105520. [CrossRef]
7. Ripari, N.; Pereira, A.F.M.; Júnior, A.F.; Rall, V.L.M.; A Aldana-Mejía, J.; Bastos, J.K.; Sforcin, J.M. Brazilian red propolis in combination with β-lactams exerts an efficient antibacterial action over methicillin-resistant *Staphylococcus aureus*(MRSA) strains. *J. Appl. Microbiol.* **2022**, *134*, lxac080. [CrossRef]
8. Silva, N.B.S.; de Souza, J.H.; Santiago, M.B.; da Silva Aguiar, J.R.; Martins, D.O.S.; da Silva, R.A.; Santos, I.d.A.; Aldana-Mejía, J.A.; Jardim, A.C.G.; Pedroso, R.d.S.; et al. Potential in vitro anti-periodontopathogenic, anti-Chikungunya activities and in vivo toxicity of Brazilian red propolis. *Sci. Rep.* **2022**, *12*, 21165. [CrossRef]
9. Conceição, M.; Gushiken, L.F.S.; Aldana-Mejía, J.A.; Tanimoto, M.H.; Ferreira, M.V.d.S.; Alves, A.C.M.; Miyashita, M.N.; Bastos, J.K.; Beserra, F.P.; Pellizzon, C.H. Histological, immunohistochemical and antioxidant analysis of skin wound healing influenced by the topical application of brazilian red propolis. *Antioxidants* **2022**, *11*, 2188. [CrossRef]
10. Squarisi, I.; De Freitas, K.S.; Lemes, D.C.; Ccapatinta, G.V.C.; Mejía, J.A.A.; Bastos, J.K.; Veneziani, R.C.S.; Ambrosio, S.R.; Tavares, D.C. Evaluation of the antiproliferative activity of red propolis hydroalcoholic extract and its fractions obtained by partition. *Biofarmasi J. Nat. Prod. Biochem.* **2020**, *18*, 70–73. [CrossRef]
11. Santiago, M.B.; Leandro, L.F.; Rosa, R.B.; Silva, M.V.; Teixeira, S.C.; Servato, J.P.S.; Ambrósio, S.R.; Veneziani, R.C.S.; Aldana-Mejía, J.A.; Bastos, J.K.; et al. Brazilian red propolis presents promising anti-H. pylori activity in in vitro and in vivo assays with the ability to modulate the immune response. *Molecules* **2022**, *27*, 7310. [CrossRef] [PubMed]
12. Santiago, K.B.; Rodrigues, J.C.Z.; de Oliveira Cardoso, E.; Conte, F.L.; Tasca, K.I.; Romagnoli, G.G.; Aldana-Mejía, J.A.; Bastos, J.K.; Sforcin, J.M. Brazilian red propolis exerts a cytotoxic action against prostate cancer cells and upregulates human monocyte functions. *Phytother. Res.* **2022**, *37*, 399–409. [CrossRef] [PubMed]
13. de Freitas, K.S.; da Silva, L.H.D.; Squarisi, I.S.; de Souza Oliveira, L.T.; Ribeiro, A.B.; Alves, B.S.; Esperandim, T.R.; de Melo, M.R.S.; Ozelin, S.D.; Lemes, D.C.; et al. Red propolis exhibits chemopreventive effect associated with antiproliferative and anti-inflammatory activities. *Toxicol. Res.* **2022**, *11*, 750–757. [CrossRef] [PubMed]
14. Boeing, T.; Mejía, J.A.A.; Ccana-Ccapatinta, G.V.; Mariott, M.; Melo Vilhena de Andrade Fonseca Da Silva, R.C.; de Souza, P.; Mariano, L.N.B.; Oliveira, G.R.; da Rocha, I.M.; da Costa, G.A.; et al. The gastroprotective effect of red propolis extract from Northeastern Brazil and the role of its isolated compounds. *J. Ethnopharmacol.* **2020**, *267*, 113623. [CrossRef] [PubMed]
15. Boeing, T.; de Oliveira, B.M.M.; Aldana-Mejía, J.A.; Ccana-Ccapatinta, G.V.; Venzon, L.; Cury, B.J.; França, T.C.S.; de Souza, P.; Junior, W.A.R.; da Silva, L.M.; et al. Brazilian red propolis accelerates gastric healing and reduces gastric submucosal layer inflammation in ultrasound-monitored rats. *Chem. Biodivers.* **2022**, *20*, e202200992. [CrossRef]
16. Silva, L.H.D.; Squarisi, I.S.; de Freitas, K.S.; Barcelos Ribeiro, A.; Ozelin, S.D.; Aldana-Mejía, J.A.; de Oliveira, L.T.S.; Rodrigues, T.E.; de Melo, M.R.S.; Nicolella, H.D.; et al. Toxicological and chemoprevention studies of Dalbergia ecastaphyllum (L.) Taub. stem, the botanical source of Brazilian red propolis. *J. Pharm. Pharmacol.* **2022**, *74*, 740–749. [CrossRef]
17. Aldana-Mejía, J.A.; Ccana-Ccapatinta, G.V.; Squarisi, I.S.; Nascimento, S.; Tanimoto, M.H.; Ribeiro, V.P.; Arruda, C.; Nicolella, H.; Esperandim, T.; Ribeiro, A.B.; et al. Nonclinical toxicological studies of brazilian red propolis and its primary botanical source *Dalbergia ecastaphyllum*. *Chem. Res. Toxicol.* **2021**, *34*, 1024–1033. [CrossRef]
18. Ccana-Ccapatinta, G.V.; Mejía, J.A.A.; Tanimoto, M.H.; Groppo, M.; de Carvalho, J.C.A.S.; Bastos, J.K. *Dalbergia ecastaphyllum* (L.) Taub. and *Symphonia globulifera* L.f.: The botanical sources of isoflavonoids and benzophenones in brazilian red propolis. *Molecules* **2020**, *25*, 2060. [CrossRef]
19. van den Boogaard, W.M.C.; Komninos, D.S.J.; Vermeij, W.P. Chemotherapy Side-Effects: Not All DNA Damage Is Equal. *Cancers* **2022**, *14*, 627. [CrossRef]
20. Russo, G.L.; Spagnuolo, C.; Russo, M. Reassessing the role of phytochemicals in cancer chemoprevention. *Biochem. Pharmacol.* **2024**, *228*, 116165. [CrossRef]
21. Aldana-Mejía, J.A.; de Miranda, A.M.; Ccana-Ccapatinta, G.V.; de Araújo, L.S.; Ribeiro, V.P.; Arruda, C.; Nascimento, S.; Squarisi, I.; Esperandim, T.; de Freitas, K.S.; et al. Genotoxicity and toxicological evaluations of Brazilian red propolis oral ingestion in a preclinical rodent model. *J. Ethnopharmacol.* **2023**, *303*, 115920. [CrossRef] [PubMed]
22. Aldana-Mejía, J.A.; Ccana-Ccapatinta, G.V.; Ribeiro, V.P.; Arruda, C.; Veneziani, R.C.; Ambrósio, S.R.; Bastos, J.K. A validated HPLC-UV method for the analysis of phenolic compounds in Brazilian red propolis and Dalbergia ecastaphyllum. *J. Pharm. Biomed. Anal.* **2021**, *198*, 114029. [CrossRef] [PubMed]
23. ANVISA. *Resolução da Diretoria Colegiada—RCD No. 166*; 24 July 2017; Ministério da Saúde—MS: Brasilia, Brazil, 2017; p. 21.
24. Basnet, R.M.; Zizioli, D.; Taweedet, S.; Finazzi, D.; Memo, M. Zebrafish larvae as a behavioral model in neuropharmacology. *Biomedicines* **2019**, *7*, 23. [CrossRef] [PubMed]
25. Prado, L.d.S.; da Silva, J.; Garcia, A.L.H.; Boaretto, F.B.M.; Grivicich, I.; Conter, L.U.; Salvi, A.d.O.; Reginatto, F.H.; Vencato, S.B.; Ferraz, A.d.B.F.; et al. Evaluation of DNA damage in HepG2 cells and mutagenicity of garcinielliptone FC, A bioactive benzophenone. *Basic Clin. Pharmacol. Toxicol.* **2017**, *120*, 621–627. [CrossRef] [PubMed]
26. Choodej, S.; Koopklang, K.; Raksat, A.; Chuaypen, N.; Pudhom, K. Bioactive xanthones, benzophenones and biphenyls from mangosteen root with potential anti-migration against hepatocellular carcinoma cells. *Sci. Rep.* **2022**, *12*, 8605. [CrossRef]

27. Crouzier, L.; Diez, C.; Richard, E.M.; Cubedo, N.; Barbereau, C.; Rossel, M.; Delaunay, T.; Maurice, T.; Delprat, B. Loss of Pde6a induces rod outer segment shrinkage and visual alterations in pde6aQ70X mutant zebrafish, a relevant model of retinal dystrophy. *Front. Cell Dev. Biol.* **2021**, *9*, 675517. [CrossRef]
28. Forero, L.L.; Narayanan, R.; Huitema, L.F.; VanBergen, M.; Apschner, A.; Peterson-Maduro, J.; Logister, I.; Valentin, G.; Morelli, L.G.; Oates, A.C.; et al. Segmentation of the zebrafish axial skeleton relies on notochord sheath cells and not on the segmentation clock. *eLife* **2018**, *7*, e33843. [CrossRef]
29. Shimojo, H.; Kageyama, R. Making waves toward the shore by synchronicity. *Dev. Cell* **2016**, *36*, 358–359. [CrossRef]
30. Fleming, A.; Keynes, R.; Tannahill, D. A central role for the notochord in vertebral patterning. *Development* **2004**, *131*, 873–880. [CrossRef]
31. Grotmol, S.; Kryvi, H.; Nordvik, K.; Totland, G.K. Notochord segmentation may lay down the pathway for the development of the vertebral bodies in the Atlantic salmon. *Anat. Embryol.* **2003**, *207*, 263–272. [CrossRef]
32. Wang, S.; Kryvi, H.; Grotmol, S.; Wargelius, A.; Krossøy, C.; Epple, M.; Neues, F.; Furmanek, T.; Totland, G.K. Mineralization of the vertebral bodies inAtlantic salmon (*Salmo salar* L.) is initiated segmentally in the form of hydroxyapatite crystal accretions in the notochord sheath. *Am. J. Anat.* **2013**, *223*, 159–170. [CrossRef] [PubMed]
33. Inohaya, K.; Takano, Y.; Kudo, A. The teleost intervertebral region acts as a growth center of the centrum: In vivo visualization of osteoblasts and their progenitors in transgenic fish. *Dev. Dyn.* **2007**, *236*, 3031–3046. [CrossRef] [PubMed]
34. Renn, J.; Büttner, A.; To, T.T.; Chan, S.J.H.; Winkler, C. A col10a1:nlGFP transgenic line displays putative osteoblast precursors at the medaka notochordal sheath prior to mineralization. *Dev. Biol.* **2013**, *381*, 134–143. [CrossRef]
35. Angeline, P.; Thomas, A.; Sankaranarayanan, S.A.; Rengan, A.K. Effect of pH on Isoliquiritigenin (ISL) fluorescence in lipo-polymeric system and metallic nanosystem. *Spectrochim. Acta Part A Mol. Biomol. Spectrosc.* **2021**, *252*, 119545. [CrossRef] [PubMed]
36. Song, Z.; Zhang, Y.; Zhang, H.; Rajendran, R.S.; Wang, R.; Hsiao, C.D.; Li, J.; Xia, Q.; Liu, K. Isoliquiritigenin triggers developmental toxicity and oxidative stress–mediated apoptosis in zebrafish embryos/larvae via Nrf2-HO1/JNK-ERK/mitochondrion pathway. *Chemosphere* **2020**, *246*, 125727. [CrossRef]
37. OECD. *Test No. 474: Mammalian Erythrocyte Micronucleus Test, OECD Guidelines for the Testing of Chemicals, Section 4*; OECD Publishing: Paris, France, 2016. [CrossRef]
38. Hagmar, L.; Strömberg, U.; Tinnerberg, H.; Mikoczy, Z. Epidemiological evaluation of cytogenetic biomarkers as potential surrogate end-points for cancer. *IARC Sci. Publ.* **2004**, *157*, 207–215.
39. ICH Topic S2[R1]. *Guidance on Genotoxicity Testing and Data Interpretation for Pharmaceuticals Intended for Human Use*; Published by the authority of the Minister of Health; Health Products and Food Branch: London, UK, 2016.
40. Silici, S.; Demiray, S.; Okan, A.; Ertuğrul, S.; Alizada, S.; Doğanyiğit, Z. Effects of short- and long-term use of propolis extracts on liver and kidney in rats. *Food Sci. Nutr.* **2024**, *12*, 5538–5547. [CrossRef]
41. Bhargava, P.; Mahanta, D.; Kaul, A.; Ishida, Y.; Terao, K.; Wadhwa, R.; Kaul, S.C. Experimental Evidence for Therapeutic Potentials of Propolis. *Nutrients* **2021**, *13*, 2528. [CrossRef]
42. Venkatachalam, K.; Vinayagam, R.; Anand, M.A.V.; Isa, N.M.; Ponnaiyan, R. Biochemical and molecular aspects of 1,2-dimethylhydrazine (DMH)-induced colon carcinogenesis: A review. *Toxicol. Res.* **2020**, *9*, 2–18. [CrossRef]
43. Darband, S.G.; Sadighparvar, S.; Yousefi, B.; Kaviani, M.; Ghaderi-Pakdel, F.; Mihanfar, A.; Rahimi, Y.; Mobaraki, K.; Majidinia, M. Quercetin attenuated oxidative DNA damage through NRF2 signaling pathway in rats with DMH induced colon carcinogenesis. *Life Sci.* **2020**, *253*, 117584. [CrossRef]
44. Takahashi, M.; Wakabayashi, K. Gene mutations and altered gene expression in azoxymethane-induced colon carcinogenesis in rodents. *Cancer Sci.* **2004**, *95*, 475–480. [CrossRef] [PubMed]
45. Li, W.; Li, C.B. Effect of oral Lactococcus lactis containing endostatin on 1, 2-dimethylhydrazine-induced colon tumor in rats. *World J. Gastroenterol.* **2005**, *11*, 7242. [CrossRef] [PubMed]
46. Walia, S.; Kamal, R.; Kanwar, S.S.; Dhawan, D.K. Cyclooxygenase as a target in chemoprevention by probiotics during 1,2-dimethylhydrazine induced colon carcinogenesis in rats. *Nutr. Cancer* **2015**, *67*, 603–611. [CrossRef] [PubMed]
47. Yuan, H.; Ma, Q.; Cui, H.; Liu, G.; Zhao, X.; Li, W.; Piao, G. How can synergism of traditional medicines benefit from network pharmacology? *Molecules* **2017**, *22*, 1135. [CrossRef] [PubMed]
48. Lai, X.; Wang, X.; Hu, Y.; Su, S.; Li, W.; Li, S. Editorial: Network pharmacology and traditional medicine. *Front. Pharmacol.* **2020**, *11*, 1194. [CrossRef]
49. Ferraz, C.R.; Carvalho, T.T.; Manchope, M.F.; Artero, N.A.; Rasquel-Oliveira, F.S.; Fattori, V.; Casagrande, R.; Verri, W.A., Jr. Therapeutic potential of flavonoids in pain and inflammation: Mechanisms of action, pre-clinical and clinical data, and pharmaceutical development. *Molecules* **2020**, *25*, 762. [CrossRef]
50. Al-Khayri, J.M.; Sahana, G.R.; Nagella, P.; Joseph, B.V.; Alessa, F.M.; Al-Mssallem, M.Q. Flavonoids as potential anti-inflammatory molecules: A review. *Molecules* **2022**, *27*, 2901. [CrossRef]
51. Santos, F.F.; Morais-Urano, R.P.; Cunha, W.R.; de Almeida, S.G.; Cavallari, P.S.D.S.R.; Manuquian, H.A.; Pereira, H.A.; Furtado, R.; Santos, M.F.C.; Amdrade, E.; et al. A review on the anti-inflammatory activities of Brazilian green, brown and red propolis. *J. Food Biochem.* **2022**, *46*, e14350. [CrossRef]
52. Westerfield, M. *The Zebrafish Book*; A guide for the laboratory use of zebrafish (*Danio rerio*); University of Oregon Press: Eugene, OR, USA, 2007.

53. Hayot, G.; Marcato, D.; von Clausbruch, C.A.C.; Pace, G.; Strähle, U.; Colbourne, J.K.; Pylatiuk, C.; Peravali, R.; Weiss, C.; Scholz, S.; et al. Evaluating Toxicity of Chemicals using a Zebrafish Vibration Startle Response Screening System. *J. Vis. Exp.* **2024**, *203*, e66153. [CrossRef]
54. Bird, R.P. Observation and quantification of aberrant crypts in the murine colon treated with a colon carcinogen: Preliminary findings. *Cancer Lett.* **1987**, *37*, 147–151. [CrossRef]
55. Furtado, R.A.; Oliveira, B.R.; Silva, L.R.; Cleto, S.S.; Munari, C.C.; Cunha, W.R.; Tavares, D.C. Chemopreventive effects of rosmarinic acid on rat colon carcinogenesis. *Eur. J. Cancer Prev.* **2015**, *24*, 106–112. [CrossRef] [PubMed]

pharmaceuticals

MDPI

Article

The Potential of Dehydrated *Geniotrigona thoracica* Stingless Bee Honey against Metabolic Syndrome in Rats Induced by a High-Carbohydrate, High-Fat Diet

Liyana Nabihah Ikhsan [1], Kok-Yong Chin [2] and Fairus Ahmad [1,*]

[1] Department of Anatomy, Faculty of Medicine, Universiti Kebangsaan Malaysia, Jalan Yaacob Latif, Bandar Tun Razak, Kuala Lumpur 56000, Malaysia

[2] Department of Pharmacology, Faculty of Medicine, Universiti Kebangsaan Malaysia, Jalan Yaacob Latif, Bandar Tun Razak, Kuala Lumpur 56000, Malaysia

* Correspondence: fairusahmad@ukm.edu.my; Tel.: +60-39-1458632

Abstract: Background/Objectives: Metabolic syndrome (MS) is diagnosed when at least three out of five key risk factors are present: obesity, high blood pressure, insulin resistance, high triglycerides (TG) and low high-density lipoprotein (HDL). MS is often associated with chronic low-grade inflammation. Recent studies have shown that raw stingless bee honey (SBH) can alleviate MS risk factors. However, the high moisture content in raw SBH predisposes it to fermentation, which can degrade its quality. Therefore, dehydrating SBH is necessary to prevent the fermentation process. This study aimed to compare the effects of dehydrated (DeGT) and raw (RGT) SBH from *Geniotrigona thoracica* species on high-carbohydrate, high-fat diet (HCHF)-induced MS in rats. Methods: Twenty-four male Wistar rats were divided into four groups: control (C), HCHF-induced MS without treatment (MS), HCHF-induced MS treated with DeGT (MS+DeGT) and HCHF-induced MS treated with RGT (MS+RGT). Group C received standard rat chow, while the other groups were fed with HCHF diet for 16 weeks. In the final eight weeks, two HCHF-induced groups received their respective SBH treatments. Results: Both DeGT and RGT treatments reduced energy intake, fat mass, high blood pressure, inflammatory (tumour necrosis factor-alpha (TNF-α)) and obesity (the leptin/adiponectin (L/A) ratio, corticosterone, 11 beta-hydroxysteroid dehydrogenase type-1 (11βHSD1)) markers, as well as prevented histomorphometry changes (prevented adipocyte hypertrophy, increased the Bowman's space area and glomerular atrophy). Additionally, DeGT increased serum HDL levels, while RGT reduced serum TG, leptin and other inflammatory markers (interleukin-6 (IL-6) and interleukin-1 beta (IL-1β)), as well as hepatosteatosis. Conclusions: While DeGT demonstrates potential as a preventive agent for MS, RGT exhibited more pronounced anti-MS effects in this study.

Keywords: honey; stingless bee honey; honey dehydration; anti-inflammatory; obesity; *Geniotrigona thoracica*; HCHF diet

1. Introduction

Metabolic syndrome (MS) is a metabolic imbalance characterized by several risk factors, including obesity, hypertension, insulin resistance and dyslipidemia. Between 2011 and 2018, approximately 35–38% of adults in the United States were diagnosed with MS [1]. In the Asia Pacific region, the prevalence of MS ranges from 11.9–37.1% among adults [2]. MS has now emerged as a worldwide public health concern due to its association with a five-fold increase in the risk of developing type II diabetes mellitus (T2DM) and a three-fold increase in developing cardiovascular diseases [3,4]. The prevalence of diabetes among individuals aged 20–79 globally was 8.8% in 2015 and is expected to reach 10.8% in 2040 [5].

The rise in MS is attributed to modern lifestyle changes. Two prominent factors contributing to this rise are the consumption of high-calorie, low-fiber fast food and a reduction in physical activity due to sedentary lifestyles [6]. The primary approach to managing MS involves adopting a healthy lifestyle, including a balanced diet, calorie control and regular physical activity. However, pharmacological or surgical interventions are necessary to manage MS risk factors effectively [7]. Pharmacological treatment often involves a combination of drugs, as no single medication can simultaneously treat all MS risk factors [8]. Consequently, this situation can lead to polypharmacy, which increases the risk of drug interactions and side effects as well as hinders patient's compliance with medication regimens [9].

In recent years, there has been growing interest in exploring the potential benefits of natural products in the treatment of MS, including green tea, cinnamon, cocoa, coffee and honey [10,11]. Honey, renowned for its various biological activities, holds promising prospects in preventing MS [12]. A study on the types of honey in Malaysia revealed that stingless bee honey (SBH) remains relatively underexplored [13]. In addition possessing high antioxidants, owing to its polyphenol [14], SBH is also rich in probiotics [15]. Unlike other honey which predominantly composed of fructose and glucose, SBH is unique because it contains trehalulose, a natural sucrose isomer as the main sugar [16,17]. Trehalulose has a low glycemic index; hence, SBH has the potential as an anti-diabetic agent [16]. Research has shown trehalose treatment on obese mice can prevent insulin resistance and adipocyte hypertrophy [18,19]. Among the various species of SBH worldwide, the most commonly domesticated species in Malaysia are the *Heterotrigona itama* (*H. itama*) and *Geniotrigona thoracica* (*G. thoracica*) species [20]. SBH had shown promising therapeutic potential in the treatment of MS. SBH from *H. itama* species can prevent obesity, hypertension and dyslipidemia [21,22]. Meanwhile, SBH from *G. thoracica* species can prevent hyperglycemia and dyslipidemia [23].

However, SBH has storage problems because of its high moisture content. Moisture content in honey is a crucial parameter because excess moisture promotes microbial contamination and fermentation process, thus shortening the lifespan of honey [24]. Fermentation also makes SBH more acidic [25]. Previous studies have shown that SBH has higher moisture and acidity than other honey types [26,27]. The dehydration process is necessary for SBH to reduce its moisture content, protecting it from microorganism contamination [25,28]. Subsequently, this can preserve the stability and beneficial properties of SBH [24]. Therefore, the fermentation process and undesirable increase in SBH acidity can be prevented, making it more palatable. However, there is a lack of studies to understand whether the dehydration process will affect the biological activities of honey.

To date, there have been no studies exploring the potential of dehydrated SBH in the treatment of MS. Therefore, this study aims to compare the potential benefits of dehydrated SBH (DeGT) with raw SBH (RGT) from *G. thoracica* species in a rat model of high-carbohydrate, high-fat diet (HCHF)-induced MS. This is to determine whether the dehydrated form of SBH exerts similar, superior or reduced effects on MS rats compared to raw SBH. If dehydrated SBH is as effective as raw SBH in preventing MS, the SBH can be dehydrated after harvesting. This will overcome storage challenges and preserve honey quality.

2. Results

2.1. Honey Analysis

2.1.1. Physicochemical Properties Analysis

Table 1 shows the physicochemical properties of DeGT and RGT. The dehydration process reduced the moisture content from 31% to 14.3%. This reduction was accompanied by a decrease in acidity, indicated by an increase in pH from 3.3 to 3.5 and a decrease in free acidity from 274.8 to 138 mEq/kg. The hydroxymethylfurfural (HMF) content was reduced from 0.3 to <0.1 mg/kg. The ash content and diastase activity remained unchanged at 0.2 g/100 g and <1 DN, respectively. For sugar content, the trehalulose, fructose and glucose level slightly decreased from 52 to 48.5, from 8.5 to 8.1 and from 11 to 7.3 g/100 g, respectively. The content of sucrose and maltose remained the same, both of which were <0.01 g/100 g.

Table 1. Physicochemical properties in DeGT and RGT.

Physicochemical Properties	Unit	DeGT	RGT
Moisture content	%	14.3	31
pH		3.5	3.3
Free acidity	mEq/kg	138	274.8
Hydroxymethylfurfural (HMF)	mg/kg	<0.1	0.3
Ash content	g/100 g	0.2	0.2
Diastase activity	DN	<1	<1
Trehalulose	g/100 g	48.5	52
Fructose	g/100 g	8.1	8.5
Glucose	g/100 g	7.3	11
Sucrose	g/100 g	<0.01	<0.01
Maltose	g/100 g	<0.01	<0.01

2.1.2. Liquid Chromatography–Mass Spectrometry (LC-MS) Analysis

Table 2 shows the bioactive compounds in DeGT and RGT. DeGT contained 33 bioactive compounds comprising 10 types of sugars, two amino acids, two phenolics, four flavonoids, five iridoid glycosides, one phenylpropanoid and nine other organic compounds. Meanwhile, RGT contained 25 bioactive compounds comprising six types of sugars, two amino acids, three phenolics, four flavonoids, three iridoid glycosides, one phenylpropanoid and six other organic compounds.

Table 2. Bioactive compounds in DeGT and RGT.

Bioactive Compounds	DeGT	RGT
Sugar	Isomaltose, mannotriose, stachyose, meso-inositol, fuzinoside	
	Raffinose, galactose, α-kojibiose, 1F-Fructofuranosylnystose, Helonioside B	2′,6′-Diacetyl-3,6-diferuloylsucrose
Amino acid	Glutamine, tyrosine	
Phenolic	Calycanthoside, dihydro-3-coumaric acid	
	-	Sinapic acid
Flavonoid	Epigallocatechin(4β,8)-gallocatechin, 6″-O-p-Hydroxybenzoyliridin, Glehlinoside B	
	Luteolin-7-O-α-D-glucoside	5′-Methoxy-bilobetin
Iridoid glycoside	Sesamoside, Geniposidic acid, Secoxyloganin	
	Rehmannioside A, Shanzhiside methyl ester	-
Phenylpropanoids	Phenylpropionic acid	
Other organic compounds	Cnideoside A, Manhuannin J, Methyl 3,4-dihydroxy-phenyllactate, 1,3,6-Trihydroxy-2-methylanthraquinone-3-O-(O-6-acetyl) neohesperidin,	
	5-Hydroxymethyl furoic acid, 1-O-Methyl-3,5-O-dicaffeoylquinic acid methyl ester, Trimethyl citrate, Meliadanoside B, 2-Hydroxy-5-methoxy acetophenone	Mudanpioside H, Sibiricaxanthone B
Total	33 bioactive compounds	25 bioactive compounds

2.2. *Energy Intake*

From week 1 to week 8, the HCHF-induced rats (MS, MS+DeGT and MS+RGT) showed a significant increase in daily energy intake compared to the C group (*, $p < 0.05$) (Figure 1). From week 9 to week 16, both DeGT and RGT treatments showed a significant reduction in daily energy intake compared to the MS group and week 1–8 (# and †, $p < 0.05$).

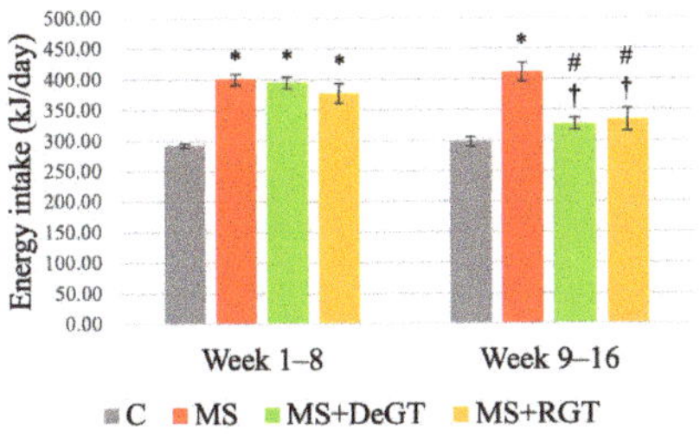

Figure 1. Energy intake at week 1–8 and week 9–16. All data are presented as mean ± SEM. Symbol '*' indicates a significant difference compared to the C group in the same week ($p < 0.05$), '#' indicates a significant difference compared to the MS group in the same week ($p < 0.05$) and '†' indicates a significant difference at week 16 compared to week 8 ($p < 0.05$). Abbreviations: C (control), MS (HCHF diet-induced rats without treatment), MS+DeGT (HCHF diet-induced rats treated with dehydrated SBH from *G. thoracica* species) and MS+RGT (HCHF diet-induced rats treated with raw SBH from *G. thoracica* species).

2.3. Anthropometric Measurements (Body Weight, Body Mass Index (BMI) and Abdominal Circumference)

Body weights of HCHF-induced rats (MS, MS+DeGT and MS+RGT) were significantly lower compared to the C group at week 8 (*, $p < 0.05$), while the body weights of the C group significantly increased at week 8 compared to the baseline (Ø, $p < 0.05$) (Figure 2a). Meanwhile, BMIs of the HCHF-induced rats (MS, MS+DeGT and MS+RGT) at week 8 were significantly lower compared to the C group and baseline (* and Ø, $p < 0.05$) (Figure 2b). Although there was a significant increase in abdominal circumference in all the groups at week 8 compared to the baseline (Ø, $p < 0.05$), there was no significant difference between all the groups at week 8 ($p > 0.05$) (Figure 2c).

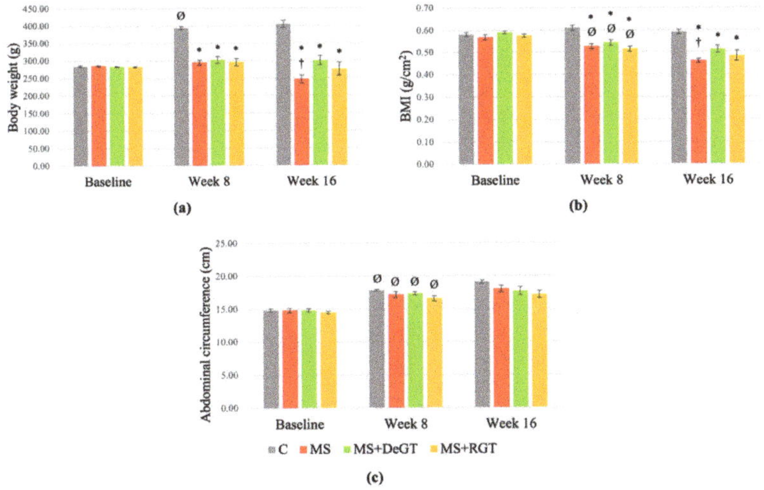

Figure 2. Anthropometric measurements comprise of (**a**) body weight, (**b**) body mass index (BMI) and (**c**) abdominal circumference at baseline, week 8 and week 16. All data are presented as mean ± SEM. Symbol '*' indicates a significant difference compared to the C group in the same week ($p < 0.05$), 'Ø' indicates a significant difference in the same group at week 8 compared to baseline ($p < 0.05$) and '†' indicates a significant difference in the same group at week 16 compared to week 8 ($p < 0.05$). Abbreviations: C (control), MS (HCHF diet-induced rats without treatment), MS+DeGT (HCHF diet-induced rats treated with dehydrated SBH from *G. thoracica* species) and MS+RGT (HCHF diet-induced rats treated with raw SBH from *G. thoracica* species).

At week 16, body weights and BMIs of the MS, MS+DeGT and MS+RGT groups were significantly lower compared to the C group (*, $p < 0.05$), and both treatments showed no significant changes in those parameters compared to the MS group ($p > 0.05$) (Figure 2a,b). Meanwhile, the MS group showed a significant decrease in body weight and BMI at week 16 compared to week 8 (†, $p < 0.05$) (Figure 2a,b). Otherwise, both DeGT and RGT treatments showed no significant changes in abdominal circumference at week 16 compared to the MS group or week 8 ($p > 0.05$) (Figure 2c).

2.4. Body Composition Based on Dual-Energy X-ray Absorptiometry (DXA) Scan (Fat Mass and Lean Mass)

At week 8, HCHF-induced rats (MS, MS+DeGT and MS+RGT) showed a significant increase in fat mass compared to the C group and baseline (* and Ø, $p < 0.05$) (Figure 3a). The lean masses of HCHF-induced rats (MS, MS+DeGT and MS+RGT) were significantly lower compared to the C group at week 8 (*, $p < 0.05$), while the lean masses of the C group significantly increased at week 8 compared to the baseline (Ø, $p < 0.05$) (Figure 3b).

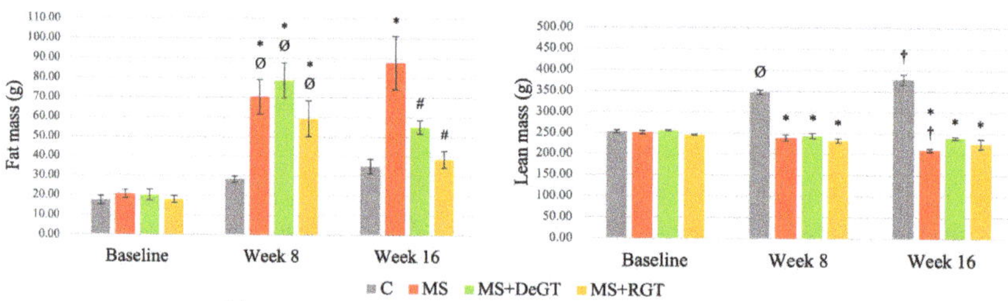

(a) (b)

Figure 3. Body composition based on Dual-Energy X-Ray Absorptiometry (DXA) scan, including (**a**) fat mass and (**b**) lean mass at baseline, week 8 and week 16. All data are presented as mean ± SEM. Symbol '*' indicates a significant difference compared to the C group in the same week ($p < 0.05$), '#' indicates a significant difference compared to the MS group in the same week ($p < 0.05$), 'Ø' indicates a significant difference in the same group at week 8 compared to baseline ($p < 0.05$) and '†' indicates a significant difference in the same group at week 16 compared to week 8 ($p < 0.05$). Abbreviations: C (control), MS (HCHF diet-induced rats without treatment), MS+DeGT (HCHF diet-induced rats treated with dehydrated SBH from *G. thoracica* species) and MS+RGT (HCHF diet-induced rats treated with raw SBH from *G. thoracica* species).

At week 16, both DeGT and RGT treatments showed a significant decrease in fat mass compared to the MS group (#, $p < 0.05$) (Figure 3a). Lean masses of the MS, MS+DeGT and MS+RGT groups were significantly lower compared to the C group at week 16 (*, $p < 0.05$), and both treatments showed no significant changes compared to the MS group at week 16 ($p > 0.05$) (Figure 3b). Meanwhile, the MS group showed a significant decrease in lean mass at week 16 compared to week 8 (†, $p < 0.05$) (Figure 3b).

2.5. Systolic and Diastolic Blood Pressure

At week 8, the HCHF-induced rats (MS, MS+DeGT and MS+RGT) showed a significant increase in systolic and diastolic blood pressure compared to the C group and baseline (* and Ø, $p < 0.05$) (Figure 4a,b). At week 16, both the DeGT and RGT treatments reduced systolic and diastolic blood pressure significantly compared to the MS group and week 8 (# and †, $p < 0.05$).

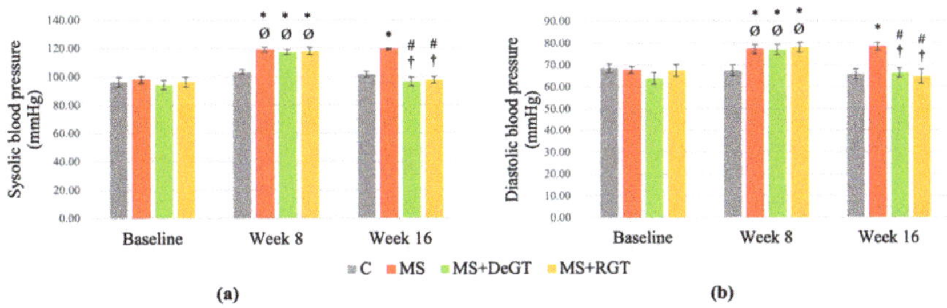

Figure 4. Blood pressure, including (**a**) systolic and (**b**) diastolic blood pressure at baseline, week 8 and week 16. All data are presented as mean ± SEM. Symbol '*' indicates a significant difference compared to the C group in the same week ($p < 0.05$), '#' indicates a significant difference compared to the MS group in the same week ($p < 0.05$), 'Ø' indicates a significant difference in the same group at week 8 compared to baseline ($p < 0.05$) and '†' indicates a significant difference in the same group at week 16 compared to week 8 ($p < 0.05$). Abbreviations: C (control), MS (HCHF diet-induced rats without treatment), MS+DeGT (HCHF diet-induced rats treated with dehydrated SBH from *G. thoracica* species) and MS+RGT (HCHF diet-induced rats treated with raw SBH from *G. thoracica* species).

2.6. Insulin Resistance

At week 8, fasting blood glucose, area under the curve of oral glucose tolerance test (AUC of OGTT), serum insulin and homeostatic model assessment for insulin resistance (HOMA-IR) of the HCHF-induced rats (MS, MS+DeGT and MS+RGT) showed no significant difference compared to the C group or baseline ($p > 0.05$) (Figure 5a–d). At week 16, both DeGT and RGT treatments showed no significant changes in fasting blood glucose, serum insulin and HOMA-IR compared to the MS group or week 8 ($p > 0.05$) (Figure 5a,c,d). Although there was a significant decrease in AUC of OGTT in all the groups at week 16 compared to week 8 (†, $p < 0.05$), there was no significant difference between all the groups at week 16 ($p > 0.05$) (Figure 5b).

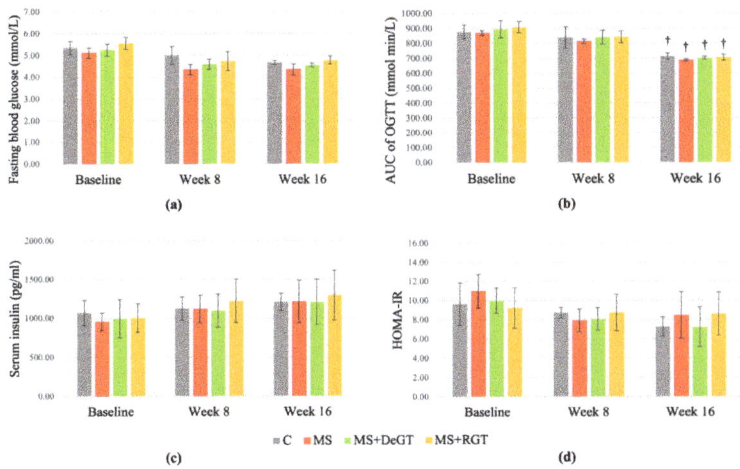

Figure 5. Insulin resistance measurements, including (**a**) fasting lipid profile, (**b**) area under the cure of oral glucose tolerance test (AUC of OGTT), (**c**) serum insulin and (**d**) Homeostatic Model Assessment for Insulin Resistance (HOMA-IR) at baseline, week 8 and week 16. All data are presented as mean ± SEM. Symbol '†' indicates a significant difference in the same group at week 16 compared to week 8 ($p < 0.05$). Abbreviations: C (control), MS (HCHF diet-induced rats without treatment), MS+DeGT (HCHF diet-induced rats treated with dehydrated SBH from *G. thoracica* species) and MS+RGT (HCHF diet-induced rats treated with raw SBH from *G. thoracica* species).

2.7. Serum Fasting Lipid Profile

At week 8, the HCHF-induced rats (MS, MS+DeGT and MS+RGT) showed a significant increase in serum triglycerides (TG) compared to the C group and baseline (* and Ø, $p < 0.05$) (Figure 6a). Although there was a significant increase in serum total cholesterol (TC) of the HCHF-induced rats (MS, MS+DeGT and MS+RGT) at week 8 compared to the baseline (Ø, $p < 0.05$), there was no significant difference compared to the C group at week 8 ($p > 0.05$) (Figure 6b). Otherwise, there were no significant differences in the serum low-density lipoprotein (LDL) and high-density lipoprotein (HDL) of HCHF-induced rats (MS, MS+DeGT and MS+RGT) at week 8 compared to the C group or baseline ($p > 0.05$) (Figure 6c,d).

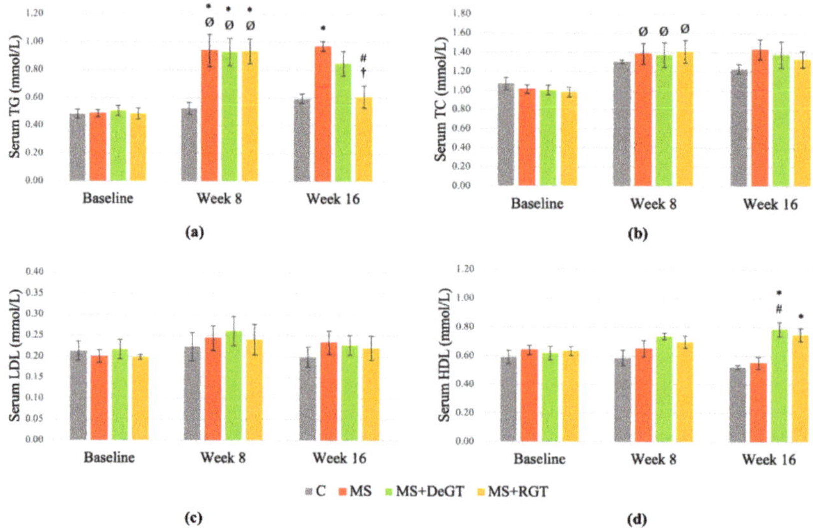

Figure 6. Serum fasting lipid profile, including (**a**) triglycerides (TG), (**b**) total cholesterol (TC), (**c**) low-density lipoprotein (LDL) and (**d**) high-density lipoprotein (HDL) at baseline, week 8 and week 16. All data are presented as mean ± SEM. Symbol '*' indicates a significant difference compared to the C group in the same week ($p < 0.05$), '#' indicates a significant difference compared to the MS group in the same week ($p < 0.05$), 'Ø' indicates a significant difference in the same group at week 8 compared to baseline ($p < 0.05$) and '†' indicates a significant difference in the same group at week 16 compared to week 8 ($p < 0.05$). Abbreviations: C (control), MS (HCHF diet-induced rats without treatment), MS+DeGT (HCHF diet-induced rats treated with dehydrated SBH from *G. thoracica* species) and MS+RGT (HCHF diet-induced rats treated with raw SBH from *G. thoracica* species).

At week 16, only RGT treatment significantly decreased serum TG compared to the MS group and week 8 (# and †, $p < 0.05$) (Figure 6a). Although both DeGT and RGT treatments showed a significant increase in serum HDL compared to the C group (*, $p < 0.05$), only DeGT treatment significantly increased serum HDL compared to the MS group (#, $p < 0.05$) (Figure 6d). Otherwise, both DeGT and RGT treatments showed no significant changes in serum TC and LDL at week 16 compared to the MS group or week 8 ($p > 0.05$) (Figure 6b,c).

2.8. Inflammatory Markers in Adipose Tissue

At week 16, this study showed a significant increase in tumor necrosis factor-alpha (TNF-α) (*, $p < 0.05$), while no significant changes were observed in interleukin-6 (IL-6) and interleukin-1 beta (IL-1β) ($p > 0.05$) in the adipose tissue of the MS group compared to the C group (Figure 7a–c). Both DeGT and RGT treatments significantly reduced TNF-α levels in adipose tissue compared to the MS group (#, $p < 0.05$) (Figure 7a). However, only

RGT treatment showed a significant reduction in IL-6 and IL-1β levels in adipose tissue compared to the MS group (#, $p < 0.05$) (Figure 7b,c).

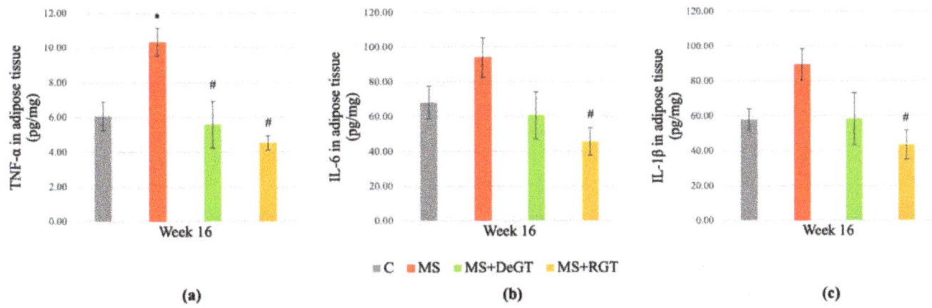

Figure 7. Inflammatory markers in adipose tissue at the end of the study consisting of (**a**) tumor necrosis factor-alpha (TNF-α), (**b**) interleukin-6 (IL-6) and (**c**) interleukin-1 beta (IL-1β). All data are presented as mean ± SEM. Symbol '*' indicates a significant difference compared to the C group ($p < 0.05$) and '#' indicates a significant difference compared to the MS group ($p < 0.05$). Abbreviations: C (control), MS (HCHF diet-induced rats without treatment), MS+DeGT (HCHF diet-induced rats treated with dehydrated SBH from *G. thoracica* species) and MS+RGT (HCHF diet-induced rats treated with raw SBH from *G. thoracica* species).

2.9. Obesity Markers in Serum and Adipose Tissue

At week 16, serum leptin and leptin/adiponectin (L/A) ratio increased significantly in the MS group compared to the C group (*, $p < 0.05$) (Figure 8a,c). Meanwhile, there were no significant differences in serum adiponectin, serum corticosterone, as well as peroxisome proliferator-activated receptor γ (PPARγ) and 11 beta-hydroxysteroid dehydrogenase type-1 (11βHSD1) levels in adipose tissue of the MS group compared to the C group ($p > 0.05$) (Figure 8b,d–f).

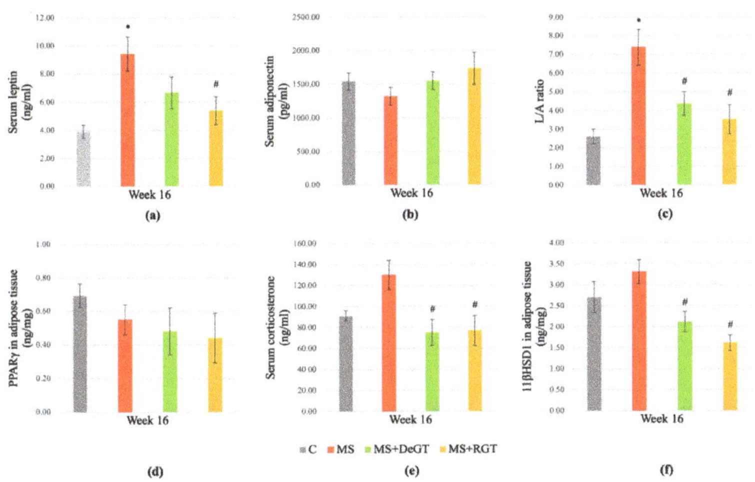

Figure 8. Obesity markers at the end of the study consisting of (**a**) serum leptin, (**b**) serum adiponectin, (**c**) leptin/adiponectin (L/A) ratio, (**d**) peroxisome proliferator-activated receptor γ (PPARγ) in adipose tissue (**e**) serum corticosterone and (**f**) 11 beta-hydroxysteroid dehydrogenase type-1 (11βHSD1) in adipose tissue. All data are presented as mean ± SEM. Symbol '*' indicates a significant difference compared to the C group ($p < 0.05$) and '#' indicates a significant difference compared to the MS group ($p < 0.05$). Abbreviations: C (control), MS (HCHF diet-induced rats without treatment), MS+DeGT (HCHF diet-induced rats treated with dehydrated SBH from *G. thoracica* species) and MS+RGT (HCHF diet-induced rats treated with raw SBH from *G. thoracica* species).

Both DeGT and RGT treatments significantly reduced serum L/A ratio, serum corticosterone and 11βHSD1 level in adipose tissue compared to the MS group at week 16 (#, $p < 0.05$) (Figure 8c,e,f). However, only RGT treatment significantly reduced serum leptin compared to the MS group at week 16 (#, $p < 0.05$) (Figure 8a). Meanwhile, both treatments showed no significant changes in serum adiponectin and PPARγ levels in adipose tissue compared to the MS group at week 16 ($p > 0.05$) (Figure 8b,d).

2.10. Histomorphometry of Adipose, Liver and Kidney Tissue

2.10.1. Adipose Tissue

At the end of the study, the MS group showed adipocyte hypertrophy, as evidenced by a significant reduction in adipocyte cell count per area as well as a significant increase in adipocyte area and perimeter compared to the C group (*, $p < 0.05$) (Figure 9a,b,e–g). Both DeGT and RGT treatments prevented adipocyte hypertrophy, as indicated by a significant increase in adipocyte cell count per area as well as a significant reduction in adipocyte area and perimeter compared to the MS group at week 16 (#, $p < 0.05$) (Figure 9b–g).

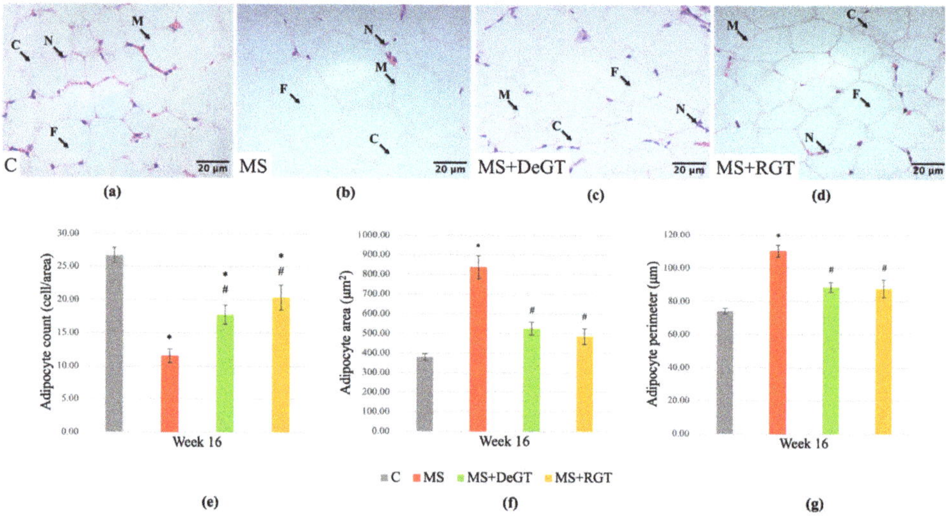

Figure 9. Photomicrograph of visceral adipose tissue in (**a**) C, (**b**) MS, (**c**) MS+DeGT and (**d**) MS+RGT rats under a light microscope at 400× magnification. Abbreviations: N (nucleus), C (cytoplasm), M (plasma membrane) and F (fat vacuole). The size of adipocytes is indicated by the measurement of (**e**) adipocyte cell count per area, (**f**) adipocyte area and (**g**) adipocyte perimeter. All data are presented as mean ± SEM. Symbol '*' indicates a significant difference compared to the C group ($p < 0.05$) and '#' indicates a significant difference compared to the MS group ($p < 0.05$). Abbreviations: C (control), MS (HCHF diet-induced rats without treatment), MS+DeGT (HCHF diet-induced rats treated with dehydrated SBH from *G. thoracica* species) and MS+RGT (HCHF diet-induced rats treated with raw SBH from *G. thoracica* species).

2.10.2. Liver Tissue

MS and MS+DeGT group showed higher hepatic macrosteatosis and microsteatosis, as confirmed by significantly higher hepatosteatosis grade compared to the C group at week 16 (@, $p < 0.05$) (Figure 10a–c,e–g,i). Meanwhile, only RGT treatment reduced hepatic macrosteatosis and microsteatosis, as indicated by a significant reduction in hepatosteatosis grade compared to the MS group (#, $p < 0.05$) (Figure 10b,d,f,h,i).

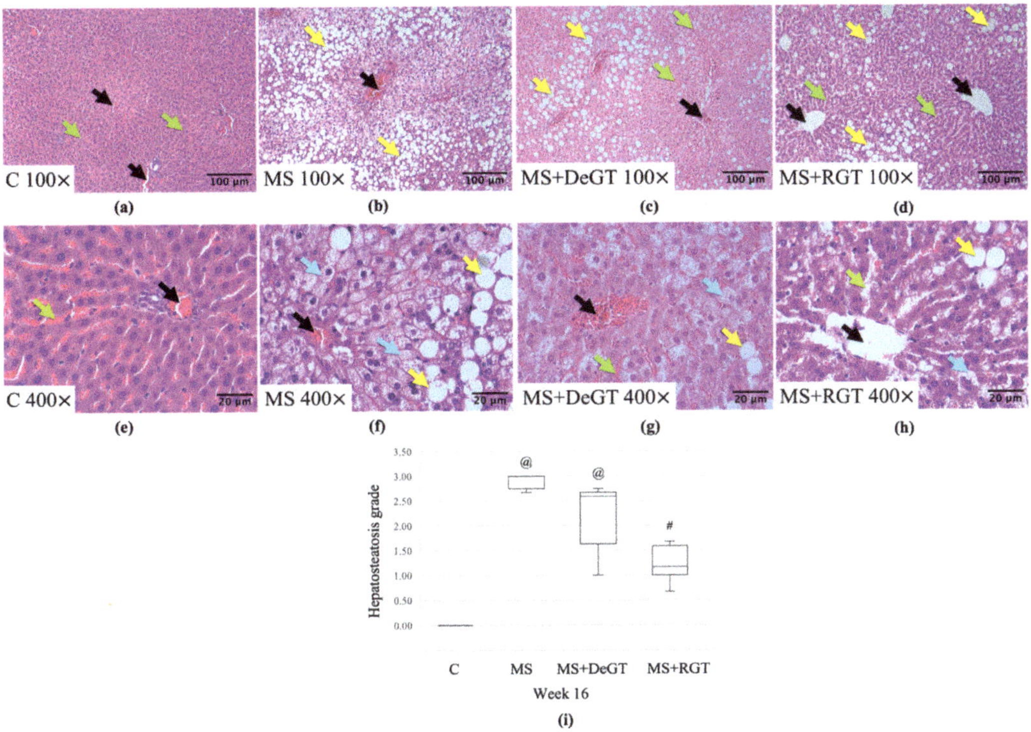

Figure 10. Photomicrograph of liver tissue in (**a**,**e**) C, (**b**,**f**) MS, (**c**,**g**) MS+DeGT and (**d**,**h**) MS+RGT rats under a light microscope at 100× and 400× magnification, respectively. Abbreviations: central vein (black arrow), sinusoids (green arrow), macrosteatosis (yellow arrow) and microsteatosis (blue arrow). The hepatosteatosis is confirmed by the measurement of (**i**) hepatosteatosis grade. The data are presented as median (IQR). Symbol '@' indicates a significant difference compared to the C group ($p < 0.05$) and '#' indicates a significant difference compared to the MS group ($p < 0.05$). Abbreviations: C (control), MS (HCHF diet-induced rats without treatment), MS+DeGT (HCHF diet-induced rats treated with dehydrated SBH from *G. thoracica* species) and MS+RGT (HCHF diet-induced rats treated with raw SBH from *G. thoracica* species).

2.10.3. Kidney Tissue

At week 16, the MS group showed a significant increase in Bowman's space area compared to the C group (*, $p < 0.05$) (Figure 11a,b,e,f,i). Histological observation at 400× magnification showed glomerular atrophy in the MS group compared to the C group (Figure 11e,f). Both DeGT and RGT treatments prevented the increase in Bowman's space area compared to the MS group at week 16 (#, $p < 0.05$) (Figure 11b–d,f–i). Based on 400× magnification histological observation, both treatments prevented glomerular atrophy compared to the MS group (Figure 11f–h).

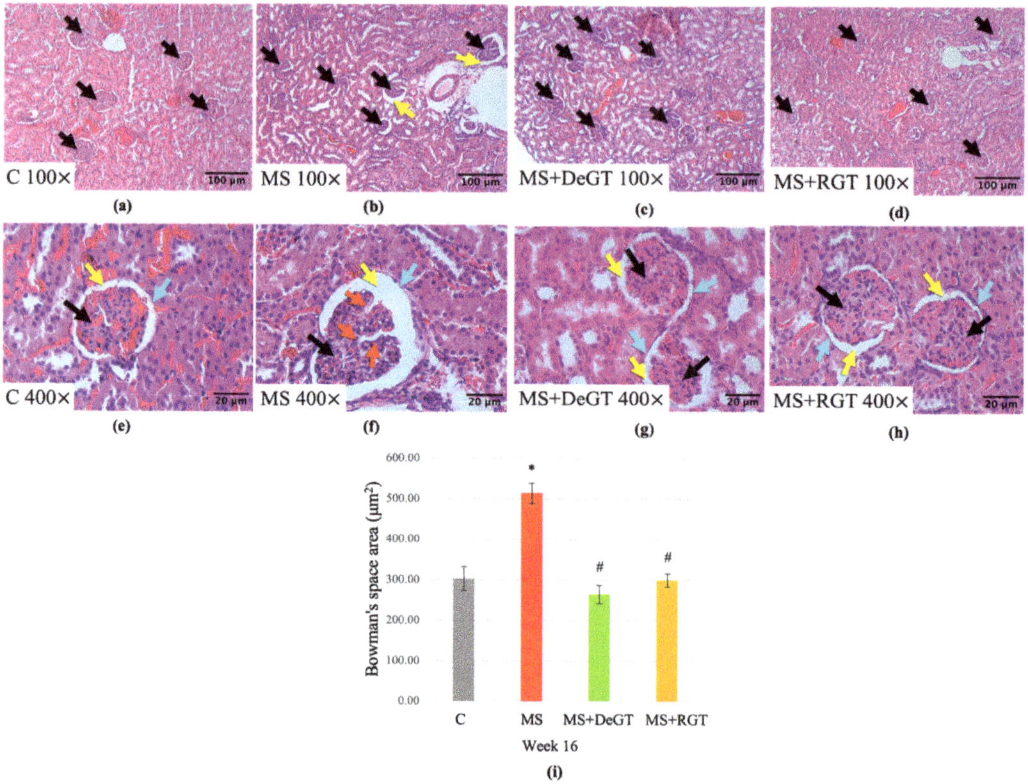

Figure 11. Photomicrograph of kidney tissue in (**a**,**e**) C, (**b**,**f**) MS, (**c**,**g**) MS+DeGT and (**d**,**h**) MS+RGT rats under a light microscope at 100× and 400× magnification, respectively. Abbreviations: glomerulus (black arrow), Bowman's space (yellow arrow), renal corpuscle (blue arrow) and glomerular atrophy (red arrow). The enlargement of Bowman's space is indicated by the measurement of (**i**) Bowman's space area. The data are presented as mean ± SEM. Symbol '*' indicates a significant difference compared to the C group ($p < 0.05$) and '#' indicates a significant difference compared to the MS group ($p < 0.05$). Abbreviations: C (control), MS (HCHF diet-induced rats without treatment), MS+DeGT (HCHF diet-induced rats treated with dehydrated SBH from *G. thoracica* species) and MS+RGT (HCHF diet-induced rats treated with raw SBH from *G. thoracica* species).

3. Discussion

The present study compared the effect of DeGT and RGT treatments on HCHF-induced MS rats. During the initial 8 weeks of HCHF induction, the rats exhibited increased energy intake, fat mass, blood pressure and serum TG. At week 16, there were increases in inflammatory (TNF-α in adipose tissue) and obesity (serum leptin, serum L/A ratio) markers. Additionally, the histomorphometry changes (adipocyte hypertrophy, hepatosteatosis, increase in Bowman's space area and glomerular atrophy) were observed. This study demonstrated that both DeGT and RGT treatments for 8 weeks effectively reduced energy intake, fat mass, high blood pressure, inflammatory (TNF-α in adipose tissue) and obesity (serum L/A ratio, serum corticosterone, 11βHSD1 in adipose tissue) markers, as well as histomorphometry changes (adipocyte hypertrophy, Bowman's space area and glomerular atrophy). Although DeGT increased serum HDL, DeGT could not reduce serum TG, IL-6 and IL-1β adipose tissue, serum leptin and hepatosteatosis in contrast to the effects observed in RGT treatment.

In this study, the HCHF diet for 8 and 16 weeks successfully induced MS by inducing at least three out of five risk factors: obesity, hypertension and hypertriglyceridemia, which are aligned with previous studies [21,22]. High-calorie intake can lead to the accumulation of excess calories in the form of body fat [29]. Excess adipose tissue oversecretes leptin, which can cause leptin resistance [30]. Leptin resistance hinders the optimal functioning of the leptin hormone in regulating satiety [31]. In this study, energy intake increased in HCHF-induced rats, which was consistent with elevated serum leptin levels. Therefore, it is hypothesized that the high energy intake in HCHF-induced rats in the study may be attributed to the development of leptin resistance.

In this study, the HCHF diet induced obesity as evidenced by an increase in fat mass. Histomorphometry results further confirmed the presence of adipocyte hypertrophy indicated by a reduction in adipocyte cell count per area, and a significant increase in adipocyte area and perimeter. Additionally, excess fat deposition in ectopic tissue was observed in the liver and confirmed by an increase in hepatosteatosis grade. However, the findings of this study showed no significant increase in anthropometric parameters: body weight, BMI and abdominal circumference in HCHF-induced rats. The lack of observable results may be attributed to the fact that the anthropometric parameters serve as a surrogate measurement for obesity and do not measure visceral fat directly [32,33]. Nevertheless, our findings suggest that the HCHF diet employed in this study can induce obesity, despite no apparent alterations in anthropometric measures.

Most of the body composition in both human and rat is contributed by lean mass compared to fat mass [34,35]. In this study, despite an increase in fat mass, no significant changes in body weight among HCHF-induced rats were observed. In contrast, the C group showed an increase in body weight along with an increase in lean mass. The difference in the outcomes may have been due to differences in the protein composition of the diet. The rat chow diet contained a higher protein content between 21 and 23%, whereas the HCHF diet contained only 3.93–4.24% protein. Protein is important for muscle growth, contributing to an increase in lean mass [36]. A previous study showed that HCHF-induced rats had significantly lower body weight collateral with lower lean mass compared to chow-fed rats [22]. Therefore, an increase in lean mass simultaneously increases body weight.

The HCHF diet induction led to fat cell accumulation in muscle tissue and the degeneration of muscle fibers in rats, as observed through histomorphometric analysis [37]. Excessive fat intake results in the infiltration of fat into the muscles (intramuscular myosteatosis), hindering muscle growth and contributing to the progression of sarcopenic obesity [38]. Sarcopenic obesity is characterized by a decrease in skeletal muscle mass accompanied by an increase in fat mass [39]. As a result, individuals with sarcopenic obesity may exhibit normal body weight, BMI and waist circumference [40,41]. While sarcopenia typically affects the elderly, obesity accelerates its onset. Moreover, previous studies have shown that inflammation can activate muscle protein degradation, causing skeletal muscle atrophy [42,43]. Therefore, the body weight, BMI and abdominal circumference that did not increase in this study could be have been due to muscle degradation in sarcopenic obesity or inflammation that may have occurred in the HCHF-induced MS rats. This was further supported by a decrease in lean mass and an increase in TNF-α observed in HCHF-induced rats in this study.

The HCHF diet induction in this study caused increases in blood pressure. Histomorphometry findings in the kidney tissue showed an increase in Bowman's space area and glomerular atrophy. The hypertension in this study can be attributed to multiple factors. Excess sodium and fructose can increase blood pressure by activating the renin–angiotensin–aldosterone system (RAAS) [44,45]. Excess adipose tissue can increase angiotensinogen secretion [46]. High leptin levels stimulate the sympathetic nervous system, which increases sodium reabsorption in the kidney [47,48]. Inflammatory marker TNF-α can stimulate the production of angiotensinogen and increase the production of reactive oxygen species (ROS) and decreasenitric oxide (NO), which acts as a vasodilator on the vascular endothelium [48,49]. Therefore, high fructose and high sodium in the HCHF diet, increased fat mass, high serum leptin and high TNF-α, which are also observed in this study, may contribute to the elevated blood pressure in the HCHF-induced rats.

Development of insulin resistance begins at the tissue level, primarily in adipose and skeletal muscle tissues, before progressing to hepatic tissue and eventually leading to systemic insulin resistance characterized by hyperinsulinemia [50]. Insulin resistance induced by the HCHF diet for 16 weeks may still be at its early stage, as suggested by previous studies [21,22]. This study further confirms the previous findings, as no systemic insulin resistance in this study occurred, as evidenced by no changes in fasting blood glucose, AUC OGTT, serum insulin and HOMA-IR. However, the study found that HCHF induced insulin resistance at the adipose tissue level, indicated by an increased L/A ratio [51]. Previous studies have shown that the HCHF diet induction for 18–20 weeks could induce insulin resistance in rats, as evidenced by increased HOMA-IR [52–54]. Therefore, it is likely that extending the period of HCHF diet induction beyond 16 weeks is necessary in this study to cause insulin resistance.

Insulin resistance is the key contributor to metabolic dyslipidemia [55]. Hepatic insulin resistance causes the failure of insulin-mediated secretion of very low-density lipoprotein (VLDL). Consequently, VLDL-rich TG increases in the blood and stimulates its conversion to LDL-rich TG and HDL-rich TG [56]. Subsequently, both are broken down by lipase enzymes into sd-LDL and sd-HDL. Sd-HDL is removed through renal clearance, reducing the HDL level [4]. However, the HCHF diet in this study increased serum TG but did not significantly alter serum TC, LDL and HDL compared to the control group. The elevation in serum TG could be attributed to the excessive intake of fructose and saturated fatty acid (SFA) in the HCHF diet, which can increase TG level in the bloodstream [57]. The lack of significant change in serum TC of the HCHF-induced rats compared to the C group could be due to the rat's natural resistance to high blood cholesterol [22,58]. Meanwhile, hepatic insulin resistance in this study might not have fully developed, which could explain the absence of significant changes in serum LDL and HDL.

Excess free fatty acids (FFA) in obesity are known to play a significant role in stimulating inflammation [59]. The inflammation, often referred to as metabolic inflammation, is characterized by chronic low-grade inflammation that occurs locally within organs [60]. A previous study by Hashim et al. (2023) [21] reported that HCHF diet induction for 16 weeks did not increase TNF-α and IL-1β levels in rat's serum. However, this study demonstrated an increase in TNF-α in adipose tissue, although no significant changes in IL-6 and IL-1β levels were observed. These findings suggest that the inflammation in MS induced by the HCHF diet is indeed a chronic low-grade inflammation detectable locally at the tissue level. Previous research has demonstrated that HCHF induction using animal fat tallow and lard oil as a source of fat could increase TNF-α, as well as IL-6 and IL-1β in adipose and liver tissue [53,61]. Therefore, substituting pure ghee with another source of fat could potentially increase all the inflammatory markers measured in this study.

Leptin levels positively correlate with increased body fat, whereas increased body fat is not correlated with serum adiponectin level [62]. This study demonstrated that the increase in fat mass was consistent with elevated serum leptin, with no significant changes in serum adiponectin and PPARγ levels in adipose tissue. PPARγ plays a crucial role in stimulating adiponectin secretion from adipose tissue [63,64]. Similar findings by a previous study that showed HCHF diet induction for 16 weeks increased serum leptin without changes in serum adiponectin [21]. Therefore, an increase in body fat will not necessarily have a suppressing effect on adiponectin levels. A previous study has revealed no correlation between serum adiponectin and body fat mass [62]. Mice fed with a high-fat diet for 30 weeks showed no changes in adiponectin expression in visceral adipose tissue and only exhibited decreased adiponectin expression in subcutaneous adipose tissue [65]. Furthermore, a human study found that metabolically obese women had lower adiponectin mRNA expression in subcutaneous compared to visceral adipose tissue [66]. These findings agree with the current study.

The 11βHSD1 enzyme plays an important role in activating corticosterone hormone [67]. Researchers have hypothesized that high corticosterone is likely to be one of the mechanisms involved in the formation of MS because both share the same metabolic effects such as obesity, hyperglycemia, dyslipidemia and hypertension [68,69]. However, HCHF induction for 16 weeks in this study could not demonstrate changes in serum corticosterone and 11βHSD1 in the adipose tissue in HCHF-induced rats. This agrees with the previous work by Hashim et al. (2023) [21]. Previous studies have shown that feeding mice a high-fat diet with 42–60% fat content could increase the expression of 11βHSD1 and plasma corticosterone [70–72]. However, the HCHF diet in the current study comprised 24.62% fat, which was significantly lower compared to previous studies. Hence, it is likely that a higher fat composition in the HCHF diet could increase corticosterone and 11βHSD1 in this study.

Treatment of DeGT and RGT in HCHF-induced rats reduced energy intake, which was consistent with a decrease in serum corticosterone observed in this study. It is well established that high corticosterone levels can increase the secretion of ghrelin, a hormone known to stimulate appetite [73,74]. Therefore, our findings suggest the treatment of DeGT and RGT reduces energy intake by lowering corticosterone levels, thereby potentially reducing ghrelin secretion.

DeGT and RGT treatments prevented obesity in rats in this study, as evidenced by a reduction in fat mass and adipocyte hypertrophy in histomorphometry findings. These findings align with the reduction in serum corticosterone and 11βHSD1 of adipose tissue in this study. It is known that corticosterone promotes fat accumulation by increasing adipogenesis [75]. A previous study also demonstrated raw SBH from *H. itama* species 1 g/kg could lower serum corticosterone and 11βHSD1 in adipose tissue [21]. However, only RGT treatment effectively reduced ectopic fat accumulation in liver tissue, as indicated by a reduction in hepatosteatosis grade.

This study demonstrated that both DeGT and RGT exerted a similar effect in lowering systolic and diastolic blood pressure. Histomorphometry of kidney tissue revealed a reduction in Bowman's space area and glomerular atrophy in both treatment groups. This effect was likely attributed to the reduction of fat mass and TNF-α in adipose tissue observed in both treatment groups. Additionally, RGT may reduce hypertension due to a reduction in serum leptin. Previous studies have shown that raw SBH from *H. itama* species 1 g/kg could lower blood pressure [21,22,76].

However, DeGT treatment could not lower serum TG levels, unlike RGT in this study. This discrepancy could have been due to the dehydration process that has been shown to reduce the phenolic content in honey [77]. Heat processing can also reduce the bioactivity of flavonoids [78]. Previous research has shown that the *Solanum nigrum* extract, which contains phenolic and flavonoid, could decrease fatty acid synthase (FASN) and sterol regulatory element binding protein 1 (SREBP-1 activity) activities, both of which are involved in TG synthesis [79]. Another study showed that the litchi flower water extract rich in phenolic and flavonoid could inhibit pancreatic enzyme lipase activity involved in postprandial TG absorption and increase the removal of triacylglycerol fat through feces [80]. Therefore, the reduction of TG by RGT was likely due to its phenolic and flavonoid compounds, which may have been lost in DeGT due to the dehydration process.

Similarly, DeGT treatment could increase HDL, while RGT did not exhibit the same effect in this study. The dehydration process in this study may enhance the bioactive compounds in DeGT, as dehydration can activate new compounds or convert the existing compounds into a more stable form [81]. A previous study showed that luteolin, a flavonoid, increased the expression of liver X receptor (LXR) and ATP binding cassette transporter G1 (ABCG1), both of which helped in the HDL maturation process [82]. Therefore, the increase in HDL by DeGT in this study was likely due to bioactive content, which may have been enhanced following the dehydration process.

This study also found that both DeGT and RGT treatments reduced inflammation, as evidenced by the reduction of TNF-α in adipose tissue. Previous studies also demonstrated the local anti-inflammatory effect of RGT 1 and 2 g/kg, as well as dried SBH from *H. itama* species in the form of bee bread 0.5 g/kg, in reducing TNF-α levels in pancreas and liver, respectively [23,83]. The reduction of inflammation in this study was likely due to the decrease in fat mass observed in both treatment groups. Excess fat could activate the adipose tissue nuclear factor-kappa B (NF-κβ) and c-Jun N-terminal kinase (JNK) pathways that initiate inflammation [84]. Previous studies have shown that RGT and bee bread from *H. itama* species decreased TNF-α along with the decrease of NF-κβ [23,83]. However, this study showed that DeGT treatment could not lower IL-6 and IL-1β in adipose tissue, unlike RGT. This could have been due to the absence of bioactive compounds in DeGT that could lower inflammatory cytokines IL-6 and IL-1β.

DeGT treatment also could not lower serum leptin, unlike RGT. However, both DeGT and RGT treatments effectively reduced the serum L/A ratio. This suggests that although DeGT did not directly impact the serum leptin level, DeGT decreased the leptin ratio per adiponectin level in rats' serum. Moreover, the L/A ratio indicates insulin resistance in adipose tissue because it accurately measures adipose tissue dysfunction [51,85]. A previous study showed that rapid and excessive adipocyte expansion caused cell hypoxia, leading to insulin resistance in adipose tissue [86]. The ability of both DeGT and RGT treatments to reduce the L/A ratio was consistent with the reduction of adipocyte hypertrophy as shown by both treatment groups, suggesting their potential in mitigating insulin resistance in adipose tissue. Figure 12 summarizes the effect of DeGT and RGT treatments observed in this study.

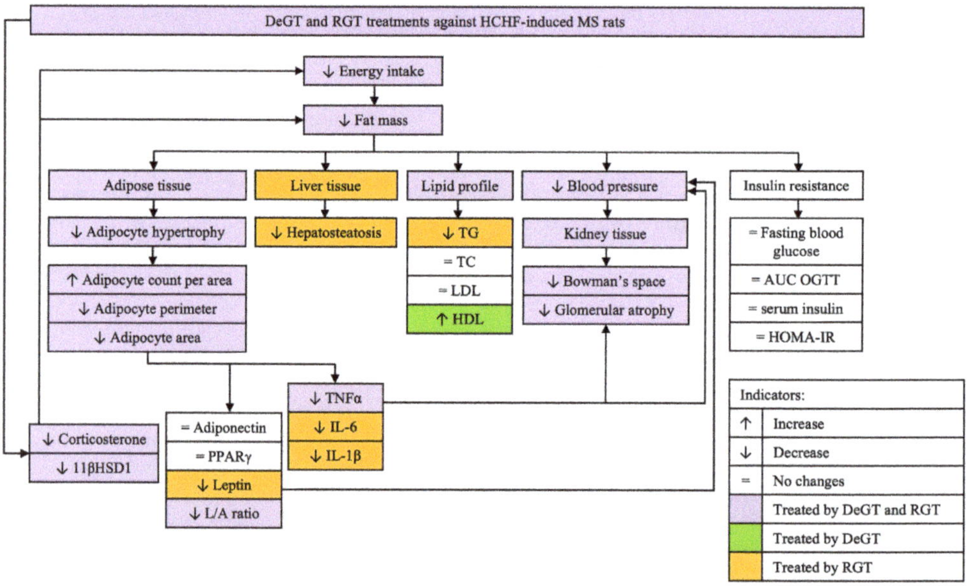

Figure 12. Summary of the effect of DeGT and RGT treatments against HCHF-induced MS.

Honey with moisture content below 17% can prevent fermentation by microorganisms [25,87]. Therefore, a dehydration process is necessary for SBH to reduce its moisture content. However, high-heat treatment can increase the HMF content in honey [88]. Excessive HMF is harmful to health due to its potential to act as a carcinogenic and genotoxic agent [89,90]. Moreover, heat treatment can cause denaturation of the diastase enzyme and a reduction in its activity [91]. Meanwhile, ash content reflects the mineral content in honey [92]. In this study, the dehydration process reduced DeGT moisture content below 17%, reduced its acidity, caused no increase in HMF and maintained diastase enzyme activity and ash content. However, there were decreased trehalulose, fructose and glucose in DeGT, while the content of sucrose and maltose remained unchanged. A previous study showed that the increased heat treatment on honey decreased its glucose content, likely due to heat causing the degradation of sugar content [93].

DeGT can treat certain MS parameters as effectively as RGT in this study, possibly due to their similar bioactive compounds. Among them are trehalulose, glutamine and epigallocatechin gallate (EGCG). Previous studies have demonstrated that these compounds have potential benefits in treating various components of MS. Trehalose can effectively treat adipocyte hypertrophy [19]. Meanwhile, glutamine can reduce body fat mass, lower high blood pressure and increase lean body mass [94]. EGCG can reduce body fat mass, serum corticosterone, 11βHSD1 in adipose tissue, high blood pressure and enlargement of Bowman's space [21,67,95].

However, DeGT was unable to treat some MS parameters like RGT, possibly due to the differences in its phenolic content. The dehydration process can reduce the phenolic content in honey [77]. Moreover, heat treatment can also reduce the bioactivity of flavonoids [78]. In this study, RGT contained sinapic acid, which was not found in DeGT. Previous studies have shown that sinapic acid can lower serum TG, leptin, IL-6 and hepatosteatosis [96–99].

DeGT can treat certain MS parameters better than RGT, possibly due to the activation of several new compounds. A previous study has shown dehydration can activate new compounds and convert existing compounds into a more stable form [81]. In this study, DeGT contained raffinose, luteolin, Rehmannioside A and quinic acid derivatives, which were not found in RGT. These compounds have been shown by previous studies to increase serum HDL [82,100–102].

To the best of our knowledge, this is the first study that compares the potential of dehydrated and raw SBH in MS treatment. The dehydration process in this study involves heat exposure, which could potentially reduce phenolic content or flavonoid bioactivity in DeGT. This factor may have caused DeGT to be less effective in treating some MS components than RGT. Using the freeze-drying method as a dehydration process could prevent honey from being exposed to heat. This may increase the probability of DeGT's potential to treat MS equally or more effectively than RGT.

4. Materials and Methods

4.1. Animals

The sample size was calculated using resource equation approach as explained by Arifin and Zahiruddin (2017) based on the following formula: $n = DF/k + 1$ (n = number of animals per group, DF = degree of freedom, k = number of groups) [103]. The DF in the formula was replaced with the minimum (10) and maximum (20) to obtain the minimum and maximum numbers of animals per group, respectively. The minimum $n = 10/k + 1 = 10/4 + 1 = 3.5$, and the maximum $n = 20/k + 1 = 20/4 + 1 = 6$. Hence, the total minimum and maximum numbers of animals (N) required were: minimum N = minimum $n \times k = 3.5 \times 4 = 14$, and maximum N = maximum $n \times k = 6 \times 4 = 24$. The maximum number of rats were adopted. Therefore, total $N = 24$ rats, with $n = 6$ rats per group.

This study has received approval from the Animal Ethics Committee, Universiti Kebangsaan Malaysia, with approval code ANAT/FP/2021/FAIRUS/24-NOV./1210-JAN.-2022-SEPT-2023. Twenty-four male Wistar rats weighing 250–300 g were obtained from the Laboratory Animal Resource Unit, Faculty of Medicine, Universiti Kebangsaan Malaysia. The rats were caged individually and acclimatized for two weeks in the Animal Laboratory Department of Anatomy, Faculty of Medicine, Universiti Kebangsaan Malaysia. The laboratory condition was standardized at 12 h of light/dark cycle and an ambient temperature of 25 ± 3 °C.

4.2. HCHF Diet Preparation

HCHF diet contains mixture of 155 g rat chow powder (Gold Coin Feedmills (M), Port Klang, Malaysia); 175 g D-(−)-Fructose fructose powder (Chemiz, Shah Alam, Malaysia); 395 g sweetened condensed milk (Gold Coin, F & N Diaries Manufacturing Sdn. Bhd.,

Malaysia); 200 g pure ghee (Enrico's Pure Ghee, RaviRaj Sdn. Bhd., Pulau Pinang, Malaysia); 25 g mixture of Hubble, Mendel and Wakeman salts (MP Biomedicals, Santa Ana, CA, USA); and 50 g tap water, as well as 25% fructose in drinking water [45].

4.3. Dehydrated and Raw SBH Preparation

Raw SBH from *G. thoracica* species (RGT) was harvested in April 2022 from a bee farm in Gombak, Selangor, Malaysia. Immediately after harvesting, 1 kg of the RGT underwent dehydration at 32–39 °C for 20 h. The dehydration process of the dehydrated SBH (DeGT) was performed using Malaysian Agricultural Research and Development Institute (MARDI) dehydration machine [104]. The treatment dosage used in this study was 1.0 g/kg/day for RGT [22] and 0.833 g/kg/day for DeGT. The calculation of the DeGT treatment dose is shown in Table 3. Both DeGT and RGT were diluted with distilled water at a 1:1 ratio during administration to rats.

Table 3. Calculation of DeGT treatment dose.

	Calculation
Moisture content	Moisture content RGT = 31%, moisture content DeGT = 14.3%. (based on honey analysis in Table 1)
Moisture reduction	Moisture reduction = moisture content RGT − moisture content DeGT $\therefore$ Moisture reduction $= 31\% - 14.3\% = 16.7\%$
Treatment dose DeGT	Treatment dose of RGT = 1.0 g/kg/day [22] Treatment dose DeGT = treatment dose RGT − (moisture reduction × treatment dose RGT) $\therefore$ Treatment dose DeGT $= 1.0 - \left(\frac{16.7}{100} \times 1.0\right) = 0.833$ g/kg/day

4.4. Honey and LC-MS Analysis

The physicochemical properties analysis of honey was conducted by UNIPEQ Sdn. Bhd. (UKM-MTDC Technology Center, Bangi, Malaysia) using the following equipment: moisture content, ATAGO® pocket refractometer (ATAGO Co., Ltd., Tokyo, Japan); pH, Sartorius PB-10 pH meter (Sartorius, Göttingen, Germany); free acidity, titration and Sartorius PB-10 pH meter (Sartorius, Germany); HMF, Waters e2695 UV Detector HPLC machine (Waters, Milford, MA, USA); ash content, carbolite furnace chamber machine (Carbolite Gero Ltd., Hope Valley, UK); diastase activity, Thermo Scientific Helios Zeta UV-Vis spectrophotometer (Thermo Fisher Scientific Inc., Waltham, MA, USA); and sugar content (trehalulose, fructose, glucose, sucrose, maltose), high-performance liquid chromatography (HPLC) Varian 385-LC ELSD machine (Varian, Inc., Palo Alto, CA, USA).

LC-MS analysis was conducted by Advanced Chemistry Solutions Company (Petaling Jaya, Selangor, Malaysia) using an ultra-high-performance liquid chromatography (UHPLC) machine, ACQUITY UPLC I-Class system (Waters, USA) and Vion IMS QTOF hybrid mass spectrometer (Waters, USA).

4.5. Study Design

The 24 male Wistar rats were assigned randomly into four groups ($n = 6$ for each group): control (C), HCHF-induced MS without treatment (MS), HCHF-induced MS treated with DeGT (MS+DeGT) and HCHF-induced MS treated with RGT (MS+RGT). Group C received rat chow, while the other groups were fed with HCHF diet ad libitum for 16 weeks. The initial eight weeks of HCHF induction aimed to ensure the successful development of MS by measuring relevant parameters before treatment. In the subsequent eight weeks (from week 9 to week 16), two groups of HCHF diet-induced MS rats (MS+DeGT and MS+RGT) received their respective supplements via oral gavage. The nutritional compositions of the rat chow [105] and HCHF diets are included in Table S1 and Table S2, respectively.

Food and drink intake for each rat were measured daily. MS parameters were taken at baseline, week 8 and week 16. The parameters for obesity were assessed by anthropometric measurements (body weight, BMI and abdominal circumference) and body composition (fat mass and lean mass). The hypertension parameter was assessed by blood pressure measurement (systolic and diastolic). The insulin resistance parameter was assessed by measurement of fasting blood glucose, OGTT, serum insulin and HOMA-IR. The levels of TG and HDL were assessed by serum fasting lipid profile (comprised of serum TG, TC, LDL and HDL). MS is diagnosed when at least three out of five key risk factors are present [21,22]. The presence of a condition was defined as a significant difference for the indices between the rats fed with HCHF diet compared to those fed with standard rat chow.

At week 16, all rats were euthanized using intravenous injection of Dorminal 20% (contains 200 mg/mL pentobarbital sodium) at a dosage of 0.7 mL/kg body weight. Serum and visceral adipose tissue were collected for enzyme-linked immunosorbent assay (ELISA) analysis to measure inflammatory and obesity markers. Organs such as visceral adipose tissue, liver and kidney were harvested for histological analysis.

4.6. Energy Intake Measurement

Energy values were calculated according to a previous study by Wong et al. (2018) [45] as follows: energy intake (kJ/day) = [food intake (g) × energy value (kJ/g)] + [drink intake (mL) × energy value (kJ/mL)]. Daily energy intakes from week 1 until week 8 were averaged (Week 1–8), and daily energy intakes from week 9 until week 16 were averaged (Week 9–16).

4.7. Anthropometric Measurement

Body weight was measured using a Nimbus® balance scale (Adam Equipment, Inc., Oxford, CT, USA). Abdominal circumference was measured at the widest area of the abdomen, and the rat's length was measured from the tip of the nose to the anus using a non-stretch plastic measuring tape (Birch Creative, Heidelberg West, VIC, Australia). BMI was calculated using the formula: BMI (g/cm^2) = weight (g)/length (cm^2).

4.8. Body Composition Measurement

Body composition, including fat and lean mass, was measured using DXA scan Hologic Discovery W and Small Animal Analysis Software 13.5.3, Hologic QDR-1000 System (Hologic Inc., Marlborough, MA, USA). Rats were anaesthetized prior DXA scan by intravenous injection of a ketamine–xylazine–Zoletil mixture at 0.1 mL/100 g of body weight.

4.9. Blood Pressure Measurement

Before the measurements, rats were placed in a holder tube and kept on a heating pad to maintain the rat's tail temperature at 33–35 °C. Systolic and diastolic blood pressure were then measured using a CODA® non-invasive blood pressure system machine (Kent Scientific Corporation, Torrington, CT, USA).

4.10. Fasting Blood Glucose and OGTT Measurement

All rats were fasted for 12 h and provided only with tap water. Prior to OGTT, minimal bleeding was done at the rat's tail. Fasting blood glucose was measured using an Accu-Chek® Instant S glucometer (Roche Diagnostics, Basel, Switzerland). Subsequently, a 40% glucose solution (D(+)-glucose, Chemiz, Shah Alam, Malaysia) at a dosage of 2.0 g/kg body weight was given to the rats via oral gavage. Blood glucose readings were then recorded at 30, 60, 90 and 120 min after glucose loading. The AUC of OGTT was calculated using the trapezoidal rule.

4.11. Serum Insulin and HOMA-IR Measurement

Before blood sampling, all rats were fasted for 12 h. Anesthesia was induced by intravenous injection of a ketamine–xylazine–Zoletil mixture at 0.1 mL/100 g body weight. Retro-orbital bleeding was performed, and blood samples were centrifuged to isolate serum using Thermo Scientific Heraeus Biofuge Primo R (Thermo Fisher Scientific Inc., USA) at

4000 rpm and 20 °C for 15 min. Serum insulin was determined using an ELISA kit (Finetest®, Wuhan, China). HOMA-IR was calculated using the formula, HOMA-IR = fasting blood glucose (mmol/L) × fasting insulin (μU/mL)/22.5 [106].

4.12. Serum Fasting Lipid Profile Measurement

The serum fasting lipid profile (TG, TC, LDL and HDL) was analyzed at the Veterinary Laboratory Services Unit (VLSU), Faculty of Veterinary Medicine, Universiti Putra Malaysia (UPM), Serdang, Malaysia using integrated chemistry system Dimension® Xpand® Plus (Siemens, Munich, Germany).

4.13. Determination of Inflammatory and Obesity Markers Using ELISA

Samples for the determination of inflammatory markers were adipose tissue homogenate, while samples for the determination of obesity markers were serum and adipose tissue homogenate. Adipose tissue homogenization was performed employing the procedures outlined in the previous study by Hashim et al. (2023) [21]. The inflammatory markers (TNF-α, IL-6 and IL-1β) and obesity markers (leptin, adiponectin and PPARγ), including corticosteroid synthesis (corticosterone and 11βHSD1), were determined using the ELISA technique (Finetest®, China). The L/A ratio was calculated by dividing the serum leptin levels (ng/mL) by serum adiponectin levels (ng/mL) [51]. Protein content in adipose was quantified using a bicinchoninic acid (BCA) protein colorimetric assay kit (Elabscience®, Houston, TX, USA).

4.14. Histomorphometry Examination and Analysis

Adipose tissue, liver and kidney were fixated in 10% formaldehyde. All tissues were processed, embedded, sectioned at 5 μm thickness, stained with hematoxylin and eosin using Autostainer XL (Leica, Wetzlar, Germany) and mounted on a glass slide. Histomorphometric examination was conducted at 100× and 400× total magnification using a Carl Zeiss Primo Star HD light microscope equipped with Zeiss ZEN Microscopy Imaging System software version 2.6 (Zeiss, Oberkochen, Germany). Histology analysis was performed using ImageJ software 1.54 (National Institutes of Health, Bethesda, MD, USA) as shown in Table 4.

Table 4. Parameters measured for histological analysis.

	Parameters
Adipose tissue	Adipocyte count, area and perimeter [22].
Liver tissue	Hepatosteatosis grading was based on the percentage of fat in liver cells [107]: Grade 0 = <5%, grade 1 = 5–33%, grade 2 = 34–66% and grade 3 = >66%
Kidney tissue	Bowman's space area calculation [108]: Area of Bowman's space = area of renal corpuscle–area of glomerulus

4.15. Statistical Analysis

All data were analyzed using the Statistical Package for the Social Science (SPSS®) version 26 software (IBM, Armonk, NY, USA), with statistical significance defined at p-value < 0.05. The normality of data distribution was assessed using the Shapiro–Wilk test. Normally distributed data were analyzed using one-way ANOVA with Tukey's post-hoc comparison. Data with a time × group design were analyzed using mixed design analysis of variance (ANOVA) with a small effect analysis as the post hoc test. Non-normally distributed data were analyzed using Kruskal–Wallis test.

5. Conclusions

DeGT is as effective as RGT in treating various MS-related factors, including energy intake, fat mass, hypertension, serum L/A ratio, serum corticosterone and 11βHSD1 in adipose tissue, TNF-α in adipose tissue, adipocyte hypertrophy, enlargement of Bowman's space area and glomerular atrophy. DeGT increased HDL levels, but DeGT was unable to reduce serum TG, IL-6 and IL-1β in adipose tissue, serum leptin and hepatosteatosis compared to RGT. In conclusion, DeGT demonstrated its potential benefits as a preventive agent for MS, but RGT showed better anti-MS agents than DeGT in this study. Prolonging the duration of HCHF diet induction or increasing its fat composition could potentially induce more MS risk factors. Meanwhile, extending the duration of DeGT treatment may increase its efficacy in treating MS. To enhance the potential of DeGT in treating MS, future research can explore alternative dehydration methods like freeze-drying, which avoids heat exposure and may yield better results than the current dehydration process. Considering the promising results in this study, we hope to explore the potential benefits in humans in the future, given that SBH is a natural product proven to be effective in preventing MS in animal studies.

Supplementary Materials: The following supporting information can be downloaded at: https://www.mdpi.com/article/10.3390/ph17111427/s1, Table S1: Nutritional composition of rat chow diet (Gold Coin Feedmills (M), Malaysia); Table S2: Nutritional composition of HCHF diet.

Author Contributions: Conceptualization, F.A. and K.-Y.C.; methodology, F.A., K.-Y.C. and L.N.I.; resources, F.A. and K.-Y.C.; investigation, L.N.I.; formal analysis, L.N.I.; software, L.N.I.; data curation, L.N.I.; visualization, L.N.I.; validation, F.A. and K.-Y.C.; supervision, F.A. and K.-Y.C.; project administration, F.A.; funding acquisition, F.A.; writing—original draft, L.N.I.; writing—review and editing, K.-Y.C. and F.A. All authors have read and agreed to the published version of the manuscript.

Funding: This work was funded by the Researcher Encouragement Grant, Center for Research and Instrumentation Management (CRIM) (GGP-2020-004), Universiti Kebangsaan Malaysia.

Institutional Review Board Statement: The animal study protocol was approved by the Animal Ethics Committee, Universiti Kebangsaan Malaysia (protocol code ANAT/FP/2021/FAIRUS/24-NOV./1210-JAN.-2022-SEPT-2023 and date of approval 24 November 2021).

Informed Consent Statement: Not applicable.

Data Availability Statement: The original contributions presented in the study are included in the article/Supplementary Material, further inquiries can be directed to the corresponding author.

Acknowledgments: We thank Department of Anatomy and Department of Pharmacology, Faculty of Medicine, Universiti Kebangsaan Malaysia, for their administrative and technical support.

Conflicts of Interest: The authors declare no conflicts of interest.

References

1. Liang, X.P.; Or, C.Y.; Tsoi, M.F.; Cheung, C.L.; Cheung, B.M.Y. Prevalence of metabolic syndrome in the United States National Health and Nutrition Examination Survey (NHANES) 2011–2018. *Eur. Heart J.* **2021**, *42* (Suppl. 1), ehab724.2420. [CrossRef]
2. Ranasinghe, P.; Mathangasinghe, Y.; Jayawardena, R.; Hills, A.P.; Misra, A. Prevalence and trends of metabolic syndrome among adults in the Asia-Pacific region: A systematic review. *BMC Public Health* **2017**, *17*, 101. [CrossRef] [PubMed]
3. Alberti, K.G.; Eckel, R.H.; Grundy, S.M.; Zimmet, P.Z.; Cleeman, J.I.; Donato, K.A.; Fruchart, J.C.; James, W.P.; Loria, C.M.; Smith, S.C., Jr. Harmonizing the metabolic syndrome: A joint interim statement of the International Diabetes Federation Task Force on Epidemiology and Prevention; National Heart, Lung, and Blood Institute; American Heart Association; World Heart Federation; International Atherosclerosis Society; and International Association for the Study of Obesity. *Circulation* **2009**, *120*, 1640–1645.
4. Fahed, G.; Aoun, L.; Bou Zerdan, M.; Allam, S.; Bou Zerdan, M.; Bouferraa, Y.; Assi, H.I. Metabolic syndrome: Updates on pathophysiology and management in 2021. *Int. J. Mol. Sci.* **2022**, *23*, 786. [CrossRef]
5. Ogurtsova, K.; da Rocha Fernandes, J.D.; Huang, Y.; Linnenkamp, U.; Guariguata, L.; Cho, N.H.; Cavan, D.; Shaw, J.E.; Makaroff, L.E. IDF diabetes atlas: Global estimates for the prevalence of diabetes for 2015 and 2040. *Diabetes Res. Clin. Pract.* **2017**, *128*, 40–50. [CrossRef]
6. Saklayen, M.G. The global epidemic of the metabolic syndrome. *Curr. Hypertens. Rep.* **2018**, *20*, 12. [CrossRef]
7. Grundy, S.M. Metabolic syndrome update. *Trends Cardiovasc. Med.* **2016**, *26*, 364–373. [CrossRef]
8. Lillich, F.F.; Imig, J.D.; Proschak, E. Multi-target approaches in metabolic syndrome. *Front. Pharmacol.* **2021**, *11*, 554961. [CrossRef]
9. Balilo, A.C.B.; Dadang, K.N.; Iguana, K.J.O.; Manabat, H.T.L.; Sumalpong, V.L.C.; Enriquez, R.J.F. Polypharmacy: Non-adherence to medication among adult. *Adv. Pharm. Res.* **2020**, *7*, 48–60. [CrossRef]

10. Mohd Ramli, E.S.; Sukalingam, K.; Kamaruzzaman, M.A.; Soelaiman, I.N.; Pang, K.-L.; Chin, K.-Y. Direct and indirect effect of honey as a functional food against metabolic syndrome and its skeletal complications. *Diabetes Metab. Syndr. Obes.* **2021**, *14*, 241–256. [CrossRef]
11. Noce, A.; Di Lauro, M.; Di Daniele, F.; Pietroboni Zaitseva, A.; Marrone, G.; Borboni, P.; Di Daniele, N. Natural bioactive compounds useful in clinical management of metabolic syndrome. *Nutrients* **2021**, *13*, 630. [CrossRef] [PubMed]
12. Ramli, N.Z.; Chin, K.-Y.; Zarkasi, K.A.; Ahmad, F. A review on the protective effects of honey against metabolic syndrome. *Nutrients* **2018**, *10*, 1009. [CrossRef] [PubMed]
13. Mohd Kamal, D.A.; Ibrahim, S.F.; Kamal, H.; Kashim, M.I.A.M.; Mokhtar, M.H. Physicochemical and medicinal properties of tualang, gelam and kelulut honeys: A comprehensive review. *Nutrients* **2021**, *13*, 197. [CrossRef] [PubMed]
14. Ranneh, Y.; Ali, F.; Zarei, M.; Md Akim, A.; Abd Hamid, H.; Khazaai, H. Malaysian stingless bee and Tualang honeys: A comparative characterization of total antioxidant capacity and phenolic profile using liquid chromatography-mass spectrometry. *LWT—Food Sci. Technol.* **2018**, *89*, 1–9. [CrossRef]
15. Zulkhairi Amin, F.A.; Sabri, S.; Ismail, M.; Chan, K.W.; Ismail, N.; Mohd Esa, N.; Mohd Lila, M.A.; Zawawi, N. Probiotic properties of *Bacillus* strains isolated from stingless bee (*Heterotrigona itama*) honey collected across Malaysia. *Int. J. Environ. Res. Public Health* **2020**, *17*, 278. [CrossRef]
16. Fletcher, M.T.; Hungerford, N.L.; Webber, D.; Carpinelli de Jesus, M.; Zhang, J.; Stone, I.S.J.; Blanchfield, J.T.; Zawawi, N. Stingless bee honey, a novel source of trehalulose: A biologically active disaccharide with health benefits. *Sci. Rep.* **2020**, *10*, 12128. [CrossRef]
17. Hungerford, N.L.; Zhang, J.; Smith, T.J.; Yates, H.S.A.; Chowdhury, S.A.; Carter, J.F.; Carpinelli de Jesus, M.; Fletcher, M.T. Feeding sugars to stingless bees: Identifying the origin of trehalulose-rich honey composition. *J. Agric. Food Chem.* **2021**, *69*, 10292–10300. [CrossRef]
18. Arai, C.; Miyake, M.; Matsumoto, Y.; Mizote, A.; Yoshizane, C.; Hanaya, Y.; Koide, K.; Yamada, M.; Hanaya, T.; Arai, S.; et al. Trehalose prevents adipocyte hypertrophy and mitigates insulin resistance in mice with established obesity. *J. Nutr. Sci. Vitaminol.* **2013**, *59*, 393–401. [CrossRef]
19. Arai, C.; Suyama, A.; Arai, S.; Arai, N.; Yoshizane, C.; Koya-Miyata, S.; Mizote, A.; Endo, S.; Ariyasu, T.; Mitsuzumi, H.; et al. Trehalose itself plays a critical role on lipid metabolism: Trehalose increases jejunum cytoplasmic lipid droplets which negatively correlated with mesenteric adipocyte size in both HFD-fed trehalase KO and WT Mice. *Nutr. Metab.* **2020**, *17*, 22. [CrossRef]
20. Jaapar, M.F.; Wan Abd Halim, W.N.M.; Muhamad, R.; Mispan, R.; Jajuli, R.; Mohd Masri, S.; Zainuddin, M.Y.; Ghazi, R.; Abd Ghani, I. The diversity and abundance of stingless bee (Hymenoptera: *Meliponini*) in peninsular Malaysia. *Adv. Environ. Biol.* **2016**, *10*, 1–8.
21. Hashim, K.-N.; Chin, K.Y.; Ahmad, F. The mechanism of kelulut honey in reversing metabolic changes in rats fed with high-carbohydrate high-fat diet. *Molecules* **2023**, *28*, 2790. [CrossRef] [PubMed]
22. Ramli, N.Z.; Chin, K.-Y.; Zarkasi, K.A.; Ahmad, F. The beneficial effects of stingless bee honey from *Heterotrigona itama* against metabolic changes in rats fed with high-carbohydrate and high-fat diet. *Int. J. Environ. Res. Public Health* **2019**, *16*, 4987. [CrossRef]
23. Aziz, M.S.A.; Giribabu, N.; Rao, P.V.; Salleh, N. Pancreatoprotective effects of *Geniotrigona thoracica* stingless bee honey in streptozotocin-nicotinamide-induced male diabetic rats. *Biomed. Pharmacother.* **2017**, *89*, 135–145. [CrossRef] [PubMed]
24. Keng, C.B.; Haron, H.; Abdul Talib, R.; Subramaniam, P. Physical properties, antioxidant content and anti-oxidative activities of Malaysian stingless kelulut (*Trigona* spp.) honey. *J. Agric. Sci.* **2017**, *9*, 32–40. [CrossRef]
25. Yap, S.K.; Chin, N.L.; Yusof, Y.A.; Chong, K.Y. Quality characteristics of dehydrated raw kelulut honey. *Int. J. Food Prop.* **2019**, *22*, 556–571. [CrossRef]
26. Kek, S.P.; Chin, N.L.; Yusof, Y.A.; Tan, S.W.; Chua, L.S. Classification of entomological origin of honey based on its physicochemical and antioxidant properties. *Int. J. Food Prop.* **2017**, *20*, S2723–S2738. [CrossRef]
27. Yap, S.K.; Chin, N.L. Identification of distinctive properties of common malaysian moneys. *Mater. Today Proc.* **2021**, *42*, 115–118. [CrossRef]
28. Mohamad Ghazali, N.S.; Yusof, Y.A.; Mohd Ghazali, H.; Chin, N.L.; Othman, S.H.; Manaf, Y.N.; Chang, L.S.; Mohd Baroyi, S.A.H. Effect of surface area of clay pots on physicochemical and microbiological properties of stingless bee (*Geniotrigona thoracica*) honey. *Food Biosci.* **2021**, *40*, 100839. [CrossRef]
29. Bluher, M. Obesity: Global epidemiology and pathogenesis. *Nat. Rev. Endocrinol.* **2019**, *15*, 288–298. [CrossRef]
30. Friedman, J.M. Leptin and the endocrine control of energy balance. *Nat. Metab.* **2019**, *1*, 754–764. [CrossRef]
31. Obradovic, M.; Sudar-Milovanovic, E.; Soskic, S.; Essack, M.; Arya, S.; Stewart, A.J.; Gojobori, T.; Isenovic, E.R. Leptin and obesity: Role and clinical implication. *Front. Endocrinol.* **2021**, *12*, 585887. [CrossRef] [PubMed]
32. Sommer, I.; Teufer, B.; Szelag, M.; Nussbaumer-Streit, B.; Titscher, V.; Klerings, I.; Gartlehner, G. The performance of anthropometric tools to determine obesity: A systematic review and meta-analysis. *Sci. Rep.* **2020**, *10*, 12699. [CrossRef] [PubMed]
33. Staynor, J.M.; Smith, M.K.; Donnelly, C.J.; Sallam, A.E.; Ackland, T.R. DXA reference values and anthropometric screening for visceral obesity in Western Australian adults. *Sci. Rep.* **2020**, *10*, 18731. [CrossRef] [PubMed]
34. Buckinx, F.; Landi, F.; Cesari, M.; Fielding, R.A.; Visser, M.; Engelke, K.; Maggi, S.; Dennison, E.; Al-Daghri, N.M.; Allepaerts, S. Pitfalls in the measurement of muscle mass: A Need for a reference standard. *J. Cachexia Sarcopenia Muscle* **2018**, *9*, 269–278. [CrossRef]

35. Veyrat-Durebex, C.; Poher, A.-L.; Caillon, A.; Somm, E.; Vallet, P.; Charnay, Y.; Rohner-Jeanrenaud, F. Improved leptin sensitivity as a potential candidate responsible for the spontaneous food restriction of the Lou/C rat. *PLoS ONE* **2013**, *8*, e73452. [CrossRef]
36. Baum, J.I.; Wolfe, R.R. The link between dietary protein intake, skeletal muscle function, and health in older adults. *Healthcare* **2015**, *3*, 529–543. [CrossRef]
37. Medhat, D.; El-Bana, M.A.; El-Daly, S.M.; Ashour, M.N.; Elias, T.R.; Mohamed, R.A.; Yassen, N.N.; Abdel-Monem, M.A.; Hussein, J. Influence of irisin on diet-induced metabolic syndrome in experimental rat model. *Complement. Integr. Med.* **2021**, *18*, 347–354. [CrossRef]
38. Li, C.W.; Yu, K.; Shyh-Chang, N.; Jiang, Z.; Liu, T.; Ma, S.; Luo, L.; Guang, L.; Liang, K.; Ma, W.; et al. Pathogenesis of sarcopenia and the relationship with fat mass: Descriptive review. *J. Cachexia Sarcopenia Muscle* **2022**, *13*, 781–794. [CrossRef]
39. Donini, L.M.; Busetto, L.; Bischoff, S.C.; Cederholm, T.; Ballesteros-Pomar, M.D.; Batsis, J.A.; Bauer, J.M.; Boirie, Y.; Cruz-Jentoft, A.J.; Dicker, D.; et al. Definition and diagnostic criteria for sarcopenic obesity: ESPEN and EASO consensus statement. *Obes. Facts* **2022**, *15*, 321–335. [CrossRef]
40. Cauley, J.A. An overview of sarcopenic obesity. *J. Clin. Densitom.* **2015**, *18*, 499–505. [CrossRef]
41. Polyzos, S.A.; Margioris, A.N. Sarcopenic obesity. *Hormones* **2018**, *17*, 321–331. [CrossRef]
42. Francaux, M.; Deldicque, L. Using polyphenol derivatives to prevent muscle wasting. *Curr. Opin. Clin. Nutr. Metab. Care* **2018**, *21*, 159–163. [CrossRef] [PubMed]
43. Lambert, K.; Coisy-Quivy, M.; Bisbal, C.; Sirvent, P.; Hugon, G.; Mercier, J.; Avignon, A.; Sultan, A. Grape polyphenols supplementation reduces muscle atrophy in a mouse model of chronic inflammation. *Nutrition* **2015**, *31*, 1275–1283. [CrossRef] [PubMed]
44. Komnenov, D.; Levanovich, P.; Rossi, N. Hypertension associated with fructose and high salt: Renal and sympathetic mechanisms. *Nutrients* **2019**, *11*, 569. [CrossRef] [PubMed]
45. Wong, S.K.; Chin, K.-Y.; Suhaimi, F.H.; Ahmad, F.; Ima-Nirwana, S. The effects of a modified high-carbohydrate high-fat diet on metabolic syndrome parameters in male rats. *Exp. Clin. Endocrinol. Diabetes* **2018**, *126*, 205–212. [CrossRef]
46. Schutten, M.T.J.; Houben, A.J.H.M.; de Leeuw, P.W.; Stehouwer, C.D.A. The link between adipose tissue renin-angiotensin-aldosterone system signaling and obesity-associated hypertension. *Physiology* **2017**, *32*, 197–209. [CrossRef]
47. Da Silva, A.A.; do Carmo, J.M.; Li, X.; Wang, Z.; Mouton, A.J.; Hall, J.E. Role of hyperinsulinemia and insulin resistance in hypertension: Metabolic syndrome revisited. *Can. J. Cardiol.* **2020**, *36*, 671–682. [CrossRef]
48. Lu, S.C.; Akanji, A.O. Leptin, obesity, and hypertension: A review of pathogenetic mechanisms. *Metab. Syndr. Relat. Disord.* **2020**, *18*, 399–405. [CrossRef]
49. Vlasova, M.; Purhonen, A.K.; Jarvelin, M.R.; Rodilla, E.; Pascual, J.; Herzig, K.H. Role of adipokines in obesity-associated hypertension. *Acta Physiol.* **2010**, *200*, 107–127. [CrossRef]
50. Fazakerley, D.J.; Krycer, J.R.; Kearney, A.L.; Hocking, S.L.; James, D.E. Muscle and adipose tissue insulin resistance: Malady without mechanism? *J. Lipid Res.* **2019**, *60*, 1720–1732. [CrossRef]
51. Agostinis-Sobrinho, C.; Vicente, S.; Norkiene, S.; Rauckienė-Michaelsson, A.; Kievisienė, J.; Dubey, V.; Razbadauskas, A.; Lopes, L.; Santos, R. Is the leptin/adiponectin ratio a better diagnostic biomarker for insulin resistance than leptin or adiponectin alone in adolescents? *Children* **2022**, *9*, 1193. [CrossRef] [PubMed]
52. Badawy, E.; El-laithy, N.A.; Morsy, S.M.; Ashour, M.N.; Elias, T.R.; Masoud, M.M.; Aly, O. Role of swimming on muscle PGC-1α, FNDC5 mRNA, and assessment of serum omentin, adropin, and irisin in high carbohydrate high fat (HCHF) diet induced obesity in rats. *Egypt. J. Med. Hum. Genet.* **2020**, *21*, 37. [CrossRef]
53. Boonloh, K.; Kukongviriyapan, V.; Kongyingyoes, B.; Kukongviriyapan, U.; Thawornchinsombut, S.; Pannangpetch, P. Rice bran protein hydrolysates improve insulin resistance and decrease pro-inflammatory cytokine gene expression in rats fed a high carbohydrate-high fat diet. *Nutrients* **2015**, *7*, 6313–6329. [CrossRef] [PubMed]
54. Palachai, N.; Wattanathorn, J.; Muchimapura, S.; Thukham-Mee, W. Antimetabolic syndrome effect of phytosome containing the combined extracts of mulberry and ginger in an animal model of metabolic syndrome. *Oxid. Med. Cell. Longev.* **2019**, *2019*, 5972575. [CrossRef]
55. Vekic, J.; Zeljkovic, A.; Stefanovic, A.; Jelic-Ivanovic, Z.; Spasojevic-Kalimanovska, V. Obesity and dyslipidemia. *Metabolism* **2019**, *92*, 71–81. [CrossRef]
56. Tomlinson, B.; Chan, P.; Lam, C. Postprandial hyperlipidemia as a risk factor in patients with type 2 diabetes. *Expert Rev. Endocrinol. Metab.* **2020**, *15*, 147–157. [CrossRef]
57. Lopez-Alvarenga, J.C.; Ebbesson, S.O.E.; Ebbesson, L.O.E.; Tejero, M.E.; Voruganti, V.S.; Comuzzie, A.G. Polyunsaturated fatty acids effect on serum triglycerides concentration in the presence of metabolic syndrome components. The Alaska-Siberia project. *Metabolism* **2010**, *59*, 86–92. [CrossRef]
58. Ness, G.C.; Gertz, K.R. Hepatic HMG-CoA reductase expression and resistance to dietary cholesterol. *Exp. Biol. Med.* **2004**, *229*, 412–416. [CrossRef]
59. Khanna, D.; Khanna, S.; Khanna, P.; Kahar, P.; Patel, B.M. Obesity: A chronic low-grade inflammation and its markers. *Cureus* **2022**, *14*, e22711. [CrossRef]
60. Van den Brink, W.; van Bilsen, J.; Salic, K.; Hoevenaars, F.P.; Verschuren, L.; Kleemann, R.; Bouwman, J.; Ronnett, G.V.; van Ommen, B.; Wopereis, S. Current and future nutritional strategies to modulate inflammatory dynamics in metabolic disorders. *Front. Nutr.* **2019**, *6*, 129. [CrossRef]

61. Elmahdy, M.K.; Helal, M.; Ebrahim, T. Potential anti-inflammatory effect of dapagliflozin in HCHF diet- induced fatty liver degeneration through inhibition of TNF-α, IL-1β, and IL-18 in rat liver. *Int. Immunopharmacol.* **2020**, *86*, 106730. [CrossRef] [PubMed]
62. Lubkowska, A.; Radecka, A.; Bryczkowska, I.; Rotter, I.; Laszczyńska, M.; Dudzińska, W. Serum adiponectin and leptin concentrations in relation to body fat distribution, hematological indices and lipid profile in humans. *Int. J. Environ. Res. Public Health* **2015**, *12*, 11528–11548. [CrossRef] [PubMed]
63. Astapova, O.; Leff, T. Chapter Six—Adiponectin and PPARγ: Cooperative and interdependent actions of two key regulators of metabolism. In *Vitamins & Hormones*; Litwack, G., Ed.; Academic Press: Cambridge, MA, USA, 2012; Volume 90, pp. 143–162. [CrossRef]
64. Woodward, L.; Akoumianakis, I.; Antoniades, C. Unravelling the adiponectin paradox: Novel roles of adiponectin in the regulation of cardiovascular disease. *Br. J. Pharmacol.* **2017**, *174*, 4007–4020. [CrossRef] [PubMed]
65. Parrasia, S.; Galletta, E.; La Spina, M.; Magrini, A.; Azzolini, M.; Salvalaio, M.; Biasutto, L. Long-term pterostilbene supplementation of a high-fat diet increases adiponectin expression in the subcutaneous white adipose tissue. *Nutraceuticals* **2022**, *2*, 102–115. [CrossRef]
66. Korac, A.; Srdic-Galic, B.; Stancic, A.; Otasevic, V.; Korac, B.; Jankovic, A. Adipokine signatures of subcutaneous and visceral abdominal fat in normal-weight and obese women with different metabolic profiles. *Arch. Med. Sci.* **2021**, *17*, 323–336. [CrossRef]
67. Hintzpeter, J.; Stapelfeld, C.; Loerz, C.; Martin, H.-J.; Maser, E. Green tea and one of Its constituents, epigallocatechine-3-gallate, are potent inhibitors of human 11β-hydroxysteroid dehydrogenase type 1. *PLoS ONE* **2014**, *9*, e84468. [CrossRef]
68. Anagnostis, P.; Athyros, V.G.; Tziomalos, K.; Karagiannis, A.; Mikhailidis, D.P. The pathogenetic role of cortisol in the metabolic syndrome: A hypothesis. *J. Clin. Endocrinol. Metab.* **2009**, *94*, 2692–2701. [CrossRef]
69. Paredes, S.; Ribeiro, L. Cortisol: The villain in metabolic syndrome? *Rev. Assoc. Médica Bras.* **2014**, *60*, 84–92. [CrossRef]
70. Kim, S.; Henneicke, H.; Cavanagh, L.L.; Macfarlane, E.; Thai, L.J.; Foong, D.; Gasparini, S.J.; Fong-Yee, C.; Swarbrick, M.M.; Seibel, M.J.; et al. Osteoblastic glucocorticoid signaling exacerbates high-fat-diet- induced bone loss and obesity. *Bone Res.* **2021**, *9*, 40. [CrossRef]
71. McManus, B.; Korpela, R.; O'Connor, P.; Schellekens, H.; Cryan, J.F.; Cotter, P.D.; Nilaweera, K.N. Compared to casein, bovine lactoferrin reduces plasma leptin and corticosterone and affects hypothalamic gene expression without altering weight gain or fat mass in high fat diet fed C57/BL6J mice. *Nutr. Metab.* **2015**, *12*, 53. [CrossRef]
72. Swierczynska, M.M.; Mateska, I.; Peitzsch, M.; Bornstein, S.R.; Chavakis, T.; Eisenhofer, G.; Lamounier-Zepter, V.; Eaton, S. Changes in morphology and function of adrenal cortex in mice fed a high-fat diet. *Int. J. Obes.* **2015**, *39*, 321–330. [CrossRef] [PubMed]
73. Azzam, I.; Gilad, S.; Limor, R.; Stern, N.; Greenman, Y. Ghrelin stimulation by hypothalamic-pituitary-adrenal axis activation depends on increasing cortisol levels. *Endocr. Connect.* **2017**, *6*, 847–855. [CrossRef] [PubMed]
74. Howick, K.; Griffin, B.T.; Cryan, J.F.; Schellekens, H. From belly to brain: Targeting the ghrelin receptor in appetite and food intake regulation. *Int. J. Mol. Sci.* **2017**, *18*, 273. [CrossRef]
75. Lee, M.-J.; Pramyothin, P.; Karastergiou, K.; Fried, S.K. Deconstructing the roles of glucocorticoids in adipose tissue biology and the development of central obesity. *Biochim. Biophys. Acta* **2014**, *1842*, 473–481. [CrossRef]
76. Kadar, N.N.M.A.; Ahmad, F.; Teoh, S.L.; Yahaya, M.F. Comparable benefits of stingless bee honey and caffeic acid in mitigating the negative effects of metabolic syndrome on the brain. *Antioxidants* **2022**, *11*, 2154. [CrossRef]
77. Zarei, M.; Fazlara, A.; Tulabifard, N. Effect of thermal treatment on physicochemical and antioxidant properties of honey. *Heliyon* **2019**, *5*, e01894. [CrossRef]
78. Gao, Y.; Xia, W.; Shao, P.; Wu, W.; Chen, H.; Fang, X.; Mu, H.; Xiao, J.; Gao, H. Impact of thermal processing on dietary flavonoids. *Curr. Opin. Food Sci.* **2022**, *48*, 100915. [CrossRef]
79. Chang, J.-J.; Chung, D.-J.; Lee, Y.-J.; Wen, B.-H.; Jao, H.-Y.; Wang, C.-J. Solanum nigrum polyphenol extracts inhibit hepatic inflammation, oxidative stress, and lipogenesis in high-fat-diet-treated mice. *J. Agric. Food Chem.* **2017**, *65*, 9255–9265. [CrossRef]
80. Wu, Y.-H.S.; Chiu, C.-H.; Yang, D.-J.; Lin, Y.-L.; Tseng, J.-K.; Chen, Y.-C. Inhibitory effects of litchi (*Litchi chinensis Sonn.*) flower-water extracts on lipase activity and diet-induced obesity. *J. Funct. Foods* **2013**, *5*, 923–929.
81. Braghini, F.; Biluca, F.C.; Gonzaga, L.V.; Vitali, L.; Costa, A.C.; Fett, R. Effect thermal processing in the honey of *Tetragonisca angustula*: Profile physicochemical, individual phenolic compounds and antioxidant capacity. *J. Apic. Res.* **2021**, *60*, 290–296. [CrossRef]
82. Park, H.S.; Lee, K.; Kim, S.H.; Hong, M.J.; Jeong, N.J.; Kim, M.S. Luteolin improves hypercholesterolemia and glucose intolerance through LXRα-dependent pathway in diet-induced obese mice. *J. Food Biochem.* **2020**, *44*, e13358. [CrossRef] [PubMed]
83. Zakaria, Z.; Othman, Z.A.; Suleiman, J.B.; Che Jalil, N.A.; Ghazali, W.S.W.; Nna, V.U.; Mohamed, M. Hepatoprotective effect of bee bread in metabolic dysfunction-associated fatty liver disease (MAFLD) rats: Impact on oxidative stress and inflammation. *Antioxidants* **2021**, *10*, 2031. [CrossRef]
84. Zatterale, F.; Longo, M.; Naderi, J.; Raciti, G.A.; Desiderio, A.; Miele, C.; Beguinot, F. Chronic adipose tissue inflammation linking obesity to insulin resistance and type 2 diabetes. *Front. Physiol.* **2020**, *10*, 1607. [CrossRef]
85. Fruhbeck, G.; Catalán, V.; Rodríguez, A.; Gómez-Ambrosi, J. Adiponectin-leptin ratio: A promising index to estimate adipose tissue dysfunction. Relation with obesity-associated cardiometabolic risk. *Adipocyte* **2018**, *7*, 57–62. [CrossRef]

86. Andrei, A.M.; Anca, B.-I.; Felix Rareş Ioan Din, A.; Camelia Elena, S.; Sorin, B.-I.; Ileana Monica, B.; Cătălina Gabriela, P. Interplay between hypoxia, inflammation and adipocyte remodeling in the metabolic syndrome. In *Hypoxia and Human Diseases*; Jing, Z., Chi, Z., Eds.; IntechOpen: Rijeka, Croatia, 2017; pp. 303–328.
87. Subramanian, R.; Umesh Hebbar, H.; Rastogi, N.K. Processing of honey: A review. *Int. J. Food Prop.* **2007**, *10*, 127–143. [CrossRef]
88. Biluca, F.C.; Della Betta, F.; de Oliveira, G.P.; Pereira, L.M.; Gonzaga, L.V.; Costa, A.C.O.; Fett, R. 5-HMF and carbohydrates content in stingless bee honey by CE before and after thermal treatment. *Food Chem.* **2014**, *159*, 244–249. [CrossRef]
89. Capuano, E.; Fogliano, V. Acrylamide and 5-hydroxymethylfurfural (HMF): A review on metabolism, toxicity, occurrence in food and mitigation strategies. *LWT—Food Sci. Technol.* **2011**, *44*, 793–810. [CrossRef]
90. Choudhary, A.; Kumar, V.; Kumar, S.; Majid, I.; Aggarwal, P.; Suri, S. 5-hydroxymethylfurfural (HMF) formation, occurrence and potential health concerns: Recent developments. *Toxin Rev.* **2021**, *40*, 545–561. [CrossRef]
91. Tosi, E.; Martinet, R.; Ortega, M.; Lucero, H.A.; Ré, E. Honey diastase activity modified by heating. *Food Chem.* **2008**, *106*, 883–887. [CrossRef]
92. Ismail, N.I. Effects of sugar adulterants on the physicochemical properties of natural honey. *J. Tomogr. Syst. Sens. Appl.* **2019**, *2*, 59–64.
93. Samira, N. The effect of heat treatment on the quality of Algerian honey. *Researcher* **2016**, *8*, 1–6.
94. Mansour, A.; Mohajeri-Tehrani, M.R.; Qorbani, M.; Heshmat, R.; Larijani, B.; Hosseini, S. Effect of glutamine supplementation on cardiovascular risk factors in patients with type 2 diabetes. *Nutrition* **2015**, *31*, 119–126. [CrossRef] [PubMed]
95. Pathak, N.M.; Millar, P.J.B.; Pathak, V.; Flatt, P.R.; Gault, V.A. Beneficial metabolic effects of dietary epigallocatechin gallate alone and in combination with exendin-4 in high fat diabetic mice. *Mol. Cell. Endocrinol.* **2018**, *460*, 200–208. [CrossRef] [PubMed]
96. El-Shial, E.M.; Kabbash, A.; El-Aasr, M.; El-Feky, O.A.; El-Sherbeni, S.A. Elucidation of natural components of *Gardenia thunbergia* Thunb. leaves: Effect of methanol extract and rutin on non-alcoholic fatty liver disease. *Molecules* **2023**, *28*, 879. [CrossRef]
97. Guo, X.; Tang, R.; Yang, S.; Lu, Y.; Luo, J.; Liu, Z. Rutin and its combination with inulin attenuate gut dysbiosis, the inflammatory status and endoplasmic reticulum stress in paneth cells of obese mice induced by high-fat diet. *Front. Microbiol.* **2018**, *9*, 2651. [CrossRef]
98. Wang, K.; Liang, C.; Cao, W.; Luo, G.; Zhong, S.; Zeng, Z.; Dai, L.; Song, J.-L. Dietary sinapic acid attenuated high-fat diet-induced lipid metabolism and oxidative stress in male syrian hamsters. *J. Food Biochem.* **2022**, *46*, e14203. [CrossRef]
99. Yoon, H.J.; Yoon, D.S.; Baek, H.J.; Kang, B.; Jung, U.J. Dietary sinapic acid alleviates adiposity and inflammation in diet-induced obese mice. *Prev. Nutr. Food Sci.* **2022**, *27*, 407. [CrossRef]
100. Dong, J.; Zheng, H.; Zeng, Q.; Zhang, X.; Du, L.; Bais, S. Protective effect of D-(-)-quinic acid as food supplement in modulating AMP-activated protein kinase signalling pathway activation in HFD induced obesity. *Hum. Exp. Toxicol.* **2022**, *41*, 09603271221119804. [CrossRef]
101. Naomi, R.; Teoh, S.H.; Rusli, R.N.M.; Embong, H.; Bahari, H.; Kumar, J. *Elateriospermum tapos* yoghurt as a therapeutic intervention for obesity-associated cognitive impairments and anxiety-like behaviour in a high fat diet maternal obese rat model. *Nutrients* **2023**, *15*, 2312. [CrossRef]
102. Stadnicka, K.; Bogucka, J.; Stanek, M.; Graczyk, R.; Krajewski, K.; Maiorano, G.; Bednarczyk, M. Injection of raffinose family oligosaccharides at 12 days of egg incubation modulates the gut development and resistance to opportunistic pathogens in broiler chickens. *Animals* **2020**, *10*, 592. [CrossRef]
103. Arifin, W.N.; Zahiruddin, W.M. Sample size calculation in animal studies using resource equation approach. *Malays. J. Med. Sci.* **2017**, *24*, 101. [PubMed]
104. Syariffuddeen, M.A.A.; Azman, H.; Yahya, S. Evaluation of performance and characteristic of stingless bee honey using MARDI's dehydrator. In Proceedings of the Konvensyen Kebangsaan Kejuruteraan Pertanian Dan Makanan, Putrajaya, Malaysia, 21 March 2019; pp. 1–4.
105. Mohamed, N.; Gwee Sian Khee, S.; Shuid, A.N.; Muhammad, N.; Suhaimi, F.; Othman, F.; Babji, A.S.; Soelaiman, I.-N. The effects of cosmos caudatus on structural bone histomorphometry in ovariectomized rats. *Evid.-Based Complement. Altern. Med.* **2012**, *2012*, 817814. [CrossRef] [PubMed]
106. Niu, Y.; He, J.; Ahmad, H.; Wang, C.; Zhong, X.; Zhang, L.; Cui, T.; Zhang, J.; Wang, T. Curcumin attenuates insulin resistance and hepatic lipid accumulation in a rat model of intra-uterine growth restriction through insulin signalling pathway and sterol regulatory element binding proteins. *Br. J. Nutr.* **2019**, *122*, 616–624. [CrossRef]
107. Wong, S.K.; Chin, K.Y.; Ahmad, F.; Ima-Nirwana, S. Biochemical and histopathological assessment of liver in a rat model of metabolic syndrome Induced by high-carbohydrate high-fat diet. *J. Food Biochem.* **2020**, *44*, e13371. [CrossRef]
108. De Souza, J.A.; Becker, L.K.; Batista, M.A.C.; de Assis Braga, D.C.; Gomes, P.M.; Alzamora, A.C.; Vieira, M.A.R.; de Lima, W.G.; Andrade, M.G.C.; de Lima Sanches, B.; et al. Swimming training improves cardiovascular autonomic dysfunctions and prevents renal damage in rats fed a high-sodium diet from weaning. *Exp. Physiol.* **2021**, *106*, 412–426. [CrossRef]

pharmaceuticals

MDPI

Article

Twenty-Week Dietary Supplementation with Beeswax Alcohol (BWA; Raydel®) Ameliorates High-Cholesterol-Induced Long-Term Dyslipidemia and Organ Damage in Hyperlipidemic Zebrafish in a Dose-Dependent Manner: A Comparative Analysis Between BWA and Coenzyme Q_{10}

Kyung-Hyun Cho *, Ashutosh Bahuguna, Yunki Lee, Sang Hyuk Lee and Ji-Eun Kim

Raydel Research Institute, Medical Innovation Complex, Daegu 41061, Republic of Korea
* Correspondence: chok@raydel.co.kr; Tel.: +82-53-964-1990; Fax: +82-53-965-1992

Abstract: Background/Objectives: Beeswax alcohol (BWA; Raydel®) is a blend of six long-chain aliphatic alcohols extracted from honeybee wax and is well known for its diverse functionality and health benefits. Herein, the efficacy of a BWA dietary intervention for 20 weeks was assessed to ameliorate high-cholesterol diet (HCD)-induced dyslipidemia and adverse effects on the vital organs of adult zebrafish. Methods: Adult zebrafish were fed different high-cholesterol diets (HCDs; final concentration of 4%, *w*/*w*) supplemented with BWA (final concentrations of 0.1%, 0.5% and 1.0%, *w*/*w*) or CoQ_{10} (final concentration of 1.0%). Following 20 weeks of supplementation, blood and different organs (liver, kidney, testes and ovaries) were collected, and biochemical, histological and immunohistochemical analyses were performed. Results: The results demonstrate a dose-dependent effect of BWA of mitigating HCD-induced mortality in zebrafish over the 20-week supplementation period, which was noticeably better than the effect exerted by coenzyme Q_{10} (CoQ_{10}). Consistently, a dose-dependent effect of BWA consumption of curtailing HCD-induced total cholesterol (TC) and triglyceride (TG) levels and increasing high-density-lipoprotein cholesterol (HDL-C) levels was noticed. Compared with CoQ_{10} (final concentration of 1.0%, *w*/*w*), BWA (final concentration of 1.0%, *w*/*w*) displayed a significantly better effect of mitigating HCD-induced dyslipidemia, as evidenced by 1.2-fold ($p < 0.05$) and 2.0-fold ($p < 0.05$) lower TC and TG levels and 2.4-fold ($p < 0.01$) higher HDL-C levels. The histological analysis revealed substantial prevention of fatty liver changes, reactive oxygen species (ROS) generation, cellular senescence and interleukin (IL)-6 production in the hepatic tissue of BWA zebrafish, which was significantly better than the effect exerted by CoQ_{10}. Consistently, compared with CoQ_{10}, significant 25% ($p < 0.05$) and 35% ($p < 0.01$) reductions in the HCD-induced elevated levels of the hepatic function biomarkers aspartate aminotransferase and alanine aminotransferase was observed in the BWA group. Likewise, BWA consumption efficiently ameliorated HCD-induced kidney, ovary and testis damage by inhibiting ROS generation, cellular senescence and lipid accumulation. Conclusion: Supplementation with BWA demonstrated higher therapeutic potential than that with CoQ_{10} to prevent dyslipidemia and organ damage associated with long-term consumption of HCDs.

Keywords: dyslipidemia; fatty liver; high-density lipoprotein (HDL); inflammation; senescence; zebrafish

1. Introduction

Beeswax is a well-known natural ingredient produced by different species of honeybees and has a varied beneficial function [1]. The majority of commercially used beeswax is obtained from the honeybee species *Apis mellifera* and *Apis cerana* [2] and contains ~67% esters, ~16% hydrocarbons and ~12% free fatty acids, along with ~1% free alcohols. Beeswax alcohol (BWA), isolated from beeswax, consists of a blend of long-chain aliphatic alcohols

(LCAAs) of C24 to C34 and is renowned for its potent antioxidant and anti-inflammatory activities [3–5]. Recently, the impact of BWA on the prevention of low-density-lipoprotein (LDL) oxidation and the functionality enhancement of high-density lipoproteins (HDLs) via augmenting HDL-associated paraoxonase (PON)-1 activity has been described [6]. Additionally, BWA substantially elevates high-density-lipoprotein cholesterol (HDL-C) levels and inhibits hepatic inflammation, leading to zebrafish protection against the stress induced by ethanol [7]. BWA entrapped in reconstituted HDL (rHDL) prevents HDL glycation and rescues zebrafish embryos from carboxymethyllysine (CML)-induced toxicity [8]. While numerous benefits have been identified, the significant impact of BWA on gastric health has been particularly highlighted in various preclinical and clinical studies [9,10]. In a preclinical study in rats, BWA supplementation was found effective against gastric ulceration induced by various stimulants without interfering with gastric acidity [10]. BWA's impacts on the quality and quantity of gastric mucosa, reduced neutrophil infiltration and improved antioxidant status in gastric mucosa are among the key events behind the gastro-protective role of BWA [10]. BWA's antioxidant effect is not confined solely to the gastric mucosa, as it also manifests as substantial modulatory effects on the antioxidant enzymes in the liver and brain [10,11], suggesting the broad applicability of BWA. In human subjects, BWA (100 mg/day) oral consumption for two months positively modulated regurgitation, bloating, sucking and flatulence scores [10]. Along with gastroprotection, BWA displayed a substantial effect on joint health on account of a noteworthy inhibitory impact on proinflammatory leukotriene B4 (LTB4), the main culprit behind the generation of superoxide and proinflammatory cytokines [10]. Based on the above-mentioned effects, the Korean Food and Drug Administration (KFDA) has approved the BWA as a functional food ingredient for gastric and joint health [12].

Coenzyme Q_{10} (CoQ_{10}) is a lipid-soluble antioxidant synthesized in the human body and has been widely used as a dietary supplement. CoQ_{10} has diverse functions in the body, including antioxidant, anti-inflammatory and obligatory components for energy production in mitochondria [13]. Under normal and healthy conditions, intrinsic CoQ_{10} is sufficient in the intracellular and blood systems; however, in certain pathological conditions, such as degenerative muscle and cardiovascular diseases [14,15], oxidative stress and ageing can deplete intrinsic CoQ_{10}, which thus needs to be supplemented externally to balance its level [16]. Nonetheless, the daily dosage range of CoQ_{10} is too wide, 30–600 mg (moderate), up to 600~3000 mg (high), depending on the requirement for curing target disorders [17]. Besides its noteworthy antioxidant role, the effect of CoQ_{10} on the lipid profile has not been observed sufficiently in animal experiments and human studies. A meta-analysis of randomized controlled trials revealed that supplementation with CoQ_{10} at around 100~300 mg for 4~48 weeks in patients with coronary artery disease (CAD) was effective in lowering total cholesterol (TC) and increasing HDL-C; however, it was not effective in improving triglyceride (TG) and low-density-lipoprotein cholesterol (LDL-C) [18]. A randomized clinical trial with type 2 diabetic patients (n = 20) showed that supplementation with CoQ_{10} at 150 mg/day for 12 weeks decreased TG but had no effect on TC. Intriguingly, a significantly negative effect of CoQ_{10} supplementation on the increase in HDL-C and reduction in LDL-C was observed [19]. Another meta-analysis on CoQ_{10} supplementation in adults revealed that a decrease in TC, LDL-C and TG levels and an increase in HDL-C levels were achieved at 400~500 mg/day, suggesting that high-dose CoQ_{10} might be associated with an improvement in the lipid profile [20]. In a comparative in vitro study, CoQ_{10} displayed a much inferior effect compared with BWA in preventing oxidative damage by LDL and was found ineffective in augmenting the functionality of HDL by modulating the activity of PON-1.

Numerous studies on BWA report on its dynamic functionality examined in vitro [6], in vivo [7] and in clinical settings [6,10]. However, studies on BWA dietary consumption's impact on high-cholesterol diet-induced dyslipidemia and associated oxidative stress and senescence in different organs remain lacking. To address this, the current study was designed to evaluate the comparative influence of 20 weeks of dietary intervention with

BWA and CoQ_{10} under the influence of a high-cholesterol diet on the plasma lipid profile, senescence and functionality of the liver, kidney and reproductive organs of hyperlipidemic zebrafish. Given that BWA is not soluble in water, for the comparative assessment, we selected lipid-soluble CoQ_{10} (as a control), which has been described as having several beneficial effects, including a substantial effect on the lipid profile [21].

2. Results

2.1. Change in Survivability and Body Weight

The results documented in Figure 1 demonstrate the survival probability during 20 weeks of consumption of the defined diets, which varied from 0.88 to 0.96 across the different groups. The HCD group exhibited the lowest survival probability (0.88), whereas the highest survival probability (0.96) was observed in the 0.1% and 1.0% BWA groups. Despite the slight difference in survival probability, the Kaplan–Meier survival analysis followed by a log-rank test revealed a non-significant difference (log-rank: χ^2 = 4.891, p = 0.229) in zebrafish survivability among the different groups.

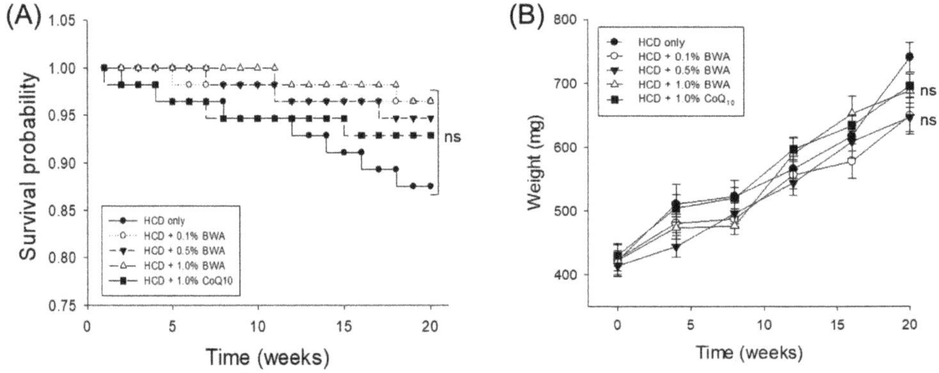

Figure 1. Survival probability (**A**) and body weight change (**B**) in zebrafish across the different groups during 20 weeks of consumption of the respective diets. HCD stands for the high-cholesterol diet, while BWA and CoQ_{10} stand for beeswax alcohol and coenzyme Q_{10}, respectively. "ns" represents the non-significant difference between the groups. The Kaplan–Meier survival analysis followed by the log-rank test was used to determine the survivable probability curve, while ANOVA followed by Tukey's post hoc analysis was used for the statistical analysis of the body weight.

Figure 1B and Table 1 display the body weight changes in the different groups following 20 weeks of consumption of the different diets. At week 20, the 0.1% BWA and 0.5% BWA groups showed 13~14% lower body weight, and the 1.0% BWA group and 1.0% coenzyme Q_{10} (CoQ_{10}) group showed 5~6% lower body weight than the HCD-only group; however, the changes in body weight were statistically non-significant ($p > 0.05$).

Table 1. Body weight (BW) of zebrafish among the different groups at the beginning and after 20 weeks supplementation of respective diets.

Diet (Total 10 mg)	HCD Alone (n = 56)	HCD+ +0.1% BWA (n = 56)	HCD +0.5% BWA (n = 56)	HCD +1.0% BWA (n = 56)	HCD +1.0% CoQ_{10} (n = 56)
BW at week 0 (mg)	421.8 ± 15.8	424.3 ± 24.2	413.5 ± 15.4	421.9 ± 25.5	429.4 ± 16.9
BW at week 20 (mg)	740.9 ± 23.3	648.7 ± 28.4	646.3 ± 22.2	688.1 ± 26.8	696.0 ± 18.1
Net increase in BW (mg)	319.1 ± 6.7	224.4 ± 9.5	232.8 ± 6.3	266.2 ± 8.9	266.6 ± 5.2
Net increase in BW (%)	175.6 ± 5.5	153.8 ± 6.7 ^{ns}	152.3 ± 5.2 ^{ns}	166.4 ± 6.5 ^{ns}	165.0 ± 4.3 ^{ns}

BW, body weight; BWA, beeswax alcohol; HCD, high-cholesterol diet; CoQ_{10}, coenzymeQ_{10}. ^{ns} represents the non-significant weight change in different groups at 20 weeks, compared with the HCD-only group.

2.2. Change in Lipid Profiles

As shown in Figure 2A,B, the highest level of total cholesterol (TC; 584 mg/dL) and triglyceride (TG; 651 mg/dL) were detected in the HCD-only group following 20 weeks of consumption. Co-consumption of BWA efficiently altered the HCD-induced high levels of TC in a dose-dependent manner. A significant reduction of 43.2% ($p < 0.001$) in TC was quantified in the 1.0% BWA group compared with the HCD-only group, while the 1.0% coenzyme Q_{10} (CoQ_{10}) group showed 27.7% lower ($p < 0.01$) TC levels than the HCD-only group. Importantly, the 1.0% BWA group exhibited 21.5% lower ($p < 0.05$) TC levels than the 1.0% CoQ_{10} group, suggesting that BWA showed higher efficacy in treating hypercholesterolemia induced by HCD supplementation.

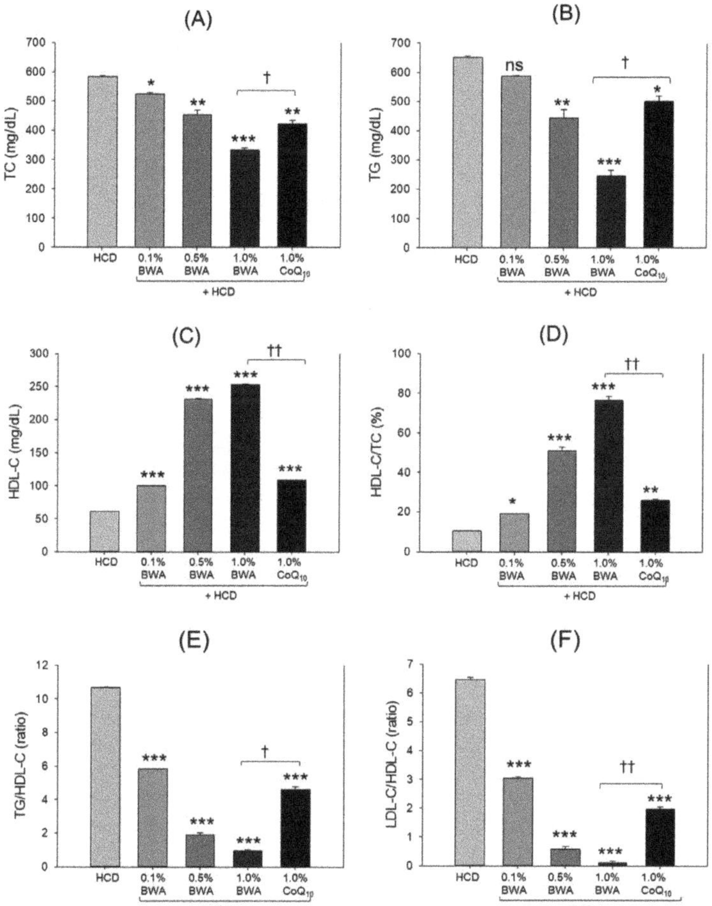

Figure 2. Quantification of (**A**) total cholesterol, (**B**) triglyceride, (**C**) HDL-C, (**D**) HDL-C/TC (%), (**E**) TG/HDL-C and (**F**) LDL-C/HDL-C among the different groups after 20 weeks of consumption of the respective diets. TC, TG, HDL-C, LDL-C, HCD, BWA and CoQ_{10} stand for total cholesterol, triglyceride, high-density-lipoprotein cholesterol, low-density-lipoprotein cholesterol, high-cholesterol diet, beeswax alcohol and coenzyme Q_{10}, respectively. * ($p < 0.05$), ** ($p < 0.01$) and *** ($p < 0.001$) depict the level of significance with respect to the HCD group, while † ($p < 0.05$) and †† ($p < 0.01$) highlight the significance between the 1.0% BWA and 1.0% CoQ_{10} groups.

Also, the co-consumption of BWA exhibited a substantial effect of lowering plasma TG levels in a dose-dependent manner, as evidenced by 31.9% ($p < 0.01$) and 62.2% lower ($p < 0.001$) TG levels detected in the 0.5% BWA and 1.0% BWA groups, respectively, compared with the HCD-only group (Figure 2B). Likewise, the 1.0% CoQ_{10} group also displayed a significant reduction of 23.1% ($p < 0.05$) in TG levels compared with the HCD-only group. However, compared with the 1.0% CoQ_{10} group, a significant reduction of 50.7% ($p < 0.05$) in TG levels was observed in the 1.0% BWA group, suggesting the higher efficacy of BWA in treating hypertriglyceridemia induced by HCD supplementation.

As shown in Figure 2C, the plasma HDL-C levels were the lowest in the HCD-only group (around 61 mg/dL) and were significantly increased by 1.6 ($p < 0.001$), 3.8 ($p < 0.001$) and 4.2 times ($p < 0.001$) in response to 0.1%, 0.5% and 1.0% BWA, respectively, indicating a substantial dose-dependent effect of BWA of increasing HCD-impaired HDL-C levels. Also, the 1.0% CoQ_{10} group displayed 1.8-fold ($p < 0.001$) higher HDL-C levels than the HCD control. Intriguingly, the effect exerted by 1.0% CoQ_{10} was nearly similar to the effect exerted by 0.1% BWA. Compared with the 1.0% BWA group, a significant 2.4-fold reduction ($p < 0.01$) in HDL-C levels was detected in the 1.0% CoQ_{10} group, suggesting a higher effectiveness of BWA in increasing HDL-C levels compared with CoQ_{10}.

Concomitantly to HDL-C, the HCD-only group showed the lowest percentage of HDL-C in TC, around 10%, which was significantly increased by 19.2% ($p < 0.05$), 51.2% ($p < 0.001$) and 76.3% ($p < 0.001$) in response to 0.1%, 0.5% and 1.0% BWA, respectively (Figure 2D). Likewise, 1.0% CoQ_{10} consumption also significantly increased ($p < 0.01$, 25.8%) the HCD-induced decrease in HDL-C/TC (%), which was nearly similar to the HDL-C/TC (%) observed in 0.1% BWA. However, compared with 1.0% CoQ_{10}, the 1.0% BWA group showed 2.9-fold higher ($p < 0.01$) HDL-C/TC (%) levels.

In contrast to HDL/TC (%), the HCD group exhibited a notably elevated TG/HDL-C ratio, which was significantly reduced ($p < 0.001$) by the consumption of BWA at concentrations ranging from 0.1% to 1.0% (Figure 2E). Similarly, 1.0% CoQ_{10} also considerably ($p < 0.001$) reduced the HCD-induced high levels of TG/HDL-C; however, compared with 1.0% BWA, 4.7-fold ($p < 0.05$) lower efficacy was noticed in the 1.0% CoQ_{10} group.

Likewise, BWA and CoQ_{10} exerted substantial effects ($p < 0.001$) of decreasing the HCD-induced increase in the LDL-C/HDL-C ratio; however, BWA, precisely at 1.0%, displayed significantly higher efficacy than 1.0% CoQ_{10} in balancing the HCD-affected LDL-C/HDL-C ratio (Figure 2F). These findings indicate that BWA co-supplementation provides significantly higher benefits than CoQ_{10} in stabilizing the lipid profile affected by HCD.

2.3. *Change in Hepatic Damage Parameters*

As shown in Figure 3, the HCD-only group showed the highest blood aspartate aminotransferase (AST) and alanine aminotransferase (ALT) levels, around 544.8 $\pm$ 3.4 IU/L and 365.7 $\pm$ 3.1 IU/L, respectively, suggesting that HCD consumption caused severe hepatic damage. Co-supplementation with BWA at 0.1%, 0.5% and 1.0% efficiently reduced the levels of AST by 14.4% ($p < 0.05$), 28.1% ($p < 0.01$) and 42.2% ($p < 0.001$), respectively, compared with the HCD-only group, testifying to the dose-dependent preventive impact of BWA against the HCD-induced increase in AST levels. Similarly, the blood ALT levels increased by the HCD decreased by 17.6% ($p < 0.01$), 26.4% ($p < 0.001$) and 45.3% ($p < 0.001$) in the 0.1%, 0.5% and 1.0% BWA groups, respectively.

The 1.0% CoQ_{10} group showed 23.5% ($p < 0.01$) and 15.9% ($p < 0.01$) lower AST and ALT levels than the HCD-only group. Compared with the 1.0% CoQ_{10} group, the 1.0% BWA group exhibited 24.5% ($p< 0.05$) and 34.9% ($p < 0.01$) reductions in AST and ALT levels, respectively. These results suggest that consumption of BWA, primarily at 1.0%, was remarkably more effective in ameliorating hepatic damage in hyperlipidemia than CoQ_{10}.

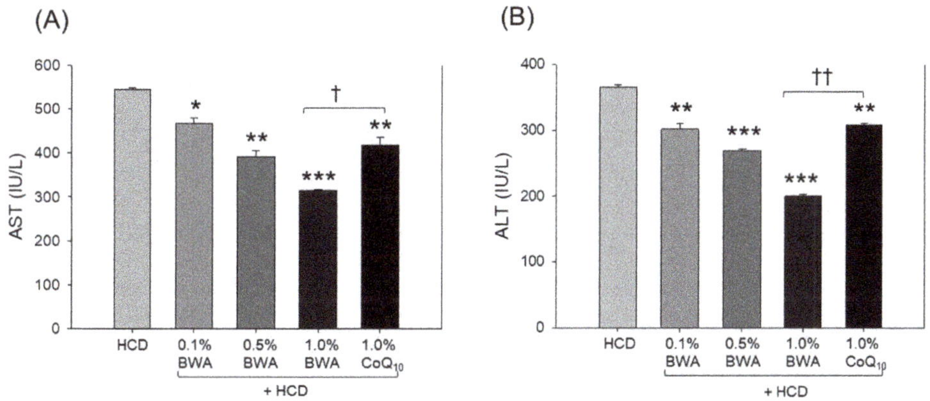

Figure 3. Quantification of the levels of the hepatic function biomarkers (**A**) aspartate aminotransferase and (**B**) alanine aminotransferase in the plasma of zebrafish after 20 weeks of consumption of different diets. HCD stands for the high-cholesterol diet, while BWA and CoQ_{10} stand for beeswax alcohol and coenzyme Q_{10}, respectively. * ($p < 0.05$), ** ($p < 0.01$) and *** ($p < 0.001$) depict the level of significance with respect to the HCD group, while † ($p < 0.05$) and †† ($p < 0.01$) highlight the significance between the 1.0% BWA and 1.0% CoQ_{10} groups.

2.4. Liver Size and Weight

The images of the whole liver collected from the zebrafish revealed a slightly enhanced liver size, indicating steatosis (fatty liver) in the HCD group. The HCD-induced large liver size was effectively averted with the consumption of BWA and CoQ_{10} (Figure 4). Consistent with these findings, liver size enlargement and increased weight were noticed in the HCD groups, which were significantly ($p < 0.05$) reduced following consumption of BWA and CoQ_{10}. Interestingly, the 0.1% BWA group showed a similar effect to the 1.0% CoQ_{10} group in preventing liver size and weight enlargement.

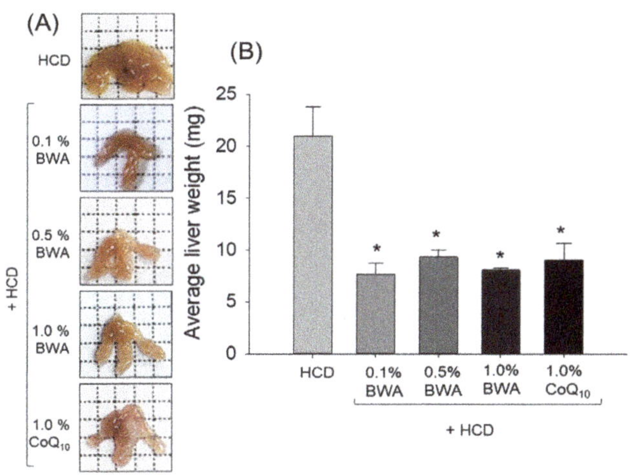

Figure 4. Comparison of liver morphology and size among zebrafish after 20 weeks of consumption of different diets. (**A**) Images of the whole liver and (**B**) liver weight of zebrafish following 20 weeks of consumption of different diets. HCD stands for the high-cholesterol diet, while BWA and CoQ_{10} stand for beeswax alcohol and coenzyme Q_{10}, respectively. * ($p < 0.05$) depicts the level of significance with respect to the HCD group.

2.5. Histological Analysis of Hepatic Inflammation

As shown in Figure 5A,E, H&E staining revealed that the HCD-only group showed the highest extent of neutrophil infiltration (indicated by the red arrows) and lipid droplet accumulation (indicated by the blue arrows). A marked accumulation of tiny lipid droplets (indicated by the green arrows) leading to vacuole formation in hepatocytes was prominently observed in the HCD-only group. Additionally, large lipid vesicles (indicated by the red arrows) caused nuclear shrinkage in certain regions, resulting in severe steatosis. In contrast, the 0.5% and 1.0% BWA groups exhibited significantly reduced infiltration of neutrophils and lipid droplet aggregation compared with the HCD group. However, the occasional presence of vacuolated hepatocytes and minor steatosis was noticed in the 0.5% and 1.0% BWA groups, though it was substantially less frequent compared with the HCD group. Furthermore, the quantification of the H&E-stained area revealed 57.8% ($p < 0.05$) and 79.2% ($p < 0.05$) smaller H&E-stained areas in the 0.5% and 1.0% BWA groups compared with the HCD-only group, suggesting a dose-dependent impact of BWA of preventing HCD-induced hepatic damage (Figure 5B,E). Interestingly, the 0.1% BWA group and the 1.0% CoQ_{10} group showed a non-significant effect ($p > 0.05$) on the inhibition of HCD-induced neutrophil infiltration and H&E-stained area, as shown in Figure 5A,B,E.

Immunohistochemistry (IHC) revealed that the HCD-only group showed the highest production of IL-6, as shown by the vital red conversion area (Figure 5C,D). At the same time, the 1.0% BWA group exhibited the lowest IL-6 levels, around 96.1% ($p < 0.01$) lower than the HCD-only group (Figure 5C,D,F). Co-consumption of 0.1% and 0.5% BWA caused significant decreases in IL-6 production of 75.1% ($p < 0.05$) and 86.6% ($p < 0.01$) compared with the HCD group, testifying to a dose-dependent effect of BWA against the inhibition of HCD-induced IL-6 production. Further, 1.0% CoQ_{10} consumption displayed a substantial IL-6 production inhibitory role, like the effect of the 0.1% BWA group. However, compared with 1.0% CoQ_{10} consumption, 6.8-fold ($p < 0.05$) higher efficacy was observed in response to 1.0% BWA consumption to curtail HCD-induced high IL-6 levels, testifying to the supremacy of BWA over CoQ_{10} in preventing hepatic inflammation measured in terms of IL-6 production.

2.6. Reactive Oxygen Species Generation and Cell Senescence in Liver

As shown in Figure 6A, the HCD-only group showed the most robust red (DHE) fluorescent intensity, depicting the utmost extent of hepatic reactive oxygen species (ROS) generation. On the contrary, the co-consumption of BWA effectively decreased ROS production, especially in the 1.0% BWA group, which exhibited around 80.2% ($p < 0.001$) less DHE fluorescent intensity than the HCD-only group (Figure 6A,C). On the other hand, the 0.1% BWA group and the 1.0% CoQ_{10} group showed a substantial preventive effect against HCD-induced ROS generation, manifested as significant reductions of 53.4% ($p < 0.01$) and 43.4% ($p < 0.05$) in DHE fluorescent intensity compared with the HCD-only group. On the other hand, compared with 1.0% CoQ_{10}, the 1.0% BWA group showed a significant reduction of 62.1% ($p < 0.05$) in the DHE-stained area, attesting to the higher efficacy BWA in restricting HCD-induced ROS generation.

As shown in Figure 6B, senescence-associated β-galactosidase (SA-β-gal) staining revealed that the HCD-only group exhibited the most severe cell senescence, around 54.5% of SA-β-gal-positive cells, suggesting that the 20 weeks of consumption of a high-cholesterol diet resulted in severe cellular senescence in the liver. The consumption of BWA and CoQ_{10} substantially prevented HCD-induced senescence (Figure 6B,D). Compared with 1.0% CoQ_{10}, 1.0% BWA exhibited a significant reduction of 84.2% ($p < 0.001$) in SA-β-gal-positive cells, demonstrating BWA enhanced efficacy over CoQ_{10} in mitigating HCD-induced cellular senescence.

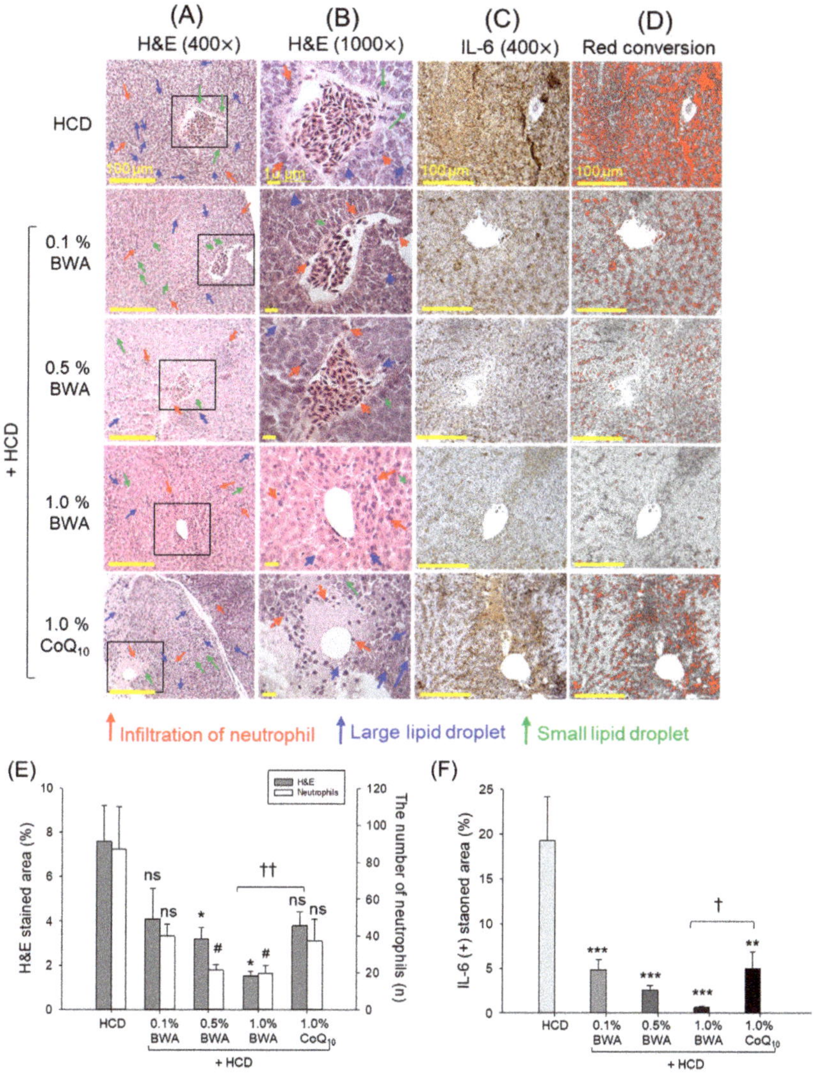

Figure 5. Hepatic histology of zebrafish after 20 weeks of consumption of different diets. (**A**,**B**) Hematoxylin and eosin (H&E) staining at 400× and 1000× magnifications; red and blue arrows indicate neutrophils and lipid droplets. (**C**) Interleukin (IL)-6-stained area examined by immunohistochemistry (IHC) and (**D**) visibility of IL-6-stained (brown color) area enhanced by its conversion into the red color (at brown color threshold of 20–120) performed by employing Image J software, version 1.53 [scale bar, 100 μm]. Quantification of (**E**) H&E-stained area and neutrophils counts and (**F**) IL-6-stained area. HCD stands for the high-cholesterol diet, while BWA and CoQ_{10} stand for beeswax alcohol and coenzyme Q_{10}, respectively. * ($p < 0.05$), ** ($p < 0.05$) and *** ($p < 0.001$) depict the level of significance for the H&E- and IL-6-stained areas, while # ($p < 0.05$) depicts the significance level for neutrophil counts with reference to the HCD group. † ($p < 0.05$) and †† ($p < 0.01$) depict the statistical difference between the 1.0% BWA and 1.0% CoQ_{10} groups; the non-significant differences between the groups are represented by "ns".

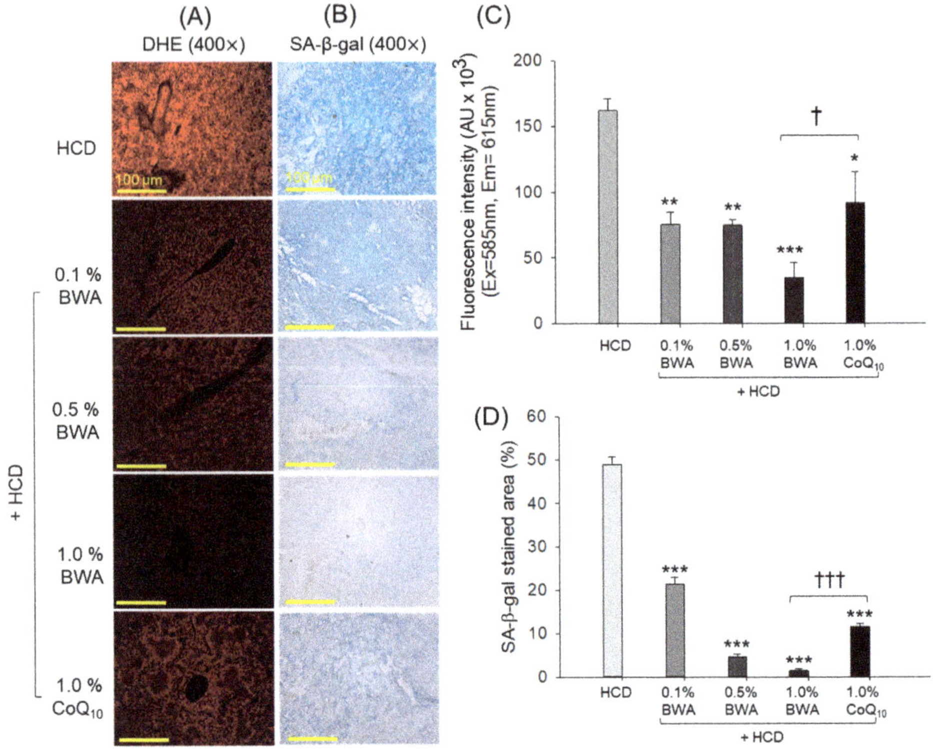

Figure 6. Detection of reactive oxygen species (ROS) generation and cellular senescence in the hepatic tissue of zebrafish following 20 weeks of consumption of different diets. (**A**) Dihydroethidium (DHE) fluorescent staining was used to detect ROS. (**B**) Senescence-associated β-galactosidase (SA-β-gal) staining [scale bar, 100 μm]. (**C**) Image J software-derived DHE fluorescent intensity quantification. (**D**) SA-β-gal-stained area quantification. HCD stands for the high-cholesterol diet, while BWA and CoQ_{10} stand for beeswax alcohol and coenzyme Q_{10}, respectively. * ($p < 0.05$), ** ($p < 0.01$) and *** ($p < 0.001$) depict the level of significance with reference to the HCD group. † ($p < 0.05$) and ††† ($p < 0.001$) highlight the significance with respect to the 1.0% BWA group.

2.7. Histological Analysis of Kidneys

As depicted in Figure 7A, the HCD group showed loosely arranged and sparsely populated proximal and distal tubular structures with frequent lumen debris (as indicated by the red arrows). On the contrary, the consumption of BWA, mainly 1.0% BWA, restored kidney histology impaired by the HCD. Likewise, 0.1% and 0.5% BWA also displayed a preventive effect against HCD-induced kidney impairment; however, the rare presence of cellular debris (as indicated by the red arrows) was observed in the tubular cast. Further, 1.0% CoQ_{10} consumption displayed a substantial preventive effect against HCD-induced kidney damage, nearly similar to that observed in the 0.5% BWA group.

DHE staining revealed massive ROS production in the HCD group, which was prevented by the consumption of 0.5% BWA, 1.0% BWA and 1.0% CoQ_{10}, evidenced by 45.6%, 57.7% and 45.1% lower DHE fluorescent intensity compared with the HCD group (Figure 7B,D). However, the difference concerning the HCD-only group was statistically non-significant.

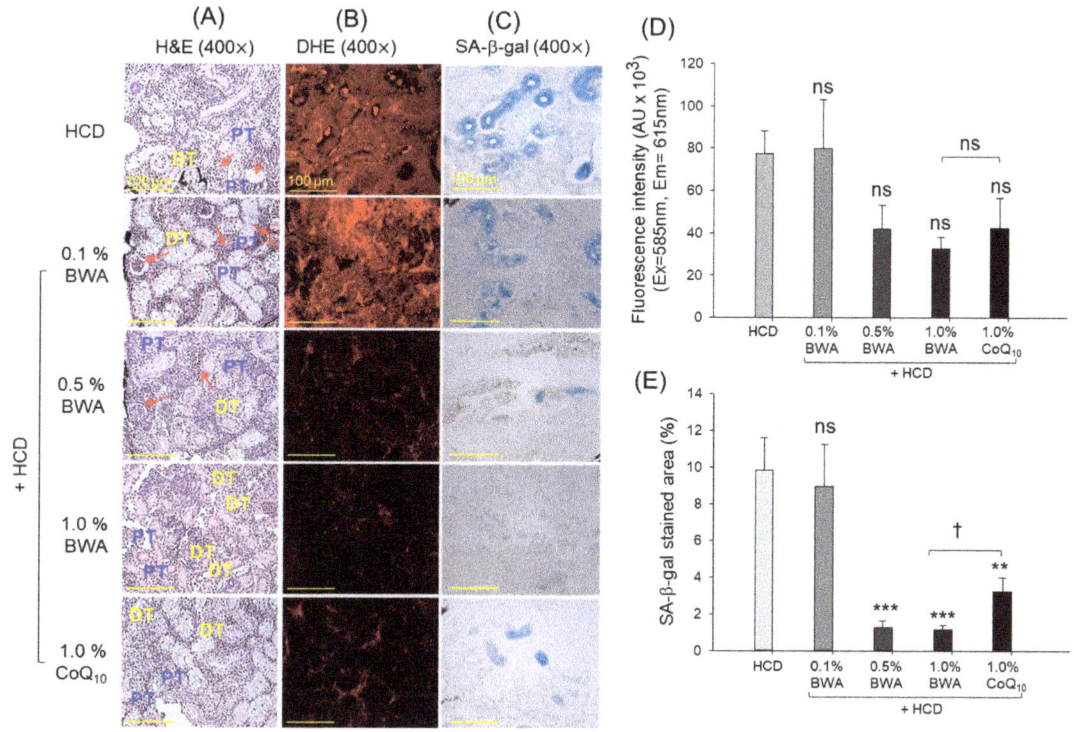

Figure 7. Analysis of kidney histology of zebrafish at 20 weeks of consumption of different diets. (**A**) Hematoxylin and eosin staining: proximal and distal tubules are represented by PT and DT, respectively, and the red arrows indicate luminal debris. (**B**) Dihydroethidium (DHE) fluorescent staining was used to detect reactive oxygen species (ROS). (**C**) Senescence-associated β-galactosidase (SA-β-gal) staining [scale bar, 100 µm]. (**D**) Image J software-derived DHE fluorescent intensity quantification. (**E**) Quantification of SA-β-gal-stained area. HCD stands for the high-cholesterol diet, while BWA and CoQ_{10} stand for beeswax alcohol and coenzyme Q_{10}, respectively. ** ($p < 0.01$) and *** ($p < 0.001$) depict the level of significance with reference to the HCD group. † ($p < 0.05$) highlights the significance between the 1.0% BWA and 1.0% CoQ_{10} groups; the non-significant differences between the groups are represented by "ns".

SA-β-gal staining suggested higher occurrence of senescent cells in the HCD group. The consumption of BWA and CoQ_{10} efficiently inhibited HCD-induced cellular senescence (Figure 7C,E). The SA-β-gal-stained area obtained from the 0.5% and 1.0% BWA groups revealed 87.1% ($p < 0.001$) and 88.3% ($p < 0.001$) lower levels of senescent cells compared with the HCD group. Also, a substantial effect, with a 67.3% ($p < 0.01$) smaller SA-β-gal-stained area, was noticed in the 1.0% CoQ_{10} group compared with the HCD group. Compared with COQ_{10}, a 64.5% smaller SA-β-gal-stained area was marked in the 1.0% BWA group, underscoring the superiority of BWA over the CoQ_{10} in mitigating HCD-induced senescence in the kidneys.

2.8. Testicular Cell Analysis

The H&E staining of the testicular sections (Figure 8A,B) showed that the HCD group had loosely arranged seminiferous tubules, occasional disruption of lamina basal membranes (indicated by the red arrows) and increased interstitial tissue area (around 33.8%) between the seminiferous tubules. Additionally, irregularly distributed spermatogonia, spermatocytes and spermatozoa were frequently observed, including void space in the lumen.

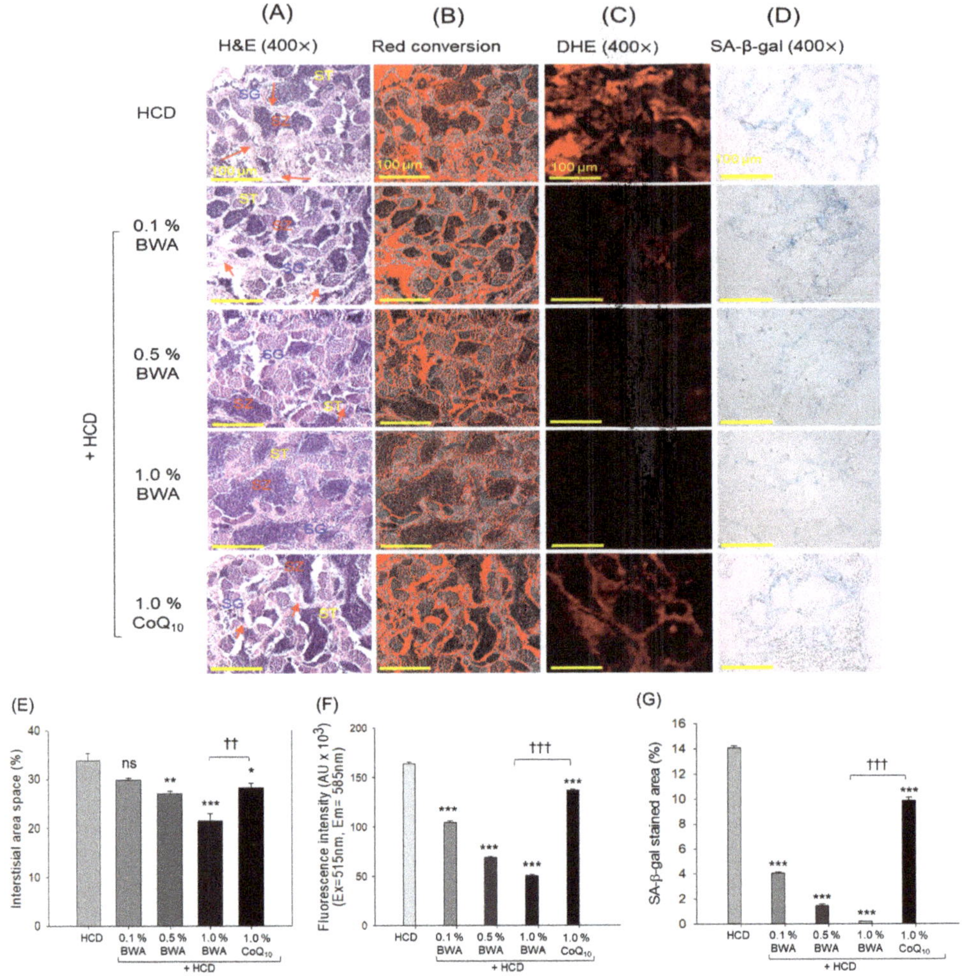

Figure 8. Histological examination of zebrafish testes following 20 weeks of consumption of different diets. (**A**) Hematoxylin and eosin (H&E) staining: spermatocytes, spermatozoa and spermatogonia are represented by ST, SZ and SG, respectively; disruption of lamina basal membranes is indicated by the red arrows. (**B**) The interstitial area was red-converted into the H&E section by using Image J software (at white color threshold of 220–255) to enhance visibility. (**C**) Dihydroethidium (DHE) fluorescent staining used to detect reactive oxygen species (ROS) and (**D**) senescence-associated-β-galactosidase (SA-β-gal) staining [scale bar, 100 μm]. (**E**) Quantification of interstitial area performed by employing Image J software. (**F**,**G**) Quantification of DHE fluorescent intensity and SA-β-gal-stained area, respectively. HCD stands for the high-cholesterol diet, while BWA and CoQ_{10} stand for beeswax alcohol and coenzyme Q_{10}, respectively. * ($p < 0.05$), ** ($p < 0.01$) and *** ($p < 0.001$) depict the level of significance with reference to the HCD group. †† ($p < 0.01$) and ††† ($p < 0.001$) highlight the significance between the 1.0% BWA and 1.0% CoQ_{10} groups; the non-significant differences between the groups are represented by "ns".

The co-consumption of BWA improved the morphological features of testicular cells, as reflected by intact seminiferous tubules with a decrease in interstitial space between the seminiferous tubules, especially in the 1.0% BWA group, which showed a noticeable 36.4% ($p < 0.001$) decrease in interstitial space area compared with the HCD group (Figure 8A,B,E). Additionally, spermatocytes, spermatozoa and spermatogonia were arranged appropriately, with the least void space in the lumen of seminiferous tubules. Notably, higher prevalence of spermatozoa (mature sperm) was noticed in the 1.0% BWA group than the HCD group.

Like the BWA effect, CoQ_{10} consumption also showed a substantial improvement in testicular cell morphology, as evidenced by a reduction of around 16.3% ($p < 0.05$) in interstitial space compared with the HCD group. However, 1.0% BWA exerted a substantially higher effect than 1.0% CoQ_{10} in terms of preventing HCD-induced testicular damage, as indicated by 24.1% ($p < 0.01$) lower interstitial space in the seminiferous tubules, indicating comparative higher efficacy of BWA compared with CoQ_{10}.

The DHE staining outcomes reveal massive ROS production in the HCD group, which was significantly ($p < 0.001$) prevented by the consumption of BWA and CoQ_{10} (Figure 8C,F). Compared with CoQ_{10}, BWA consumption at 0.1%, 0.5% and 1.0% displayed 23.7%, 49.4% and 63.3% lower DHE fluorescent intensity, suggesting the functional superiority of BWA over CoQ_{10} in maintaining HCD-induced high oxidative stress.

SA-β-gal staining revealed that the HCD-only group showed the highest blue color intensity and blue color-stained area corresponding to SA-β-gal-positive senescent cells, which was substantially prevented by the consumption of BWA in a dose-dependent manner (Figure 8D,G). As shown in Figure 8D,G, the HCD-only group showed an SA-β-gal-stained area of 14.1%, which was reduced to 4.0%, 1.4% and 0.2% by the consumption of 0.1% BWA, 0.5% BWA and 1.0% BWA, respectively. Likewise, CoQ_{10} also significantly prevented HCD-induced cellular senescence. However, compared with the BWA, the efficacy of CoQ_{10} in preventing HCD-induced cellular senescence was much lower. As depicted in Figure 8D,G, a 49-fold ($p < 0.001$) smaller senescent area was detected in the 1.0% BWA group compared with the 1.0% CoQ_{10} group, attesting to the higher potency of BWA in mitigating HCD-induced testis senescence.

2.9. Ovarian Cell Analysis

As shown in Figure 9A,D, the HCD-only group showed the highest previtellogenic oocyte content (~93%) and the lowest mature-vitellogenic oocyte content (~2%), indicating the adverse effect of HCD supplementation on the impairment of oocyte development. The co-consumption of BWA improved HCD-impaired oocyte development in a dose-dependent manner, especially at 1.0%. The BWA group showed the lowest previtellogenic oocyte content (~73%) and the highest mature-vitellogenic oocyte content (~10%). Also, CoQ_{10} consumption substantially affected the restoration of HCD-altered oocyte counts. Between the 1.0% consumption of BWA and CoQ_{10}, BWA displayed a significant 12.1% ($p < 0.05$) reduction in previtellogenic oocyte content, indicating the superior functionality of BWA in addressing HCD-induced ovary impairment.

The findings of DHE staining show the influential role of BWA in overcoming HCD-induced ROS production (Figure 9B,E). Significant reductions of 31.2%, 43.4% and 51.5% in DHE-stained area in response to 0.1%, 0.5% and 1.0% BWA compared with the HCD-only group testify to the dose-dependent effect of BWA of diminishing HCD-induced ROS production. Also, CoQ_{10} consumption displayed a substantial preventive effect on HCD-induced ROS production; however, compared with 1.0% BWA, the effect exerted by 1.0% CoQ_{10} was significantly 41.1% lower ($p < 0.001$), indicating comparatively lower efficacy of CoQ_{10} with respect to BWA in reducing ROS production.

SA-β-gal staining suggested higher prevalence of cellular senescence in the ovarian section of the HCD group, which was efficiently mitigated by the co-consumption of both BWA and CoQ_{10} (Figure 9C,F). However, compared with BWA, the efficacy of CoQ_{10} was lower in preventing HCD-induced senescence in the ovaries. Compared with 1.0% CoQ_{10}, significant reductions of 80.1% ($p < 0.001$) and 61.5% ($p < 0.001$) in SA-β-gal-stained area were found in the 1.0% BWA group, attesting to its importance in mitigating HCD-induced ovary impairment.

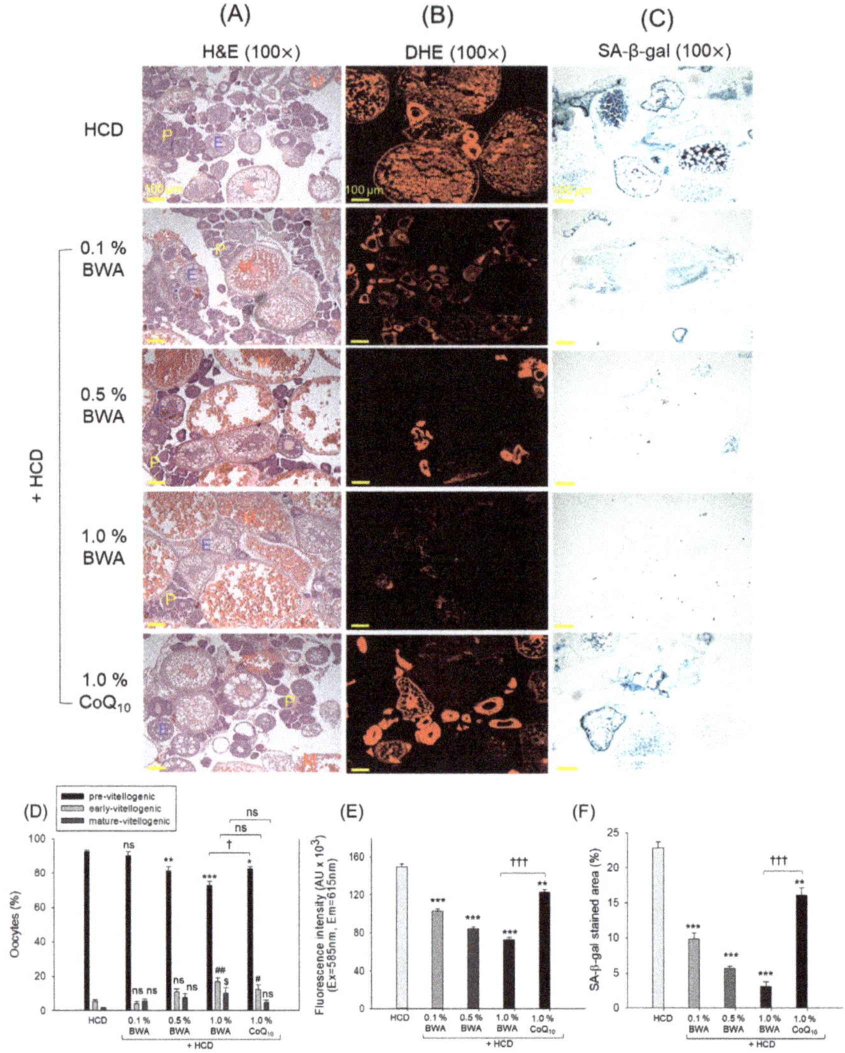

Figure 9. Histological examination of zebrafish ovaries following 20 weeks of consumption of different diets. (**A**) Hematoxylin and eosin (H&E) staining: premature, early and mature vitellogenic oocytes are represented by P, E and M, respectively. (**B**) Dihydroethidium (DHE) fluorescent staining for detecting reactive oxygen species (ROS). (**C**) Senescence-associated β-galactosidase (SA-β-gal) staining [scale bar, 100 μm]. (**D**) Different oocyte population quantification. (**E**) Quantification of DHE fluorescent intensity by employing Image J software. (**F**) Quantification of SA-β-gal-stained area. HCD stands for the high-cholesterol diet, while BWA and CoQ_{10} stand for beeswax alcohol and coenzyme Q_{10}, respectively. * ($p < 0.05$), ** ($p < 0.01$) and *** ($p < 0.001$) depict the level of significance for the previtellogenic oocytes, DHE and SA-β-gal-stained area, while # ($p < 0.05$) and ## ($p < 0.01$) depict the significance level for early-vitellogenic oocytes with respect to the HCD group. † ($p < 0.05$), ††† ($p < 0.001$) highlights the significance between the 1.0% BWA and 1.0% CoQ_{10} groups; the non-significant differences between the groups are represented by "ns".

3. Discussion

In the present study, the comparative effects of BWA and CoQ_{10} consumption were examined on the blood lipid profile, body weight, survivability and function of vital organs of hyperlipidemic zebrafish. Zebrafish was selected as a model organism due to its high genome similarity to humans [22]. Also, the key events and essential receptors and enzymes of lipid metabolism in zebrafish are very similar to those in human beings, thus making it an excellent model organism for assessing the impact of drugs and nutraceuticals on dyslipidemia [23].

The established role of HCD supplementation in dyslipidemia in zebrafish [7,24,25] and other model organisms has been well elucidated [26,27]. Consistently, we have also noticed the impact of the HCD on the increase in TC, TG and LDL-C and decrease in HDL-C levels in zebrafish. Supplementation with both BWA and CoQ_{10} was found to be adequate to counter HCD-induced dyslipidemia by effectively managing the altered TC, TG, LDL-C and HDL-C levels. Nevertheless, the comparative analysis suggested a much inferior effect of CoQ_{10} compared with BWA in managing the disrupted plasma lipid profile caused by the HCD. A noteworthy 2.3-fold increase in HDL-C levels was observed in response to the consumption of 1.0% BWA compared with that observed in CoQ_{10}. The outcomes enforced the functional superiority of BWA over CoQ_{10} in the management of HCD-induced dyslipidemia. The results are aligned with the accumulating literature depicting the impact of CoQ_{10} on decreasing TC, TG and LDL-C levels and increasing HDL-C levels [28]. However, the literature has revealed a variation in the countering of the dyslipidemic effect of CoQ_{10} in response to the used dose of CoQ_{10}. Moreover, studies have documented the non-effectiveness of CoQ_{10} at the tested concentration of 150 mg/day in diabetic patients [19]. Contrary to the available literature for CoQ_{10}, a limited study describes the effect of BWA on the plasma lipid profile. In that study, BWA displayed a substantial impact on the increase in HDL-C levels hampered by exposure to ethanol [7], supporting the present finding concerning BWA's positive effect on the increase in HDL-C levels. The presence of LCAAs, such as hexacosanol, triacontanol and octacosanol, in BWA is the key contributor responsible for the beneficial effect of BWA on the management of the HCD-affected plasma lipid profile. This notion is supported by the previous finding depicting the inhibitory role of triacontanol [29] and hexacosanol [30] in cholesterol biosynthesis. Research has been documented the visible effect of hexacosanol on the activation of AMP-activated protein kinase (AMPK), which induced the inactivation of 3-hydroxy-3-methyl-glutaryl-coenzyme A reductase (HMG-CoA), a principal rate-limiting enzyme for cholesterol biosynthesis [30]. Additionally, hexacosanol has a negative impact on the nuclear translocation of sterol regulatory element-binding protein-2 (SREBP-2), which regulates the production of HMG-CoA at the transcriptional level, thus inhibiting cholesterol biosynthesis [30]. A similar effect of octacosanol (a major constituent of BWA) of inhibiting cholesterol biosynthesis has been observed [31,32].

Beyond improving the plasma lipid profile, BWA demonstrated a notable ability to protect the liver from damage associated with the HCD. Substantially reduced neutrophil infiltration, prevention of fatty liver changes and hepatic IL-6 generation were observed in the BWA group in a dose-dependent manner. Specifically, 1.0% BWA displayed a substantial hepatoprotective role, significantly higher than the effect exerted by the consumption of 1.0% CoQ_{10}. Also, compared with CoQ_{10}, BWA displayed higher efficacy in preventing HCD-induced oxidative stress and cellular senescence in the liver. The findings are consistent with previous studies that have demonstrated the hepatoprotective effect of BWA [11,33]. In one such study, BWA consumption for 6 months substantially improved fatty liver changes and insulin resistance in patients with non-alcoholic fatty liver disease (NAFLD) [33].

BWA's antioxidant and anti-inflammatory effect, demonstrated in several preclinical and clinical studies, ascribe a gastro-protective role to this substance [10,34–36]. The antioxidant role of BWA mediated by the scavenging of hydroxyl radicals and by modulating cellular antioxidant catalase, superoxide dismutase (SOD) and glutathione peroxidase

(GSH-PX) has been found to be a key event in protecting the gastric mucosa from a variety of stimuli [9,35]. The better hepatoprotective activity of BWA compared with CoQ_{10} can be justified by earlier findings documenting a higher antioxidant impact of BWA compared with CoQ_{10} on the scavenging of free radicals and the inhibition of oxidative damage of lipoproteins [6]. Moreover, compared with CoQ_{10}, BWA efficiently inhibits CML-induced oxidative stress and protects zebrafish embryos from apoptotic cell death [6], indicative of BWA's better cellular antioxidant role compared with CoQ_{10}. It has also been described that BWA substantially enhances the activity of the HDL-associated antioxidant paraoxonase (PON)-1, while CoQ_{10} failed to display any such effect [6]. This might be an additional reason behind the better antioxidant role of BWA compared with CoQ_{10} in mitigating HCD-induced challenges and oxidative stress. Furthermore, BWA consumption (100 mg BWA/day for 12 weeks) showed substantial potential to reduce malondialdehyde (MDA) and total hydroperoxide levels and augmenting total antioxidant status in humans, strengthening the remarkable antioxidant impact of BWA [6].

Increased liver size is commonly linked to fatty liver disease [37], and in our study, we observed a similar increase in liver size following HCD consumption. However, BWA treatment notably reduced this increase, indicative of its hepatoprotective effect, as further supported by hepatic histological results. The hepatoprotective nature of BWA, as observed from the histological analysis, is also confirmed by the diminished plasma AST and ALT levels, which are important hepatic function biomarkers [38–40].

The lower prevalence of AST and ALT in the 1.0% BWA group compared with CoQ_{10} suggests a greater hepatoprotective function of BWA, consistent with the findings of the hepatic histological outcomes. We believe that the reduced AST and ALT levels could be correlated with elevated HDL-C and low TC levels in response to BWA. This notion is in accordance with earlier findings that establish a negative correlation between elevated HDL-C [40] and low TC levels [41] and AST and ALT levels, strengthening the current findings that suggest that BWA, compared with CoQ_{10}, has substantial effects on the increase in HDL-C, decrease in TG levels and consequently lower AST and ALT levels, indicating better hepatic health.

BWA prevents the fatty liver changes induced by an HCD; this may be attributed to the presence of hexacosanol, which has been identified to stimulate autophagy commenced by the upregulation of an autophagy-related gene (ATG16L) and anti-microtubule-associated protein 1A/1B light chain 3 (LC3-II) [30], resulting in the inhibition of hepatic lipid accumulation and subsequent fatty liver changes [30,42]. Elevated levels of IL-6 in response to HCD consumption may be associated with excessive ROS generation, as several reports depict the induction of the inflammatory pathway induced by oxidative stress [43]. Also, the induction of IL-6 might be a major contributor that aggravates HCD-induced dyslipidemia. The notion is supported by the findings disclosing elevated TG levels in response to IL-6 production [44]. Further, many inflammatory disorders, such as rheumatoid arthritis (RA), systemic lupus erythematosus (SLE) and psoriasis, substantially affect the blood lipid profile, indicating the tight association between inflammation and an altered lipid profile [45–47]. As BWA showed higher effectiveness than CoQ_{10} in restricting HCD-induced high IL-6 production, it might be a key component of the mechanism behind a high degree of hepatic protection and the management of the plasma lipid profile. Our results are in line with earlier studies describing BWA's potential as an anti-inflammatory agent that prevents inflammatory disorders (arthritis) in mice [48] and humans [49].

The association of ROS/oxidative stress with cellular senescence has already been described [50,51]. BWA, owing to its better inhibitory impact than CoQ_{10} on cellular ROS generation, exerts an ameliorating effect on oxidative stress and leads to subsequent prevention of cellular senescence.

HCD-induced adverse effects have been described as damage to the kidneys [52] and reproductive system [20,53]. The adverse impact of HCDs on the testicular structures, precisely on the seminiferous tubules and the interstitial area, has been documented [54], and we have also observed a similar detrimental effect in zebrafish. Noticeable superior kidney, testis and ovary protective effects exerted by BWA compared with CoQ_{10} by curtailing HCD-induced ROS generation and cellular senescence were observed in zebrafish during the 20 weeks of the consumption study. We believe that kidney protection against HCD-induced damage is attributed to BWA's higher antioxidant efficacy, which maintains cellular oxidative stress, which has been described as a key event in preventing cellular senescence [55] in a variety of organs. Additionally, the critical role of hexacosanol (a component of BWA) has been illustrated as the modulation of nitric oxide synthetase and protein kinase C (PKC), leading to the prevention of glomerular sclerosis and improvement in diabetic nephropathy [56,57]. To the best of our knowledge, this is the first study describing the protective effect of BWA against cholesterol-induced impairment of the liver, kidney and reproductive organs.

4. Materials and Methods

4.1. Materials

A typical blend of six long-chain aliphatic alcohols (LCAAs; C24-C34) containing beeswax alcohol (BWA; Raydel®) was extracted from a block of wax of honeybees (mainly mellifera linage), which was complementary provided by Raydel® Pty, Ltd., Thornleigh, NSW, Australia. The BWA (Batch#: 330020123) was >86% pure and contained 6.1% tetracosanol, 10.7% hexacosanol, 13.8% octacosanol, 30.5% triacontanol, 22.1% dotriacontanol and 2.9% tetratriacontanol. A certificate of chemical analysis is provided in Supplementary Figure S1. All the other chemicals and reagents used in the present study were of analytical grade and used as supplied unless otherwise stated. Supplementary Materials contain a detailed list of the chemicals and reagents used.

4.2. Zebrafish Maintenance

The adult (~16 weeks aged) wild zebrafish (*Danio rerio*) AB strain of mixed gender (male and female) was procured from a local market and fed normal tetrabit (ND; Gmbh D49304, Melle, Germany). The ND was composed of 47.5% crude protein, 6.5% crude fat, 2.0% crude fiber, 10.5% crude ash, vitamin A (29.77 IU/g), vitamin D3 (1.86 IU/g), vitamin E (0.2 mg/g) and vitamin C (0.13 mg/g). The zebrafish were housed in an aerated water tank maintained at 28 °C with constant water supply and a photoperiod of 10 h of darkness and 14 h of light. The zebrafish were maintained following the prescribed rules of care and use of laboratory animals [58], and the study protocols were approved by the Committee of Animal Care and Use of Raydel Research Institute (approval code RRI-23-001; approval date 27 July 2023).

4.3. Preparation of Different Diets

The different BWA or CoQ_{10} formulated diets were prepared by incorporating BWA or CoQ_{10} in a high-cholesterol diet (HCD). To prepare the HCD, normal tetrabit (ND) was mixed with cholesterol (final concentration of 4%, *w*/*w*) [59]. In brief, the ND (800 g) was supplemented with 32 g of cholesterol (equivalent to 4% *w*/*w*) and mixed (by spatula) to distribute the cholesterol. Subsequently, an organic solvent (chloroform) was added to the mixture (ND + cholesterol) and agitated mechanically to properly distribute the cholesterol. The chloroform was completely evaporated in the fume hood to obtain ND supplemented with cholesterol, which was named the HCD. The HCD (25 mg) from three different locations was collected to ascertain nearly similar cholesterol distribution. The cholesterol was extracted from the samples by vigorous agitation with chloroform. The extracted cholesterol was quantified by using a commercial cholesterol diagnostic kit (cholesterol, T-CHO, Clean TS-S; Walko Pure Chemicals, Osaka, Japan).

The HCD was individually supplemented with BWA (final concentration of 0.1%, 0.5% and 1.0%, *w*/*w*) to form three different BWA-enriched diets named HCD + 0.1% BWA, HCD + 0.5% BWA and HCD + 1.0% BWA, respectively. Similarly, CoQ_{10} (final concentration of 1.0%, *w*/*w*) was mixed with the HCD to prepare a CoQ_{10}-enriched diet named HCD + 1.0% CoQ_{10}. Detailed proportions of the tetrabit, cholesterol, BWA and

CoQ_{10} used to prepare different diets are included in Table 2. The selection of the used diets (0.1–1.0%, *w*/*w*) was based on preliminary studies, where we tested the effect of different amounts of BWA and found that 1.0% BWA as a maximum diet addition exerted beneficial effects on hyperlipidemia zebrafish [60].

Table 2. Composition of different zebrafish diets prepared by mixing cholesterol, beeswax alcohol and coenzyme Q_{10} (CoQ_{10}).

Diet (Total: 10 mg)	HCD Only	HCD+ +0.1% BWA	HCD +0.5% BWA	HCD +1.0% BWA	HCD +1.0% CoQ_{10}
Tetrabit	9.6	9.59	9.55	9.5	9.5
Cholesterol	0.4	0.4	0.4	0.4	0.4
BWA	0	0.01	0.5	0.1	0
CoQ_{10}	0	0	0	0	0.1
Total (mg)	10	10	10	10	10

BWA, beeswax alcohol; HCD, high-cholesterol diet; CoQ_{10}, coenzyme Q_{10}.

4.4. Consumption of Different Diets by Zebrafish

All the zebrafish (~16 weeks old) were exclusively fed the HCD for 4 weeks before segregation into different groups. After four weeks of feeding on the HCD, the zebrafish (n = 280) were arbitrarily allocated to five distinct groups (n = 56/group) (Figure 10). The zebrafish in group I were continuously fed only the HCD. The zebrafish in groups II, III and IV were fed HCD + 0.1% BWA, HCD + 0.5% BWA and HCD + 1.0% BWA, respectively. The group V zebrafish were fed HCD + 1.0% CoQ_{10}. Each group's zebrafish (n = 56) were divided into four sets (n = 14/tank) and fed the specified diets for 20 weeks. Each set (n = 14) of different groups received 140 mg of the respective diets/tank twice a day in the morning and evening (i.e., a total of 280 mg/day, ~equivalent to 20 mg/day/zebrafish). Over the 20-week consumption period, zebrafish survivability was monitored every day.

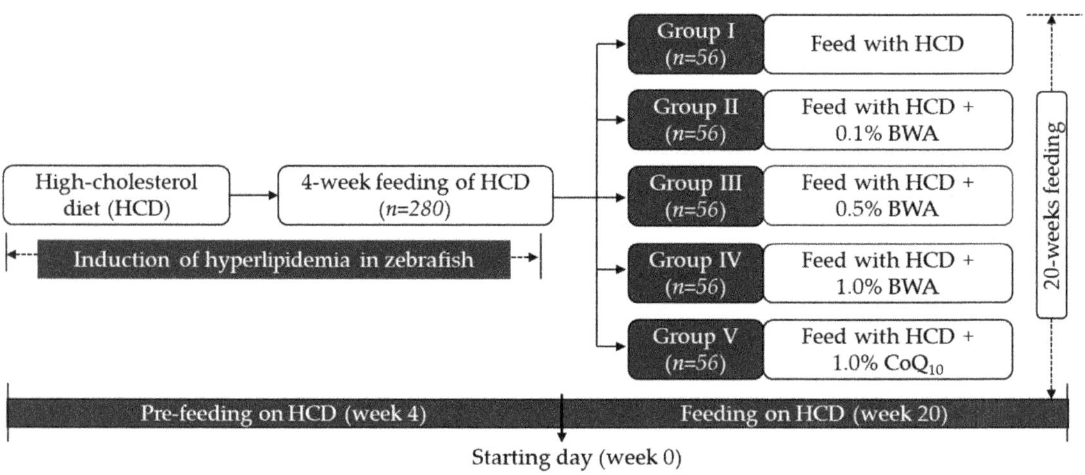

Figure 10. A layout of the experimental plan of the 20-week consumption study. HCD stands for the high-cholesterol diet, while BWA and CoQ_{10} stand for beeswax alcohol and coenzyme Q_{10}.

The body weight of zebrafish in different groups was measured at 0, 4, 8, 12, 16 and 20 weeks by using the gravimetric method. Body weight was analyzed after anesthetizing the zebrafish by submerging them into 0.1% 2-phenoxyethanol. The surface of the anathematized zebrafish was dried by using filter paper, and the weight was measured with an electronic weighing balance (Ohaus, Parsippany-Troy Hills, NJ, USA); immediately, the zebrafish were transferred into their tank. For the body weight analysis, one set of zebrafish (n = 14) from each group were used. Notably, at different time points (0–20 weeks), similar sets of the respective groups were used to analyze body weight.

4.5. Collection of Blood and Organs

After 20 weeks of consumption of different diets, the zebrafish were sacrificed by using hypothermic shock [59], and blood was immediately collected in EDTA-prewashed tubes and subjected to centrifugation to obtain plasma. The plasma obtained from the different groups was analyzed by utilizing commercial kits to assess total cholesterol, triglyceride, HDL and the hepatic function enzymatic markers AST and ALT. Supplementary Method S1 provides the detailed blood analysis procedure. The organs (liver, kidney, testes and ovaries) of the sacrificed zebrafish were surgically removed under an optical microscope (at 10× magnification) and preserved separately in 10% formalin.

4.6. Histology and Immunohistochemistry (IHC)

The tissue sections (liver, kidney, testes and ovaries) were embedded in FSC22 clear frozen compound (Leica) and subsequently processed for cryo-tissue sectioning by using a Leica CM 1510S cryo-microtome (Leica Biosystem, Nussloch, Germany). A thin section (7 μm) was sliced and processed for hematoxylin and eosin (H&E) staining [61]. The histological changes in the different H&E-stained tissue sections were analyzed under a microscope (Motic microscopy PA53MET; Hong Kong, China) equipped with a digital camera to examine neutrophil infiltration, vacuolation due to small lipid droplets accumulation in the hepatocytes, hepatic ballooning and steatosis (fatty liver changes). The H&E images of the hepatic tissue captured were processed by using Image J software (http://rsb.info.nih.gov/ij; accessed on 16 January 2023; version 1.53) to quantify the number of neutrophils (stained dark violet to blue) and the H&E-stained area.

For the testis sections, the H&E-stained area was visualized to examine spermatogenesis, seminiferous tubules and interstitial space between the seminiferous tubules [62,63]. The interstitial space in the H&E-stained images was quantified by using Image J software after converting the images into RGB stack according to a threshold level [of lower limit (220) and upper limit (255)]. A minimum of three images from each group were examined for the histological analysis of testicular tissue.

For the ovary sections, the previtellogenic, early-vitellogenic and mature-vitellogenic stages, as described previously [64,65], were analyzed. The classification for the previtellogenic stage is follicles measuring 250 μm in diameter or smaller, including the smallest previtellogenic follicles and those in the peri-nucleolar stage. Follicles of 250–500 μm in diameter were classified as being in the early-vitellogenic stage. Follicles of 500 μm in diameter or larger were assigned to the mature-vitellogenic stage, including follicles characterized by yolk-filled alveoli distributed throughout the ooplasm and vitellogenic follicles.

Cellular senescence in the tissue sections was examined by the senescence-associated β-galactosidase (SA-β-gal) assay [66]. In brief, the tissue section (7 μm thick) was covered with 5-bromo-4-chloro-3-indolyl-β-D-galactopyranoside (X-gal) overnight (16 h) and visualized microscopically for the detection of blue-stained senescent-positive cells.

Interleukin (IL)-6 in the hepatic section was detected by IHC staining employing an anti-IL-6 primary antibody and enzyme-linked anti-IL-6 antibodies following an earlier described method [67]. IL-6 quantification was performed by employing image J software by converting IL-6-stained images into RGB stack according to threshold levels [of lower limit (20) and upper limit (120)] to minimize the inclusion of background staining. All the images were processed at the same threshold values. The detailed procedure for IHC staining is provided in Supplementary Method S1.

4.7. Dihydroethidium (DHE) Fluorescent Staining

The tissue sections (7 μm thick) were stained for 30 min with DHE (final concentration of 30 μM) [68]. Subsequently, the stained sections were washed with phosphate-buffered saline (PBS) and visualized under a fluorescent microscope at the excitation and emission wavelengths of 585 nm and 615 nm.

4.8. Statistical Analysis

One-way analysis of variance (ANOVA) followed by Tukey's post hoc analysis, performed by employing SPSS software (version 29.0; Chicago, IL, USA), was used to establish the statistical difference between the groups. The experimental values for each experiment were obtained from three replicate experiments and presented as the average values ± standard errors of the mean (SEM).

5. Conclusions

This study compared the functional difference between BWA and CoQ_{10} against the detrimental effects caused by the consumption of an HCD. After 20 weeks of consumption, BWA (final concentration of 1.0%, w/w) showed a significantly better effect than CoQ_{10} (final concentration of 1.0%, w/w) in preventing HCD-induced high TC and TG levels. Consistently, BWA increased HDL-C levels more than CoQ_{10}. A substantially better effect compared with CoQ_{10} in preventing HCD-induced liver, kidney and reproductive organ damage was observed in response to BWA consumption. Also, higher efficacy of BWA compared with CoQ_{10} was noticed in countering HCD-induced ROS generation, which lead to the protection of liver, kidney and reproductive organs. Compared with CoQ_{10}, BWA displayed substantially higher anti-inflammatory activity by curtailing HCD-induced hepatic IL-6 production and preventing fatty liver changes. This study confirms the functional superiority of BWA over CoQ_{10}; the former can be used as a nutraceutical to prevent dyslipidemia and associated adverse disorders.

Supplementary Materials: The following supporting information can be downloaded at: https://www.mdpi.com/article/10.3390/ph17111434/s1, Figure S1: Certificate of analysis and composition of beeswax alcohol (BWA), Method S1: List of chemicals used and detailed methodology for quantification of plasma lipid profile and hepatic function biomarkers and immunohistochemical (IHC) analysis.

Author Contributions: Conceptualization, K.-H.C.; methodology, A.B., J.-E.K., Y.L. and S.H.L.; data curation and writing—original draft preparation, K.-H.C.; writing—review and editing, K.-H.C., supervision, K.-H.C. All authors have read and agreed to the published version of the manuscript.

Funding: This research study received no external funding.

Institutional Review Board Statement: The animal study protocol was approved by the Committee of Animal Care and Use of Raydel Research Institute (approval code RRI-23-001; approval date 27 July 2023).

Informed Consent Statement: Not applicable.

Data Availability Statement: The data used to support the findings of this study are available from the corresponding author upon reasonable request.

Conflicts of Interest: The authors declare no conflicts of interest.

References

1. Bradbear, N. *Bees and Their Role in Forest Livelihoods: A Guide to the Services Provided by Bees and the Sustainable Harvesting, Processing and Marketing of Their Products*; Food and Agriculture Organization of the United Nations: Rome, Italy, 2009.
2. Fratini, F.; Cilia, G.; Turchi, B.; Felicioli, A. Beeswax: A minireview of its antimicrobial activity and its application in medicine. *Asian Pacif. J. Tropic. Med.* **2016**, *9*, 839–843. [CrossRef] [PubMed]
3. Menéndez, R.; Amor, A.; González, R.; Jiménez, S.; Mas, R. Inhibition of rat microsomal lipid peroxidation by the oral administration of D002. *Braz. J. Med. Biol. Res.* **2000**, *33*, 85–90. [CrossRef] [PubMed]
4. Rodriguez, I.; Illnait, J.; Molina, V.; Oyarzabal, A.; Fernandez, L.; Mesa, M.; Más, R.; Mendoza, S.; Gámez, R.; Jiménez, S. Comparison of the antioxidant effects of D-002 (beeswax alcohols) and grape seed extract (GSE) on plasma oxidative variables in healthy subjects. *Lat. Am. J. Pharm.* **2010**, *29*, 255–262.

5. Lopez, E.; Illnait, J.; Molina, V.; Oyarzabal, A.; Fernandez, L.; Perez, Y.; Mas, R.; Mesa, M.; Fernandez, J.; Mendoza, S. Effects of D-002 (beeswax alcohols) on lipid peroxidation in middle-aged and older subjects. *Lat. Am. J. Pharm.* **2008**, *27*, 695–703.
6. Cho, K.-H.; Baek, S.-H.; Nam, H.-S.; Bahuguna, A.; López-González, L.E.; Rodríguez-Cortina, I.; Illnait-Ferrer, J.; Fernández-Travieso, J.C.; Molina-Cuevas, V.; Pérez-Guerra, Y.; et al. Beeswax alcohol prevents low-density lipoprotein oxidation and demonstrates antioxidant activities in zebrafish embryos and human subjects: A clinical study. *Curr. Issues Mol. Biol.* **2024**, *46*, 409–429. [CrossRef]
7. Han, Y.; Zee, S.; Cho, K.-H. Beeswax alcohol and fermented black rice bran synergistically ameliorated hepatic injury and dyslipidemia to exert antioxidant and anti-inflammatory activity in ethanol-supplemented zebrafish. *Biomolecules* **2023**, *13*, 136. [CrossRef]
8. Cho, K.-H.; Baek, S.-H.; Nam, H.-S.; Bahuguna, A. Enhancement of antioxidant and anti-glycation properties of beeswax alcohol in reconstituted high-density lipoprotein: Safeguarding against carboxymethyllysine toxicity in zebrafish. *Antioxidants* **2023**, *12*, 2116. [CrossRef]
9. Pérez, Y.; Oyárzabal, A.; Mas, R.; Molina, V.; Jiménez, S. Protective effect of D-002, a mixture of beeswax alcohols, against indomethacin-induced gastric ulcers and mechanism of action. *J. Nat. Med.* **2013**, *67*, 182–189. [CrossRef]
10. Molina, V.; Mas, R.; Carbajal, D. D-002 (beeswax alcohols): Concurrent joint health benefits and gastroprotection. *Indian J. Pharm. Sci.* **2015**, *77*, 127–134. [CrossRef]
11. Mendoza, S.; Noa, M.; Pérez, Y.; Mas, R. Preventive effect of D-002, a mixture of long-chain alcohols from beeswax, on the liver damage induced with CCl4 in rats. *J. Med. Food* **2007**, *10*, 379–383. [CrossRef]
12. Korean Food and Drug Administration (KFDA). Available online: https://www.foodsafetykorea.go.kr/portal/healthyfoodlife/searchHomeHFDetail.do?prdlstReportLedgNo=2023021000330706 (accessed on 16 May 2023).
13. Farsi, F.; Nezhad, P.A.; Morshedzadeh, N. The Hepatoprotective Effects of Coenzyme Q10 Against Oxidative Stress. In *The Liver*; Academic Press: Cambridge, MA, USA, 2018; pp. 281–294.
14. Potgieter, M.; Pretorius, E.; Pepper, M.S. Primary and secondary coenzyme Q10 deficiency: The role of therapeutic supplementation. *Nutr. Rev.* **2013**, *71*, 180–188. [CrossRef] [PubMed]
15. Brandmeyer, E.A.; Shen, Q.; Thimmesch, A.R.; Pierce, J.D. Using coenzyme Q10 in clinical practice. *Nursing* **2014**, *44*, 63–66. [CrossRef] [PubMed]
16. Bhagavan, H.N.; Chopra, R.K. Coenzyme Q10: Absorption, tissue uptake, metabolism and pharmacokinetics. *Free Radic. Res.* **2006**, *40*, 445–453. [CrossRef]
17. Raizner, A.E. Coenzyme Q10. *Methodist Debakey Cardiovasc. J.* **2019**, *15*, 185–191. [CrossRef]
18. Jorat, M.V.; Tabrizi, R.; Mirhosseini, N.; Lankarani, K.B.; Akbari, M.; Heydari, S.T.; Mottaghi, R.; Asemi, Z. The effects of coenzyme Q10 supplementation on lipid profiles among patients with coronary artery disease: A systematic review and meta-analysis of randomized controlled trials. *Lipids Health Dis.* **2018**, *17*, 230. [CrossRef] [PubMed]
19. Zahedi, H.; Eghtesadi, S.; Seifirad, S.; Rezaee, N.; Shidfar, F.; Heydari, I.; Golestan, B.; Jazayeri, S. Effects of CoQ_{10} supplementation on lipid profiles and glycemic control in patients with Type 2 diabetes: A randomized, double blind, placebo-controlled trial. *J. Diabetes Metab. Disord.* **2014**, *13*, 81. [CrossRef]
20. Liu, C.-Y.; Chang, T.-C.; Lin, S.-H.; Wu, S.-T.; Cha, T.-L.; Tsao, C.-W. Metformin ameliorates testicular function and spermatogenesis in male mice with high-fat and high-cholesterol diet-induced obesity. *Nutrients* **2020**, *12*, 1932. [CrossRef]
21. Zou, J.; Tian, Z.; Zhao, Y.; Qiu, X.; Mao, Y.; Li, K.; Shi, Y.; Zhao, D.; Liang, Y.; Ji, Q.; et al. Coenzyme Q10 supplementation improves cholesterol efflux capacity and antiinflammatory properties of high-density lipoprotein in Chinese adults with dyslipidemia. *Nutrition* **2022**, *101*, 111703. [CrossRef]
22. Patton, E.E.; Zon, L.I.; Langenau, D.M. Zebrafish disease models in drug discovery: From preclinical modelling to clinical trials. *Nat. Rev. Drug Discov.* **2021**, *20*, 611–628. [CrossRef]
23. Fang, L.; Liu, C.; Miller, Y.I. Zebrafish models of dyslipidemia: Relevance to atherosclerosis and angiogenesis. *Transl. Res.* **2014**, *163*, 99–108. [CrossRef]
24. Tang, D.; Geng, F.; Yu, C.; Zhang, R. Recent application of zebrafish models in atherosclerosis research. *Front. Cell Dev. Biol.* **2021**, *9*, 643697. [CrossRef] [PubMed]
25. Jin, Y.; Kozan, D.; Anderson, J.L.; Hensley, M.; Shen, M.C.; Wen, J.; Moll, T.; Kozan, H.; Rawls, J.F.; Farber, S.A. A high-cholesterol zebrafish diet promotes hypercholesterolemia and fasting-associated liver triglycerides accumulation. *bioRxiv* **2023**. [CrossRef]
26. Udomkasemsab, A.; Prangthip, P. High fat diet for induced dyslipidemia and cardiac pathological alterations in Wistar rats compared to Sprague Dawley rats. *Clin. Investig. Arterioscler.* **2019**, *31*, 56–62. [PubMed]
27. Puska, L.G.; Nagy, Z.B.; Giricz, Z.; Onody, A.; Csonka, C.; Kitajka, K.; Hackler, L., Jr.; Zvara, A.; Ferdinandy, P. Cholesterol diet-induced hyperlipidemia influences gene expression pattern of rat hearts: A DNA microarray study. *FEBS Lett.* **2004**, *562*, 99–104. [CrossRef] [PubMed]
28. Liu, Z.; Tian, Z.; Zhao, D.; Liang, Y.; Dai, S.; Liu, M.; Hou, S.; Dong, X.; Zhaxinima; Yang, Y. Effects of coenzyme Q_{10} supplementation on lipid profiles in adults: A meta-analysis of randomized controlled trials. *J. Clin. Endocrinol. Metab.* **2023**, *108*, 232–249. [CrossRef]
29. Singh, D.K.; Li, L.; Porter, T.D. Policosanol inhibits cholesterol synthesis in hepatoma cells by activation of AMP-kinase. *J. Pharmacol. Exp. Ther.* **2006**, *318*, 1020–1026. [CrossRef]

30. Lee, J.H.; Jia, Y.; Thach, T.T.; Han, Y.; Kim, B.; Wu, C.; Kim, Y.; Seo, W.D.; Lee, S.J. Hexacosanol reduces plasma and hepatic cholesterol by activation of AMP-activated protein kinase and suppression of sterol regulatory element-binding protein-2 in HepG2 and C57BL/6J mice. *Nutr. Res.* **2017**, *43*, 89–99. [CrossRef]
31. Taylor, J.C.; Rapport, L.; Lockwood, G.B. Octacosanol in human health. *Nutrition* **2003**, *19*, 192–195. [CrossRef] [PubMed]
32. Bai, J.; Yang, T.; Zhou, Y.; Xu, W.; Han, S.; Guo, T.; Zhu, L.; Qin, D.; Luo, Y.; Hu, Z.; et al. Octacosanol modifies obesity, expression profile and inflammation response of hepatic tissues in high-fat diet mice. *Foods* **2022**, *11*, 1606. [CrossRef]
33. Fernandez-Travieso, J.C.; Rodriguez-Perez, I.; Ruenes-Domech, C.; Fernandez-Dorta, L.; Mendoza-Castano, S. Benefits of the therapy with abexol in patients with non-alcoholic fatty liver disease. *Gastroenterol. Res.* **2020**, *13*, 73. [CrossRef]
34. Molina, V.; Valdés, S.; Carbajal, D.; Arruzazabala, L.; Menéndez, R.; Más, R. Antioxidant effects of D-002 on gastric mucosa of rats with experimentally-induced injury. *J. Med. Food.* **2001**, *4*, 79–83. [CrossRef] [PubMed]
35. Molina, V.; Ledón, T.; Ravelo, Y.; Zamora, Z.; Mena, L. Effects of D-002 (Beeswax alcohols) on concentrations of prostaglandin E2 in rat gastric mucosa. *J. Pharm. Pharm. Res.* **2017**, *1*, 2.
36. Molina, V.; Ravelo, Y.; Zamora, Z.; Mas, R. Effects of D-002 on Non-steroidal anti-inflammatory drugs-induced gastric ulcer in rats. *Int. J. Pharm. Sci. Rev. Res.* **2015**, *30*, 253–257.
37. Dorostghol, M.; Gharibvand, M.M.; Hanafi, M.G.; Motamedfar, A. Comparison of size of the liver between patients with non-alcoholic fatty liver disease and healthy controls. *J. Fam. Med. Prim. Care* **2024**, *13*, 425–430. [CrossRef]
38. Kew, M.C. Serum aminotransferase concentration as evidence of hepatocellular damage. *Lancet* **2000**, *355*, 591–592. [CrossRef]
39. Herrera, J.L. Abnormal liver enzyme levels: The spectrum of causes. *Postgrad. Med.* **1993**, *93*, 113–116. [CrossRef]
40. Esteghamati, A.; Jamali, A.; Khalilzadeh, O.; Noshad, S.; Khalili, M.; Zandieh, A.; Morteza, A.; Nakhjavani, M. Metabolic syndrome is linked to a mild elevation in liver aminotransferases in diabetic patients with undetectable non-alcoholic fatty liver disease by ultrasound. *Diabetol. Metab. Syndr.* **2010**, *2*, 65. [CrossRef]
41. Deb, S.; Puthanveetil, P.; Sakharkar, P. A population-based cross-sectional study of the association between liver enzymes and lipid levels. *Int. J. Hepatol.* **2018**, *2018*, 1286170. [CrossRef] [PubMed]
42. Christian, P.; Sacco, J.; Adeli, K. Autophagy: Emerging roles in lipid homeostasis and metabolic control. *Biochim. Biophys. Acta* **2013**, *1831*, 819–824. [CrossRef]
43. Hussain, T.; Tan, B.; Yin, Y.; Blachier, F.; Tossou, M.C.; Rahu, N. Oxidative stress and inflammation: What polyphenols can do for us? *Oxid. Med. Cell. Longev.* **2016**, *2016*, 7432797. [CrossRef]
44. Qiao, Q.; Bouwman, F.G.; van Baak, M.A.; Roumans, N.J.T.; Vink, R.G.; Mariman, E.C.M. Plasma levels of triglycerides and IL-6 are associated with weight regain and fat mass expansion. *J. Clin. Endocrinol. Metab.* **2022**, *107*, 1920–1929. [CrossRef] [PubMed]
45. Agca, R.; Heslinga, S.C.; Rollefstad, S.; Heslinga, M.; McInnes, I.B.; Peters, M.J.; Kvien, T.K.; Dougados, M.; Radner, H.; Atzeni, F.; et al. EULAR recommendations for cardiovascular disease risk management in patients with rheumatoid arthritis and other forms of inflammatory joint disorders: 2015/2016 update. *Ann. Rheum. Dis.* **2017**, *76*, 17–28. [CrossRef] [PubMed]
46. Steiner, G.; Urowitz, M.B. Lipid profiles in patients with rheumatoid arthritis: Mechanisms and the impact of treatment. *Semin. Arthritis Rheum.* **2009**, *38*, 372–381. [CrossRef]
47. Feingold, K.R.; Grunfeld, C. The effect of inflammation and infection on lipids and lipoproteins. In *Endotext*; Feingold, K.R., Anawalt, B., Boyce, A., Chrousos, G., Dungan, K., Grossman, A., Hershman, J.M., Kaltsas, G., Koch, C., Kopp, P., et al., Eds.; MDText.com, Inc.: South Dartmouth, MA, USA, 2000.
48. Puig, M.N.; Castaño, S.M.; Ferreiro, R.M.; Clara, M.V.; Hernansez, N.M. Effects of oral administration of D-002 (Beeswax alcohols) on histological and functional outcomes in a rat model of antigen-induced arthritis: Preliminary study. *Int. J. Pharmacol. Phytochem. Ethnomed.* **2016**, *5*, 60–68.
49. Puente, R.; Illnait, J.; Mas, R.; Carbajal, D.; Mendoza, S.; Fernández, J.C.; Mesa, M.; Gámez, R.; Reyes, P. Evaluation of the effect of D-002, a mixture of beeswax alcohols, on osteoarthritis symptoms. *Korean J. Intern. Med.* **2014**, *29*, 191–202. [CrossRef]
50. Khosla, S.; Farr, J.N.; Tchkonia, T.; Kirkland, J.L. The role of cellular senescence in ageing and endocrine disease. *Nat. Rev. Endocrinol.* **2020**, *16*, 263–275. [CrossRef]
51. Flensted-Jensen, M.; Oró, D.; Rørbeck, E.A.; Zhang, C.; Madsen, M.R.; Madsen, A.N.; Norlin, J.; Feigh, M.; Larsen, S.; Hansen, H.H. Dietary intervention reverses molecular markers of hepatocellular senescence in the GAN diet-induced obese and biopsy-confirmed mouse model of NASH. *BMC Gastroenterol.* **2024**, *24*, 59. [CrossRef]
52. Sahadevan, M.; Kasiske, B.L. Hyperlipidemia in kidney disease causes and consequences. *Curr. Opin. Nephrol. Hypertens.* **2002**, *11*, 323–329. [CrossRef] [PubMed]
53. Çiftci, G.; Tuna, E. Effects of cholesterol and *Lactobacillus acidophilus* on testicular function. *Clin. Exp. Reprod. Med.* **2021**, *48*, 229. [CrossRef]
54. Jing, J.; Ding, N.; Wang, D.; Ge, X.; Ma, J.; Ma, R.; Hung, X.; Jueraitetibaike, K.; Liang, K.; Wang, S.; et al. Oxidized-LDL inhibits testosterone biosynthesis by affecting mitochondrial function and the p38 MAPK/COX-2 signaling pathway in Leydig cells. *Cell Death Dis.* **2020**, *11*, 626. [CrossRef]
55. Nousis, L.; Kanavaros, P.; Barbouti, A. Oxidative stress-induced cellular senescence: Is labile iron the connecting link? *Antioxidants* **2023**, *12*, 1250. [CrossRef] [PubMed]
56. Okada, S.; Saito, M.; Kazuyama, E.; Hanada, T.; Kawaba, Y.; Hayashi, A.; Satoh, K.; Kanzaki, S. Effects of *N*-hexacosanol on nitric oxide synthase system in diabetic rat nephropathy. *Mol. Cell. Biochem.* **2008**, *315*, 169–177. [CrossRef]

57. Saito, M.; Kinoshita, Y.; Satoh, I.; Shinbori, C.; Kono, T.; Hanada, T.; Uemasu, J.; Suzuki, H.; Yamada, M.; Satoh, K. *N*-hexacosanol ameliorates streptozotocin-induced diabetic rat nephropathy. *Eur. J. Pharmacol* **2006**, *544*, 132–137. [CrossRef]
58. (NRC) National Research Council of the National Academy of Sciences. *Guide for the Care and Use of Laboratory Animals*; National Academy Press: Washington, DC, USA, 2010.
59. Cho, K.-H.; Kim, J.-E.; Bahuguna, A.; Kang, D.-J. Long-term supplementation of ozonated sunflower oil improves dyslipidemia and hepatic inflammation in hyperlipidemic zebrafish: Suppression of oxidative stress and inflammation against carboxymethyllysine toxicity. *Antioxidants* **2023**, *12*, 1240. [CrossRef]
60. Cho, K.-H.; Bahuguna, A.; Kim, J.-E.; Lee, Y.; Lee, S.H. Comparative Assessment of Beeswax Alcohol and Coenzyme Q_{10} (CoQ_{10}) to Prevent Liver Aging, Organ Damage, and Oxidative Stress in Hyperlipidemic Zebrafish Exposed to D-Galactose: A 12-Week Dietary Intervention. *Pharmaceuticals* **2024**, *17*, 1250. [CrossRef] [PubMed]
61. Fischer, A.H.; Jacobson, K.A.; Rose, J.; Zeller, R. Hematoxylin and eosin staining of tissue and cell sections. *Cold Spring Harb. Protoc.* **2008**, *2008*, prot4986. [CrossRef] [PubMed]
62. Lee, E.-Y.; Cho, K.-H. High-dose consumption of NaCl resulted in severe degradation of lipoproteins associated with hyperlipidemia, hyperglycemia, and infertility via impairment of testicular spermatogenesis. *Toxicol. Res.* **2016**, *5*, 557–569. [CrossRef]
63. Koc, N.D.; Teksöz, N.; Ural, M.; Akbulut, C. Histological structure of zebrafish (*Danio rerio*, Hamilton, 1822) testicles. *Elixir Aquacult.* **2012**, *46*, 8117–8120.
64. Sutha, J.; Anila, P.A.; Gayathri, M.; Ramesh, M. Long term exposure to tris (2-chloroethyl) phosphate (TCEP) causes alterations in reproductive hormones, vitellogenin, antioxidant enzymes, and histology of gonads in zebrafish (*Danio rerio*): In vivo and computational analysis. *Comp. Biochem. Physiol. Toxicol. Pharmacol. CBP* **2022**, *254*, 109263.
65. Patel, U.N.; Patel, U.D.; Khadayata, A.V.; Vaja, R.K.; Modi, C.M.; Patel, H.B. Long-term exposure of the binary mixture of cadmium and mercury damages the developed ovary of adult zebrafish. *Environ. Sci. Pollut. Res. Int.* **2022**, *29*, 44928–44938.
66. Cho, K.-H.; Bahuguna, A.; Kang, D.-J.; Kim, J.-E. Prolonged supplementation of ozonated sunflower oil bestows an antiaging effect, improves blood lipid profile and spinal deformities, and protects vital organs of zebrafish (*Danio rerio*) against age-related degeneration: Two-years consumption study. *Antioxidants* **2024**, *13*, 123. [CrossRef] [PubMed]
67. Al-Ghamdi, T.H.; Atta, I.S. Efficacy of interleukin-6 in the induction of liver cell proliferation after hemi-hepatectomy: Histopathologic and immunohistochemical study. *Int. J. Clin. Exp. Pathol.* **2020**, *13*, 1540–1549. [PubMed]
68. Owusu-Ansah, E.; Yavari, A.; Mandal, S.; Banerjee, U. Distinct mitochondrial retrograde signals control the G1-S cell cycle checkpoint. *Nat. Genet.* **2008**, *40*, 356–361. [CrossRef] [PubMed]

pharmaceuticals

MDPI

Article

An Advanced Combinatorial System from *Vitis vinifera* Leaves and Propolis Enhances Antioxidants' Skin Delivery and Fibroblasts Functionality

Sophia Athanasopoulou [1], Eleni Spanidi [1], Eleni Panagiotidou [1], Andrea Cavagnino [2], Anaïs Bobier [2] and Konstantinos Gardikis [1,3,*]

[1] Research and Development Department, APIVITA SA, Industrial Park Markopoulo Mesogaias, 19003 Athens, Greece; sofia.athanasopoulou@puig.com (S.A.); eleni.spanidi@puig.com (E.S.); eleni.panagiotidou@puig.com (E.P.)

[2] OxiProteomics SAS, 2 Rue Antoine Etex, 94000 Creteil, France; contact@oxiproteomics.fr (A.C.)

[3] Department of Pharmacy, Frederick University, Nicosia 1036, Cyprus

* Correspondence: konstantinos.gardikis@puig.com

Abstract: Background/Objectives: Vine leaves are a bulky by-product that are disposed of and treated as waste in the wine production process. In the present study polyphenols from vine leaves were extracted and simultaneously encapsulated in a new delivery system consisting of liposomes and cyclodextrins. This system was further combined with propolis polyphenols encapsulated in cyclodextrins, resulting in a colloidal suspension for the release of antioxidants in a time-controlled way, the rate of which depends on the ratio of the materials. The result is a raw material that exhibits antioxidant and ECM protective effects when administered in skin fibroblasts (NHDFs). **Methods**: The antioxidant and ECM promoting efficacy of the produced raw material was assessed by the Folin–Ciocalteu method, DPPH assay, and in cellulo assays in fibroblasts, such as the cell viability assay, scratch assay, cell migration assay, gene expression analysis, and immunofluorescence analysis, for the detection, visualization, and quantification of collagen-I, collagen-IIIa, and elastin signals and collagenase assay. **Results**: Treatment of NHDFs with the combinatorial delivery system promoted collagen and elastin synthesis and deposition in normal conditions and, upon induced external stress, as assessed by in vitro transcriptomic and proteomic analysis. A significant inhibition of collagenase was also observed, suggesting a multitargeted efficacy of the active ingredients also by preventing collagen degradation. **Conclusions**: Therefore, this liposome–cyclodextrin encapsulated polyphenol complex represents a novel bioactive ingredient with promising skin applications.

Keywords: polyphenols; collagen; elastin; skin delivery system

1. Introduction

Skin aging is a complex process that involves various biological mechanisms, including oxidative stress, inflammation, and degradation of the extracellular matrix (ECM) components. Age-dependent deterioration of the ECM involves alterations in collagen turnover and decreased levels of elastin—two essential proteins for healthy skin tissue. In young skin, collagen provides structure and support to the skin, while elastin helps it to stay flexible and elastic. As skin ages, the production of collagen and elastin by fibroblasts naturally declines, leading to wrinkles, sagging skin, and other signs of aging. Collagen crosslinks stabilize, while collagen bundles become disorganized. Polyphenols are a group of natural compounds widely found in plants and have been reported to exhibit strong antioxidant activity [1]. Polyphenols deriving from natural sources, have been shown to help reverse this decline by stimulating the production of functional collagen and elastin in skin cells [2–5].

Vine leaves are a bulky by-product which is generated during winemaking and viticulture processes, often considered as agricultural waste, and discarded or burned, leading to environmental pollution. Their applications to date have been limited, at best, to a small number of edible products and at worst to the creation of a soil enhancer. However, recent research has shed light on the potential of upcycling waste from vine leaves into valuable cosmeceutical ingredients [6,7]. Grapes and grape products, as sources of bioactive chemicals applied in cosmetic manufacture, constitute an environmentally friendly alternative for generated residues. The active ingredients from these sources are potentially very valuable to the cosmetics industry, which is always in search of new and sustainable sources for effective raw materials. Vine leaves are rich in various bioactive compounds, including polyphenols, flavonoids, and organic acids, which are known for their antioxidant, anti-inflammatory, and anti-aging properties [8]. Flavonoids are a type of polyphenol that have been shown to possess anti-inflammatory properties and protect the skin from UV radiation-induced damage [9,10]. Organic acids, such as tartaric acid and malic acid, are also present in vine leaves, and have been reported to exhibit exfoliating and brightening effects on the skin [11]. These bioactive compounds make waste from vine leaves a promising source of cosmeceutical ingredients.

Polyphenols are the most abundant and the most studied class of bioactive compounds present in *Vitis vinifera* leaves. They represent secondary metabolites and include phenolic acids, coumarins, flavonoids, stilbenes, and lignans [8]. Previous studies from our lab on vine leaf extracts from the area of Santorini, Greece, have indicated significant transcriptional and epigenetic effect on UVA stressed fibroblasts. The specific extract was shown to activate two genes with important roles in the anti-aging and ECM organization processes, namely SIRT-1 and HSP-47, via their transcriptional upregulation, which has been shown to be mechanistically linked with an observed demethylation of their promoters.

Propolis is another natural product that demonstrates important antioxidant, anti-aging and anti-inflammatory activities [12–14]. Raw propolis, a natural resinous substance produced by honeybees (*Apis mellifera* L.), results from the combination of their saliva containing enzymes, beeswax, and resins from plant sources. Its main constituents include 50–60% resins, 30–40% waxes and fatty acids, 5–10% essential oils, approximately 5% pollen, and 5% other compounds, such as amino acids and vitamins. The chemical composition, colors, and biological activities of propolis vary based on bee race, geographical origin, and the specific plant or tree species used by bees for collecting pollen and exudates, as well as the sampling season [15–18]. According to a plethora of studies, the main secondary metabolites in propolis are phenolic substances, especially flavonoids, belonging to different sub-classes such as flavanones, flavones, flavonols, and dihydroflavonols, which constitute more than 50% of the propolis weight. Other phenolic compounds found in abundance in propolis are hydroquinones, caffeic acids and related esters, and phenolic aldehydes [19].

In recent years, the interest in the potential use of propolis polyphenols in cosmeceutical applications, including skincare products has increased, due to their beneficial effects on skin health and appearance.

Several studies have investigated the anti-aging effects of propolis polyphenols in cosmeceutical applications [20,21]. For instance, a study by González-Masís et al. (2020) found that propolis polyphenols increased cell metabolic activity and cell proliferation in human skin fibroblasts, mechanisms that are responsible for synthesizing ECM components, such as collagen and elastin [22]. Another study by Franchin et al. (2016) evaluated in vivo, in mammalian model organisms the effects of isoflavonoids of propolis, in acute and chronic inflammation and found a potential anti-inflammatory activity that could alleviate skin tissue aging due to chronic inflammation [23,24].

Complementary to the anti-aging effect of propolis, several studies have demonstrated the antioxidant effects of propolis polyphenols in cosmeceutical applications. For example, a study by Lagouri et al. (2014) found that propolis polyphenols extracted from Greek propolis exhibited strong antioxidant activity, as evidenced by their ability to scavenge reactive oxygen species (ROS) [25]. Another in vitro study has demonstrated the antioxidant activity of propolis polyphenols by inhibiting lipid peroxidation in human skin cells [26]. The antioxidant effects of a propolis-based cream in human volunteers were evaluated by Diniz et al. (2019) who found that the cream significantly reduced biomarkers of oxidative stress cell damage in healthy humans, with increased antioxidant enzymatic capacity, especially of superoxide dismutase (SOD) [27]. Previous studies have identified that propolis extracts collected from different geographical areas in Greece demonstrate significant differentiation on their chromatographic profile and concentration of bioactive components, with this diversity also being reflected in their biological activity [28,29]. For instance, samples originating from Central Greece are characterized as very rich in flavonoids, compared to samples from other regions of Greece, and show high antioxidant and anti-collagenase activity [30].

Studies from our lab on a specific propolis extract from Olympus Mountain (Central Greece) have demonstrated that it confers significant protection against the cytotoxic effects of UVB radiation by remarkably reducing DNA and protein oxidation damage levels in human immortalized keratinocytes (HaCaT). It also demonstrated significant anti-aging efficacy, as it decreased histological damage and also decreased the induced expression of certain metalloproteinases (MMPs) following exposure to UVB in a reconstituted skin model [9].

To address a complex issue, such as UV-induced dermal cell damage, our target was to develop a combinatorial delivery system incorporating polyphenols from different sources and of different types, called the vine propolis delivery system (VPDS), aiming at specific molecular targets. Propolis and *Vitis vinifera* leaves were chosen as polyphenol sources due to the high concentration of different polyphenols they contain, and due to the significant efficacy of those specific extracts in mechanisms that support skin cell functionality. Our analytical results were in line with the literature [31,32].

More specifically, polyphenols from vine leaves were extracted and simultaneously encapsulated in a new combinatorial system for cosmeceutical use, consisting of liposomes and cyclodextrins. In parallel, polyphenols from propolis collected from Mount Olympus, Greece, were encapsulated in the system resulting in a colloidal suspension that releases polyphenols in a time-controlled way.

In the present study, which presents the results of research concerning an innovative approach to natural anti-aging biomaterials, we focused on the antioxidant activity of the combinatorial system of vine leaves and propolis polyphenols and its potential to synergistically increase the functionality of fibroblasts in protein levels, by stimulating collagen and elastin protein production, along with its effect in cell proliferation, cell migration, and the transcriptional regulation of genes implicated in cellular growth, cell adhesion and contractility.

2. Results

2.1. Experimental Results

2.1.1. Phytochemical Assays

The encapsulation efficiency of polyphenols in the VPDS 91% ± 4% when the initial materials contain total polyphenol compounds exceeded 16 μg GA/mL, as described in the Materials and Methods section.

Table 1 depicts the mean hydrodynamic diameter, polydispersity index, and ζ-potential of the system at day 1, and after 1 month at various temperatures. The values remain practically stable except for the temperature of 38 °C, where there is a statistically significant increase in particle size, possibly attributed to particle aggregation.

The initial concentration of total phenols was 709 ± 22 μg GA/mL, while the antioxidant capacity was 5.23 ± 2.39 mM Trolox equivalents. Over the course of 24 weeks, both the antioxidant capacity and total polyphenols remained stable without significant fluctuations (Table 2).

The values of phytochemical parameters, such as pH value, refractive index, and density, were stable at different temperatures and time points for 24 weeks. The in vitro controlled release of the VPDS system was studied using only cyclodextrins and prior to the addition of the liposome (Figure 1).

Table 1. Hydrodynamic diameter, polydispersity index, and ζ-potential of the system at day 1, and after 1 month at various temperatures.

Time	Conditions	z-Average Diameter (nm)	SD	PI	SD	ζ-pot (mV)	SD
T (0)	25 °C	444	63	0.455	0.059	−18	5.2
Day 30	6 °C	501	50	0.477	0.084	−16	3.0
Day 30	38 °C	821	199	0.616	0.105	−21	2.9
Day 30	25 °C	609	111	0.516	0.099	−22	3.2

Table 2. Evaluation of stability test of DPPH: Antioxidant activity (± SD) and TPCs (± SD) of the VPDS.

Time	Conditions	TPC (μg GA/mL)			DPPH (mM Trolox Equivalent)		
T(0)		709	±	22	5.23	±	2.36
Day 30	RT	640	±	38	4.75	±	2.20
	6 °C	535	±	44	4.96	±	2.16
	38 °C	550	±	31	4.59	±	1.63
	25 °C	502	±	28	4.73	±	1.67

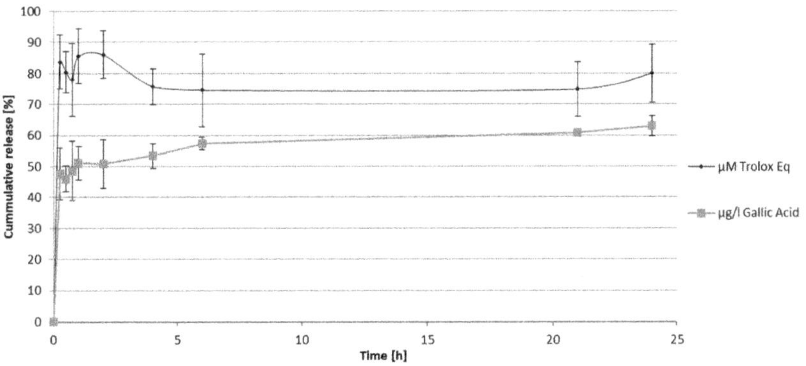

Figure 1. In vitro release profile of vine leaves and propolis combinational extract in cyclodextrins measuring antioxidant activity against DPPH free radical (μM Trolox Eq.) (± SD) and total phenolic content-TPC (μg/L gallic acid) (± SD).

As shown in Figure 1, about 80% of the antioxidant activity is released in the first 15 min and, at the same time, about 50% of the total phenolic compounds are released.

The in vitro release profile of VPDS system as a function of time is presented below in Figure 2. The release of the antioxidant activity reaches practically a plateau at 4 h and the content of the total phenolic compounds are reached at 6 h.

2.1.2. Cell Viability and Migration Assay

To assess the effect of the active ingredients on cell viability, an MTT Assay using three different concentrations of VPDS (0.1% *v*/*v*, 0.2% *v*/*v* and 0.5% *v*/*v*) was performed in NHDFs. An increase in cell metabolism and proliferation by 20% was demonstrated with the concentration of active ingredients at 0.1% *v*/*v*. This effect was not observed when the concentration was doubled or 5 times higher (Figure 3A).

Following the cell viability assay that determined the optimal concentration of the active, we performed a cell migration assay (scratch assay) in a confluent monolayer of NHDFs to assess the potential wound healing action of the active ingredients. The in vitro cell migration assay (scratch assay) that was conducted in NHDFs demonstrated a significant closure (−33%) of the "wound" after 24 h of treatment with VPDS 0.1% v/v (Figure 3B).

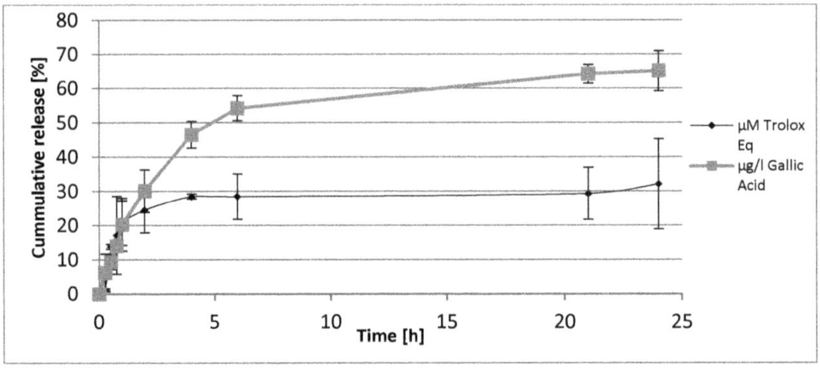

Figure 2. In vitro release of antioxidant activity with free radical DPPH (μM Trolox Eq.) (±SD) and total phenolic content -TPC (μg/L gallic acid) (±SD) of VPDS for time 0 to 24 h.

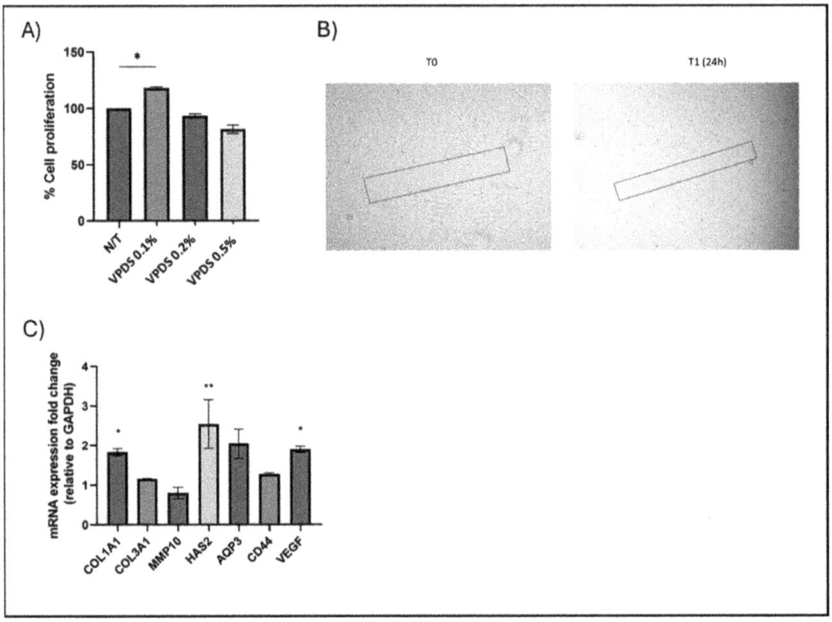

Figure 3. (**A**). Cell viability assay showing that VPDS 0.1% v/v increased cell metabolism and proliferation by +20%; (**B**). Cell migration assay. Representative images from the wound healing assay of NHDF cell cultures treated with the active ingredients demonstrated that cell invasion into the cell-free region (outlined) after 24 h of treatment with VPDS 0.1% v/v (decreasing the cell free area by 33%); (**C**). Transcriptional regulation of key genes of fibroblasts' functionality showing that VPDS 0.1% v/v increased the expression of key genes: +80% for Col1A1, +150% for HAS2, and +90% for VEGF. (* p-value < 0.05,** p-value < 0.01).

2.1.3. Transcriptomic Assays

To further examine the observed increase in cell proliferation and wound healing, we tested potential transcriptional changes in key genes of fibroblast functionality, related with ECM remodeling, hyaluronan synthesis, and a major orchestrator of tissue repair and wound healing, VEGF. A real time PCR analysis demonstrated that VPDS 0.1% *v*/*v* increased the expression of key genes of fibroblasts' functionality: +80% for Col1A1; +150% for hyaluronan synthase-2 (HAS2); and +90% for VEGF (Figure 3C).

2.1.4. Immunofluorescence Assays

The efficacy of VPDS 0.1% *v*/*v* was additionally tested upon exposure of fibroblasts to a combination of stressors, namely UVA irradiation and the addition of particulate matter (ERMCZ100 PM10-like—PAHs; 1 $\mu g/cm^2$), mimicking the condition of stress from urban pollution.

VPDS 0.1% *v*/*v* counteracted the changes induced by the UVA/pollution stress in dermal fibroblasts, restoring the levels of collagen and elastin. More specifically, in situ analyses of collagen-I, collagen-IIIa, and elastin were performed by epi-fluorescence microscopy via specific immunofluorescence detection. As shown in Figure 4, the presence of the active ingredient cancelled out the effects of stress exposure.

The quantification of collagen-I levels was carried out by integrating the intensity of the specific signal over the surface of evaluation, normalized by the number of cells. Three images per condition were analyzed and the results are reported as histograms (Figure 4A(i),B(i)). The levels of collagen-I decreased upon pollution exposure. The presence of VPDS 0.1% *v*/*v* contrasted with the stress-induced decrease of collagen-I.

Quantification of the collagen-IIIa levels was carried out by integrating the intensity of the specific signal over the surface of evaluation, normalized by the number of cells. Three images per condition were analyzed, and the results are reported as histograms (Figure 4A(ii),4B(ii)). The levels of collagen-IIIa increased upon pollution exposure. The presence of VPDS 0.1% *v*/*v* counteracted the stress-induced increase of collagen-IIIa.

Similarly, for elastin levels, their quantification was carried out by integrating the intensity of the specific signal over the surface of evaluation, normalized by the number of cells. Three images per condition were analyzed and the results are reported as histograms (Figure 4A(iii),B(iii)).

A significant decrease of the collagen-I levels was observed in NHDFs, where pollution stress was applied in comparison with unstressed NHDFs. For collagen-IIIa, a significant increase of its levels was detected upon stress, in comparison with both unstressed NHDFs, but also with cells treated with the active ingredients for 24 h, where the increase was efficiently counteracted.

2.1.5. ELISA-Enzymatic Assays

After having confirmed that the active ingredients counteracted the changes induced by the UVA/pollution stress in dermal fibroblasts by restoring levels of collagen and elastin, we further investigated its effects in collagen and elastin production in late passage fibroblasts. A statistically significant increase in elastin levels was confirmed in treated NHDFs with a 4-fold change, compared to untreated cells. Moreover, we measured the levels of the two types of collagen and their ratio in untreated and treated with the active ingredients in late passage NHDFs, in comparison with the levels from young passage NHDFs, as the immunofluorescence experiments had shown an increase of collagen-IIIa upon exposure to pollution stress and a decrease of collagen-I levels. A statistically significant difference was observed between the ratio of young passage dermal fibroblasts and untreated late passage fibroblasts for the two types of collagen, with the ratio of the latter being 3-fold lower than the ratio of young passage fibroblasts.

Additionally, we tested the inhibitory effect of the VPDS, along with its different components (*Vitis vinifera* leaves and propolis extracts) in the enzyme collagenase. The complex showed a statistically significant inhibition of collagenase at the same rate with the propolis extract, leading to the assumption that the inhibitory action is mainly attributable to the latter.

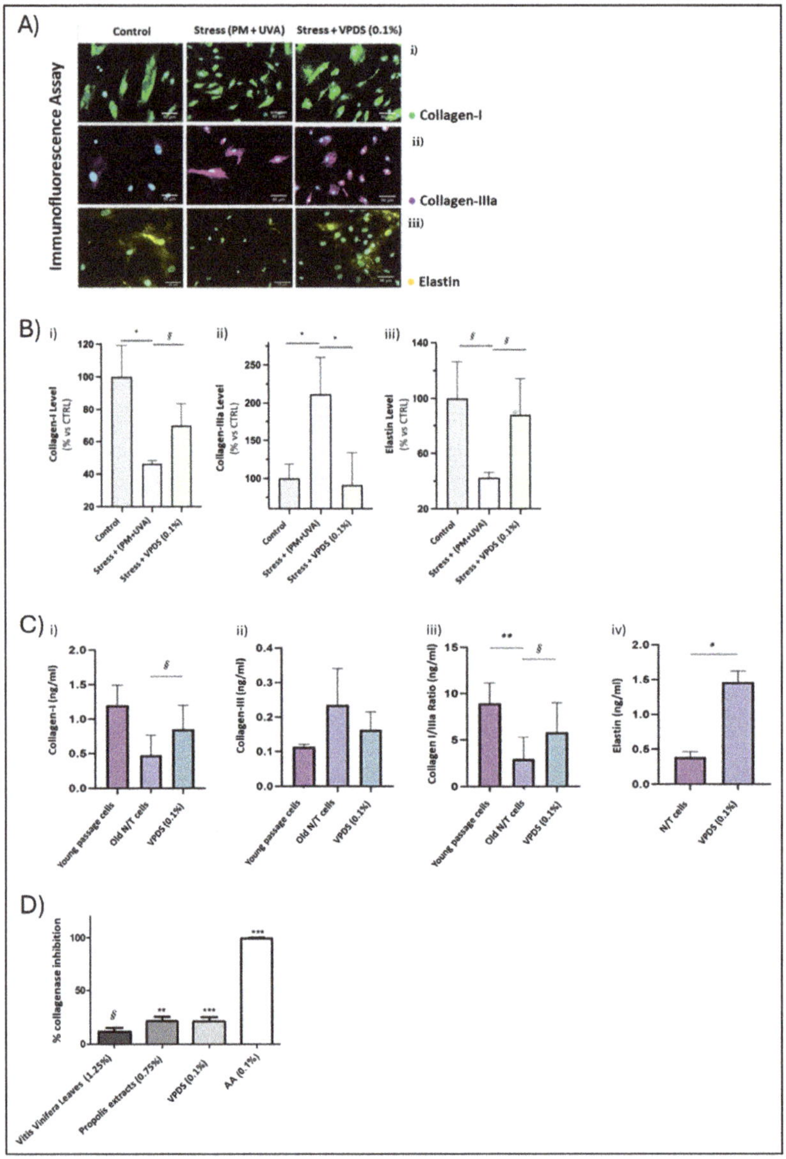

Figure 4. (**A**) (**i**) In situ visualization of Collagen-I (in green). The specific signal of collagen-I immunofluorescence detection is visualized in green and superposed to cell nuclei (DAPI, in cyan). (**ii**) In situ visualization of collagen-IIIa (in purple). The specific signal of collagen-IIIa immunofluorescence detection is visualized in purple and superposed to cell nuclei (DAPI, in cyan). (**iii**) In situ visualization of elastin (in yellow). The specific signal of elastin immunofluorescence detection is visualized in yellow and superposed to cell nuclei (DAPI, in cyan). (**B**) (**i**) Graph bar representation of the quantification of collagen-I by detection of specific signal normalized by the number of cells and on the control group * $p < 0.05$ § $p < 0.1$—*t*-test for binary comparisons versus stress group (unpaired, two-ways). (**ii**) Graph bar representation of the quantification of collagen-IIIa by detection of specific signal normalized by the number of cells and on the control group * $p < 0.05$—*t*-test for binary comparisons versus stress group (unpaired, two-ways). (**iii**) Graph bar

representation of the quantification of elastin by detection of specific signal normalized by the number of cells and on the control group § $p < 0.1$—t-test for binary comparisons versus stress group (unpaired, two-ways). (**C**) (**i**) Graph bar representation of the quantification of collagen-I by detection of protein level in NDHFs § $p < 0.1$—t-tests for comparison of young passage fibroblasts untreated, old passage untreated and old passage treated. (**ii**) Graph bar representation of the quantification of collagen-IIIa by detection of protein level in NDHFs § $p < 0.1$—t-tests for comparison of young passage fibroblasts untreated, old passage untreated and old passage treated. (**iii**) Graph bar representation of the ratio of collagen-I/-IIIa in young passage cells and upon replicative senescence of treated and untreated NHDFs. (**iv**) Graph bar representation of the quantification of elastin by detection of protein level in NDHFs * $p < 0.05$ t-tests for comparison old passage fibroblasts untreated and treated. (**D**) Inhibition of collagenase. Mean (±SEM, N = 4), *** $p < 0.001$ ** $p < 0.01$ § $p < 0.1$—one-way ANOVA (Dunnett's multiple comparisons test).

3. Discussion

Combining vine leaves polyphenols with propolis polyphenols may have several potential benefits due to their individual and synergistic effects. We here focused on the combination's beneficial effects in dermal fibroblast's functionality for potential use as a cosmeceutical with anti-aging and antioxidant properties.

Using a high diversity of polyphenols has been previously shown to increase the potential biological benefits of those molecules [4], and our screening in vitro results proved this assumption).

To overcome the issue of polyphenol degradation over time, vine leaves and propolis polyphenols were encapsulated in two distinct delivery systems: liposomes/cyclodextrins and cyclodextrins, respectively [33,34]. The reasoning behind the choice of those materials was initially the already demonstrated ability of combinatorial liposome/cyclodextrin systems to achieve controlled release of encapsulated substances. The use of the combination of liposomes and cyclodextrins is based on the concept of advanced drug delivery nanosystems [35]. In such systems, materials of a different nature are used aiming to modulate the release rate of encapsulated molecules, as well as to increase entrapment efficiency and low leakage of drugs. Specifically on the interaction of cyclodextrins with liposomes, several successful attempts have been performed [33,34,36]. Such drug-in-cyclodextrin-in-liposome (DCL) systems are based on the physicochemical interactions between cyclodextrins and phospholipids resulting in creating membranes of altered fluidity that can prove beneficial for controlled delivery of bioactive molecules [37].

For propolis polyphenols, a propolis–cyclodextrin complex was designed, achieving an almost instant release of polyphenols, polyphenol stability, as well as solubility in highly polar solvents.

This technological platform that can deliver a wide diversity of polyphenols to the human skin in a time-controlled way was assessed against various factors of skin aging.

Aging skin is known to have an impaired barrier function, which leads to a dry appearance and increased sensitivity to external aggressors, increasing the risk for skin problems [38]. The principal changes in aging skin, aside from the uneven texture and pigmentation of the epidermis, take place at the level of the dermal connective tissue and primarily manifest as the loss of mature collagen and modifications to the elastic network [39]. Elastases and matrix metalloproteinases (MMPs) are two of the enzymes that break down ECM. These endopeptidases play significant roles in several physiological processes, including tissue repair and remodeling, cell migration and differentiation, or wound healing [40,41]. They are responsible for the turnover of several ECM components, including all types of collagen and elastin, while increased levels of their enzymatic activities have been associated with a variety of pathological conditions and adverse effects, including accelerated skin aging.

It is well recognized that phenolic chemicals, such as the primary phenolics found in red grapes called anthocyanins, not only have well-known antioxidant characteristics but have the power to directly inhibit skin-aging enzymes, such as collagenase (MMP-1). In this regard, it was expected and finally proven that these bioactive compounds encountered in the winery residues used, let alone in their combination with propolis polyphenols, exhibited potential ECM protecting properties.

To assess the bioactivity of this in-house produced new combinatorial polyphenol release system, we first examined the effects of different concentrations of VPDS on cellular proliferation and metabolic activity via an MTT assay. Given the important observed increase in cell viability and metabolism of NHDFs treated with VPDS in the concentration of 0.1%, we assessed the molecular activity of the active ingredients by targeting a panel of genes representative of ECM structural proteins, in association with regulatory genes involved in pathways that modulate growth factors, cell adhesion, and contractility.

We observed an enhanced expression of collagen-I, one of the most important providers of structural support to the ECM and a well-known activator of dermal fibroblasts [42,43]. The levels of the ECM protein elastin also increased upon treatment with VPDS. This outcome, in association with the upregulated expression of the Col1A1 gene is indicative of a regulatory role of the system in normal ECM remodeling. Interestingly, the increase in elastin protein levels is confirmed not only upon treatment of NHDFs exposed in UV and pollution stress, but in fibroblasts that had undergone replicative senescence.

More specifically, a statistically significant increase in elastin levels was confirmed in old passage NHDFs treated with VPDS. Moreover, we observed a decrease in collagen-I protein levels accompanied by a simultaneous increase in collagen-IIIa in NHDFs that had undergone pollution stress (exposure to UVA and particulate matter). Interestingly, we show that collagen-I and collagen-IIIa protein levels were reversed after 24 h treatment with VPDS. Thus, we evaluated and compared the ratio of the protein levels of collagen-I and collagen IIIa (collagen type I/III) in untreated and treated late passage NHDFs with the ratio of untreated young passage NHDFs. A statistically significant difference was observed between the collagen ratio of young passage dermal fibroblasts and untreated late passage fibroblasts. Interestingly, in a translational approach of these findings, a similar observation in the ratio of the two types of collagen has also been reported in vivo and more specifically in the skin of patients where skin deformation type of facial aging was assessed. Early development of ptosis has been more rapid in patients with a reduced collagen type I/III ratio. Histological examination of these patients indicated the immaturity of connective tissue, suggesting a prognostic value of the collagen-I/IIIa ratio [44].

Fibrillar collagen-IIIa is found in abundance in the skin of the fetus, while less is found in adult skin. Moreover, it can be found in fibers along with type I collagen fibrils in the reticular organs and blood vessel walls [45]. Collagen-IIIa is abundant in hollow organs, such as vocal cords, but it also interacts with platelets during blood coagulation (through specific glycoproteins and non-integrin receptors) and is a crucial signaling molecule in tissue regeneration (by taking part in cellular adhesion, migration, proliferation, and differentiation through interaction with receptors on the cell surface, including integrins) [46]. In the transcriptional study, the expression of the Col3A1 gene did not present upregulation, suggesting that in normal conditions collagen type IIIa is beneficial when expressed in steady levels.

A significant upregulation of HAS2 expression was also demonstrated, suggesting the implication of the ingredient in hyaluronic acid (HA) synthesis. HA is a basic linear polymer that results in a massive hydrophilic molecule that imparts a significant amount of moisture and supports the turgor and flexibility of healthy skin. Yet HA serves vital metabolic and physiological purposes that were previously largely underappreciated, in addition to aesthetic ones. By its interaction with the important cell-surface receptor CD44, extracellular HA regulates the fibroblasts' physiology. Via CD44 interactions with the cytoskeleton, EGF, and TGF receptors, this relationship promotes intracellular signaling for cellular proliferation both directly and indirectly [47]. Stress conditions, either UVB exposure or serum starvation, have been shown to reduce HAS2 expression in human primary skin fibroblasts, resulting in an increased susceptibility to stress-induced apoptosis [48]. Increase in HAS-2 expression, therefore, may contribute to efficient HA generation for the development of a pericellular HA coat and supporting and stimulating ECM molecule production [47]. An increasing trend was also demonstrated in both the CD44 gene that encodes the receptor of HA, along with the Aquaporin-3 (AQP-3) gene. HA is a natural regulator of AQP-3, a protein responsible for transmembrane water transport in human skin, with an important role in the epithelial barrier structure; thus, it is possible that HAS2 upregulation may trigger in a latter phase an increase also in this protein, as they have a synergetic function in the skin ECM [49].

Interestingly, and in accordance with the wound healing effect of the bioactive ingredient, an increase in the expression of VEGF was also detected. As the latter has been shown to orchestrate the expression of growth factor genes and cell migration, its upregulation is coherent with previous studies that have emphasized the role of known vine polyphenols also in wound healing in vitro and in model organisms [50]. VEGF is also a factor that, apart from being a key mediator in vascular remodeling, has also been demonstrated to promote specific ECM synthesis and fibroblast activation [51]. Moreover, regarding wound healing processes, collagen-I, which plays a crucial function in enhancing connective tissue by maintaining tissue health and providing an ECM outline for cellular adhesion and migration, is also involved. Collagen's role in wound healing is to attract fibroblasts and make the deposition of newly formed collagen easier [23]. Massive MMPs are produced by chronic wounds, which hinder the normal healing process [52]. The ECM's excessive MMPs are pickled and arrested by collagen. Hence the extract's induction of the relative expression of type I collagen can also support wound healing by preventing chronic inflammation [52].

In addition to the demonstrated upregulation in the expression of collagen-I, a significant inhibition of collagenase was also observed, suggesting a multitargeted efficacy of the active both by enhancing the formation of new collagen and by preventing its degradation in the ECM.

Overall, our obtained results demonstrate that the innovative combinatorial system of polyphenols from vine leaves encapsulated in cyclodextrins and liposomes along with propolis polyphenols in cyclodextrins shows significant effects in the functionalities of dermal fibroblasts for an effective ECM remodeling.

These results are in line with the DPPH assay that demonstrated significant antioxidant activity, which was furthermore stable after accelerated aging for one month.

4. Materials and Methods

4.1. Preparation of Combinatorial Delivery System

To produce the VPDS, *Vitis vinifera* leaves cultivated on Santorini Island in Greece were used at a concentration of 1.5% (*w*/*w*). Additionally, organic certified raw propolis sourced from Greek cultivation, specifically from the Olympus Mountain region (30% *w*/*w*), was incorporated. To optimize encapsulation efficiency, the raw materials—*Vitis vinifera* leaves and raw propolis—should contain total polyphenol compounds exceeding 16 µg GA/mL. This involves dissolving 5% (*v*/*w*) of the raw materials in methanol (PanReac, AppliChem, Darmstadt, Germany) and measuring the resulting solution using a spectrophotometer via the Folin–Ciocalteu method. As solvents, ultrapure water produced at APIVITA with a Reverse Osmosis System and 1.3 propanediol (Connect Chemicals, Vimercate (MB), Italy) in a 60/40 ratio were used. Additionally, 6% (*w*/*w*) hydroxypropyl-β-cyclodextrin (Gangwal Chemicals Pvt. Ltd., Mumbai, India) was dispersed in the solvent system. After seven days, the resulting mixture underwent filtration using a 25 µm nylon bag. Intense stirring at 3000 rpm facilitated the addition of 3% *w*/*w* liposomes (Pro-Lipo™ Neo), which contained propanediol (75.0% *w*/*w*), lecithin (25.0% *w*/*w*), tocopherol (0.25% *w*/*w*), and Helianthus annuus (sunflower) seed Oil (0.15% *w*/*w*). These liposomes were provided by *Generex pharmacist* Pvt. Ltd., Mumbai, India/Lucas Meyer Cosmetics, Massy, France. Following three days of storage at 6 °C, the mixture underwent further filtration through a 0.22 µm Millipore membrane filter and aliquots were stored at 25 °C, 6 °C and 38 °C.

4.2. Physicochemical Characterization of VPDS

The VPDS was characterized as described by Spanidi et al. (2021) [33]. The hydrodynamic diameter of the CRPP system was measured by light scattering. Then, 100 μL of the liposomal suspension was diluted 30-fold immediately after preparation or after reconstitution and z-average mean and ζ-potential of the formulations were measured. Samples were scattered (633 nm) at 90° angle, and measurements were made at 25 °C in a photon correlation spectrometer (Zetasizer Pro, Malvern Instruments, Malvern, UK).

4.3. VPDS Encapsulation Efficiency

The encapsulation efficiency was calculated by the equation:

$$EE = \text{entrapped polyphenols}/\text{initial polyphenols} \times 100$$

Entrapped polyphenols is the total phenolic content measured in the final system, as described in the TPC section. Initial polyphenols refer to the total phenolic content of the initial materials when dissolved in methanol, as described by Spanidi et al. [33].

4.4. Total Phenolic Content (TPC)

The TPC was determined using the Folin-Ciocalteu method according to the method by Arnous et al. [53].

4.5. Antioxidant Activity by 2,2-Diphenylpicrylhydrazyl (DPPH)

The antioxidant activity of the colloidal systems was determined by using 2,2-diphenylpicrylhydrazyl (DPPH) free radical as described by Brand-Williams et al. (1995) [54].

4.6. In Vitro Release Studies of VPDS

The release rate of the polyphenols of VPDS was measured in a buffer solution at pH 7.2 at 37 °C. An in vitro study of the release of the polyphenols of the extract was performed by using dialysis sacks. A total of 1 mL of the VPDS was placed in the dialysis sacks of a MWCO = 1000 (Pur-A-Lyzer, Midi Dialysis Kit, Sigma-Aldrich, St. Louis, MO, USA). The sack was placed in a buffer pH = 7.2 (CARLO ERBA Reagents, Val-de-Reuil, France) which was constantly stirred with a magnetic bar and thermostated at 37 °C throughout the experiments (hot plate magnetic stirrer, IKA® Werke GmbH & Co., Staufen im Breisgau, Germany). At specific time points (15′, 30′, 45′, and 1, 2, 4, 6, 21, and 24 h), samples were taken, and their polyphenol concentration and antioxidant activity were measured. The buffer quantity removed is replaced by buffer pH = 7.2 at temperature of 37 °C to maintain the sink conditions.

4.7. MTT Cell Viability Assay

Cell viability was determined using an MTT colorimetric assay kit Vybrant®, Thermo Fisher Scientific, Waltham, MA, USA), following the manufacturer's protocol.

4.8. Cell Migration Assay

Dermal fibroblasts' monolayer was scraped with a p200 pipet tip to create a "scratch" (T0). Dermal fibroblasts (NHDFs) were then treated for 24 h with 0.1% *v*/*v* VPDS upon serum starvation conditions. Photos were taken at T0 and after 24 h with ZEN Microscopy Software (Zen lite 2012 blue edition, Zeiss, Vienna, Austria).

4.9. Collagenase Assay

The assay was based on spectrophotometric methods reported in the literature with some modifications for use in a microplate reader (150 μL total volume of the final reaction mixture) [55]. The assay was performed in a 50 mM tricine buffer with 10 mM calcium chloride and 400 mM sodium chloride, pH 7.5. Collagenase from *Clostridium histolyticum* (EC.3.4.24.3) was dissolved in a buffer at an initial concentration of 0.8 U/mL (0.1 U/mL final concentration). The synthetic substrate N-[3-(2-furyl) acryloyl]-Leu-Gly-Pro-Ala (FALGPA) was dissolved in a buffer at an initial concentration of 2 mM (final concentration 1 mM). The tested compounds were incubated with the enzyme in a buffer for 15 min. After the incubation the substrate is added. The absorbance was measured immediately after the addition of the substrate, at 345 nm and then every 1 min for 10 min using microplate reader (infinite 200 M Pro, Tecan, Männedorf, Switzerland). Ascorbic acid (AA) was used as a positive control.

4.10. Gene and Protein Expression Analysis

For the isolation of total RNA (400 ng), as well as for cDNA synthesis, the NucleoSpin RNA kit Macherey-Nagel, Germany and the PrimeScript RT reagent kit (Takara Bio, Kusatsu shi, Japan), were used, respectively. The qPCR method, as well as the process of gene analysis, was conducted as previously described. For the relative gene expression, the comparative threshold cycle method was used. GAPDH was used as normalization control.

Collagen and elastin expression was quantified by ELISA (Fine tests) in 450 μg/mL protein lysates, according to the manufacturer's protocol.

4.11. Immunofluorescence Analysis

Human dermal fibroblasts at initial density of 10.000 cells/well and maintained in optimal growing conditions for 2 days. At day 1, particulate matters (ERMCZ100 PM10-like—PAHs; 1 μg/cm^2) were added to the cells belonging from "Stress" groups and "Stress + VPDS" groups. After 1 h of contact the cells were irradiated with UVA (LED source, 365 nm, 3 J/cm^2) in an irradiation chamber.

Immediately after the irradiation, the culture medium was renewed, the active ingredient added to the cells (0.1%) and left in contact for 24 h. The control group did not receive any treatment, except from the renewal of the culture medium. After 24 h of incubation, the cells were fixed on the plate and analyzed by in situ immunofluorescence detection, visualization and quantification of collagen-I, collagen-IIIa, and elastin signals.

4.12. Statistical Analysis

Results are expressed as the mean ± SEM of two different experiments. Statistical analysis between two individual groups was performed by Student's *t*-test and one-way ANOVA (Dunnett's multiple comparisons test). A $p \leq 0.05$ was considered statistically significant. Statistical analysis and graphs were performed with Sigma Plot Software v.10 and GraphPad Prism 9 (GraphPad software Inc., San Diego, CA, USA).

5. Conclusions

The new raw material presents a novel, controlled way of dealing with antioxidants delivery to human skin for anti-aging reasons. It exhibits antioxidant and ECM protective effects when administered in skin fibroblasts (NHDFs). Treatment of NHDFs with the combinatorial delivery system for vine extract and propolis polyphenols promoted collagen end elastin synthesis and deposition under normal and stressed conditions. Therefore, this liposome–cyclodextrin encapsulated polyphenol system represents a novel bioactive and sustainable approach for cosmetics production with promising skin applications.

6. Patents

Patent WO/2023/222267 is based on the results of this publication.

Author Contributions: S.A. and K.G., conceptualization; S.A., E.S. and E.P., formal analysis; K.G., funding acquisition; S.A., E.S., E.P., A.C., A.B. and K.G., investigation; S.A., E.S., E.P., A.C., A.B. and K.G., methodology; K.G., resources; K.G., supervision; S.A., E.S. and E.P., visualization; S.A., E.S., and E.P., writing—original draft preparation; K.G., A.C. and A.B., writing—review and editing. All authors have read and agreed to the published version of the manuscript.

Funding: This research received no external funding.

Data Availability Statement: All study data available upon request.

Acknowledgments: The authors would like to thank all the R&D team for their collaboration.

Conflicts of Interest: The authors declare no conflicts of interest.

Abbreviations

AQP-3, Aquaporin-3; CD44, cluster of differentiation 44; DPPH, 2,2-Diphenyl-1-picrylhydrazyl; ECM, extracellular matrix; EGF, epidermal growth factor; GA, gallic acid; HA, hyaluronic acid; HAS-2, hyaluronan synthase-2; MTT, methylthiazolyldiphenyl-tetrazolium bromide; NHDFs, normal human diploid fibroblasts; ROS, reactive oxygen species; SOD, superoxide dismutase; TGF, transforming growth factor; TPC, total phenolic content; VEGF, vascular endothelial growth factor; VPDS, vine propolis delivery system.

References

1. Hano, C.; Tungmunnithum, D. Plant Polyphenols, more than Just Simple Natural Antioxidants: Oxidative Stress, Aging and Age-Related Diseases. *Medicines* **2020**, *7*, 26. [CrossRef]
2. Anunciato, T.P.; da Rocha Filho, P.A. Carotenoids and Polyphenols in Nutricosmetics, Nutraceuticals, and Cosmeceuticals. *J. Cosmet. Dermatol.* **2012**, *11*, 51–54. [CrossRef]
3. Chiang, H.-M.; Lin, T.-J.; Chiu, C.-Y.; Chang, C.-W.; Hsu, K.-C.; Fan, P.-C.; Wen, K.-C. Coffea Arabica Extract and Its Constituents Prevent Photoaging by Suppressing MMPs Expression and MAP Kinase Pathway. *Food Chem. Toxicol.* **2011**, *49*, 309–318. [CrossRef]
4. Chowdhury, A.; Nosoudi, N.; Karamched, S.; Parasaram, V.; Vyavahare, N. Polyphenol Treatments Increase Elastin and Collagen Deposition by Human Dermal Fibroblasts; Implications to Improve Skin Health. *J. Dermatol. Sci.* **2021**, *102*, 94–100. [CrossRef] [PubMed]
5. Lyu, J.-L.; Liu, Y.-J.; Wen, K.-C.; Chiu, C.-Y.; Lin, Y.-H.; Chiang, H.-M. Protective Effect of Djulis (*Chenopodium Formosanum*) Extract against UV- and AGEs-Induced Skin Aging via Alleviating Oxidative Stress and Collagen Degradation. *Molecules* **2022**, *27*, 2332. [CrossRef] [PubMed]
6. Baroi, A.M.; Popitiu, M.; Fierascu, I.; Sărdărescu, I.-D.; Fierascu, R.C. Grapevine Wastes: A Rich Source of Antioxidants and Other Biologically Active Compounds. *Antioxidants* **2022**, *11*, 393. [CrossRef] [PubMed]
7. Chakka, A.K.; Babu, A.S. Bioactive Compounds of Winery By-Products: Extraction Techniques and Their Potential Health Benefits. *Appl. Food Res.* **2022**, *2*, 100058. [CrossRef]
8. Nzekoue, F.K.; Kouamo Nguefang, M.L.; Alessandroni, L.; Mustafa, A.M.; Vittori, S.; Caprioli, G. Grapevine Leaves (*Vitis Vinifera*): Chemical Characterization of Bioactive Compounds and Antioxidant Activity during Leave Development. *Food Biosci.* **2022**, *50*, 102120. [CrossRef]
9. Karapetsas, A.; Voulgaridou, G.-P.; Konialis, M.; Tsochantaridis, I.; Kynigopoulos, S.; Lambropoulou, M.; Stavropoulou, M.-I.; Stathopoulou, K.; Aligiannis, N.; Bozidis, P.; et al. Propolis Extracts Inhibit UV-Induced Photodamage in Human Experimental In Vitro Skin Models. *Antioxidants* **2019**, *8*, 125. [CrossRef]
10. Menaa, F.; Menaa, A. Chapter 64—Skin Photoprotection by Polyphenols in Animal Models and Humans. In *Polyphenols in Human Health and Disease*; Watson, R.R., Preedy, V.R., Zibadi, S., Eds.; Academic Press: San Diego, CA, USA, 2014; pp. 831–838. ISBN 978-0-12-398456-2.
11. Tang, S.-C.; Yang, J.-H. Dual Effects of Alpha-Hydroxy Acids on the Skin. *Molecules* **2018**, *23*, 863. [CrossRef]
12. Kalogeropoulos, N.; Konteles, S.J.; Troullidou, E.; Mourtzinos, I.; Karathanos, V.T. Chemical Composition, Antioxidant Activity and Antimicrobial Properties of Propolis Extracts from Greece and Cyprus. *Food Chem.* **2009**, *116*, 452–461. [CrossRef]
13. Pasupuleti, V.R.; Sammugam, L.; Ramesh, N.; Gan, S.H. Honey, Propolis, and Royal Jelly: A Comprehensive Review of Their Biological Actions and Health Benefits. *Oxid. Med. Cell. Longev.* **2017**, *2017*, 1259510. [CrossRef] [PubMed]
14. Acito, M.; Varfaj, I.; Brighenti, V.; Cengiz, E.C.; Rondini, T.; Fatigoni, C.; Russo, C.; Pietrella, D.; Pellati, F.; Bartolini, D.; et al. A Novel Black Poplar Propolis Extract with Promising Health-Promoting Properties: Focus on Its Chemical Composition, Antioxidant, Anti-Inflammatory, and Anti-Genotoxic Activities. *Food Funct.* **2024**, *15*, 4983–4999. [CrossRef]
15. Bonamigo, T.; Campos, J.F.; Alfredo, T.M.; Balestieri, J.B.P.; Cardoso, C.A.L.; Paredes-Gamero, E.J.; de Picoli Souza, K.; Dos Santos, E.L. Antioxidant, Cytotoxic, and Toxic Activities of Propolis from Two Native Bees in Brazil: Scaptotrigona Depilis and Melipona Quadrifasciata Anthidioides. *Oxid. Med. Cell. Longev.* **2017**, *2017*, 1038153. [CrossRef]
16. Boisard, S.; Le Ray, A.-M.; Gatto, J.; Aumond, M.-C.; Blanchard, P.; Derbré, S.; Flurin, C.; Richomme, P. Chemical Composition, Antioxidant and Anti-AGEs Activities of a French Poplar Type Propolis. *J. Agric. Food Chem.* **2014**, *62*, 1344–1351. [CrossRef]
17. Sforcin, J.M.; Fernandes, A.J.; Lopes, C.A.; Bankova, V.; Funari, S.R. Seasonal Effect on Brazilian Propolis Antibacterial Activity. *J. Ethnopharmacol.* **2000**, *73*, 243–249. [CrossRef] [PubMed]
18. Silici, S.; Kutluca, S. Chemical Composition and Antibacterial Activity of Propolis Collected by Three Different Races of Honeybees in the Same Region. *J. Ethnopharmacol.* **2005**, *99*, 69–73. [CrossRef]

19. Hossain, R.; Quispe, C.; Khan, R.A.; Saikat, A.S.M.; Ray, P.; Ongalbek, D.; Yeskaliyeva, B.; Jain, D.; Smeriglio, A.; Trombetta, D.; et al. Propolis: An Update on Its Chemistry and Pharmacological Applications. *Chin. Med.* **2022**, *17*, 100. [CrossRef] [PubMed]
20. Barros, K.B.N.T.; de França Fonteles, M.M. Propolis and Its Cosmetic Applications: A Technological Prospection. *J. Young Pharm.* **2019**, *11*, 350–352. [CrossRef]
21. Segueni, N.; Akkal, S.; Benlabed, K.; Nieto, G. Potential Use of Propolis in Phytocosmetic as Phytotherapeutic Constituent. *Molecules* **2022**, *27*, 5833. [CrossRef] [PubMed]
22. González-Masís, J.; Cubero-Sesin, J.M.; Corrales-Ureña, Y.R.; González-Camacho, S.; Mora-Ugalde, N.; Baizán-Rojas, M.; Loaiza, R.; Vega-Baudrit, J.R.; Gonzalez-Paz, R.J. Increased Fibroblast Metabolic Activity of Collagen Scaffolds via the Addition of Propolis Nanoparticles. *Materials* **2020**, *13*, 3118. [CrossRef]
23. Felician, F.F.; Yu, R.-H.; Li, M.-Z.; Li, C.-J.; Chen, H.-Q.; Jiang, Y.; Tang, T.; Qi, W.-Y.; Xu, H.-M. The Wound Healing Potential of Collagen Peptides Derived from the Jellyfish *Rhopilema esculentum*. *Chin. J. Traumatol.* **2019**, *22*, 12–20. [CrossRef] [PubMed]
24. Pilkington, S.M.; Bulfone-Paus, S.; Griffiths, C.E.M.; Watson, R.E.B. Inflammaging and the Skin. *J. Invest. Dermatol.* **2021**, *141*, 1087–1095. [CrossRef]
25. Lagouri, V.; Prasianaki, D.; Krysta, F. Antioxidant Properties and Phenolic Composition of Greek Propolis Extracts. *Int. J. Food Prop.* **2014**, *17*, 511–522. [CrossRef]
26. Bae, I.A.; Ha, J.W.; Choi, J.Y.; Boo, Y.C. Antioxidant Effects of Korean Propolis in HaCaT Keratinocytes Exposed to Particulate Matter 10. *Antioxidants* **2022**, *11*, 781. [CrossRef]
27. Diniz, D.P.; Lorencini, D.A.; Berretta, A.A.; Cintra, M.A.C.T.; Lia, E.N.; Jordão, A.A.J.; Coelho, E.B. Antioxidant Effect of Standardized Extract of Propolis (EPP-AF®) in Healthy Volunteers: A "Before and After" Clinical Study. *Evid. Based Complement. Altern. Med.* **2020**, *2020*, 7538232. [CrossRef] [PubMed]
28. Pyrgioti, E.; Graikou, K.; Cheilari, A.; Chinou, I. Assessment of Antioxidant and Antimicrobial Properties of Selected Greek Propolis Samples (North East Aegean Region Islands). *Molecules* **2022**, *27*, 8198. [CrossRef]
29. Pyrgioti, E.; Graikou, K.; Aligiannis, N.; Karabournioti, S.; Chinou, I. Qualitative Analysis Related to Palynological Characterization and Biological Evaluation of Propolis from Prespa National Park (Greece). *Molecules* **2022**, *27*, 7018. [CrossRef]
30. Stavropoulou, M.I.; Stathopoulou, K.; Cheilari, A.; Benaki, D.; Gardikis, K.; Chinou, I.; Aligiannis, N. NMR Metabolic Profiling of Greek Propolis Samples: Comparative Evaluation of Their Phytochemical Compositions and Investigation of Their Anti-Ageing and Antioxidant Properties. *J. Pharm. Biomed. Anal.* **2021**, *194*, 113814. [CrossRef]
31. Kasiotis, K.M.; Anastasiadou, P.; Papadopoulos, A.; Machera, K. Revisiting Greek Propolis: Chromatographic Analysis and Antioxidant Activity Study. *PLoS ONE* **2017**, *12*, e0170077. [CrossRef] [PubMed]
32. Singh, J.; Rasane, P.; Kaur, R.; Kaur, H.; Garg, R.; Kaur, S.; Ercisli, S.; Choudhary, R.; Skrovankova, S.; Mlcek, J. Valorization of Grape (*Vitis Vinifera*) Leaves for Bioactive Compounds: Novel Green Extraction Technologies and Food-Pharma Applications. *Front. Chem.* **2023**, *11*, 1290619. [CrossRef]
33. Spanidi, E.; Karapetsas, A.; Voulgaridou, G.P.; Letsiou, S.; Aligiannis, N.; Tsochantaridis, I.; Kynigopoulos, S.; Lambropoulou, M.; Mourtzinos, I.; Pappa, A.; et al. A New Controlled Release System for Propolis Polyphenols and Its Biochemical Activity for Skin Applications. *Plants* **2021**, *10*, 420. [CrossRef]
34. Spanidi, E.; Athanasopoulou, S.; Liakopoulou, A.; Chaidou, A.; Hatziantoniou, S.; Gardikis, K. Royal Jelly Components Encapsulation in a Controlled Release System—Skin Functionality, and Biochemical Activity for Skin Applications. *Pharmaceuticals* **2022**, *15*, 907. [CrossRef]
35. Demetzos, C. Advanced Drug Delivery Nanosystems: Perspectives and Regulatory Issues. *Adv. Exp. Med. Biol.* **2015**, *822*, 195–198. [CrossRef]
36. Levet, G.; Krykun, S.; Cornelio, B.; Pilato, S.; Moffa, S.; Fontana, A.; Gouhier, G.; Estour, F. Drugs in Cyclodextrin in Liposomes: How a Suitable Formulation of an Active Substance Can Improve Its Efficiency? *Processes* **2024**, *12*, 478. [CrossRef]
37. Hammoud, Z.; Khreich, N.; Auezova, L.; Fourmentin, S.; Elaissari, A.; Greige-Gerges, H. Cyclodextrin-Membrane Interaction in Drug Delivery and Membrane Structure Maintenance. *Int. J. Pharm.* **2019**, *564*, 59–76. [CrossRef]
38. Tončić, R.J.; Kezić, S.; Hadžavdić, S.L.; Marinović, B. Skin Barrier and Dry Skin in the Mature Patient. *Clin. Dermatol.* **2018**, *36*, 109–115. [CrossRef] [PubMed]
39. Wlaschek, M.; Maity, P.; Makrantonaki, E.; Scharffetter-Kochanek, K. Connective Tissue and Fibroblast Senescence in Skin Aging. *J. Invest. Dermatol.* **2021**, *141*, 985–992. [CrossRef] [PubMed]
40. Fisher, G.J.; Wang, B.; Cui, Y.; Shi, M.; Zhao, Y.; Quan, T.; Voorhees, J.J. Skin Aging from the Perspective of Dermal Fibroblasts: The Interplay between the Adaptation to the Extracellular Matrix Microenvironment and Cell Autonomous Processes. *J. Cell. Commun. Signal.* **2023**, *17*, 523–529. [CrossRef]
41. Wittenauer, J.; Mäckle, S.; Sußmann, D.; Schweiggert-Weisz, U.; Carle, R. Inhibitory Effects of Polyphenols from Grape Pomace Extract on Collagenase and Elastase Activity. *Fitoterapia* **2015**, *101*, 179–187. [CrossRef] [PubMed]
42. Edgar, S.; Hopley, B.; Genovese, L.; Sibilla, S.; Laight, D.; Shute, J. Effects of Collagen-Derived Bioactive Peptides and Natural Antioxidant Compounds on Proliferation and Matrix Protein Synthesis by Cultured Normal Human Dermal Fibroblasts. *Sci. Rep.* **2018**, *8*, 10474. [CrossRef]
43. Katsnelson, A. Cosmetics: Molecular Beauty. *Nature* **2015**, *526*, S4–S5. [CrossRef]
44. Manturova, N.E.; Smirnova, G.O.; Stupin, V.A.; Silina, E.V. The Ratio of Collagen Types I/III as a Marker of Skin Aging and Prognosis of Aesthetic Facial Surgery Results. *J. Pharm. Sci. Res.* **2018**, *10*, 2543–2546.

45. Kuivaniemi, H.; Tromp, G. Type III Collagen (COL3A1): Gene and Protein Structure, Tissue Distribution, and Associated Diseases. *Gene* **2019**, *707*, 151–171. [CrossRef] [PubMed]
46. Wulandari, E.; Jusman, S.W.A.; Moenadjat, Y.; Jusuf, A.A.; Sadikin, M. Expressions of Collagen I and III in Hypoxic Keloid Tissue. *Kobe. J. Med. Sci.* **2016**, *62*, E58–E69.
47. Maytin, E. V Hyaluronan: More than Just a Wrinkle Filler. *Glycobiology* **2016**, *26*, 553–559. [CrossRef]
48. Wang, Y.; Lauer, M.E.; Anand, S.; Mack, J.A.; Maytin, E. V Hyaluronan Synthase 2 Protects Skin Fibroblasts against Apoptosis Induced by Environmental Stress. *J. Biol. Chem.* **2014**, *289*, 32253–32265. [CrossRef] [PubMed]
49. Zhang, H.; Cai, W.; Shao, X. Regulation of Aquaporin-3 Water Permeability by Hyaluronan. *Phys. Chem. Chem. Phys.* **2021**, *23*, 25706–25711. [CrossRef]
50. Al-Warhi, T.; Zahran, E.M.; Selim, S.; Al-Sanea, M.M.; Ghoneim, M.M.; Maher, S.A.; Mostafa, Y.A.; Alsenani, F.; Elrehany, M.A.; Almuhayawi, M.S.; et al. Antioxidant and Wound Healing Potential of *Vitis Vinifera* Seeds Supported by Phytochemical Characterization and Docking Studies. *Antioxidants* **2022**, *11*, 881. [CrossRef]
51. Westergren-Thorsson, G.; Bagher, M.; Andersson-Sjöland, A.; Thiman, L.; Löfdahl, C.-G.; Hallgren, O.; Bjermer, L.; Larsson-Callerfelt, A.-K. VEGF Synthesis Is Induced by Prostacyclin and TGF-β in Distal Lung Fibroblasts from COPD Patients and Control Subjects: Implications for Pulmonary Vascular Remodelling. *Respirology* **2018**, *23*, 68–75. [CrossRef] [PubMed]
52. Rohani, M.G.; Parks, W.C. Matrix Remodeling by MMPs during Wound Repair. *Matrix Biol.* **2015**, *44–46*, 113–121. [CrossRef] [PubMed]
53. Arnous, A.; Makris, D.P.; Kefalas, P. Correlation of Pigment and Flavanol Content with Antioxidant Properties in Selected Aged Regional Wines from Greece. *J. Food Compos. Anal.* **2002**, *15*, 655–665. [CrossRef]
54. Brand-Williams, W.; Cuvelier, M.E.; Berset, C. Use of a Free Radical Method to Evaluate Antioxidant Activity. *LWT—Food Sci. Technol.* **1995**, *28*, 25–30. [CrossRef]
55. Van Wart, H.E.; Steinbrink, D.R. A Continuous Spectrophotometric Assay for Clostridium Histolyticum Collagenase. *Anal. Biochem.* **1981**, *113*, 356–365. [CrossRef] [PubMed]

pharmaceuticals

Article

Polyphenol Profile and Antioxidant, Antityrosinase, and Anti-Melanogenesis Activities of Ethanol Extract of Bee Pollen

Qiang He †, Jie Wang †, Jingjing Li and Wenchao Yang *

College of Bee Science and Biomedicine, Fujian Agriculture and Forestry University, Fuzhou 350002, China; h3077ang@163.com (Q.H.); wangjie01092023@163.com (J.W.); lijingjing000407@163.com (J.L.)
* Correspondence: beesyang@gmail.com
† These authors contributed equally to this work.

Abstract: Background/Objective: Bee pollen, a rich nutritional food, was employed to develop a raw material for skin whitening. **Methods:** The polyphenol profile and antioxidant, antityrosinase, and anti-melanogenesis activities of the ethanol extracts of five species of bee pollens (EEBPs) were determined. **Results:** The results showed that there were a total of 121 phenolic compounds in these EEBPs. Each type of bee pollen had unique substances. The best anti-melanogenesis activity was observed for sunflower EEBP, about 25% at a concentration of 25 μg/mL BEEP. The anti-melanogenesis activities of EEBPs from high to low were sunflower, apricot, camellia, rapeseed, and lotus EEBPs. The anti-melanogenesis activity in B16F10 cells was positively correlated with the antityrosinase activity and total phenol content, with coefficients of 0.987 and 0.940. The Kyoto Encyclopedia of Genes and Genomes enrichment analysis results of untargeted proteomics revealed that sunflower EEBP inhibited melanogenesis in B16F10 cells by reducing the expression of the proteins MAP2K1, NFKB2, RELB, RPS6KA3, CASP3, TRAF6, MAP2K5, MAPKAPK3, STRADA, CCNA2, and FASN involved in the cAMP, MAPK, and TNF signaling pathways, even though these pathways were not significantly different from the control group. **Conclusions:** The sunflower EEBP has high inhibition effect on melanogenesis than other species EEBPs. The results provide a basis for the future industrial development of a raw material for skin whitening.

Keywords: polyphenols; antioxidant; antityrosinase; anti-melanogenesis; bee pollen

1. Introduction

Bee pollen is composed of copious amounts of pollen grains, which were foraged by workers using the weak electrostatic field generated between the negatively charged flower and the positively charged body, mixed with a small dose of the secretions from salivary glands or nectar, and placed in specific baskets situated on the tibia of their hind legs [1,2]. There are many biological substances, including carbohydrates, proteins, vitamins, minerals, polyphenols, dietary fiber, volatile compounds, and lipids, in bee pollen. The moisture content ranges from 1.82 to 7.33% in commercial bee pollen [3] and 20 to 30% in the original bee pollen [4]. Bee pollen contains approximately 40–85% carbohydrates, including 15.2–22.4% fructose, 7.0–21.9% glucose, 14–19.8% sucrose, and others (W/W, dry weight, DW) [5]. There are approximately 13.6–26.8% (W/W, DW) protein with a total of 20 amino acids, 1–10% total lipids, 0.0019–0.0344% vitamin B, 0.0015% vitamin A, 0.0062% vitamin E (α-tocopherol), and trace amounts of vitamin C in bee pollen [5,6]. It contains rich micronutrients such as potassium (K), sodium (Na), calcium (Ca), magnesium (Mg), phosphorus (P), zinc (Zn), iron (Fe), copper (Cu), and manganese (Mn) [5]. There is also a very diverse group of yellow-to-red-color polyenes, polyphenols, dietary fiber, and volatile compounds, among which polyphenols include 19 phenolic acids, 25 flavonoids, and seven glycosylated flavonoids [3–8]. The chemical compositions of diverse bee pollens vary from different botanical origins, geographic origins, entomological origins, processing methods, and storage conditions [2–8]. These chemical compositions decide the functional effects of bee pollen, such as antioxidant, antifungal, antimicrobial, antiviral, anti-inflammatory, hepatoprotective, anticancer, immunostimulatory, radical-scavenging, gut-microbiota-modulating, and local analgesic activities [5,9–11].

The antioxidant capability is one of the significant bioactivities of bee pollen. This primarily depends on the presence of various compounds, including 4-hydroxybenzoic, *p*-coumaric, phenyllactic, caffeic, transcinnamic, syringic, 3,4 dimethoxycinnamic (acid), chlorogenic, rosmarinic, and vanillic acids; apigenin; caffeic acid phenethyl ester (CAPE); chrysin; epicatechin; hesperetin; taxifolin; myricetin; catechin; genistein; isorhamnetin; kaempferol; luteolin; pinocembrin; quercetin; and rutin [8]. Enzymes like catalase and superoxide dismutase (SOD), along with glutathione (GSH), also play roles in the antioxidant effects of bee pollen [12]. The antioxidant capability is influenced by several factors, including the processing method [13–15], botanical origin [8,16], storage [17], geographical origin [18], and extraction solvents [14,19].

In addition to the in vitro antioxidant activity, in vivo studies have reported benefits. *Cistaceae* bee pollen modulates the expression of antioxidant enzymes in the liver, brain, and lysate of erythrocytes and reduces hepatic lipid peroxidation levels in mice [20]. The water and methanol extracts of bee pollen increase the SOD level and the total antioxidant capacity and significantly reduce the malondialdehyde (MDA) content in mice and rats [12,21]. Bee pollen relieves the oxidative stress on hepatocytes [22], oxidative damage and reactive oxygen species produced by propionic acid [23,24], and NaF-induced oxidative stress in rats [25]. Furthermore, bee pollen alleviates oxidative stress in hepatocytes and both oxidative damage and reactive oxygen species produced by propionic acid and sodium fluoride in rats [26].

Beyond the antioxidant activity, polyphenols also possess the ability to inhibit tyrosinase [27], which is a biofunctional copper-containing enzyme that plays a crucial role in the melanin biosynthesis pathway within melanocytes. Tyrosinase catalyzes the hydroxylation of monophenols and the oxidation of diphenols to form quinines [28]. Melanin is the primary determinant of skin color and a vital substance to prevent skin damage caused by UV radiation and oxidative stress [29]. However, the excessive accumulation of melanin might result in hyperpigmentation diseases, such as lentigo, ephelides, melasma, freckles and nevus, and melanomas, which may increase the risks of both cancer and Parkinson's disease [30–33]. Consequently, tyrosinase inhibitors are being widely studied as treatments for pigmentation issues and for the development of skin-whitening agents [27,28,34–39]. Examples of natural compounds with antityrosinase activity include a quercetin-loaded olive oil nanoemulsion [34], flavonoids from *Trifolium nigrescens* subsp. petrisavi [36], citrus essential oils [37], mango seed kernel extract [38], and safflospermidines separated from the bee pollen of *Helianthus annuus* L. [39]. Notably, safflospermidines exhibit higher antityrosinase activity than kojic acid in vitro. Traditional tyrosinase inhibitors, such as kojic acid, aloesin, hydroquinone, and α- and β-arbutins, have been used as skin-whitening agents [27]. However, there is a need for more effective and safer tyrosinase inhibitors, as cytotoxicity or side effects may be caused by irritation, peeling, redness, or stinging in daily life [40].

There are limited research reports on the antityrosinase and antioxidant activities of bee pollen harvested in China. In this paper, the polyphenol profiles and antioxidant, antityrosinase, and anti-melanogenesis activities of sunflower bee pollen extract in B16F10 melanoma cells were determined to discover an effective and safer tyrosinase inhibitor for further utilization as a raw material for skin-whitening agents.

2. Results

2.1. Components in Ethanol Extracts of Bee Pollens

2.1.1. TPCs and TFCs in Ethanol Extracts of Bee Pollens

There were significant differences among the TPCs and TFCs of ethanol extracts of various species of bee pollen (EEBP) (Table 1). The TPCs and TFCs of bee pollen samples ranged from 5.36 to 132.57 mg GAE/g and 1.99 to 109.06 mg RE/g calculated by the equations of the standard curves y = 0.00567x + 0.07371 (r^2 = 0.9929) and y = 0.00148x + 0.05319 (r^2 = 0.9929), respectively.

Table 1. Total phenolic and flavonoid contents of ethanol extracts of bee pollens.

Bee Pollen	TPC (mg GAE/g)	TFC (mg RE/g)
Rapeseed	64.80 ± 1.34 ^{c}	79.81 ± 1.62 ^{b}
Apricot	79.00 ± 1.14 ^{b}	66.55 ± 4.72 ^{c}
Camellia	64.29 ± 1.64 ^{c}	64.1 9± 1.77 ^{c}
Lotus	5.36 ± 0.50 ^{d}	1.99 ± 0.45 ^{d}
Sunflower	132.57 ± 1.41 ^{a}	109.06 ± 1.35 ^{a}

Different lowercase characters in the same column mean statistically significant differences ($p < 0.05$).

2.1.2. The Polyphenols in Ethanol Extracts of Bee Pollens

The ion spectra of ethanol extracts of bee pollens were shown in Figure 1. A diverse variety of polyphenols has been identified in five species of EEBPs. In total, 71 polyphenolic compounds were found, with significant variation across different bee pollen samples (Table 2).

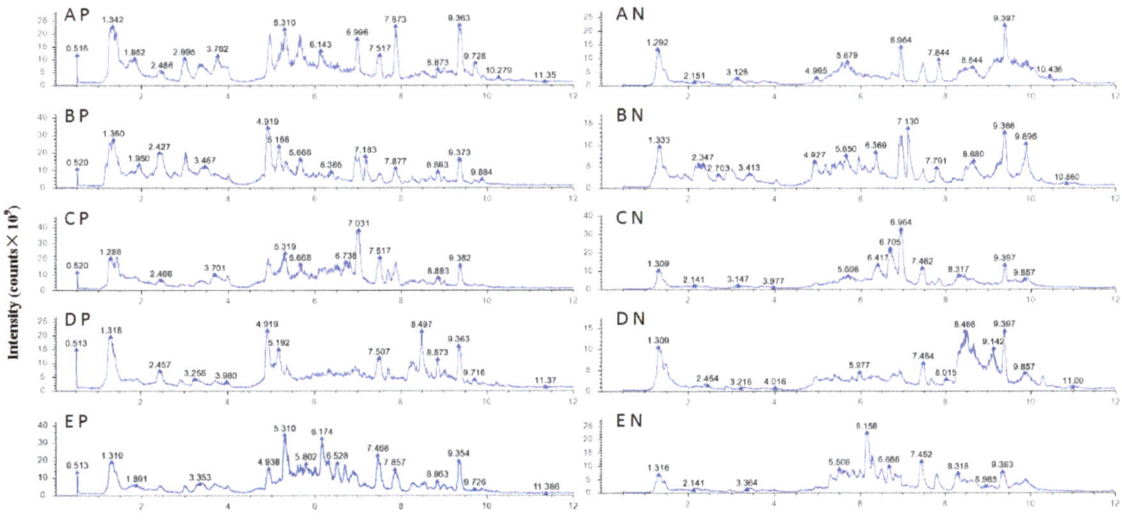

Figure 1. UHPLC–MS/MS ion spectra of ethanol extracts of bee pollens: A, B, C, D, and E represent rapeseed, apricot, camellia, lotus, and sunflower bee pollens, respectively. P and N represent positive ion mode and negative ion mode, respectively.

EEBPs of rapeseed, camellia, sunflower, lotus, and apricot bee pollens contain 56, 46, 45, 42, and 35 polyphenolic compounds, respectively. Certain flavonoids are unique to specific types of bee pollen: orientin, (−)-catechin gallate, methyl hesperidin, hesperidin, and epicatechin are found only in rapeseed bee pollen; chloropelargonidin is exclusive to camellia bee pollen; violacein and tricin-O-malonylhexoside are present only in sunflower bee pollen; and heptamethoxyflavonoids, isovitexin, chlorocyanidin, and baohuoside I are unique to lotus bee pollen. In terms of the relative content, camelliaside A is the most abundant flavonoid in rapeseed bee pollen; rutin is the most prevalent in both lotus and apricot bee pollens; kaempferol has the highest relative content in camellia bee pollen; and quercetin-3β-D-glucoside is the dominant flavonoid in sunflower bee pollen.

Table 2. Flavonoids in ethanol extracts of bee pollens.

Name	Formula	Molecular Weight	Retention Time (min)	m/z	Relative Quantitative Value #					Polarity Mode
					A	B	C	D	E	
4′,7-Dihydroxyflavanone	$C_{15}H_{12}O_4$	256.07342	6.011	257.0807	ND *	421,160,345.9	2,761,299.049	2,878,041.662	ND	pos
Paracetamol	$C_8H_9NO_2$	151.06328	5.696	152.0706	43,034,369.2	76,811,021.73	376,365,295.8	147,656,556.3	388,854,376.3	pos
Diosmetin	$C_{16}H_{12}O_6$	300.06318	6.039	301.0705	214,452,989	191,074,539.2	52,141,965.55	24,221,989	32,956,884.01	pos
Galangin	$C_{15}H_{10}O_5$	270.05258	6.642	271.0599	71,935,041.1	78,118,724.65	39,386,575.66	20,616,903.96	ND	pos
Isorhamnetin	$C_{16}H_{12}O_7$	316.0581	5.561	317.0654	684,415,707	2,700,227,153	848,073,257	1,339,085,340	410,416,525.5	pos
Kaempferol	$C_{15}H_{10}O_6$	286.04762	5.783	287.0549	421,485,230	542,513,047.8	1,083,001,678	3,746,952,740	4,545,692,793	pos
Apigenin	$C_{15}H_{10}O_5$	270.05266	6.035	271.0599	59,073,999	492,996,321.1	34,174,186.03	103,121,637.5	15,609,215.28	pos
Chrysin	$C_{15}H_{10}O_4$	254.05766	6.584	255.0649	386,526,326	472,417,967.1	187,207,714.9	146,964,633.5	25,581,440.96	pos
Hesperetin	$C_{16}H_{14}O_6$	302.07906	5.396	303.0863	ND	1,206,039,601	5,768,035.731	70,706,093.49	19,793,290.76	pos
4-Ethylphenol	$C_8H_{10}O$	122.07331	7.007	123.0805	232,956,283	219,609,736.9	581,174,572.1	848,615,029.3	744,324,047.7	pos
3-Hydroxyphenylacetic acid	$C_8H_8O_3$	152.04652	3.448	153.0538	1,258,417,229	495,499,205.9	32,153,838.89	178,078,042.9	156,571,841.1	pos
DL-Metanephrine	$C_{10}H_{15}NO_3$	197.1052	1.438	198.1125	44,608,165.2	14,591,930.83	25,372,108.46	174,820,069.1	493,116,291	pos
Robinetin	$C_{15}H_{10}O_7$	132.04349	5.472	303.0501	7,228,439.57	192,17,361,011	347,711,367.3	295,845,940.9	113,126,228.6	pos
Isoeugenol	$C_{10}H_{12}O_2$	164.08379	5.872	165.0911	121,446,929	168,376,512.1	507,361,781.8	664,056,676.7	257,748,794.5	pos
N-Oleoyl dopamine	$C_{26}H_{43}NO_3$	439.30561	7.476	440.3129	ND	186,795,049.6	ND	7,434,264.734	ND	pos
4′-O-Glucosylvitexin	$C_{27}H_{30}O_{15}$	594.15738	5.303	595.1647	137,988,745	201,390,496.8	12,019,090.94	123,593,071.6	21,336,459.52	pos
Epicatechin	$C_{15}H_{14}O_6$	308.08945	5.238	291.0861	ND	ND	ND	158,962,728.2	ND	pos
Dihydrocapsaicin	$C_{18}H_{29}NO_3$	307.21458	5.781	308.2219	13,025,748.8	5,255,758.773	28,698,096.6	33,645,843.33	58,189,390.76	pos
Vanillin	$C_8H_8O_3$	170.05787	5.896	188.0917	18,507,044.3	39,733,515.43	23,754,186	16,790,489.85	23,462,102.25	pos
Antiarol	$C_9H_{12}O_4$	184.07359	5.897	185.0811	ND	34,692,677.88	33,181,916.55	11,779,943.87	13,883,890.37	pos
Rhoifolin	$C_{27}H_{30}O_{14}$	616.11857	11.184	617.1259	ND	ND	ND	83,619,032.81	115,639,570.7	pos
Narcissoside	$C_{28}H_{32}O_{16}$	624.17131	5.543	625.1786	12,927,457.8	6,672,526.705	3,798,041.678	4,862,624.146	ND	pos
Neodiosmin	$C_{28}H_{32}O_{15}$	646.12896	10.452	647.1362	10,404,117.8	7,699,224.206	ND	227,282,528.5	222,436,152.3	pos
(+)-Catechin	$C_{15}H_{14}O_6$	290.0791	5.095	291.0864	ND	1,884,259.734	ND	62,231,803.58	ND	pos
Isovanillin	$C_8H_8O_3$	152.04737	4.003	170.0812	43,279,880.4	36,658,145.71	57,981,490.76	49,821,480.76	43,032,161.47	pos
Olivetol	$C_{11}H_{16}O_2$	180.11491	6.118	181.1222	1,579,855,301	219,826,697.2	1,867,879,237	7,178,979,570	4,250,002,794	pos
N-Sinapoylputrescine	$C_{15}H_{22}N_2O_4$	294.15804	5.245	295.1653	223,796,341	85,396,936	2,034,501,055	114,756,689.9	642,065,079.6	pos
m-Cresol	C_7H_8O	108.05771	6.987	109.065	453,056,628	492,797,783.9	760,132,605.4	934,468,079.3	1,352,699,960	pos
N-Feruloylspermidine	$C_{17}H_{27}N_3O_3$	321.20493	5.311	322.2122	16,227,369.5	ND	ND	388,149,239	291,830,830.8	pos
Syringetin	$C_{17}H_{14}O_8$	346.06869	5.989	347.076	213,797,430	36,006,183.47	83,525,509.69	56,476,876.03	2,790,118.961	pos
10-Gingerol	$C_{21}H_{34}O_4$	350.24526	6.449	351.2525	63,159,023.2	31,907,273.33	85,237,129.4	59,818,272.11	185,615,026	pos
Synephrine	$C_9H_{13}NO_2$	167.09488	5.367	168.102	11,473,821.2	10,736,209.71	32,505,178.53	29,179,639.69	37,779,114.95	pos
Homovanillic acid	$C_9H_{10}O_4$	182.0578	6.121	165.0545	36,791,534.7	53,843,338.18	98,234,762.32	79,103,854.53	64,102,700.09	pos
3-Hydroxy-glabrol	$C_{25}H_{28}O_5$	408.19311	2.638	409.2004	15,627,920.5	7,577,848.342	12,982,293.77	2,144,060.696	65,127,151.99	pos

Table 2. *Cont.*

Name	Formula	Molecular Weight	Retention Time (min)	*m/z*	Relative Quantitative Value [#]					Polarity Mode
					A	B	C	D	E	
Eupatilin	$C_{18}H_{16}O_7$	344.08942	6.993	345.0967	ND	55,836,940	28,821,311.22	ND	ND	pos
Cyanin chloride	$C_{27}H_{31}ClO_{16}$	646.12943	7.508	647.1367	ND	ND	ND	80,724,006.14	78,662,587.44	pos
N-Caffeoylagmatine	$C_{14}H_{20}N_4O_3$	292.15315	5.011	585.3145	7,508,559.99	ND	24,444,379.22	ND	31,458,991.44	pos
Capsaicin	$C_{18}H_{27}NO_3$	305.19874	6.452	306.206	12,087,681.5	2,776,542.382	25,089,124.12	17,821,873.15	15,588,985.07	pos
(−)-Epigallocatechin	$C_{15}H_{14}O_7$	306.07351	5.599	307.0808	ND	ND	ND	53,832,441.21	13,548,177.99	pos
Tangeretin	$C_{20}H_{20}O_7$	372.12075	5.423	355.1177	ND	ND	ND	5,917,055.075	ND	pos
Tyrosol	$C_8H_{10}O_2$	138.06757	5.138	299.1232	ND	5,068,007.118	6,256,197.387	3,557,810.413	5,186,575.09	pos
Epigallocatechin gallate	$C_{22}H_{18}O_{11}$	458.0842	5.285	457.0769	ND	ND	ND	33,786,926.33	2,234,317.434	neg
Luteolin	$C_{15}H_{10}O_6$	286.04732	10.293	285.04	40,846,755.4	35,743,531.6	65,613,907.63	22,530,517.56	33,920,595.23	neg
Quercetin-3β-D-glucoside	$C_{21}H_{20}O_{12}$	464.09462	5.497	463.0873	7,811,562.25	31,223,348,577	424,844,619.2	93,067,914.68	49,376,059.55	neg
Quercetin	$C_{15}H_{10}O_7$	302.04189	6.168	301.0346	50,861,607.5	3,456,250,485	167,546,683.1	100,938,577	9,389,005.75	neg
Naringenin	$C_{15}H_{12}O_5$	272.06788	5.811	271.0606	696,497,190	2,964,782,677	26,471,899.02	157,562,617.8	15,620,342.86	neg
Trifolin	$C_{21}H_{20}O_{11}$	448.09963	5.586	447.0924	15,251,810.2	3,616,379,862	219,125,099.9	768,635,754.3	672,018,938.1	neg
Myricetin	$C_{15}H_{10}O_8$	318.03709	11.206	317.0298	ND	3,028,274.129	ND	19,796,260.72	8,338,753.585	neg
Catechin	$C_{15}H_{14}O_6$	290.07854	5.233	289.0713	ND	11,479,131.28	ND	362,680,090	21,989,649.4	neg
Rutin	$C_{27}H_{30}O_{16}$	610.15255	5.406	609.1453	4,896,680,579	11,032,993,617	4,297,271,375	391,130,440.3	181,767,093.3	neg
Camelliaside A	$C_{33}H_{40}O_{20}$	756.21056	5.419	755.2033	1,856,076,137	152,399,114.1	9,105,591.564	4,331,242,550	2,044,379,996	neg
Vitexin	$C_{21}H_{20}O_{10}$	432.10434	5.582	477.1025	25,549,827.3	3,047,473,762	142,276,104.5	693,348,490.6	225,742,072.2	neg
Quercetin-3-O-beta-glucopyranosyl-6′-acetate	$C_{23}H_{22}O_{13}$	506.10501	5.508	505.0977	3,746,894.48	1,951,523,698	22,777,582.34	5,963,197.709	ND	neg
(−)-Gallocatechin	$C_{15}H_{14}O_7$	306.07093	1.48	305.0636	426,513,401	202,996,217.7	352,989,760.4	778,605,608.9	197,179,065.1	neg
C-pentosyl-apeignin O-feruloylhexoside	$C_{36}H_{36}O_{17}$	740.19445	5.658	739.1872	ND	ND	4,277,967.468	482,030,561.8	398,168,515.7	neg
Lysionotin	$C_{18}H_{16}O_7$	344.08877	6.465	343.0815	5,045,809.68	366,547,540.5	ND	ND	ND	neg
Morin Hydrate	$C_{15}H_{12}O_8$	320.05248	5.669	319.0452	40,211,091.5	ND	ND	9,452,094.08	6,808,868.601	neg
Laricitrin	$C_{16}H_{12}O_8$	332.05252	5.702	331.0452	30,519,617	24,396,606.59	15,799,130.1	313,192,808.2	5,637,949.068	neg
Liquiritigenin	$C_{15}H_{12}O_4$	256.07285	5.724	255.0656	ND	222,165,135.5	ND	ND	ND	neg
Scutellarin	$C_{21}H_{18}O_{12}$	462.07957	5.554	461.0723	ND	5,717,791.241	264,675,766.2	ND	ND	neg
Astragaloside I	$C_{45}H_{72}O_{16}$	868.48566	9.474	867.4784	192,740,828	ND	9,275,827.199	ND	ND	neg
Procyanidin B2	$C_{30}H_{26}O_{12}$	578.1422	5.083	577.1349	ND	ND	ND	148,408,865.7	5,040,187.901	neg
Dihydromyricetin	$C_{15}H_{12}O_8$	320.05263	5.306	319.0454	ND	ND	ND	85,023,185.27	2,195,644.614	neg
Typhaneoside	$C_{34}H_{42}O_{20}$	770.21135	5.284	769.2041	159,063,911	1,31,733,637.6	34,066,220.05	231,660,164.2	63,182,732.09	neg
Flavanone	$C_{15}H_{12}O_2$	224.08876	3.351	223.0815	20,038,004.3	1,65,971,467.7	9,437,481.559	19,717,896.64	8,643,483.933	neg
Epicatechin-3-O-gallate	$C_{22}H_{18}O_{10}$	442.08902	5.363	441.0817	ND	ND	ND	42,171,533.16	3,743,314.08	neg

Table 2. *Cont.*

Name	Formula	Molecular Weight	Retention Time (min)	*m/z*	Relative Quantitative Value #					Polarity Mode
					A	B	C	D	E	
Theaflavin	$C_{29}H_{24}O_{12}$	564.12608	5.844	563.1188	ND	ND	ND	28,600,078.21	33,086,570.62	neg
Casticin	$C_{19}H_{18}O_8$	374.09987	6.383	373.0926	ND	26,391,447.21	ND	ND	ND	neg
Tricin O-malonylhexoside	$C_{26}H_{26}O_{15}$	578.12501	5.27	577.1177	ND	29,288,856.87	ND	ND	ND	neg
Wogonoside	$C_{22}H_{20}O_{11}$	460.09926	5.694	459.092	ND	ND	ND	17,955,043.79	13,013,533.49	neg
Methyl Hesperidin	$C_{29}H_{36}O_{16}$	640.20009	5.25	639.1928	ND	ND	ND	7,345,122.487	ND	neg
Isosilybin	$C_{25}H_{22}O_{10}$	482.12057	5.762	481.1133	ND	ND	18,684,411.97	ND	ND	neg
Engeletin	$C_{21}H_{22}O_{10}$	434.12086	5.569	433.1136	ND	13,637,214.15	10,381,819.84	ND	ND	neg
Heptamethoxyflavone	$C_{22}H_{24}O_9$	432.14137	5.495	431.1341	ND	ND	7,644,360.736	ND	ND	neg
Isovitexin	$C_{21}H_{20}O_{10}$	432.10562	6.007	431.0983	ND	ND	3,278,357.703	ND	ND	neg
Pelargonidin chloride	$C_{15}H_{11}ClO_5$	306.02892	6.223	305.0217	ND	ND	ND	ND	ND	neg
Pectolinarin	$C_{29}H_{34}O_{15}$	622.1918	10.469	621.1845	1,634,093.99	3,236,392.594	1,918,622.412	ND	981,732.339	neg
Astilbin	$C_{21}H_{22}O_{11}$	450.11592	4.901	449.1086	ND	ND	ND	3,294,421.57	ND	neg
Cyanidin chloride	$C_{15}H_{11}ClO_6$	322.0258	5.564	321.0185	ND	ND	2,971,429.103	ND	ND	neg
(−)-Catechin Gallate	$C_{22}H_{18}O_{10}$	442.08978	4.971	423.0719	ND	ND	ND	3,956,997.454	ND	neg
6-Shogaol	$C_{17}H_{24}O_3$	276.17204	7.294	275.1649	ND	ND	1,419,321.159	ND	ND	neg
Orientin	$C_{21}H_{20}O_{11}$	448.10042	4.997	447.0931	ND	ND	ND	ND	ND	neg
Baohuoside I	$C_{27}H_{30}O_{10}$	514.18345	1.851	513.1762	ND	ND	479,069.6341	ND	ND	neg
Tulipanin	$C_{27}H_{31}O_{16}$	611.16334	4.729	610.1561	ND	ND	ND	1,155,753.351	807,483.1285	neg
Kuwanon A	$C_{25}H_{24}O_6$	420.1573	1.995	419.15	ND	124,712.2319	ND	154,082.8984	ND	neg
Vitexin-2-O-rhaMnoside	$C_{27}H_{30}O_{14}$	578.16401	2.963	577.1567	ND	ND	ND	341,012.0014	245,379.7201	neg
Quercetin 3-O-sophoroside	$C_{27}H_{30}O_{17}$	626.14729	5.308	625.14	12,969,050	5,464,610,685	22,465,559.36	385,733,174.2	62,948,432.34	neg
Sinapyl Alcohol	$C_{11}H_{14}O_4$	210.08836	5.613	209.0811	ND	ND	3,982,772.239	58,595,380.89	93,954,803.85	neg
Pyrogallol	$C_6H_6O_3$	126.03056	3.136	125.0233	52,253,814.5	50,876,134.5	54,751,955.84	5,056,863,601	4,650,663,073	neg
Cyanidin 3-rutinoside	$C_{27}H_{31}O_{15}$	595.16789	4.9	594.1606	ND	ND	ND	78,888,627.46	3,570,249.836	neg
Eriodictyol	$C_{15}H_{12}O_6$	288.06298	6.017	269.0451	37,755,502.9	151,216,709.3	18,272,926.02	41,340,090.1	4,827,039.11	neg
Vaccarin	$C_{32}H_{38}O_{19}$	726.19982	5.289	725.1928	ND	63,646,196.73	ND	ND	5,883,643.504	neg
6-Paradol	$C_{17}H_{26}O_3$	278.1878	5.89	323.186	185,053,697	305,250,229.3	295,294,310.1	275,009,885.5	659,984,250.6	neg
Epigallocatechin	$C_{15}H_{14}O_7$	306.07363	4.832	305.0664	ND	ND	ND	37,577,124.11	3,325,753.027	neg
Taxifolin	$C_{15}H_{12}O_7$	304.05811	5.441	303.0505	3,570,091.41	16,824,267.62	21,717,034.58	7,035,144.266	2,900,749.473	neg
Quercetin 3-alpha-L-arabinofuranoside (Avicularin)	$C_{20}H_{18}O_{11}$	434.08376	5.554	433.0765	ND	72,544,130.62	2,043,273.191	5,471,247.624	ND	neg
Ferulaldehyde	$C_{10}H_{10}O_3$	178.06273	7.239	355.1183	20,749,154.8	22,025,828.83	4,208,647.71	7,550,227.058	ND	neg

* ND means that the substance was not detected in the ethanol extract of the bee pollen. A, B, C, D, and E represent rapeseed, apricot, camellia, lotus, and sunflower bee pollens, respectively. # The relative quantitative value of each component can be compared among different EEBPs, but it cannot be compared among different components.

2.2. Antioxidant and Tyrosinase Inhibitory Capacities of Ethanol Extracts of Bee Pollens

The antioxidant capacities of EEBPs are shown in Table 3. The antioxidant capacities of sunflower EEBP were highest among those of the other four species EEBPs determined by the DPPH, FRAP, and ABTS assays.

Table 3. Antioxidant capacities of ethanol extracts of bee pollens.

Bee Pollen	DPPH (μg TE/mg)	FRAP (μg TE/mg)	ABTS (μg TE/mg)
Rapeseed	76.03 ± 1.17 [b]	123.82 ± 3.79 [b]	177.31 ± 1.39 [b]
Apricot	31.36 ± 1.44 [d]	56.04 ± 2.22 [d]	174.30 ± 1.88 [b]
Camellia	60.03 ± 1.49 [c]	96.34 ± 2.41 [c]	166.14 ± 2.80 [b]
Lotus	2.50 ± 0.18 [e]	8.29 ± 0.48 [e]	13.80 ± 0.52 [c]
Sunflower	119.26 ± 2.17 [a]	156.83 ± 4.62 [a]	204.88 ± 1.89 [a]

Different superscript lowercase characters in the same column mean statistically significant differences ($p < 0.05$).

The tyrosinase inhibitory capacities of EEBP are shown in Figure 2. The five EEBPs inhibited the activity of tyrosinase in a concentration-dependent manner. There were significant differences in the inhibition rate among different species of EEBPs. The sunflower EEBP had much higher inhibition rates for tyrosinase activity than the EEBPs of apricot, rapeseed, camellia, and lotus. At a concentration of 50 μg/mL, the inhibition rate of the sunflower EEBP was higher than 50%, while those of the other EEBPs were lower than 50%.

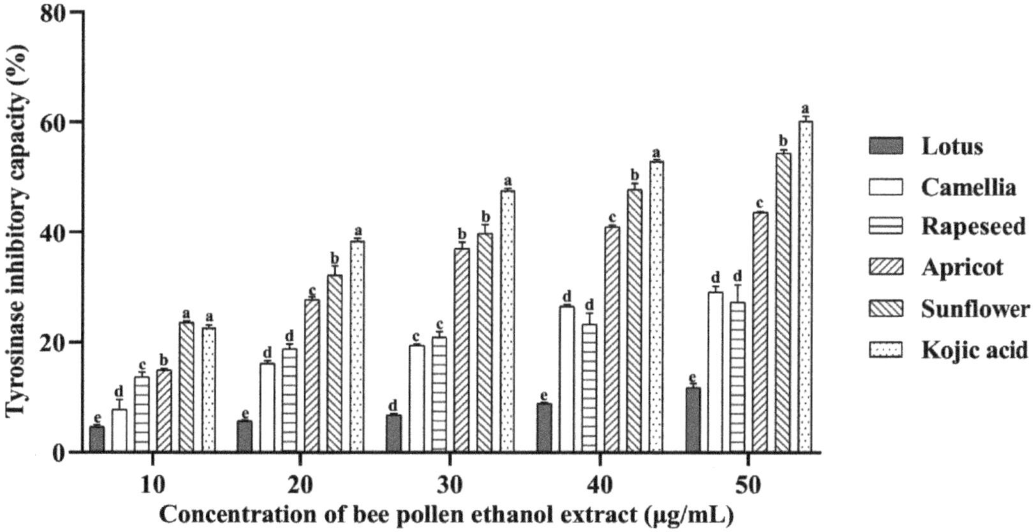

Figure 2. The antityrosinase activities of ethanol extracts of bee pollens. Note: Different lowercase characters above the same concentration mean significant differences ($p < 0.05$).

2.3. Anti-Melanogenesis Activity of Ethanol Extracts of Bee Pollens on Melanin Production in Mouse B16F10 Melanoma Cells

The relative melanin contents in B16F10 cells treated with EEBPs decreased in a concentration-dependent manner (Figure 3). The highest anti-melanogenesis activity was observed for sunflower EEBP, which was about 25% at 25 μg/mL BEEP, followed by apricot, camellia, rapeseed, and lotus EEBPs.

The correlation coefficients among DPPH, FRAP, ABTS, TPC, TFC, tyrosinase inhibitory, and anti-melanogenesis activities showed that the anti-melanogenesis activity was highly dependent on the TPCs in the EEBPs ($p < 0.05$, Table 4).

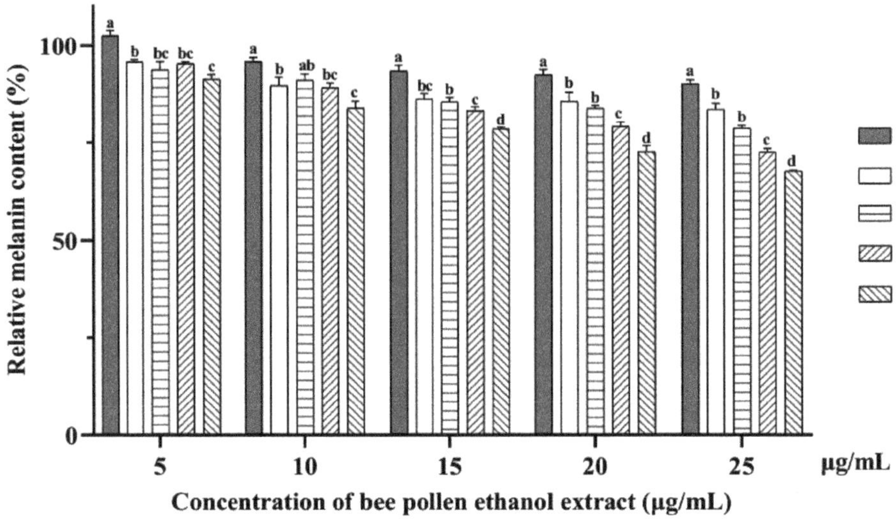

Figure 3. The relative melanin content in B16F10 cells treated with ethanol extracts of bee pollens. Note: Different lowercase characters above the same concentration mean significant differences ($p < 0.05$).

Table 4. The correlation coefficients among DPPH, FRAP, ABTS, TPC, TFC, tyrosinase inhibitory, and anti-melanogenesis activities.

	DPPH	FRAP	ABTS	TPC	TFC	Tyrosinase Inhibitory	Anti-Melanogenesis
DPPH	1						
FRAP	0.986 **	1					
ABTS	0.800	0.849	1				
TPC	0.879 *	0.885	0.849 *	1			
TFC	0.924 *	0.939 *	0.959 **	0.953 *	1		
Tyrosinase Inhibitory	0.722	0.682	0.827	0.964 *	0.866	1	
Anti-Melanogenesis	0.675	0.633	0.811	0.940 *	0.826	0.987 **	1

Characters "*" and "**" mean significant differences at $p < 0.05$ and $p < 0.01$, respectively.

2.4. Anti-Melanogenesis Mechanism of the Ethanol Extract of Sunflower Bee Pollen on Melanin Production in Mouse B16F10 Melanoma Cells

The DIA quantitative proteomics analysis identified a total of 7555 proteins. Compared to the control group, 272 proteins were differentially expressed, consisting of 171 up-regulated and 101 down-regulated differentially expressed proteins (DEPs). The volcano map of differentially expressed proteins in B16F10 cells (sunflower EEBP vs. control) is shown in Figure S2. Analyzing the subcellular localization of these differentially expressed proteins revealed that 28.35% were located in the cytoplasm, 27.84% in the nucleus, and 11.34% in the mitochondria. The Gene Ontology (GO) enrichment analysis indicated that the differentially expressed proteins primarily participated in metabolic processes, catalytic activities, redox processes, and calcium ion binding. Additionally, the KEGG enrichment analysis suggested that the sunflower EEBP inhibited melanogenesis in B16F10 cells by reducing the expression of proteins associated with the cAMP, MAPK, and TNF signaling pathways (Table 5), which are highly related to melanogenesis, even though these pathways were not significantly different from the control group.

Table 5. The differentially expressed proteins enriched in pathways highly related to melanogenesis in mouse B16F10 melanoma cells treated with the ethanol extract of sunflower bee pollen compared with the control group.

Pathway	Up-Regulated Proteins	Down-Regulated Proteins
MAPK		MAP2K1, NFKB2, RELB, RPS6KA3, CASP3, TRAF6, MAP2K5, MAPKAPK3
cAMP	ADCY7, GRIN2A	MAP2K1
AMPK	CPT1A	STRADA, CCNA2, FASN

3. Discussion

The polyphenol components varied mainly depending on the botanic source. In this experiment, the TPC of bee pollen samples ranged from 5.39 to 132.51 mg GAE/g EEBP. This range is similar to other research if the extraction rate was included, which were 9.41 to 27.49 [41], 4.64 to 17.93 [42], and 12.60 to 84.22 mg GAE/g bee pollen [43], and 15.73 to 26.92 [44], 4.2 to 29.6 GAE mg/g extract of bee pollen [45]. The EEBP with the highest TPC was sunflower bee pollen, which was different from previous reports, which were 12.29 mg GAE/g dried bee pollen from Hungary [41], 7.56 mg GAE/g dried bee pollen from Romania [42], and 2.907 mg GAE/g of dried bee pollen harvested from Serbia [46]. Meanwhile, the EEBP with the lowest TPC was lotus bee pollen, which was similar to the reported values [47] of 1.81 mg PAE/g bee pollen from China extracted with 75% ethanol/water solvents and determined by protocatechuic acid (PA) as the standard solution. The EEBP with a medium TPC was rapeseed, 12.57 mg GAE/g dried bee pollen from China [48] and calculated by free and bound phenolic extracts and measured by the same method as this paper. There was 12.90 mg PAE/g bee pollen from China extracted by 75% ethanol/water solvents [47]. This difference in the TPC may be related to the different geographic origins, extraction solvents, and storage conditions of bee pollen.

The TPC mainly depends on the polyphenols in bee pollen. EEBPs of rapeseed, camellia, sunflower, lotus, and apricot bee pollens contain 56, 46, 45, 42, and 35 polyphenols. Reports showed that there were 37 phenolic compounds in sunflower bee pollen from Serbia [46], 35 phenolic compounds in eight bee pollen samples from Morocco [49], and 258 phenolic compounds in thirty-two bee pollen samples from Italy [44]. The different phenolic compounds in bee pollen depend on the geographic and botanical origins, storage conditions, extraction solvent, and determination methods of bee pollen.

The antioxidant activities of various species of bee pollen are mostly attributed to their polyphenols. Consistency exists in the antioxidant activities from the DPPH, FRAP, and ABTS assays. There is a consistency in the DPPH (IC_{50}) and ABTS assays [47]. EEBPs from five of a total of fourteen species from high to low were rapeseed = camellia > apricot > sunflower > lotus [47], which were similar to sunflower > rapeseed > camellia > apricot > lotus in this experiment. This different result was caused by the different expression method, TE per bee pollen or EEBPs. The phenolic compounds can directly participate in antioxidant activity [50]. This is consistent with the results of this study, where the correlation coefficients between the phenolic content and antioxidant activity were higher than 0.858.

Tyrosinase is the key enzyme for melanin production in the human body. Inhibiting tyrosinase can effectively reduce melanin synthesis, thereby achieving a whitening effect on the skin [51]. Some studies have found that phenolamide in bee pollen is a component that affects the tyrosinase activity [52]. In this study, the five EEBPs inhibited tyrosinase in a concentration-dependent manner. The inhibitory activity of sunflower EEBP toward tyrosinase was the highest. Sunflower bee pollen from Thailand also showed inhibition of tyrosinase activity after extraction with methanol [39], which is consistent with the results of this study. However, some studies have shown that apricot bee pollen, after extraction with ethyl acetate, has a better inhibitory effect on tyrosinase activity than sunflower bee pollen [52]. This difference may be the difference in extraction methods and solvents. The bee pollen in this study was extracted with ethanol, while it was first extracted with ethanol followed by ethyl acetate in the previous studies. A study analyzed the tyrosinase inhibitory properties of 14 types of single-flower bee pollens from China. The results showed that almost all the samples had different tyrosinase inhibitory activities due to the plant sources of bee pollen and extraction solvents. The apricot, camellia, and sunflower extracts showed excellent tyrosinase inhibitory activity [47]. In this study, the five EEBPs inhibited melanin synthesis in the mouse B16F10 melanoma cells within the concentration ranges that did not affect cellular activity. Some studies have also shown that the phenolic substances extracted from rapeseed bee pollen inhibited tyrosinase activity, thereby inhibiting melanin production [48]. DIA quantitative proteomics was used to detect the in vitro inhibitory effect of sunflower EEBP on melanin production in B16F10 cells. DEPs STAT1, caspase-3, FASN, and METTL3 were significantly up-regulated, and Heme oxygenase 1 (HO-1), Cytochrome c, and Melanophilin (MLPH) were significantly down-regulated. They were enriched in pathways related to melanin production.

The protein STAT1 usually exists in the form of a functional dimer. When STAT1 is up-regulated, it may be closely related to tumorigenesis. The biological forms of STAT1 include activated phosphorylated forms and the less active non-phosphorylated form [53]. The expression of phosphorylation STAT1 increased when normal human melanocytes (NHMs) [54] and B16F10 cells [55] were treated with the cytokine IFN-γ. In this study, expression of STAT1 in B16F10 cells was also significantly increased. Sunflower EEBP inhibits melanin production through the up-regulation of STAT1.

Caspase-3 is a cysteine–aspartic protease commonly involved in pyroptosis and apoptosis [56], but it is also involved in the processing and production of melanin. Rhododendrol inhibits tyrosinase with a decrease in melanin synthesis in mouse B16 melanoma cells and an increase in caspase-3 levels [57]. In the study of epidermal functional melanocytes and melanin loss, caffeic acid derivatives down-regulated caspase-3 in PIG1 cells, thereby protecting against melanin loss [58]. In this study, the caspase-3 protein was up-regulated after EEBP acted on B16F10 cells. Sunflower EEBP destroyed the protection of melanin loss, thereby inhibiting melanin production.

Fatty acid synthase (FASN) is an important protein that can synthesize fatty acids in cells [59]. During this process, the overexpression of METTL3 can increase the expression of FASN [60]. Different types of fatty acids can inhibit melanin production [61–64]. Both FASN and METTL3 were significantly up-regulated in this study. Sunflower EEBP increased the synthesis of fatty acids in cells and further inhibited melanin production.

Heme oxygenase 1 (HO-1) is a ubiquitous protein in most human tissues and is involved in many physiological processes [65]. Kaempferol can promote melanin synthesis and the expression of HO-1 in PIG1 cells [66] and reduce the production of ROS in the cells and the damage caused by H_2O_2. HO-1 was significantly down-regulated in B16F10 cells treated with EEBP. Sunflower EEBP decreased HO-1 levels and blocked the melanin synthesis pathway.

Cytochrome c is an intermembrane mitochondrial protein that interacts in the peroxidation process of various molecules. Cytochrome c can oxidize catecholamines and their S-cysteinyl derivatives, producing melanin as the final product [67]. Cytochrome c was down-regulated by the sunflower EEBP thereby reducing the synthesis of the final product melanin.

Melanophilin (MLPH) is a protein involved in the formation and transfer of melanin [68]. MLPH expression in B16F10 cells was significantly reduced after wogonin treatment [69], consistent with the down-regulation of MLPH in this study when B16F10 cells were treated with the sunflower EEBP.

4. Materials and Methods

4.1. Samples and Chemical Reagents

Rapeseed bee pollen, apricot bee pollen, camellia bee pollen, lotus bee pollen, and sunflower bee pollen were produced in Luoping County of Yunnan Province, Qinglong County of Hebei Province, Fuzhou City of Fujian Province, Jianyang County of Fujian Province, and Xuchang County of Henan Province, China, respectively. All bee pollen samples were harvested in 2023 and stored at −30 °C. The identification of the botanical origins and purities of bee pollen samples was determined by counting the percent of the matching types of pollen grains using a conventional inverted microscope (Nikon TS-100f, Tokyo, Japan) [3]. The purities of bee pollen samples are shown in Table S1. The morphologies of pollen gains are shown in Figure S1.

Dulbecco's modified Eagle's medium (DMEM) with high glucose, double antibiotics, and serum-free non-programmed cell freezing solution were purchased from Wuhan Pricella Biotechnology Co., Ltd. (Wuhan, China). LC-MS-grade methanol and formic acid were purchased from Thermo Fisher Scientific (Waltham, MA, USA). LC-MS-grade water was purchased from Merck, Germany. Analytical grade anhydrous ethanol and ferric chloride were purchased from Aladdin Scientific (Riverside, CA, USA). Trolox, 1,1-diphenyl-2-trinitrophenylhydrazine (DPPH), 2,2-azino-bis(3-ethyl-benzothiazole-6-sulfonic acid) diammonium salt (ABTS), petroleum ether, 2,4,6-tripyridyltriazine (TPTZ), PBS powder, mushroom tyrosinase, kojic acid, anhydrous ethanol, and sodium acetate were purchased from Shanghai Macklin Biochemical Technology Co., Ltd. (Shanghai, China). Acetic acid, PBS (pH 7.2–7.4), and hydrochloric acid were purchased from Sinopharm (Beijing, China). Trypan blue dye (0.4%) was purchased from Beijing Solarbio Science & Technology Co., Ltd. (Beijing, China). The CCK-8 kit was purchased from DOJINDO (Kumamoto, Japan). Trypsin was purchased from Hyclone Co., Logan, UT, USA. The B16F10 cell line was purchased from the China Center for Type Culture Collection (Wuhan, China).

4.2. Methods

4.2.1. Extraction of Bee Pollen

EEBPs were prepared according to reference [52], with some modifications. Bee pollen (50 g) was crushed. The lipids of the powder were removed with 100 mL of petroleum ether at 25 °C for 30 min with ultrasonic assistance (40 kHz) two times. Then, the residue was extracted with 200 mL of 80% ethanol at 25 °C for 30 min with ultrasonic assistance two times. Subsequently, the mixture was concentrated using a rotary evaporator after filtration. It was then dried using a vacuum freeze dryer (DGJ-500H, Shanghai Boden Biotechnology Co., Ltd., Shanghai, China) to obtain the EEBP, which was then stored at −30 °C (Haier Biomedical, Qingdao, China) for further experiments.

4.2.2. Determination of the Components in the Ethanol Extracts of Bee Pollens

The total phenolic contents (TPCs) of EEBPs were determined by the Folin–Ciocalteu (FC) colorimetric method [70]. Briefly, the EEBP was dissolved in ethanol and diluted to a concentration of 500 μg/mL. Then, 0.5 mL of the EEBP solution was mixed thoroughly with 2.5 mL of a 10% Folin phenol reagent in a 10 mL centrifuge tube. After 5 min, 2 mL of a 7.5% sodium carbonate solution (Na_2CO_3) was added to the mixture. The tube was placed in the dark at 25 °C for 60 min. The absorbance at 765 nm was measured by an ultraviolet spectrophotometer (T6, Beijing Puxi General Instrument Co., Ltd., Beijing, China). Gallic acid solutions (0.5 mL) of 10, 20, 40, 80, and 160 μg/mL were employed to establish a standard curve. The TPC is expressed as the gallic acid equivalent (mg GAE/g) contained in the EEBP.

The total flavone contents (TFCs) of EEBPs were determined using rutin standards and the $NaNO_2$-$Al(NO_3)_3$-NaOH colorimetric method [43]. The EEBP was dissolved in anhydrous ethanol and diluted to 500 μg/mL. The EEBP solution (1 mL) was added to a 10 mL centrifuge tube, 0.25 mL of a 5% $NaNO_2$ solution was added to mix and react for 6 min, then 0.25 mL of a 10% $Al(NO_3)_3$ solution was added to mix and react for 6 min, and finally, 2 mL of a 4% NaOH solution and 1.5 mL of ethanol were added. After standing for 15 min, the absorbance was measured at 510 nm. Rutin working solutions (1 mL) at 10, 20, 40, 80, and 160 μg/mL were used to establish the standard curve. The total flavonoid content is expressed as the rutin equivalent (mg RE/g) contained in the EEBP.

The chemical components of EEBPs were determined using a UHPLC-MS/MS system (Vanquish UHPLC system (Thermo Fisher Scientific Inc., Germering, Germany) coupled with an Orbitrap Q ExactiveTM HF-X mass spectrometer (ThermoFisher, Germering, Germany) by an untargeted metabolomic method performed by Novogene Co., Ltd. (Beijing, China) [71]. EEBP (25 mg) and 5000 μL of an 80% methanol aqueous solution were added to a 10 mL EP tube. It was whirled and centrifuged at 15,000× g at 4 °C for 20 min. A certain amount of the supernatant was diluted with mass spectrometry-grade water to a methanol content of 53%. It was centrifuged again for the UHPLC-MS/MS analysis. The chromatographic column was a Hypesil Gold column (C18) at 40 °C. Solutions of 0.1% formic acid and methanol were mobile phases A and B, respectively. The chromatographic gradient elution program was 0–1.5 min, 98% A; 3 min 15% A; 10 min 0% A; and 10.1–12 min 2% A at 0.2 mL/min. The mass spectrometry conditions were as follows: scan range of 100–1500 m/z; ESI source spray voltage of 3.5 kV; sheath gas flow rate of 35 psi; aux gas flow rate of 10 L/min; capillary temperature of 320 °C; s-lens RF level of 60; aux gas heater temperature of 350 °C; positive and negative polarity; and data-dependent MS/MS secondary scans.

4.2.3. Antioxidant and Tyrosinase Inhibitory Capacities of Ethanol Extracts of Bee Pollens

The DPPH radical scavenging activity, FRAP total antioxidant capacity, and ABTS cation radical scavenging activity of EEBPs were determined at 517, 593, and 734 nm using an ultraviolet spectrophotometer [72]. The results are shown in Trolox equivalents (TE), μg TE/mg EEBP.

The tyrosinase inhibitory capacities were determined according to reference [3], with some modifications. EEBPs were dissolved in ethanol (2 mg/mL) and then diluted to different concentrations (10–50 μg/mL) with PBS buffer (pH 6.8). A sample solution of 25 μL and 25 μL of tyrosinase solution (200 U/mL) were added to a 96-well plate and pre-incubated at 37 °C for 2 min, and then 200 μL of L-DOPA (0.5 mM) was added to each well for the reaction. The absorbance of the mixture was measured at 475 nm every 20 s at 37 °C for a total of 20 times. The inhibition rate was calculated as follows:

$$\text{Inhibition rate (\%)} = (1 - \text{k1}/\text{k0}) \times 100 \tag{1}$$

where k1 is the slope of the kinetic equation of the sample group and the positive control group, and k0 is the slope of the kinetic equation of the blank control group.

4.2.4. Anti-Melanogenesis Activities of Ethanol Extracts of Bee Pollens on Melanin Production in Mouse B16F10 Melanoma Cells

Mouse B16F10 melanoma cells were cultured in high-glucose DMEM (containing 10% FBS fetal bovine serum and 1% double antibiotics) in a 5% CO_2 incubator at 37 °C (C150, Binder, Tuttlingen, Germany). The cell number in suspension (100 μL) was counted with the assistance of trypan blue staining (100 μL). The concentration of cells was diluted to 5 × 10^4 cells/mL with the culture medium. Add 100 μL of cell suspension to each well of the 96-well plate. These cells were cultured for 24 h. The culture medium was removed and 100 μL of sterile PBS was added to each well for washing. Culture medium (100 μL) containing 5, 10, 15, 20, or 25 μg/mL EEBPs were added to 6 wells for each dose. Wells containing whole culture medium were the control group. Cells were continuously cultured in the incubator for 48 h. These cells were washed with sterile PBS. And then, 110 μL of culture medium containing the CCK-8 solution was added in a dark place. The cells were cultured for 2 h. Then, the absorbance at 450 nm was measured.

$$\begin{gathered}\text{Cell proliferation activity (\%)} = [(\text{OD of the experimental group} - \text{OD of the} \\ \text{blank group})/(\text{OD of the control group} - \text{OD of the blank group})] \times 100\end{gathered} \tag{2}$$

The determination of the anti-melanogenesis effect of EEBPs was performed according to the method of Sim et al. [73], with slight changes. Cells at a concentration of 1 × 10^4 cells/mL were transferred into 6-well plates. After treatment with 5, 10, 15, 20, or 25 μg/mL EEBP for 48 h, the cells in each group were collected into centrifuge tubes and counted. After centrifugation, 0.5 mL of a 1 mM NaOH solution (containing 10% DMSO) was added and heated in a water bath at 80 °C for 2 h. The absorbance at 405 nm was measured using an ELISA reader.

$$\text{Relative melanin content (\%)} = \text{(OD of experimental group/number of cells in the experimental group)/(OD of blank group/number of blank cells)} \times 100 \quad (3)$$

The correlations among DPPH, FRAP, ABTS, TPC, TFC, antityrosinase, and anti-melanogenesis activities were analyzed.

4.2.5. Analysis of the Anti-Melanogenesis Mechanism of the Ethanol Extract of Sunflower Bee Pollen on Melanin Production in Mouse B16F10 Melanoma Cells by Label-Free Proteomics

Differentially expressed proteins in mouse melanoma cells (B16F10) treated with sunflower EEBP, compared to a control group, were determined using DIA quantitative proteomics. In brief, 2 mL of cells at a concentration of 1×10^5 cells/mL were added to a 6-well plate and cultured for 24 h. After removing the culture medium, the cells were rewashed with 2 mL of PBS (pH 7.2–7.4). The cells were then incubated with 2 mL of culture medium containing 25 μg/mL sunflower EEBP (resulting in a final concentration of 25 μg/mL) for 48 h. Following this, the cells were washed twice with pre-cooled PBS at 4 °C and then digested with trypsin (0.25%). The collected cells were washed again with pre-cooled PBS and centrifuged (TDZ4K, Hunan Xiangyi Laboratory Instrument Development Co., Ltd., Changsha, China) at 137× g for 5 min twice. The cells were frozen in liquid nitrogen for 15 min and stored at −80 °C in a Haier Biomedical refrigerator (Qingdao, China). The extraction and determination of the total protein concentration, as well as the protein spectral analysis, were performed as outlined in a previous report [71].

4.2.6. Statistical Analysis

All experiments except for the chemical substance determination were performed in triplicate. Except for the proteomic experiment, one-way ANOVA was used to analyze the differences using GraphPad Prism 8.4.3 for Windows (GraphPad Software, Inc. San Diego, CA, USA), where $p < 0.01$ means an extremely statistically significant difference between the treatment group and the control group, and $p < 0.05$ means a statistically significant difference. The results are expressed as means ± standard errors.

The offline data files for the chemical substance determination were imported into CD 3.3 library search software for processing. Each metabolite was screened by parameters such as the retention time and mass-to-charge ratio. Then, the peak area was corrected with the first QC to make the identification more accurate. Then, the mass deviation was set to 5 ppm, the signal intensity deviation was 30%, and the minimum signal intensity, the adduct ion, and other information were set for peak extraction. At the same time, the peak area was quantified, and the target ion was integrated. The molecular formula was predicted by the molecular ion peak and fragment ion and compared with the mzCloud (https://www.mzcloud.org/, accessed on 10 August 2024), mzVault, and Masslist databases. A blank sample was employed to remove the background ions, and the original quantitative results were standardized to obtain the relative peak area. The compounds with a relative peak area CV higher than 30% in the QC sample were deleted, and, finally, the metabolite identification and relative quantitative values were obtained using the following formula: sample metabolite original quantitative value/(sum of sample metabolite quantitative values/sum of QC1 sample metabolite quantitative values). The data processing was based on the Linux operating system (CentOS v6.6) and R (R-3.4.3) and Python (Python-3.5.0) software.

The spectra obtained from LC-MS/MS were analyzed as described in a previous report [74]. The proteins whose quantities were significantly different between the experimental and control groups ($p \leq 0.05$ and fold change (FC) > 1.2 or FC < 0.83) were defined as differentially expressed proteins (DEPs).

5. Conclusions

Each type of bee pollen has unique substances. The antityrosinase activity of sunflower EEBP and anti-melanogenesis activity in B16F10 cells were the highest among the rapeseed, apricot, camellia, lotus, and sunflower EEBPs. The anti-melanogenesis activities of bee pollens were positively correlated with their antityrosinase activities and total phenol contents. The sunflower EEBP inhibited melanogenesis in B16F10 cells by reducing the expression of related proteins in the cAMP, MAPK, and TNF signaling pathways. This result provides a basis for the future industrial development of a raw material for skin whitening using sunflower bee pollen.

Supplementary Materials: The following supporting information can be downloaded at https://www.mdpi.com/article/10.3390/ph17121634/s1: Table S1. The purity of bee pollen samples. Figure S1. Morphology of bee pollen grains. Figure S2. Volcano map of proteins in B16F10 cells (sunflower EEBP vs. control).

Author Contributions: Conceptualization, methodology, software, W.Y.; data curation, Q.H., J.W. and J.L.; writing—original draft preparation, Q.H. and J.W.; writing—review and editing, W.Y. All authors have read and agreed to the published version of the manuscript.

Funding: This research received no external funding.

Institutional Review Board Statement: Not applicable.

Informed Consent Statement: Not applicable.

Data Availability Statement: Data are contained within this article.

Conflicts of Interest: The authors declare no conflicts of interest.

References

1. Clarke, D.; Morley, E.; Robert, D. The bee, the flower, and the electric field: Electric ecology and aerial electroreception. *J. Comp. Physiol. A Neuroethol. Sens. Neural. Behav. Physiol.* **2017**, *203*, 737–748. [CrossRef] [PubMed]
2. Campos, M.G.; Frigerio, C.; Lopes, J.; Bogdanov, S. What is the future of Bee-Pollen? *J. ApiProd. ApiMed. Sci.* **2010**, *2*, 131–144. [CrossRef]
3. Yang, K.; Wu, D.; Ye, X.; Liu, D.; Chen, J.; Sun, P. Characterization of chemical composition of bee pollen in China. *J. Agric. Food Chem.* **2013**, *61*, 708–718. [CrossRef]
4. Campos, M.G.; Bogdanov, S.; de Almeida-Muradian, L.B.; Szczęsna, T.; Mancebo, Y.; Frigerio, C.; Ferreira, F. Pollen composition and standardisation of analytical methods. *J. Apic. Res.* **2008**, *47*, 154–161. [CrossRef]
5. Li, Q.; Wang, K.; Marcucci, M.C.; Sawaya, A.C.; Hu, L.; Xue, X.; Wu, L.; Hu, F. Nutrient-rich bee pollen: A treasure trove of active natural metabolites. *J. Funct. Foods* **2018**, *49*, 472–484. [CrossRef]
6. Nogueira, C.; Iglesias, A.; Feás, X.; Estevinho, L.M. Commercial bee pollen with different geographical origins: A comprehensive approach. *Int. J. Mol. Sci.* **2012**, *13*, 11173–11187. [CrossRef]
7. Qiao, J.; Feng, Z.; Zhang, Y.; Xiao, X.; Dong, J.; Haubruge, E.; Zhang, H. Phenolamide and flavonoid glycoside profiles of 20 types of monofloral bee pollen. *Food Chem.* **2023**, *405*, 134800. [CrossRef] [PubMed]
8. Çobanoğlu, D.N. Assessing monofloral bee pollens from Türkiye: Palynological verification, phenolic profile, and antioxidant activity. *J. Food Sci.* **2024**, *89*, 1711–1726. [CrossRef] [PubMed]
9. Kalaycıoğlu, Z.; Kaygusuz, H.; Döker, S.; Kolaylı, S.; Erim, F.B. Characterization of Turkish honeybee pollens by principal component analysis based on their individual organic acids, sugars, minerals, and antioxidant activities. *LWT–Food Sci. Technol.* **2017**, *84*, 402–408. [CrossRef]
10. Cheng, N.; Chen, S.; Liu, X.; Zhao, H.; Cao, W. Impact of schisandrachinensis bee pollen on nonalcoholic fatty liver disease and gut microbiota in highfat diet induced obese mice. *Nutrients* **2019**, *11*, 346. [CrossRef]
11. Tao, Y.; Zhou, E.; Li, F.; Meng, L.; Li, Q.; Wu, L. Allergenicity alleviation of bee pollen by enzymatic hydrolysis: Regulation in mice allergic mediators, metabolism, and gut microbiota. *Food* **2022**, *11*, 3454. [CrossRef] [PubMed]
12. Khalil, F.; El-Sheikh, N.M. The effects of dietary Egyptian propolis and bee pollen supplementation against toxicity if sodium fluoride in rats. *Vet. Med. J. Giza* **2010**, *11*, 310–316. [CrossRef]
13. Kaškonienė, V.; Adaskeviciute, V.; Kaškonas, P.; Mickienė, R.; Maruška, A.S. Antimicrobial and antioxidant activities of natural and fermented bee pollen. *Food Biosci.* **2020**, *34*, 100532. [CrossRef]
14. Lawag, I.L.; Yoo, O.; Lim, L.Y.; Hammer, K.; Locher, C. Optimisation of bee pollen extraction to maximise extractable antioxidant constituents. *Antioxidants* **2021**, *10*, 1113. [CrossRef] [PubMed]

15. De-Melo, A.A.; Estevinho, M.L.; Sattler, J.A.; Souza, B.R.; Freitas, A.D.; Barth, O.M.; Almeida-Muradian, L.B. Effect of processing conditions on characteristics of dehydrated bee-pollen and correlation between quality parameters. *LWT–Food Sci. Technol.* **2016**, *65*, 808–815. [CrossRef]
16. Gercek, Y.C.; Celik, S.; Bayram, S. Screening of plant pollen sources, polyphenolic compounds, fatty acids and antioxidant/antimicrobial activity from bee pollen. *Molecules* **2022**, *27*, 117. [CrossRef] [PubMed]
17. Orvalho, T.; Vaz, D.C.; Ribeiro, V.; Campos, M.J. Storage procedures influence the antioxidant capacity of bee pollen. In Proceedings of the 1st International Conference on Water Energy Food and Sustainability (ICoWEFS 2021), Leiria, Portugal, 10–12 May 2021. [CrossRef]
18. Leblanc, B.; Davis, O.K.; Boue, S.M.; DeLucca, A.; Deeby, T. Antioxidant activity of Sonoran Desert bee pollen. *Food Chem.* **2009**, *115*, 1299–1305. [CrossRef]
19. Özcan, M.M.; Aljuhaimi, F.; Babiker, E.E.; Uslu, N.; Ceylan, D.A.; Ghafoor, K.; Özcan, M.M.; Dursun, N.; Ahmed, I.A.; Jamiu, F.G.; et al. Determination of antioxidant activity, phenolic compound, mineral contents and fatty acid compositions of bee pollen grains collected from different locations. *J. Apic. Sci.* **2019**, *63*, 69–79. [CrossRef]
20. Sarić, A.; Balog, T.; Sobocanec, S.; Kusić, B.; Sverko, V.; Rusak, G.; Likić, S.; Bubalo, D.; Pinto, B.; Reali, D.; et al. Antioxidant effects of flavonoid from *Croatian Cystus incanus* L. rich bee pollen. *Food Chem. Toxicol.* **2009**, *47*, 547–554. [CrossRef]
21. Jin, T.; Saravanakumar, K.; Wang, M. In vitro and in vivo antioxidant properties of water and methanol extracts of linden bee pollen. *Biocatal. Agric. Biotechnol.* **2018**, *13*, 186–189. [CrossRef]
22. Yıldız, O.; Can, Z.; Saral, O.; Yuluğ, E.; Oztürk, F.; Aliyazıcıoğlu, R.; Canpolat, S.; Kolaylı, S. Hepatoprotective potential of chestnut bee pollen on carbon tetrachloride-induced hepatic damages in rats. *Evid. Based Complement. Alternat. Med.* **2013**, *2013*, 461478. [CrossRef] [PubMed]
23. Al-Salem, H.S.; Al-Yousef, H.M.; Ashour, A.E.; Ahmed, A.F.; Amina, M.; Issa, I.S.; Bhat, R.S. Antioxidant and hepatorenal protective effects of bee pollen fractions against propionic acid-induced autistic feature in rats. *Food Sci. Nutr.* **2020**, *8*, 5114–5127. [CrossRef] [PubMed]
24. Aabed, K.; Shafi Bhat, R.; Moubayed, N.; Al-Mutiri, M.; Al-Marshoud, M.; Al-Qahtani, A.; Ansary, A. Ameliorative effect of probiotics (Lactobacillus paracaseii and Protexin®) and prebiotics (propolis and bee pollen) on clindamycin and propionic acid-induced oxidative stress and altered gut microbiota in a rodent model of autism. *Cell. Mol. Biol.* **2019**, *65*, 1–7. [CrossRef]
25. Al-daihan, S.; Bhata, R.S. Protective effect of bee pollen against sodium fluoride induced hepatonephrotoxicity and serum electrolyte changes in rats. *Fluoride* **2019**, *52*, 9–17.
26. Oyarzún, J.E.; Andia, M.E.; Uribe, S.; Núñez Pizarro, P.; Núñez, G.; Montenegro, G.; Bridi, R. Honeybee pollen extracts reduce oxidative stress and steatosis in hepatic cells. *Molecules* **2020**, *26*, 6. [CrossRef]
27. Pham, T.N.; Cazier, E.A.; Gormally, E.; Lawrence, P. Valorization of biomass polyphenols as potential tyrosinase inhibitors. *Drug Discov. Today* **2024**, *29*, 103843. [CrossRef] [PubMed]
28. Gou, L.; Lee, J.; Hao, H.; Park, Y.D.; Zhan, Y.; Lü, Z.R. The effect of oxaloacetic acid on tyrosinase activity and structure: Integration of inhibition kinetics with docking simulation. *Int. J. Biol. Macromol.* **2017**, *101*, 59–66. [CrossRef]
29. Brenner, M.; Hearing, V.J. The protective role of melanin against UV damage in human skin. *Photochem. Photobiol.* **2008**, *84*, 539–549. [CrossRef]
30. Wang, N.; Hebert, D.N. Tyrosinase maturation through the mammalian secretory pathway: Bringing color to life. *Pigm. Cell Res.* **2006**, *19*, 3–18. [CrossRef]
31. Saud, A.; Sagineedu, S.R.; Ng, H.S.; Stanslas, J.; Lim, J.C.W. Melanoma metastasis: What role does melanin play? *Oncol. Rep.* **2022**, *48*, 217. [CrossRef]
32. Bose, A.; Petsko, G.A.; Eliezer, D. Parkinson's disease and melanoma: Co-occurrence and mechanisms. *J. Park. Dis.* **2018**, *8*, 385–398. [CrossRef] [PubMed]
33. Krainc, T.; Monje, M.H.G.; Kinsinger, M.; Bustos, B.I.; Lubbe, S.J. Melanin and neuromelanin: Linking skin pigmentation and Parkinson's disease. *Mov. Disord.* **2023**, *38*, 185–195. [CrossRef]
34. Silva, C.C.; Benati, R.B.; Massaro, T.N.; Pereira, K.D.; Gaspar, L.R.; Marcato, P.D. Antioxidant and anti-tyrosinase activities of quercetin-loaded olive oil nanoemulsion as potential formulation for skin hyperpigmentation. *J. Dispers. Sci. Technol.* **2022**, *44*, 2628–2638. [CrossRef]
35. Şöhretoğlu, D.; Sari, S.; Barut, B.; Özel, A. Tyrosinase inhibition by some flavonoids: Inhibitory activity, mechanism by in vitro and in silico studies. *Bioorg. Chem.* **2018**, *81*, 168–174. [CrossRef]
36. Demirkiran, O.; Sabudak, T.; Ozturk, M.; Topcu, G. Antioxidant and tyrosinase inhibitory activities of flavonoids from *Trifolium nigrescens* Subsp. *petrisavi*. *J. Agric. Food Chem.* **2013**, *61*, 12598–12603. [CrossRef]
37. Matsuura, R.; Ukeda, H.; Sawamura, M. Tyrosinase inhibitory activity of citrus essential oils. *J. Agric. Food Chem.* **2006**, *54*, 2309–2313. [CrossRef] [PubMed]
38. Maisuthisakul, P.; Gordon, M.H. Antioxidant and tyrosinase inhibitory activity of mango seed kernel by product. *Food Chem.* **2009**, *117*, 332–341. [CrossRef]
39. Khongkarat, P.; Ramadhan, R.; Phuwapraisirisan, P.; Chanchao, C. Safflospermidines from the bee pollen of *Helianthus annuus* L. exhibit a higher in vitro antityrosinase activity than kojic acid. *Heliyon* **2020**, *6*, e03638. [CrossRef] [PubMed]
40. O'Donoghue, J.L. Hydroquinone and its analogues in dermatology-a risk-benefit viewpoint. *J. Cosmet. Dermatol.* **2006**, *5*, 196–203. [CrossRef]

41. Végh, R.; Sipiczki, G.; Csóka, M. Investigating the antioxidant and color properties of bee pollens of various plant sources. *Chem. Biodivers.* **2023**, *20*, e202300126. [CrossRef]
42. Oroian, M.; Dranca, F.; Ursachi, F. Characterization of romanian bee pollen—An important nutritional source. *Foods* **2022**, *11*, 2633. [CrossRef] [PubMed]
43. De Arruda, V.A.S.; dos Santos, A.V.; Sampaio, D.F.; Araújo, E.D.S.; Peixoto, A.L.D.C.; Estevinho, L.M.; de Almeida-Muradian, L.B. Brazilian bee pollen: Phenolic content, antioxidant properties and antimicrobial activity. *J. Apic. Res.* **2021**, *60*, 775–783. [CrossRef]
44. Alimoglu, G.; Guzelmeric, E.; Yuksel, P.I.; Celik, C.; Deniz, I.; Yesilada, E. Monofloral and polyfloral bee pollens: Comparative evaluation of their phenolics and bioactivity profiles. *LWT–Food Sci. Technol.* **2021**, *142*, 110973. [CrossRef]
45. Rocchetti, G.; Castiglioni, S.; Maldarizzi, G.; Carloni, P.; Lucini, L. UHPLC-ESI-QTOF-MS phenolic profiling and antioxidant capacity of bee pollen from different botanical origin. *Int. J. Food Sci. Technol.* **2018**, *54*, 335–346. [CrossRef]
46. Kostić, A.Ž.; Milinčić, D.D.; Gašić, U.M.; Nedić, N.; Stanojević, S.P.; Tešić, Ž.L.; Pešić, M.B. Polyphenolic profile and antioxidant properties of bee-collected pollen from sunflower (*Helianthus annuus* L.) plant. *LWT* **2019**, *112*, 108244. [CrossRef]
47. Zhang, H.; Wang, X.; Wang, K.; Li, C. Antioxidant and tyrosinase inhibitory properties of aqueous ethanol extracts from monofloral bee pollen. *J. Apic. Sci.* **2015**, *59*, 119–128. [CrossRef]
48. Sun, L.; Guo, Y.; Zhang, Y.; Zhuang, Y. Antioxidant and anti-tyrosinase activities of phenolic extracts from rape bee pollen and inhibitory melanogenesis by cAMP/MITF/TYR pathway in b16 mouse melanoma cells. *Front. Pharmacol.* **2017**, *8*, 104. [CrossRef]
49. Aylanc, V.; Larbi, S.; Calhelha, R.; Barros, L.; Rezouga, F.; Rodríguez-Flores, M.S.; Seijo, M.C.; El Ghouizi, A.; Lyoussi, B.; Falcão, S.I.; et al. Evaluation of antioxidant and anticancer activity of mono- and polyfloral moroccan bee pollen by characterizing phenolic and volatile compounds. *Molecules* **2023**, *28*, 835. [CrossRef]
50. Duh, P.D.; Tu, Y.Y.; Yen, G.C. Antioxidant activity of water extract of Harng Jyur (*Chrysanthemum morifolium* Ramat). *Food Sci. Technol.* **1999**, *32*, 269–277. [CrossRef]
51. Zhang, H.; Zhu, X.; Huang, Q.; Zhang, L.; Liu, X.; Liu, R.; Lu, Q. Antioxidant and anti-inflammatory activities of rape bee pollen after fermentation and their correlation with chemical components by ultra-performance liquid chromatography-quadrupole time of flight mass spectrometry-based untargeted metabolomics. *Food Chem.* **2023**, *409*, 135342. [CrossRef]
52. Zhang, X.; Yu, M.; Zhu, X.; Liu, R.; Lu, Q. Metabolomics reveals that phenolamides are the main chemical components contributing to the anti-tyrosinase activity of bee pollen. *Food Chem.* **2022**, *389*, 133071. [CrossRef] [PubMed]
53. Bonham, A.J.; Wenta, N.; Osslund, L.M.; Prussin, A.J., 2nd; Vinkemeier, U.; Reich, N.O. STAT1: DNA sequence-dependent binding modulation by phosphorylation, protein: Protein interactions and small-molecule inhibition. *Nucleic Acids Res.* **2013**, *41*, 754–763. [CrossRef] [PubMed]
54. Choi, H.; Choi, H.; Han, J.; Jin, S.H.; Park, J.Y.; Shin, D.W.; Lee, T.R.; Kim, K.; Lee, A.Y.; Noh, M. IL-4 inhibits the melanogenesis of normal human melanocytes through the JAK2-STAT6 signaling pathway. *J. Investig. Dermatol.* **2013**, *133*, 528–536. [CrossRef]
55. Han, N.R.; Park, H.J.; Ko, S.G.; Moon, P.D. Stigmasterol exerts an anti-melanoma property through down-regulation of reactive oxygen species and programmed cell death ligand 1 in melanoma cells. *Antioxidants* **2024**, *13*, 380. [CrossRef] [PubMed]
56. Bhat, A.A.; Thapa, R.; Afzal, O.; Agrawal, N.; Almalki, W.H.; Kazmi, I.; Alzarea, S.I.; Altamimi, A.S.A.; Prasher, P.; Singh, S.K.; et al. The pyroptotic role of Caspase-3/GSDME signalling pathway among various cancer: A Review. *Int. J. Biol. Macromol.* **2023**, *242*, 124832. [CrossRef]
57. Sasaki, M.; Kondo, M.; Sato, K.; Umeda, M.; Kawabata, K.; Takahashi, Y.; Suzuki, T.; Matsunaga, K.; Inoue, S. Rhododendrol, a depigmentation-inducing phenolic compound, exerts melanocyte cytotoxicity via a tyrosinase-dependent mechanism. *Pigm. Cell Melanoma Res.* **2014**, *27*, 754–763. [CrossRef]
58. Jin, R.; Hu, W.; Zhou, M.; Lin, F.; Xu, A. Caffeic acid derivative WSY6 protects melanocytes from oxidative stress by reducing ROS production and MAPK activation. *Heliyon* **2024**, *10*, e24843. [CrossRef]
59. Günenc, A.N.; Graf, B.; Stark, H.; Chari, A. Fatty acid synthase: Structure, function, and regulation. In *Macromolecular Protein Complexes IV*; Springer: Cham, Switzerland, 2022; Volume 99, pp. 1–33. [CrossRef]
60. Xie, W.; Ma, L.L.; Xu, Y.Q.; Wang, B.H.; Li, S.M. METTL3 inhibits hepatic insulin sensitivity via N6-methyladenosine modification of Fasn mRNA and promoting fatty acid metabolism. *Biochem. Biophys. Res. Commun.* **2019**, *518*, 120–126. [CrossRef]
61. Ando, H.; Ryu, A.; Hashimoto, A.; Oka, M.; Ichihashi, M. Linoleic acid and alpha-linolenic acid lightens ultraviolet-induced hyperpigmentation of the skin. *Arch. Dermatol. Res.* **1998**, *290*, 375–381. [CrossRef]
62. Kose, A. Chemical composition and tyrosinase inhibitory activities of fatty acids obtained from Heterotrophic Microalgae, *S. limacinum* and *C. cohnii*. *Appl. Biochem. Biotechnol.* **2023**, *195*, 369–385. [CrossRef]
63. Diwakar, G.; Rana, J.; Saito, L.; Vredeveld, D.; Zemaitis, D.; Scholten, J. Inhibitory effect of a novel combination of Salvia hispanica (chia) seed and Punica granatum (pomegranate) fruit extracts on melanin production. *Fitoterapia* **2014**, *97*, 164–171. [CrossRef] [PubMed]
64. Jeong, H.S.; Yun, H.Y.; Baek, K.J.; Kwon, N.S.; Park, K.C.; Kim, D.S. Okadaic acid suppresses melanogenesis via proteasomal degradation of tyrosinase. *Biol. Pharm. Bull.* **2013**, *36*, 1503–1508. [CrossRef] [PubMed]
65. Consoli, V.; Sorrenti, V.; Grosso, S.; Vanella, L. Heme Oxygenase-1 signaling and redox homeostasis in physiopathological conditions. *Biomolecules* **2021**, *11*, 589. [CrossRef] [PubMed]
66. Xie, Y.; Mei, X.; Shi, W. Kaempferol promotes melanogenesis and reduces oxidative stress in PIG1 normal human skin melanocytes. *J. Cell. Mol. Med.* **2023**, *27*, 982–990. [CrossRef]

67. Rosei, M.A.; Blarzino, C.; Coccia, R.; Foppoli, C.; Mosca, L.; Cini, C. Production of melanin pigments by cytochrome c/H_2O_2 system. *Int. J. Biochem. Cell Biol.* **1998**, *30*, 457–463. [CrossRef] [PubMed]
68. Wang, F.; Ma, W.; Fan, D.; Hu, J.; An, X.; Wang, Z. The biochemistry of melanogenesis: An insight into the function and mechanism of melanogenesis-related proteins. *Front. Mol. Biosci.* **2024**, *11*, 1440187. [CrossRef]
69. Kudo, M.; Kobayashi-Nakamura, K.; Tsuji-Naito, K. Bifunctional effects of O-methylated flavones from Scutellaria baicalensis Georgi on melanocytes: Inhibition of melanin production and intracellular melanosome transport. *PLoS ONE* **2017**, *12*, e0171513. [CrossRef]
70. Sánchez-Rangel, J.C.; Benavides, J.; Heredia, J.B.; Cisneros-Zevallos, L.; Jacobo-Velázquez, D.A. The Folin-Ciocalteu assay revisited: Improvement of its specificity for total phenolic content determination. *Anal. Methods* **2013**, *5*, 5990–5999. [CrossRef]
71. Zhang, C.; Tian, Y.; Yang, A.; Tan, W.; Liu, X.; Yang, W. Antitumor effect of poplar propolis on human cutaneous squamous cell carcinoma A431 cells. *Int. J. Mol. Sci.* **2023**, *24*, 16753. [CrossRef]
72. Tan, W.; Tian, Y.; Zhang, Q.; Miao, S.; Wu, W.; Miao, X.; Kuang, H.; Yang, W. Antioxidant and antibacterial activity of Apis laboriosa honey against *Salmonella enterica serovar* Typhimurium. *Front. Nutr.* **2023**, *10*, 1181492. [CrossRef]
73. Sim, M.; Choi, I.; Cho, J.; Shin, H.M.; Cho, H. Anti-melanogenesis and anti-oxidant of Salix pseudo-lasiogyne water extract in α-MSH-induced B16F10 melanoma cells. *Food Agric. Immunol.* **2017**, *28*, 1003–1016. [CrossRef]
74. Liu, X.; Tian, Y.; Yang, A.; Zhang, C.; Miao, X.; Yang, W. Antitumor effects of poplar propolis on DLBCL SU-DHL-2 Cells. *Foods* **2023**, *12*, 283. [CrossRef] [PubMed]

pharmaceuticals

MDPI

Article

Improved Antibacterial Properties of Fermented and Enzymatically Hydrolyzed Bee Pollen and Its Combined Effect with Antibiotics

Vaida Damulienė [1], Vilma Kaškonienė [1,*], Paulius Kaškonas [2], Rūta Mickienė [1] and Audrius Maruška [1]

[1] Instrumental Analysis Open Access Centre, Vytautas Magnus University, LT-44404 Kaunas, Lithuania; vaida.damuliene@vdu.lt (V.D.); ruta.mickiene@vdu.lt (R.M.); audrius.maruska@vdu.lt (A.M.)

[2] Institute of Metrology, Kaunas University of Technology, LT-51368 Kaunas, Lithuania; paulius.kaskonas@ktu.lt

* Correspondence: vilma.kaskoniene@vdu.lt

Abstract: Background/Objectives: A variety of phytochemicals from different plants are collected by bees into bee pollen granules. This research focused on evaluating the effects of lactic acid fermentation and enzymatic hydrolysis on the antibacterial activity of bee pollen and its interaction with antibiotics. There is limited knowledge regarding the interactions between treated bee pollen extracts and antibiotics, and this study contributes to the field by providing new insights into the antibacterial activity of pollen subjected to eight distinct treatment methods. **Methods**: Bee pollen's bacterial fermentation using a *Lacticaseibacillus rhamnosus* culture and spontaneous fermentation were performed. Bee pollen hydrolysis was performed using commercial enzymes, including enzyme mixtures as well as pure enzymes. The agar well diffusion assay was employed to assess the antibacterial activity against *Staphylococcus aureus*, *Listeria monocytogenes*, and *Salmonella enterica* serovars Enteritidis and Typhimurium, as well as their interaction with antibiotics (ceftazidime, ciprofloxacin, oxytetracycline dihydrate, and erythromycin). **Results**: This study showed an enhancement in bee pollen's antibacterial activity after both fermentation and enzymatic hydrolysis. The increase varied with the pollen's origin, treatment type, and culture used for antimicrobial tests. More than 77% of bee pollen extracts demonstrated a synergistic effect with antibiotics across all tested bacterial strains, while antagonistic interactions were comparatively rare. **Conclusions**: The applied treatment methods can improve the antibacterial properties of bee pollen. Bee pollen extracts, in combination with antibiotics, can enhance their effectiveness. These findings provide new insights into the potential use of bee pollen in combating bacterial infections.

Keywords: European bee pollen; antimicrobial activity; solid-state fermentation; *Viscozyme®* *L*; *Clara-diastase*; cellulase

1. Introduction

Since ancient times, many diseases have been treated using medicines made from natural products. Over the years, many of these have been replaced by synthetic chemicals; nevertheless, interest in natural substances is growing again [1]. Various pharmaceutical companies are conducting increasing research to discover new sources of biologically active compounds and evaluate their properties. Detailed studies have determined that the resistance of pathogenic microorganisms to antimicrobial agents is rapidly increasing, prompting the search for new therapeutic compounds that not only have healing properties but also fewer harmful side effects [2].

A significant portion of published studies relate to evaluating the positive biological properties or chemical components of various plants or their parts. Plants are among the best sources of natural products, especially various bioactive compounds [3,4]. These extracts can be used as antimicrobial agents to treat diseases caused by various pathogenic organisms. Furthermore, most of them exhibit active pharmacological effects, such as antibacterial, antifungal, antiparasitic, or anticancer properties [5–9].

The diverse chemical composition of plants and their parts, especially biologically active substances extracted from essential oils, increasingly encourages the investigation of the synergistic effects of plant extracts with antibiotics, which can help reduce the quantities of pharmaceutical drugs used [10,11]. Based on the available data in the literature, it has been reported that only a specific subset of plant extracts enhances the effectiveness of antibiotics [12]. Furthermore, the combination of synthetically derived and natural compounds not only leads to fewer side effects on living organisms but also contributes to reducing bacterial resistance.

It is not surprising that bee-collected pollen also exhibits various biological activities, as it is part of the plant that worker bees collect and mix with nectar and salivary secretions [13]. Bee pollen in the recent decade was re-discovered, and many studies revealing their impact on human health as food or a natural source remedy indicate its potential in promoting health, preventing disease, and improving quality of life [14–16]. Bee pollen is one of the most easily accessible natural products receiving considerable attention in the field of pharmaceutical applications. Its diverse chemical composition contributes to its potent antibacterial, antifungal, anti-inflammatory, and anticancer properties [15,16]. Studies have identified rutin, vanillic acid, gallic acid, quercetin, p-coumaric acid, hesperidin, kaempferol, apigenin, luteolin, and isorhamnetin as the main compounds responsible for these properties. More detailed analysis of these compounds revealed their effectiveness against specific pathogenic organisms, such as *S. aureus*, *E. coli*, *Streptococcus viridans*, and *Pseudomonas aeruginosa* [17,18]. Moreover, the antimicrobial activity of bee pollen is exceptionally influenced by highly active lactic acid bacteria. The uniqueness of these bacteria lies in the production of specific substances called bacteriocins, which halt the growth and development of pathogenic bacteria by disrupting their membranes [19]. The activity of bacteriocins produced by lactic acid bacteria against *Listeria monocytogenes*, *Listeria innocua*, *S. aureus*, *E. coli*, *Micrococcus luteus*, *P. aeruginosa*, *B. subtilis*, and *Salmonella* serovars Enteritidis and Typhimurium has been proven [20,21].

Bee pollen is one of the most popular natural products used commercially. However, its outer wall, composed of sporopollenin, is exceptionally resilient, elastic, chemically resistant, and provides protection from external damage. Consequently, bee pollen has limited bioavailability due to difficulties in digestion by humans [22–24]. Therefore, it is crucial to discover straightforward ways to enhance its bioavailability [23,25]. Mechanical treatment involving shear forces that generate heat [26], physical treatment using supercritical fluids [27], lactic acid fermentation [28–30], or enzymatic hydrolysis [31,32] have been studied for this purpose.

The available literature on the impact of bee pollen on antibiotic efficacy is scarce. Honey and propolis are the most frequently tested bee products in combination with antibiotics [33,34]. There are only a few studies investigating the use of bee pollen as an enhancer of drug effects. For example, research by Hanafy et al. [35] suggests that bee pollen can synergize with chemotherapy drugs, specifically Avastin® (bevacizumab), enhancing their anti-cancer efficacy. Extracts of bee pollen phenolic compounds and nanoparticles have shown enhanced anti-proliferative activity against cancer cell lines, such as MCF-7 breast cancer cells and A549 lung cancer cells, when combined with these drugs. This synergy likely arises from bee pollen's high flavonoid and polyphenol content, which contributes to cancer cell apoptosis and the inhibition of cancer-promoting signaling pathways. Araque and Vit [36] highlighted the antimicrobial potential of bee pollen and its ability to synergize with conventional treatments after analyzing *Tetragonisca angustula* (stingless bee) pot-pollen in combination with amikacin and meropenem against extensively drug-resistant bacteria. Additionally, the study by Ilie et al. [37] demonstrated a synergistic inhibitory effect when bee pollen extracts were combined with soluble compounds from two lactic acid bacterial strains, *L. rhamnosus* MF9 and *E. faecalis* 2M17, against two clinical pathogenic bacteria.

These studies reveal the potential of bee pollen extracts and suggest that interactions between bee pollen and antibiotics or other drugs can vary, depending on the specific application, the organism involved, the botanical origin of the bee pollen, or even the treatment method used, as demonstrated in the present study.

While bee pollen is valued for its antibacterial properties and high nutritional content, it is important to acknowledge that bees may also bring hazardous materials into the hive from the fields. These materials include pesticides, pyrrolizidine alkaloids, heavy metals, and even mycotoxins. Currently, European Commission regulations on bee pollen safety are less stringent than those for honey, likely due to its lower consumption levels. However, scientific studies confirm that the presence of these contaminants in bee pollen is a significant concern [38,39]. Existing regulations, such as EU 2023/915 [40] and EC 366/2005 [41], primarily focus on honey. For bee pollen, safety regulations are limited to specific pesticides and pyrrolizidine alkaloids.

There is optimism that in the future, potential risks associated with pesticides, pyrrolizidine alkaloids, heavy metals, and mycotoxins in bee pollen will be more comprehensively addressed and corresponding regulations will be improved. Therefore, when considering the practical application of bee pollen in health, pharmacy, or the food industry, it is essential to first ensure that the bee pollen used is free from contaminants. The aim of this research was to evaluate the effects of solid-state lactic acid fermentation and enzymatic hydrolysis on the antibacterial activity of bee pollen and its interaction with antibiotics.

2. Results and Discussion

Nine samples of bee pollen from different regions of Europe were subjected to spontaneous fermentation, bacterial fermentation using *L. rhamnosus* culture, and enzymatic hydrolysis with *Clara-diastase*, *Viscozyme® L*, lipase, protease, amyloglucosidase, and cellulase. The enzymes were selected based on their ability to degrade certain structural components of the pollen wall present in the exine, intine, or both [42,43]. The impact of fermentation on antibacterial activity against *Staphylococcus aureus*, *Listeria monocytogenes*, and *Salmonella enterica* serovars Enteritidis and Typhimurium was evaluated. Additionally, in vitro interactions of natural, fermented, and enzymatically hydrolyzed bee pollen in combination with antibacterial agents were assessed against each bacterial strain analyzed. Antibiotics from different classes were selected for the study based on their chemical structure: cephalosporins (ceftazidime pentahydrate), fluoroquinolones (ciprofloxacin), tetracyclines (oxytetracycline), and macrolides (erythromycin). The experimental design is presented in Figure 1.

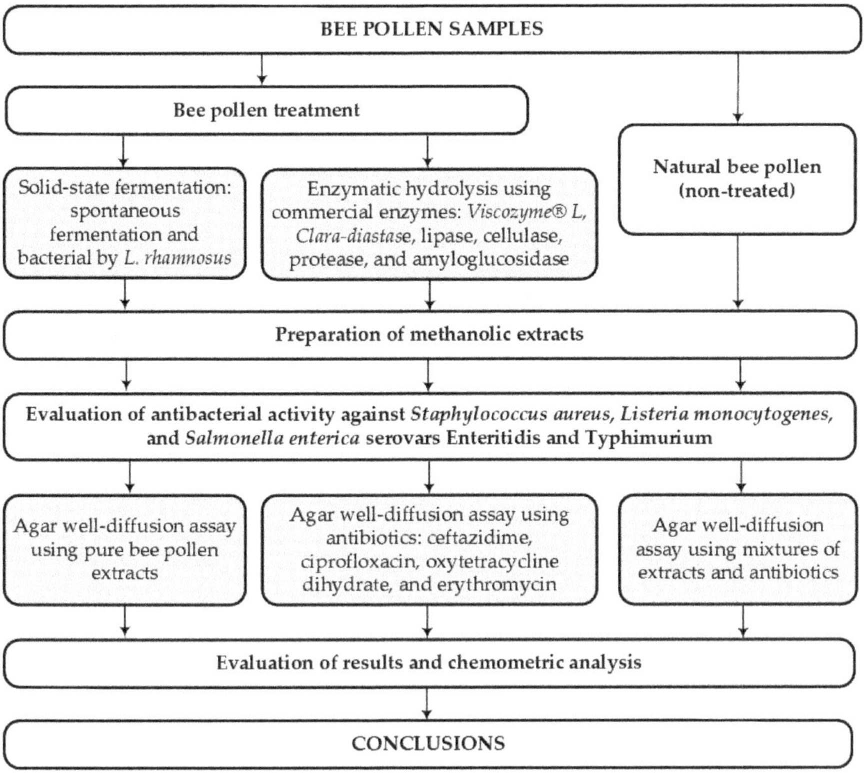

Figure 1. Design of experimental research.

First of all, to determine the impact of methanol on antibacterial activity, the antibacterial activity of 80% methanol alone was independently evaluated as part of this study. The results indicated that the effect of methanol was negligible, with the clear zone radius around the wells not exceeding 1 mm (the highest average clear zone was 0.75 mm). Additionally, the extracts were diluted with water at a 1:1 ratio or mixed with an aqueous antibiotic solution before analysis, effectively reducing the concentration of methanol by half. Therefore, the impact of methanol on the observed antibacterial activity was considered minimal and unlikely to interfere with the findings. This conclusion aligns with the literature data showing that methanol has weak bactericidal properties compared to other alcohols [44]. Methanol is rarely used as a disinfectant in healthcare settings due to its limited effectiveness against microorganisms [45].

2.1. Antimicrobial Activity of Treated Bee Pollen

The results of the antimicrobial activity of differently treated and untreated bee pollen extracts, as well as their combinations with antibiotics, are presented in Table 1 and expressed as the average diameter of the inhibition zone in millimeters.

Table 1. An impact of fermentation and enzymatic hydrolysis on antibacterial activity of tested bee pollen and interaction with antibiotics (n = 10; SY—synergistic effect, AN—antagonistic effect; *i*—observed significant changes after effect with antibiotics are labeled as "*i*" (increased) when $p \leq 0.05$).

Treatment	Used Antibiotic	Against *Salmonella* Typhimurium				Against *Salmonella* Enteritidis				Against *L. monocytogenes*				Against *S. aureus*			
		Inhibition Zone, mm	MIN–MAX, mm	SY	AN	Inhibition Zone, mm	MIN–MAX, mm	SY	AN	Inhibition Zone, mm	MIN–MAX, mm	SY	AN	Inhibition Zone, mm	MIN–MAX, mm	SY	AN
Natural	Without antibiotic	4.00 ± 2.98	0.91–9.14	–	–	7.79 ± 4.09	2.13–15.31	–	–	7.68 ± 2.71	5.10–12.90	–	–	8.09 ± 4.27	2.21–15.42	–	–
	Ceftazidime	11.76 ± 5.32 ^{i}	5.15–20.80	9	0	20.61 ± 9.19 ^{i}	9.70–36.00	9	0	19.43 ± 4.10 ^{i}	13.60–26.65	9	0	20.59 ± 7.84 ^{i}	8.35–32.85	9	0
	Ciprofloxacin	11.38 ± 4.12 ^{i}	6.30–17.40	9	0	15.04 ± 6.10 ^{i}	7.95–24.25	7	2	13.87 ± 4.14 ^{i}	7.05–20.00	8	1	20.25 ± 5.95 ^{i}	11.80–30.60	9	0
	Oxytetracycline	15.37 ± 5.84 ^{i}	7.90–22.60	9	0	19.63 ± 8.70 ^{i}	8.85–33.10	9	0	22.28 ± 6.35 ^{i}	11.90–31.15	9	0	22.73 ± 7.18 ^{i}	10.35–31.25	9	0
	Erythromycin	16.64 ± 6.76 ^{i}	8.85–25.90	9	0	20.11 ± 8.49 ^{i}	8.55–33.45	9	0	24.16 ± 7.94 ^{i}	11.00–37.50	9	0	20.25 ± 7.93 ^{i}	4.30–32.00	8	1
Spontaneous fermentation	Without antibiotic	5.16 ± 2.98	1.51–10.56	–	–	10.95 ± 3.82	5.49–18.95	–	–	9.31 ± 2.91	6.00–14.27	–	–	11.28 ± 3.83	5.59–19.05	–	–
	Ceftazidime	17.27 ± 5.24 ^{i}	9.80–27.05	9	0	30.91 ± 5.20 ^{i}	22.55–38.30	9	0	22.50 ± 4.47 ^{i}	15.85–29.30	9	0	23.56 ± 6.63 ^{i}	15.85–35.20	9	0
	Ciprofloxacin	16.12 ± 4.21 ^{i}	8.95–22.65	9	0	21.69 ± 5.80 ^{i}	12.95–29.80	9	0	20.57 ± 3.48 ^{i}	14.25–25.15	9	0	23.87 ± 6.71 ^{i}	14.55–34.70	9	0
	Oxytetracycline	21.37 ± 5.35 ^{i}	13.55–28.20	9	0	27.35 ± 7.43 ^{i}	14.90–37.40	9	0	25.87 ± 6.32 ^{i}	16.30–35.65	9	0	25.89 ± 7.39 ^{i}	14.60–37.80	9	0
	Erythromycin	23.47 ± 8.76 ^{i}	9.30–37.85	9	0	26.09 ± 6.40 ^{i}	16.25–36.50	9	0	30.29 ± 8.85 ^{i}	18.05–39.65	9	0	23.63 ± 9.35 ^{i}	6.65–39.10	8	1
Bacterial fermentation	Without antibiotic	6.06 ± 3.17	1.62–11.94	–	–	12.84 ± 4.81	7.07–21.54	–	–	10.23 ± 2.96	6.54–15.58	–	–	13.16 ± 4.85	7.12–21.62	–	–
	Ceftazidime	20.90 ± 6.50 ^{i}	12.50–30.50	9	0	36.44 ± 7.34 ^{i}	29.10–45.25	9	0	23.61 ± 4.47 ^{i}	17.55–30.35	9	0	26.64 ± 6.20 ^{i}	18.95–38.05	9	0
	Ciprofloxacin	21.15 ± 6.57 ^{i}	10.95–29.35	9	0	27.08 ± 5.30 ^{i}	20.45–35.10	9	0	22.12 ± 3.95 ^{i}	15.40–27.60	9	0	26.67 ± 6.42 ^{i}	18.50–36.70	9	0
	Oxytetracycline	26.95 ± 6.18 ^{i}	17.15–36.70	9	0	31.71 ± 7.94 ^{i}	20.10–43.75	9	0	26.81 ± 6.06 ^{i}	16.40–35.95	9	0	29.68 ± 6.52 ^{i}	21.40–41.55	9	0
	Erythromycin	29.13 ± 11.09 ^{i}	10.90–41.85	9	0	32.16 ± 9.33 ^{i}	18.90–41.30	9	0	32.67 ± 9.47 ^{i}	20.65–44.20	9	0	26.09 ± 9.77 ^{i}	9.90–43.70	8	1
Enzymatic hydrolysis with protease	Without antibiotic	7.77 ± 2.51	3.50–11.45	–	–	10.72 ± 3.34	7.25–16.60	–	–	11.37 ± 1.56	9.55–14.80	–	–	13.64 ± 3.98	9.15–21.70	–	–
	Ceftazidime	8.27 ± 3.15	3.95–14.10	2	7	12.80 ± 5.18	5.65–20.45	2	7	13.54 ± 2.99	6.80–16.65	4	4	16.05 ± 4.93	8.10–22.55	3	6
	Ciprofloxacin	7.84 ± 4.02	2.65–15.95	1	7	9.77 ± 4.45	2.40–16.15	1	8	11.63 ± 3.14	6.25–15.75	1	8	15.41 ± 5.85	9.00–27.00	5	4
	Oxytetracycline	9.87 ± 4.43	3.15–19.50	1	8	12.16 ± 3.70	5.55–16.40	3	6	15.62 ± 3.81	8.05–20.00	6	3	17.21 ± 6.14	6.95–26.95	5	4
	Erythromycin	11.30 ± 4.36	3.95–18.60	4	5	11.89 ± 4.55	3.10–17.30	2	6	19.92 ± 6.26	11.20–32.90	8	1	14.97 ± 6.60	2.90–24.50	2	7
Enzymatic hydrolysis with lipase	Without antibiotic	6.48 ± 2.16	3.35–9.75	–	–	9.12 ± 3.42	5.30–15.95	–	–	10.42 ± 1.58	9.00–13.85	–	–	12.47 ± 4.52	5.95–21.05	–	–
	Ceftazidime	7.86 ± 5.20	2.50–18.45	3	6	11.92 ± 5.69	5.60–21.95	2	7	11.98 ± 2.83	8.85–16.50	2	7	15.14 ± 6.26	3.90–23.50	5	4
	Ciprofloxacin	9.18 ± 4.20	2.55–15.95	3	5	9.47 ± 3.45	5.45–15.45	3	6	11.37 ± 3.01	6.40–15.90	1	8	15.05 ± 5.64	5.70–23.05	5	4
	Oxytetracycline	10.19 ± 4.53	3.90–15.55	5	4	12.09 ± 6.73	5.50–25.05	2	7	14.96 ± 4.01	8.40–19.65	6	3	17.75 ± 7.33	7.30–28.20	6	3
	Erythromycin	13.23 ± 7.48	3.50–24.95	6	3	14.44 ± 6.40	5.40–25.65	6	3	17.35 ± 5.44	9.80–26.85	7	2	14.42 ± 6.18	4.45–22.55	2	7
Enzymatic hydrolysis with cellulase	Without antibiotic	11.40 ± 4.19	5.75–18.50	–	–	17.86 ± 4.26	12.20–23.35	–	–	16.74 ± 4.02	13.55–26.65	–	–	20.68 ± 5.56	13.50–26.85	–	–
	Ceftazidime	19.64 ± 4.96 ^{i}	12.45–26.90	9	0	32.54 ± 6.04 ^{i}	23.15–42.00	9	0	25.77 ± 2.52 ^{i}	22.60–30.35	8	1	30.19 ± 7.21 ^{i}	19.00–38.45	9	0
	Ciprofloxacin	19.29 ± 4.47 ^{i}	11.90–23.90	9	0	24.66 ± 3.74 ^{i}	19.45–29.15	9	0	24.73 ± 1.75 ^{i}	22.05–27.65	8	1	29.01 ± 6.07 ^{i}	18.45–36.95	8	1
	Oxytetracycline	22.21 ± 4.40 ^{i}	16.00–29.55	9	0	29.02 ± 7.17 ^{i}	20.10–41.65	9	0	29.06 ± 3.50 ^{i}	25.35–36.00	9	0	32.73 ± 7.16 ^{i}	21.35–41.50	9	0
	Erythromycin	26.89 ± 7.46 ^{i}	18.00–38.85	9	0	30.75 ± 8.74 ^{i}	18.95–42.90	9	0	34.91 ± 8.26 ^{i}	27.90–42.25	9	0	30.55 ± 9.45 ^{i}	9.85–41.70	8	1
Enzymatic hydrolysis with *Clara-diastase*	Without antibiotic	9.39 ± 3.57	4.25–15.45	–	–	13.79 ± 3.24	10.60–18.60	–	–	12.46 ± 1.37	9.40–14.50	–	–	15.38 ± 4.34	9.75–22.20	–	–
	Ceftazidime	17.87 ± 5.83 ^{i}	9.00–28.40	8	1	29.41 ± 6.26 ^{i}	22.55–40.10	9	0	26.25 ± 5.12 ^{i}	22.15–36.25	9	0	25.54 ± 7.40 ^{i}	14.25–41.05	9	0
	Ciprofloxacin	18.81 ± 8.51 ^{i}	11.60–39.85	9	0	21.57 ± 3.75 ^{i}	15.95–28.00	9	0	21.09 ± 4.05 ^{i}	16.05–29.80	9	0	25.36 ± 7.90 ^{i}	17.30–42.80	9	0
	Oxytetracycline	22.10 ± 11.44 ^{i}	10.75–43.10	9	0	25.39 ± 9.06 ^{i}	11.90–37.35	8	1	26.86 ± 3.98 ^{i}	20.45–32.35	9	0	27.09 ± 9.27 ^{i}	13.00–41.55	9	0
	Erythromycin	25.41 ± 8.81 ^{i}	10.80–41.95	9	0	26.91 ± 9.33 ^{i}	11.50–41.30	8	1	33.00 ± 9.86 ^{i}	17.65–44.85	9	0	24.07 ± 8.98 ^{i}	5.90–37.30	8	1
Enzymatic hydrolysis with *Viscozyme® L*	Without antibiotic	10.16 ± 4.03	4.90–17.50	–	–	15.48 ± 4.15	9.75–21.30	–	–	14.12 ± 1.47	12.30–15.95	–	–	17.32 ± 4.85	11.35–25.65	–	–
	Ceftazidime	21.24 ± 11.73 ^{i}	9.75–45.40	9	0	32.38 ± 6.41 ^{i}	25.55–43.45	9	0	25.63 ± 5.26 ^{i}	20.70–37.85	9	0	29.62 ± 9.34 ^{i}	15.80–45.90	9	0
	Ciprofloxacin	19.76 ± 10.11 ^{i}	8.95–43.60	9	0	22.01 ± 4.20 ^{i}	14.50–28.25	9	0	22.36 ± 2.17 ^{i}	19.20–25.10	9	0	26.38 ± 6.88 ^{i}	14.45–35.50	9	0
	Oxytetracycline	20.79 ± 5.44 ^{i}	13.70–28.25	9	0	28.70 ± 6.79 ^{i}	17.45–37.40	9	0	28.77 ± 10.68 ^{i}	21.25–40.80	9	0	28.86 ± 9.15 ^{i}	14.60–39.90	9	0
	Erythromycin	23.09 ± 8.50 ^{i}	9.35–37.10	9	0	27.27 ± 6.48 ^{i}	19.50–36.55	9	0	35.47 ± 9.64 ^{i}	23.05–44.50	9	0	26.33 ± 9.73 ^{i}	6.75–39.05	8	1
Enzymatic hydrolysis with amyloglucosidase	Without antibiotic	5.29 ± 2.83	0.95–9.55	–	–	8.64 ± 3.80	4.70–16.00	–	–	9.77 ± 1.92	7.65–13.50	–	–	10.89 ± 4.01	5.35–17.95	–	–
	Ceftazidime	7.44 ± 3.30	1.85–12.40	2	7	13.48 ± 5.89	7.10–25.65	6	3	12.69 ± 3.67	7.30–17.45	5	4	14.89 ± 6.30	6.85–25.50	7	2
	Ciprofloxacin	8.05 ± 3.43	2.65–12.95	4	5	9.14 ± 4.02	3.60–16.95	1	8	9.92 ± 2.75	6.45–13.50	0	8	12.77 ± 6.30	4.80–24.10	3	6
	Oxytetracycline	11.84 ± 7.40	4.35–28.35	6	2	12.47 ± 5.05	5.55–20.20	4	5	15.93 ± 3.34	9.05–19.90	8	1	17.98 ± 7.22	5.25–28.05	8	1
	Erythromycin	12.48 ± 4.35	6.35–18.70	9	0	14.12 ± 5.83	6.40–21.80	6	3	21.46 ± 5.29	10.25–28.40	8	1	16.20 ± 5.53	3.55–21.30	7	2

A positive effect of both solid-state fermentation and enzymatic hydrolysis on bee pollen antibacterial activity was observed. Antibacterial activity after spontaneous fermentation significantly ($p \leq 0.05$) increased by 1.04–2.18 times against *S. aureus*, 1.09–1.38 times against *L. monocytogenes*, 1.18–2.22 times against *Salmonella* Enteritidis, and 1.07–2.92 times against *Salmonella* Typhimurium. Antibacterial activity after bacterial fermentation significantly ($p \leq 0.05$) increased by 1.18–2.31 times against *S. aureus*, 1.21–1.61 times against *L. monocytogenes*, 1.26–2.34 times against *Salmonella* Enteritidis, and 1.21–4.08 times against *Salmonella* Typhimurium. Higher antibacterial activity compared to natural or spontaneously fermented bee pollen was observed after bacterial fermentation with *L. rhamnosus*. These results may be influenced by the superior breakdown of the pollen cell wall by *L. rhamnosus* or its capability to release bacteriocins, as suggested by some studies [46].

Moreover, a significant intensification of antibacterial activity was observed after enzymatic hydrolysis of bee pollen against cultures of pathogenic bacteria. Antibacterial activity showed statistically significant ($p \leq 0.05$) differences in all enzymatically hydrolyzed bee pollen samples collected from different regions of Europe. Overall, the antibacterial efficacy following enzymatic hydrolysis showed a significant ($p \leq 0.05$) increase in activity by 1.14–6.42 times against *S. aureus*, 1.05–3.31 times against *L. monocytogenes*, 1.04–6.06 times against *Salmonella* Enteritidis, and 1.04–7.56 times against *Salmonella* Typhimurium. The most significant increases in antibacterial activity were observed after enzymatic hydrolysis with *Clara-diastase* (1.09 to 5.98 times) and *Viscozyme*® *L* (1.21 to 6.50 times), while the smallest increases were determined with amyloglucosidase (1.04 to 3.51 times). The substantial increases in antibacterial activity following enzymatic hydrolysis reveal that it would be advisable to treat bee pollen enzymatically with *Clara-diastase* and *Viscozyme*® *L* before use in any applications where antibacterial properties are desired, such as in food preservation, natural health supplements, cosmetic formulations, or antimicrobial coatings for packaging materials.

By comparison, the antimicrobial activity of natural (spontaneous) fermentation and enzymatic hydrolysis can be observed to depend on the type of bee pollen, the enzyme used, and the bacterial strain tested. However, in most cases, enzymatic hydrolysis resulted in better antimicrobial activity compared to spontaneous fermentation. For instance, bee pollen extracts hydrolyzed with cellulase showed 1.2 to 4.3 times stronger inhibition, which was statistically significant ($p \leq 0.05$), compared to those subjected to spontaneous fermentation. Similarly, extracts treated with enzyme mixtures such as *Viscosyme*® *L* and *Clara-diastase* exhibited higher antimicrobial activity (1.1–3.7 times), with a few exceptions where the difference was not statistically significant ($p \leq 0.05$). In contrast, for *Salmonella* Enteritidis inhibition, extracts from spontaneous fermentation demonstrated 1.2–1.9 times higher inhibition, which was statistically significant ($p \leq 0.05$), compared to pollen hydrolyzed with lipase or amyloglucosidase in 12 out of 18 cases; in the remaining cases, the results were not statistically different ($p \leq 0.05$). In summary, while the antimicrobial activity of bee pollen increased following both spontaneous fermentation and enzymatic hydrolysis, the highest activity was generally observed with enzymatic hydrolysis, particularly when cellulase was used. However, it is important to note that the differences can vary depending on the specific conditions.

Variations in the obtained results suggest that geographical origins, likely closely linked to the botanical origin of bee pollen, as well as climatic conditions, play an extremely important role in the antibacterial activity of natural or treated pollen. The palynological analysis was not performed in this study; however, a visual inspection of the bee pollen indicates that the samples have a diverse range of colors, which suggests the presence of pollen from different botanical origins (Figure S1). The most significant differences in antibacterial activity against both *Salmonella* Enteritidis and *L. monocytogenes* were observed in pollen from Lithuania, Sweden, and Slovakia when comparing the results obtained after bacterial fermentation and spontaneous fermentation. The representation of antibacterial activity depending on bee pollen's geographical origin has been added to the supplementary file (Table S1). In contrast, the differences in antibacterial activity between different fermentation types were not substantial in pollen from other countries. However, after spontaneous fermentation, the antibacterial activity against *S. aureus* bacterial cultures in pollen samples from various origins appears to be quite similar, with Lithuanian pollen standing out the most (with activity differences between Lithuanian and other samples reaching 1.5–3.4 times).

The literature highlights that the antibacterial activity of bee pollen has been actively studied in recent years. Kacaniova et al. [47] reported a positive effect of bee pollen from Slovakia on antibacterial activity against *L. monocytogenes*, *P. aeruginosa*, *S. aureus*, *S. enterica*, and *E. coli*. Additionally, studies in various countries have identified antibacterial activity of bee pollen against *S. aureus*, *E. faecalis*, *P. aeruginosa*, *S. enterica*, and *S. pyogenes* [18,37,48,49]. However, the antibacterial activity of fermented bee pollen remains an underexplored area in scientific research by other authors. In our previous study, it was found that the antibacterial activity against *S. aureus* increased by 1.4–2.0 times after spontaneous fermentation of Latvian pollen and by 1.2–2.2 times after fermentation with *L. rhamnosus*. Furthermore, the antibacterial activity of fermented bee pollen was assessed against *M. luteus* and *E. coli* [30].

2.2. Antimicrobial Activity of Treated Bee Pollen and Antibiotics Mixtures

This study demonstrated interactions between bee pollen extracts and antibiotics, predominantly synergistic (SY), although some cases showed antagonistic (AN) or additive effects (Table 1). These interactions depended on the treatment method, tested bacteria, antibacterial agent, and the origin of bee pollen, which may be closely correlated with botanical origin and phytochemical composition—both of which were analyzed in this study.

Among the 324 combinations evaluated against *Salmonella* Typhimurium, 261 (80.56%) were synergistic, while 60 (18.52%) showed antagonistic effects. Against *Salmonella* Enteritidis, there were 250 (77.16%) synergistic and 73 (22.53%) antagonistic combinations. For *L. monocytogenes*, 269 (83.02%) combinations were synergistic and 53 (16.36%) were antagonistic. Similarly, against *S. aureus*, 267 (82.41%) combinations were synergistic and 57 (17.59%) were antagonistic. Only six additive interactions across all combinations were detected. It is difficult to determine the best combination of treatment methods and antibiotics. However, it is worth mentioning that the mixtures with bee pollen extracts obtained after spontaneous fermentation, *L. rhamnosus* fermentation, or enzymatic hydrolysis by *Viscozyme*® *L* showed a synergistic effect, except for the mixtures with erythromycin against *S. aureus* (bee pollen sample was obtained from Malta). Promising results were obtained after blending antibiotics with extracts hydrolyzed by cellulase or *Clara-diastase*, with only 4 antagonistic cases detected out of 171. Plant extracts (and possibly bee pollen as well) can interact with antibiotics through various mechanisms, including changing bacterial cell permeability, blocking bacterial resistance mechanisms like efflux pumps, modifying active sites on bacterial cells, inhibiting enzymes that degrade antibiotics in bacterial cell walls, and preventing bacterial biofilm formation [50]. The antibacterial mechanisms of antibiotics themselves also vary, which may impact their interaction with plant extracts. Antibiotics can inhibit cell wall synthesis, damage the cytoplasmic membrane, hinder nucleic acid and protein synthesis, or target specific enzyme systems [51]. However, further comprehensive studies are necessary to ascertain the functioning of these particular mechanisms. At the moment, the main goal of this study was aimed to evaluate whether the bacterial fermentation or enzymatic hydrolysis has an impact on the antibacterial activity of bee pollen, if there are differences between bee pollen from different geographical origins (geographical region is related to botanical origin), and whether bee pollen may affect the activity of antibiotics.

The strongest effect on *S. aureus* was observed when bee pollen was subjected to enzymatic hydrolysis with *Viscozyme®* L and combined with ceftazidime (15.80 ± 2.45 to 45.90 ± 1.20 mm). The most significant impact on *L. monocytogenes* was noted when bee pollen was enzymatically hydrolyzed with *Clara-diastase* or *Viscozyme®* L and combined with erythromycin (up to 44.85 ± 1.27 and 44.50 ± 1.33 mm, respectively). The highest activity against *Salmonella* Enteritidis was observed when bee pollen underwent bacterial fermentation and was combined with ceftazidime (29.10 ± 0.57 to 45.25 ± 1.05 mm). The greatest effect on *Salmonella* Typhimurium was observed when bee pollen was enzymatically hydrolyzed with *Viscozyme®* L and combined with ceftazidime (9.75 ± 1.16 to 45.40 ± 1.33 mm).

However, antagonistic interactions were detected between antibiotics and bee pollen extracts after enzymatic hydrolysis with lipase, protease, and amyloglucosidase. Antibacterial activity against *S. aureus* decreased by 0.45–0.99 times when bee pollen extract after enzymatic hydrolysis with lipase was combined with antibiotics, against *L. monocytogenes* by 0.46–0.99 times, against *Salmonella* Enteritidis by 0.37–0.98 times, and against *Salmonella* Typhimurium by 0.40–0.99 times. Antibacterial activity against *S. aureus* decreased by 0.46–0.97 times when bee pollen extract after enzymatic hydrolysis with protease was combined with antibiotics, against *L. monocytogenes* by 0.44–0.98 times, against *Salmonella* Enteritidis by 0.22–0.98 times, and against *Salmonella* Typhimurium by 0.38–0.99 times. When bee pollen extracts after hydrolysis with amyloglucosidase were combined with antibiotics, antibacterial activity decreased by 0.31–0.99 times against *S. aureus*, 0.42–0.99 times against *L. monocytogenes*, 0.20–0.99 times against *Salmonella* Enteritidis, and 0.36–0.99 times against *Salmonella* Typhimurium.

According to the literature, the bee pollen wall consists of two layers: the exine (outer) and the intine (inner). The exine is made of polysaccharides and serves as the primary storage for glycoproteins, lipids, and phenols. The intine is composed of cellulose, hemicellulose, and pectin [52]. The structure of the bee pollen wall is more easily broken down by cellulase, *Viscozyme®* L (an enzyme mixture of cellulase, xylanase, arabanase, and glucanase), and *Clara-diastase* (an enzyme mixture of amylase, cellulase, invertase, and peptidase) compared to lipase, protease, or amyloglucosidase due to its main wall components.

From the perspective of bee pollen collection regions, bee pollen from colder climate regions (Lithuania, Sweden, and Poland) demonstrated better antibacterial performance, whereas pollen from southern European countries (Malta, Italy, and Spain) showed lower activity against the tested pathogenic bacteria. The improvement in antibacterial activity after adding antibiotics between samples from Lithuania (highest) and Malta (lowest) reached 75%.

A recent study identified naringenin, quercetin, luteolin, and rutin as the main flavonoids, and ferulic and ellagic acids as the principal phenolic acids, in both natural and fermented bee pollen [28]. Based on the available data in the literature, flavonoids and phenolic acids in bee pollen exhibit antibacterial activity against Gram-negative, Gram-positive bacteria, and even pathogenic fungi [24]. Flavonoids have been shown to potentially enhance the efficacy of antibiotics against pathogenic bacteria by disrupting bacterial cytoplasmic membranes, inhibiting nucleic acid synthesis, or blocking the fatty acid synthesis pathway [5,53]. Meanwhile, ferulic and ellagic acids increase the production of superoxide ions, which disrupt bacterial energy metabolism, alter cell membrane properties, and induce the formation of pores in cell membranes, resulting in leakage of vital intracellular components [54,55].

Some compounds show significant efficacy only when combined with an antibiotic. Identifying the specific compound within an extract responsible for the synergistic interaction is challenging. Additionally, some compounds exhibit synergistic activity through mechanisms beyond their inherent antimicrobial properties due to polyvalent effects [56].

2.3. Chemometric Analysis

The acquired measurement data were structured into a data matrix of size of $9 \times 4 \times 5 \times 90$, representing the countries of bee pollen collection, the bacteria against which antibacterial activity was assessed, the tested antibiotics, and the treatment ways. Therefore, each tested fermented or enzymatically hydrolyzed bee pollen sample supplemented with antibiotics was characterized by an antibiotic activity profile, composed of 16 variables (4 different antibiotics and 4 different bacteria). The control samples were defined by four variables, elucidating antibacterial activity of the fermented or enzymatically hydrolyzed pollen against tested bacteria without antibiotics.

Prior to statistical analyses, a data standardization procedure was applied to remove bias by subtracting the average value of each variable and scaling the scatter (variance), dividing each variable by its standard deviation. The procedure allowed us to achieve data scattered around a zero value with unified variance.

Firstly, this research was directed to estimation of antibacterial activity differences among tested bee pollen treatments and improvement of this characteristic after addition of antibiotics, processing each country's data independently. The PCA was performed on the structured data matrix to extract principal orthogonal and uncorrelated components, explaining the largest portion of the data variance. The decision about number of principle components to retain was based on the Kaiser criterion and Cattell's scree test. The analysis of the measurement results from 9 counties allowed us to reduce input data matrix dimensions from 16 variables to 3 principal components, retaining from 92.70% to 97.27% of the initial data variance. The principal components obtained were utilized as an input for hierarchical clustering analysis, employing the following HCA parameters: squared Euclidean distance served as the similarity metric, and the linkage rule was set to average. The samples from Denmark and Lithuania are presented in Figure 2, as samples from other countries performed similarly. The clustering results are presented as a heatmap with dendrogram, which was cut to form clusters at the 60% level of the maximum observed distance. Abbreviations are used in Figure 2; for example, A4B1 represents erythromycin's (A4) impact on *Salmonella* Typhimurium (B1) after blending with specifically treated bee pollen (vertical axis).

The statistical significance of the formed clusters after HCA was tested, applying Student's *t*-test. It was assumed that the variables of all samples falling to the same cluster were drawn from the same Gaussian distributions, and hypotheses testing about equality of the means between clusters was performed. The results revealed that observed differences between samples assigned to the distinct clusters were statistically significant at level $\alpha < 0.05$. Clustering of the samples according to the antibacterial profile revealed two distinct clusters exhibiting antibacterial activity performance differences: the first "high performance antibacterial activity" group included mixtures of antibiotics and spontaneous and bacterial fermentation samples together with samples enzymatically hydrolyzed using enzymes—cellulase, *Clara-diastase*, and *Viscozyme® L*. The samples containing antibiotics with natural bee pollen from Sweden, Poland, and Lithuania also were attributed to this group. The second "low performance antibacterial activity" cluster encompassed the rest of the samples, including control samples without antibiotics and mixtures of antibiotics with enzymatically hydrolyzed pollen using lipase, protease, and amyloglucosidase.

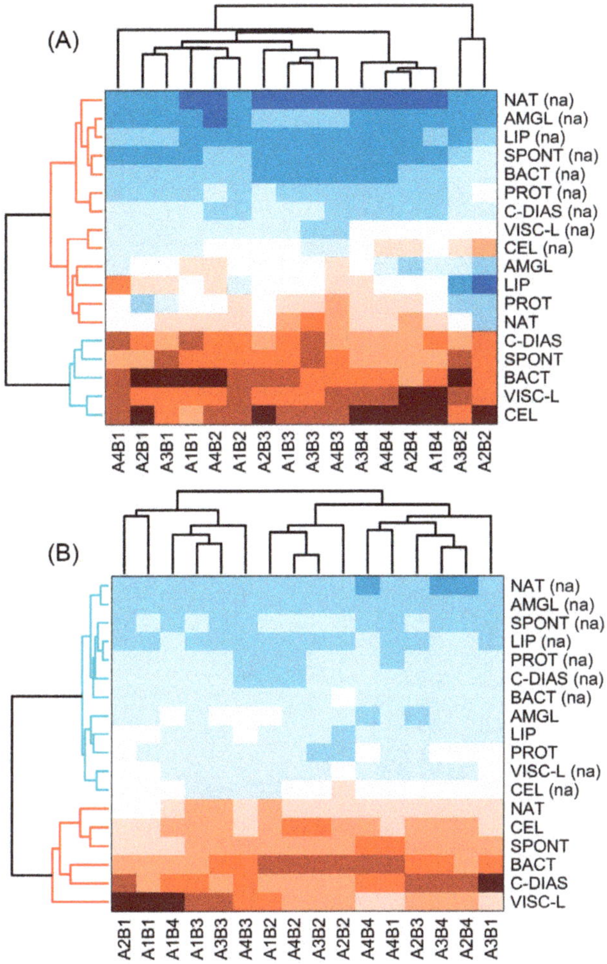

Figure 2. Heatmaps with dendrograms of hierarchical clustering analysis of Denmark (**A**) and Lithuanian (**B**) bee pollen samples. Bacteria: B1—*Salmonella* Typhimurium, B2—*Salmonella* Enteritidis, B3—*Listeria monocytogenes*, B4—*Staphylococcus aureus*; antibiotics: A1—ceftazidime, A2—ciprofloxacin, A3—oxytetracycline, A4—erythromycin; treatment: NAT—natural bee pollen (without treatment), SPONT—spontaneous fermentation, BACT—lactis acid fermentation, PROT—enzymatic hydrolysis by protease, LIP—hydrolysis by lipase, CEL—hydrolysis by cellulase, C-DIAS—hydrolysis by *Claradiastase*, VISC-L—hydrolysis by *Viscozyme® L*, AMGL—hydrolysis by amyloglucosidase. Control samples are denoted as (na). The red–blue color scheme is used to visualize observed distances between samples to reveal clusters: dark blue represents the smallest, while dark red represents the largest distance values.

To expose improvements of tested pollen treatments and treated pollen mixtures with antibiotics on antibacterial activity, Euclidean distance calculation was employed. Euclidean distance can be used as a measure of similarity of objects in the N dimension space described by the same set of variables. The calculated Euclidean distance was expressed as the average value of bee pollen samples from nine countries. The sorted results in ascending order are presented in Figure 3.

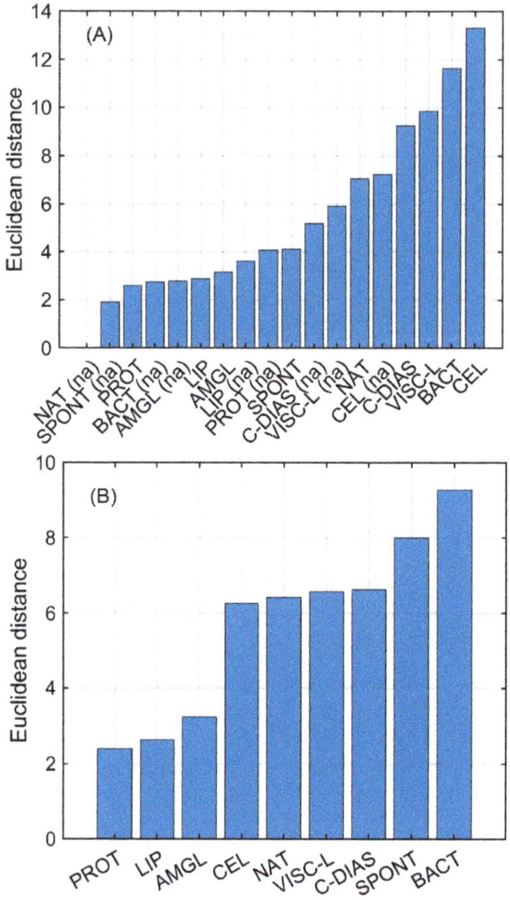

Figure 3. Evaluated Euclidean distance reveals antibacterial activity performance scatter among tested samples: (**A**)—distance of each tested sample from natural pollen sample; (**B**)—distance between a control fermentation sample and the same sample after addition of antibiotics (NAT—natural bee pollen (without treatment), SPONT—spontaneous fermentation, BACT—lactis acid fermentation, PROT—enzymatic hydrolysis by protease, LIP—hydrolysis by lipase, CEL—hydrolysis by cellulase, C-DIAS—hydrolysis by *Clara-diastase*, VISC-L—hydrolysis by *Viscozyme® L*, AMGL—hydrolysis by amyloglucosidase). Control samples are denoted as (na).

Looking at Figure 3A, it is clearly seen that the best antibacterial activity performance improvement comparing to the natural bee pollen control sample is exhibited by the mixture of antibiotics and bee pollen hydrolyzed with cellulase enzyme, while the mixture of bacterial pollen fermentation with antibiotics is not far behind. The worst performances among samples mixed with antibiotics are shown by enzymatic hydrolysis with protease, lipase, and amyloglucosidase. Figure 3B shows the calculated Euclidean distance between the same bee pollen samples before (control sample) and after (mixture sample) addition of antibiotics. The bar plot reveals a non-uniform increase in antibacterial activity in the tested samples after adding antibiotics, which reaches up to 270%. These uneven changes in the antibacterial activity profile indicate a synergistic effect, which is highly demonstrated in spontaneous and bacterial fermentation. The synergism effect is weakly exposed in pollen samples enzymatically hydrolyzed with protease, lipase, and amyloglucosidase.

The successive analysis was aimed at clustering antibacterial activity data according to pollen collection region, processing each pollen treatment type independently. Following the same analysis pattern, PCA was performed and 2–4 principal components out of 16 were retained, explaining from 97.08% to 84.12% of the initial data variance. HCA with the same settings was employed to cluster the results, which are presented in Figure 4. The clustering results are presented as a heatmap with dendrogram, which was cut to form clusters at the 60% level of the maximum observed distance. Differences between samples in the formed clusters were statistically significant at $\alpha < 0.05$ according to the hypotheses testing.

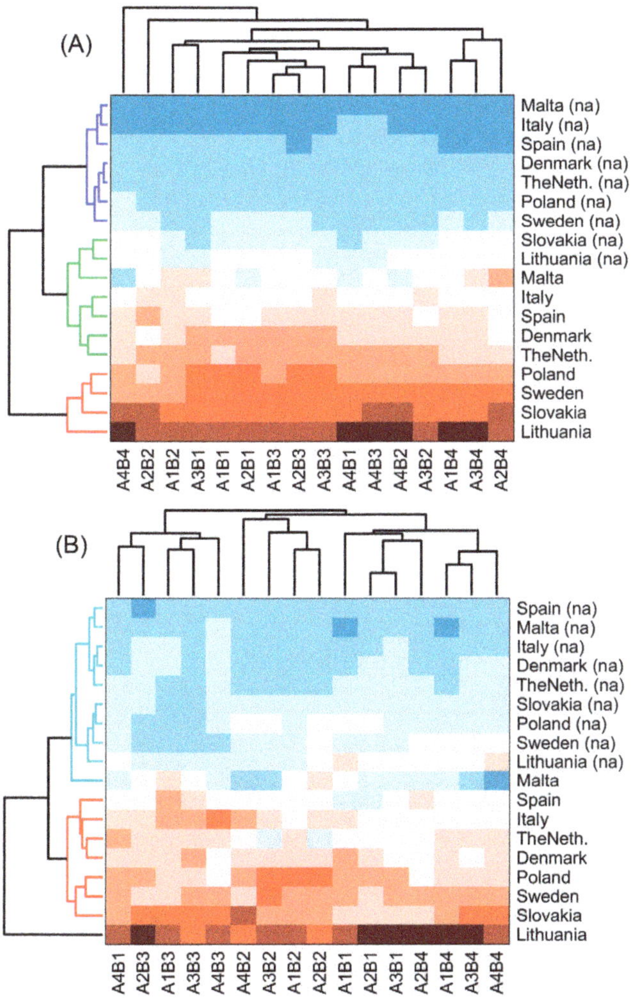

Figure 4. Heatmaps with dendrograms of hierarchical clustering analysis of bacterial fermentation application (**A**) and *Clara-diastase* enzyme application (**B**). Bacteria: B1—*Salmonella* Typhimurium, B2—*Salmonella* Enteritidis, B3—*Listeria monocytogenes*, B4—*Staphylococcus aureus*; antibiotics: A1—ceftazidime, A2—ciprofloxacin, A3—oxytetracycline, A4—erythromycin. Control samples are denoted as (na). The red-blue color scheme is used to visualize observed distances between samples to reveal clusters: dark blue represents the smallest, while dark red represents the largest distance values.

Figure 4A is very similar for natural pollen, bacterial and spontaneous fermentations, and also enzymatic hydrolysis using cellulase. Three clusters are suggested by the analysis according to the underlying data structure: a "high performance" cluster including Lithuanian, Polish, Slovakian and Swedish pollen, a "medium performance" cluster that included pollen samples collected in Malta, Italy, Spain, the Netherlands, and Denmark, and a "low performance" group that mainly was composed of control bee pollen samples. It is interesting to note that Lithuanian and Slovakian pollen control samples were attributed to the "medium performance" group, revealing that the antibacterial activity of these samples is very high and similar to the mixtures of southern Europe pollen samples (e.g., Malta) with antibiotics. Enzymatic hydrolysis using *Clara-diastase* and *Viscozyme® L* enzymes showed another picture, presented in Figure 4B. In this case, all samples were grouped to two groups, expect the Lithuanian sample, who's antibacterial profile was distinct from all the tests. The first cluster contained all control samples together with Malta pollen with antibiotics, while the second group included the rest of the countries' treated pollen samples and antibiotics mixtures. The results presented in Figure 4 revealed that pollen from southern countries (Malta, Spain, and Italy) performed weaker than pollen from colder climate regions (Lithuania, Sweden, and Poland).

The clustering results of samples enzymatically hydrolyzed with lipase, protease, and amyloglucosidase did not reveal a clear clustering pattern, and the grouping was rather chaotic. Many samples were treated as separate unique clusters, which indicated that there was no expressed trend in the antibacterial activity profile and minor differences in pollen origin played a role in clustering. Clear separation of control samples and samples with antibiotics was also not observed.

The Euclidean distance measure to examine pollen origin impact on antibacterial activity was calculated and expressed as the average value of nine bee pollen samples with fermentations applied. The sorted results in ascending order are presented in Figure 5, which shows the calculated Euclidean distance between bee pollen samples, collected in the same country, before (control sample) and after (mixture sample) addition of antibiotics. The bar plot affirms a non-uniform increase in antibacterial activity in the tested samples after adding antibiotics; however, the non-uniformity is not as strongly expressed as in the case of treatments.

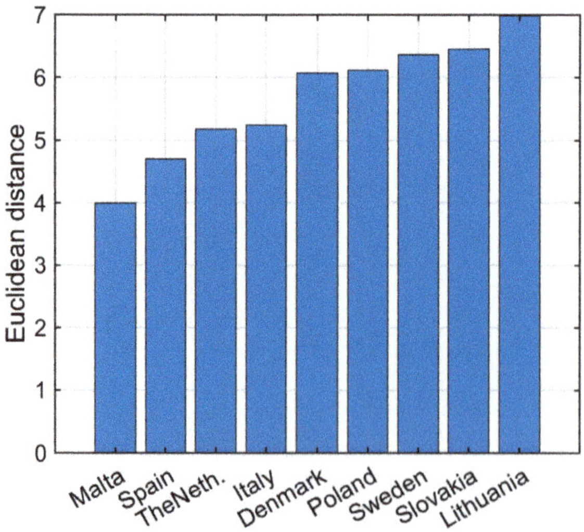

Figure 5. Evaluated Euclidean distance reveals antibacterial activity performance between a control country sample and the same sample after addition of antibiotics.

The difference between Malta and Lithuania samples reaches 75%. Again, these uneven changes in the antibacterial activity profile indicate a synergistic effect. The synergism in the Lithuanian sample is expressed the most, while in the Malta sample it is the weakest.

The present study demonstrates the potential of various bee pollen treatment methods to enhance antibacterial activity and suggests possible synergistic effects with certain antibiotics against specific bacteria. Fermented or hydrolyzed pollen itself can be used as a natural preservative to extend the shelf life of food products or as a functional food. These preliminary findings indicate that combining bee pollen extracts with antibiotics may have potential for treating infectious diseases and addressing emerging drug resistance issues. After the selection of the most promising treatment method, this study may be expanded to include an analysis of a higher content of samples from different geographical regions and monofloral bee pollen samples, as environmental factors and local flora can significantly influence bee pollen's composition and bioactivity. As the study was limited to a specific set of bacterial strains and antibiotics, future work should expand to a broader range of pathogens, especially antibiotic-resistant organisms, as well as a higher variety of antibacterial agents from different classes. However, further in vivo experiments are necessary to validate the efficacy of this combination in combating bacterial infections. Future research should also focus on evaluating the stability of bee pollen and antibiotic mixtures during storage, the reproducibility and optimization of these methods for industrial-scale production, and, of course, the economic feasibility of these findings.

3. Materials and Methods

3.1. Bee Pollen Samples

Nine dried bee pollen samples from various regions of Europe were collected during the flowering season, from May to August 2018, for this study. The samples included Lithuanian bee pollen from the Šiauliai region, Kuršėnai (55°59′ N 22°55′ E); Swedish bee pollen from the Hagfors region (60°02′ N 13°39′ E); Polish bee pollen from Bialystok (53°08′ N 23°08′ E); Danish bee pollen from the Alsgarde region (56°04′ N 12°32′ E); Dutch bee pollen from South Holland, Gouda (52°0′ N 4°42′ E); Slovak bee pollen from the Trnava region (48°22′ N 17°35′ E); Maltese bee pollen from the Northern region, Mellieha (35°57′ N 14°21′ E); Spanish bee pollen from the Valencia region (39°28′ N 0°22′ W); and Italian bee pollen from the Bibbiena region (43°42′ N 11°49′ E). All samples were stored at +5 °C in a dry environment, following ISO 24382:2023 [57] recommendations, for a maximum of 6 months. Prior to analysis or processing, the bee pollen samples were homogenized using a pestle and porcelain mortar.

3.2. Solid-State Fermentation of Bee Pollen

Solid-state fermentation of bee pollen was conducted using an inoculum of *Lacticaseibacillus rhamnosus* GG (ATCC 53103) (Gefilus, Valio Ltd., Helsinki, Finland) for bacterial fermentation and without the addition of bacteria for spontaneous fermentation. Bacterial culture viability was restored in MRS broth with Tween 80 (Biolife Italiana S.r.l., Milan, Italy) at 37 °C until reaching a cell density of 0.730 at 600 nm, determined spectrophotometrically using a Spectronic 1201 spectrophotometer (Milton Roy Co., Frederick, MD, USA).

Spontaneous and bacterial fermentations of non-pasteurized bee pollen were performed following the methodology described by Adaškevičiūtė et al. [28]. Briefly, 10 g of each bee pollen sample was moistened with 2 mL of sterile distilled water (Thermo Scientific, Fremont, CA, USA), followed by the addition of a mixture of honey and water (1.5 g honey with 2.5 mL water) after 2 h. For spontaneous fermentation, 800 µL of MRS broth with Tween 80 was added, while for bacterial fermentation, 800 µL of *L. rhamnosus* suspension (2.9×10^9 colony-forming units (CFU)/mL) was added. Control samples were prepared using bidistilled water instead of bacteria or MRS broth.

The vials were placed in an incubator (Biosan, Riga, Latvia) and fermented at +37 °C for 11 and 9 days, respectively [58]. After the bioprocess, solid-state samples were extracted with 80% methanol as described in Section 3.4.

3.3. Enzymatic Hydrolysis of Bee Pollen

Enzymatic hydrolysis of bee pollen was conducted using six commercial enzymes: two enzyme mixtures—*Clara-diastase* and *Viscozyme® L*—and four pure enzymes—lipase from *Aspergillus oryzae*, protease from *Bacillus* species, amyloglucosidase from *A. niger*, and cellulase from *A. niger* (Sigma-Aldrich Corporation, Taufkirchen, Germany). The bioprocess followed the methodology of our previous study [31]. Briefly, 1 g of bee pollen was mixed with 0.5 mL of sterile distilled water and treated at 121 °C for 15 min. The resulting mixture was supplemented with the optimal amount of each enzyme (175 μL of cellulase, *Viscozyme® L*, and *Clara-diastase*; 200 μL of protease, lipase, and amyloglucosidase) and incubated for the optimal duration (3 h 15 min for cellulase, *Viscozyme® L*, and *Clara-diastase*; 3 h 45 min for protease, lipase, and amyloglucosidase) [31]. Control samples were prepared using the corresponding buffer instead of the tested enzyme.

Vials containing the samples were boiled for 2 min to terminate the bioprocess, and the resulting mixtures were extracted using 80% methanol as described in Section 3.4.

3.4. Extraction of Bee Pollen Samples

Natural bee pollen samples were moistened with bidistilled water in order to achieve the appropriate consistency. All samples (natural, after fermentation or enzymatic hydrolysis) were extracted in a 1:10 ratio with 80% methanol (Sigma-Aldrich Corporation, Taufkirchen, Germany) [29]. After extraction, samples were filtered through 7–10 μm paper filter (Labbox, Barcelona, Spain) and 0.22 μm polyvinylidene fluoride (PVDF) membrane filter (BGB Analytik, Alexandria, VA, USA).

3.5. Antibacterial Activity and Interaction with Antibiotics Evaluation

The antibacterial activity of bee pollen extracts, antibiotics, or bee pollen and antibiotic mixtures was evaluated using the agar well diffusion method [29]. The inhibition of growth of four pathogenic bacteria was tested, including Gram-positive *Staphylococcus aureus* ATCC 6538 (LGC Standards, Lomianki, Poland) and *Listeria monocytogenes* ATCC 7644, as well as Gram-negative *Salmonella enterica* subsp. *enterica* serovar Enteritidis ATCC 13076 and *Salmonella enterica* subsp. *enterica* serovar Typhimurium ATCC 14028. Revitalization of indicator strains was performed using LB medium (Carl Roth, Karlsruhe, Germany). Succinctly, an overnight-grown bacterial inoculum in sterile LB-agar medium was spread onto Petri dishes. The following antibiotics were used during the analysis: ceftazidime pentahydrate (98%), ciprofloxacin (98%), oxytetracycline dihydrate (95%) (Acros Organics, Geel, Belgium), and erythromycin (≥93%) (Carl Roth Gmbh & Co. Kg, Karlsruhe, Germany).

Before the antibacterial test, three series of samples were prepared: (1) bee pollen extract were diluted with sterile water (1:1); (2) 30 μg/mL aqueous antibiotic solutions were diluted with sterile water (1:1); and (3) bee pollen extract mixed with 30 μg/mL corresponding antibiotic in a ratio (1:1). The prepared solutions were tested for antibacterial activity as described below.

Three wells were cut in each dish, and a drop of liquid agar was used at the bottom to prevent extract leakage. Wells were filled with 100 μL of 0.9% NaCl, 80% methanol, or testing solution. Ten repetitions were performed for each sample (bee pollen, antibiotics, or their mixture).

Antibacterial activity was evaluated by inhibition zone expressed by millimeters after incubation for 24 h at +37 °C. In vitro interactions ($I_{combination}$) between bee pollen extracts and antibacterial agents were determined and evaluated using the subsequent formula:

$$I_{combination} = A_e + A_a, \quad (1)$$

where A_e—inhibition zone (mm) of bee pollen extract, A_a—inhibition zone (mm) of antibiotics. The results were interpreted as follows:

- Synergistic, when the combined antibacterial activity was greater than the sum of the bee pollen extract and antibiotic antibacterial activity.
- Additive, when the combined antibacterial activity was equal to the sum of the bee pollen extract and antibiotic antibacterial activity.
- Antagonistic, when the combined antibacterial activity was weaker than the sum of the bee pollen extract and antibiotic antibacterial activity.

3.6. *Statistical Analysis*

The data were systematized using MS Excel 15.11.2 (2015, Microsoft, Redmond, WA, USA) software, and the results were subjected to analysis through linear regression modeling. Subsequently, chemometric analysis was carried out using MATLAB v23.2.0—R2023b Update 6 (2023, MathWorks, Natick, MA, USA) software.

Measured data were organized into a multidimensional matrix, representing 9 countries (Denmark, Sweden, Poland, Lithuania, Slovakia, the Netherlands, Italy, Spain, and Malta), 4 bacteria (*Salmonella* Typhimurium (B1), *Salmonella* Enteritidis (B2), *Listeria monocytogenes* (B3), and *Staphylococcus aureus* (B4)), 4 antibiotics (ceftazidime (A1), ciprofloxacin (A2), oxytetracycline (A3), and erythromycin (A4)), and 9 treatments (natural bee pollen (NAT), spontaneous (SPONT) and bacterial (BACT) fermentation, and enzymatic hydrolysis using enzymes—protease (PROT), lipase (LIP), cellulase (CEL), *Clara-diastase* (C-DIAS), *Viscozyme*® *L* (VISC-L), amyloglucosidase (AMGL)) conducting 10 repeated inhibition zone measurements. The dataset also included the results of 10 measurements of control samples for each fermentation and enzymatic hydrolysis, conducted without antibiotics. The final size of the data matrix prepared for chemometric analysis was 9 × 4 × 5 × 90. The data were analyzed from the perspective of pollen treatment (fermentation, enzymatic hydrolysis) and pollen origin (country) to determine treatment ways and pollen collection regions contributing the most to the antibiotic activity, emphasizing the synergistic effect.

Data preprocessing involved standardizing the variables by subtracting the mean and then dividing by the standard deviation. ANOVA was used for hypothesis testing to identify statistically significant changes in antibacterial activity values after fermentation or enzymatic hydrolysis, as well as following the addition of antibiotics, with a significance level of $p \leq 0.05$.

Clustering analysis involved a data standardization procedure, principal component analysis (PCA), hierarchical clustering analysis (HCA), and Euclidean distance between samples estimation. PCA was aimed at removing correlation in the initial variables and reducing the number of data dimensions. Applied HCA allowed us to group tested samples to clusters according to similarities among them according to the antibacterial activity profile. For statistical power improvement, hypotheses testing was employed to test statistical significance of the clusters formed by HCA. Student's t statistic was used to test statistically significant differences between variables, describing samples assigned to distinct clusters.

The statistical analysis was aimed to reveal optimal treatment ways and pollen collection regions in Europe, exposing better antibacterial performance and emphasizing the effect of added antibiotics. Euclidean distance calculation was employed to investigate antibacterial activity improvements between bee pollen samples before and after addition of antibiotics and evaluate the synergistic effect. The *ED* value was calculated in an orthogonal variable space after PCA (i.e., principal component space) using the following equation:

$$ED = \sqrt{\sum_{i=1}^{N} (S_{control\_i} - S_i)^2} \quad (2)$$

where $S_{control}$ denotes a control pollen sample, *S* denotes a sample, for which Euclidean distance is being evaluated, *N* is the number of variables, describing the samples.

4. Conclusions

Solid-state fermentation of bee pollen positively impacts antibacterial activity. Spontaneous fermentation significantly ($p \leq 0.05$) increased antibacterial activity by 1.04–2.92 times, while bacterial fermentation increased it by 1.18–4.08 times across all tested bee pollen samples. Additionally, interactions of natural and treated bee pollen extracts in combination with antibiotics were studied. Among all combinations tested against four Gram-positive and Gram-negative pathogenic bacteria, bee pollen extracts combined with four different antimicrobial agents exhibited 80.79% synergistic, 18.75% antagonistic, and 0.46% additive properties. These findings suggest that bee pollen extracts contain natural inhibitors operating through various mechanisms, potentially enhancing the effectiveness of antibiotics.

Chemometric analysis revealed that the highest antibacterial activity was achieved through bacterial fermentation and enzymatic hydrolysis with cellulolytic enzymes (cellulase, *Clara-diastase*, and *Viscozyme® L*), while the weakest activity was observed in samples enzymatically hydrolyzed with lipase, protease, and amyloglucosidase. The most pronounced synergistic effects after adding antibiotics were observed in samples from spontaneous and bacterial fermentation. Pollen from southern countries (Malta, Spain, and Italy) exhibited weaker antibacterial activity and less interaction with antibiotics compared to pollen from colder regions (Lithuania, Sweden, and Poland).

Supplementary Materials: The following supporting information can be downloaded at: https://www.mdpi.com/article/10.3390/ph18010015/s1, Figure S1: Tested bee pollen samples from various European countries; Table S1: An impact of fermentation and enzymatic hydrolysis on antibacterial activity of tested bee pollen and interaction with antibiotics.

Author Contributions: Conceptualization, V.K.; Investigation, V.D.; Validation, V.D.; Methodology, V.D. and P.K.; Formal analysis, P.K.; Writing—original draft, V.D. and P.K.; Supervision, V.K., P.K., and A.M.; Visualization, V.K.; Data curation, V.K.; Writing—review and editing, V.K., R.M., and A.M. All authors have read and agreed to the published version of the manuscript.

Funding: This research was funded by the Research Council of Lithuania, grant number 09.3.3-LMT-K-712-10-0232 and 09.3.3-LMT-K-712-16-0030. Instrumental analysis hardware, resources, and consumables were funded and provided by the Instrumental Analysis Open Access Centre of Vytautas Magnus University.

Institutional Review Board Statement: Not applicable.

Informed Consent Statement: Not applicable.

Data Availability Statement: Data will be made available on request.

Conflicts of Interest: The authors declare no conflicts of interest.

References

1. Atanasov, A.G.; Waltenberger, B.; Pferschy-Wenzig, E.V.; Linder, T.; Wawrosch, C.; Uhrin, P.; Temml, V.; Wang, L.; Schwaiger, S.; Heiss, E.H.; et al. Discovery and resupply of pharmacologically active plant-derived natural products: A review. *Biotechnol. Adv.* **2015**, *33*, 1582–1614. [CrossRef] [PubMed]
2. Atanasov, A.G.; Zotchev, S.B.; Dirsch, V.M.; the International Natural Product Sciences Taskforce; Supuran, C.T. Natural products in drug discovery: Advances and opportunities. *Nat. Rev. Drug Discov.* **2021**, *20*, 200–216. [CrossRef]
3. Molyneux, R.J.; Lee, S.T.; Gardner, D.R.; Panter, K.E.; James, L.F. Phytochemicals: The good, the bad and the ugly? *Phytochemistry* **2007**, *68*, 2973–2985. [CrossRef]
4. Yuan, H.; Ma, Q.; Ye, L.; Piao, G. The traditional medicine and modern medicine from natural products. *Molecules* **2016**, *21*, 559. [CrossRef]
5. Cushnie, T.P.; Lamb, A.J. Antimicrobial activity of flavonoids. *Int. J. Antimicrob. Agents* **2005**, *26*, 343–356. [CrossRef] [PubMed]
6. David, E.; Elumalai, E.K.; Sivakumar, C.; Therasa, S.V. Evaluation of antifungal activity and phytochemical screening of *Solanum surattense* seeds. *J. Pharm. Res.* **2010**, *3*, 684–687.
7. Egamberdieva, D.; Wirth, S.; Behrendt, U.; Parvaiz, A.; Berg, G. Antimicrobial activity of medicinal plants correlates with the proportion of antagonistic endophytes. *Front. Microbiol.* **2017**, *8*, 199. [CrossRef] [PubMed]
8. Gnat, S.; Majer-Dziedzic, B.; Nowakiewicz, A.; Trościańczyk, A.; Ziolkowska, G.; Jesionek, W.; Choma, I.; Dziedzic, R.; Zięba, P. Antimicrobial activity of some plant extracts against bacterial pathogens isolated from feces of red deer (*Cervus elaphus*). *Pol. J. Vet. Sci.* **2017**, *20*, 697–706. [PubMed]
9. Wazir, A.; Mehjabeen, J.N.; Sherwani, S.K.; Ahmad, M. Antibacterial, antifungal and antioxidant activities of some medicinal plants. *Pak. J. Pharm. Sci.* **2014**, *6*, 2145–2152.
10. Machado, A.; Zamora-Mendoza, L.; Alexis, F.; Álvarez-Suarez, J.M. Use of plant extracts, bee-derived products, and probiotic-related applications to fight multidrug-resistant pathogens in the post-antibiotic era. *Future Pharmacol.* **2023**, *3*, 535–567. [CrossRef]
11. Silva, D.M.; Costa, P.A.D.; Ribon, A.O.B.; Purgato, G.A.; Gaspar, D.M.; Diaz, M.A.N. Plant extracts display synergism with different classes of antibiotics. *An. Acad. Bras. Cienc.* **2019**, *91*, e20180117. [CrossRef]
12. Jouda, M.M.; Elbashiti, T.; Masad, A. The antibacterial effect of some medicinal plant extracts and their synergistic effect with antibiotics. *World J. Pharm. Pharm. Sci.* **2016**, *46*, 59–69.
13. Algethami, J.S.; El-Wahed, A.A.A.; Elashal, M.H.; Ahmed, H.R.; Elshafiey, E.H.; Omar, E.M.; Naggar, Y.A.; Algethami, A.F.; Shou, Q.; Alsharif, S.M.; et al. Bee pollen: Clinical trials and patent applications. *Nutrients* **2022**, *14*, 2858. [CrossRef] [PubMed]
14. Agrawal, P.; Kaur, J.; Rasane, P. Bee pollen: A superfood with health benefits and digestibility challenges. *J. Food Chem. Nanotechnol.* **2023**, *9*, S483–S489. [CrossRef]
15. Denisow, B.; Denisow-Pietrzyk, M. Biological and therapeutic properties of bee pollen: A review. *J. Sci. Food Agric.* **2016**, *96*, 4303–4309. [CrossRef] [PubMed]
16. Komosinska-Vassev, K.; Olczyk, P.; Kaźmierczak, J.; Mencner, L.; Olczyk, K. Bee pollen: Chemical composition and therapeutic application. *eCAM* **2015**, *2015*, 297425. [CrossRef] [PubMed]
17. Aličić, D.; Šubarić, D.; Jašić, M.; Pašalić, H.; Ačkar, D. Antioxidant properties of pollen. *Hrana Zdr. Boles. Znan. Stručni Časopis Za Nutr. Dijetetiku* **2014**, *3*, 6–12.
18. Velásquez, P.; Rodríguez, K.; Retamal, M.; Giordano, A.; Valenzuela, L.; Montenegro, G. Relation between composition, antioxidant and antibacterial activities, and botanical origin of multi-floral bee pollen. *J. Appl. Bot. Food Qual.* **2017**, *90*, 306–314. [CrossRef]
19. Savadogo, A.; Ouattara, C.A.T.; Bassole, I.H.N.; Traore, S.A. Bacteriocins and lactic acid bacteria—A minireview. *Afr. J. Biotechnol.* **2006**, *5*, 678–683.
20. Chen, J.; Pang, H.; Wang, L.; Ma, C.; Wu, G.; Liu, Y.; Guan, Y.; Zhang, M.; Qin, G.; Tan, Z. Bacteriocin-producing lactic acid bacteria strains with antimicrobial activity screened from *Bamei* pig feces. *Foods* **2022**, *11*, 709. [CrossRef] [PubMed]
21. Kaškonienė, V.; Stankevičius, M.; Bimbiraitė-Survilienė, K.; Naujokaitytė, G.; Šernienė, L.; Mulkytė, K.; Malakauskas, M.; Maruška, A. Current state of purification, isolation, and analysis of bacteriocins produced by lactic acid bacteria. *Appl. Microbiol. Biotechnol.* **2017**, *101*, 1323–1335. [CrossRef] [PubMed]
22. Benavides-Guevara, R.M.; Quicazan, M.C.; Ramirez-Toro, C. Digestibility and availability of nutrients in bee pollen applying different pretreatments. *Ing. Compet.* **2017**, *19*, 119–128.
23. Zuluaga, C.M.; Serrato-Bermudez, J.C.; Cecilia Quicazán, M. Bee-pollen structure modification by physical and biotechnological processing: Influence on the availability of nutrients and bioactive compounds. *Chem. Eng. Trans.* **2015**, *43*, 79–84. [CrossRef]
24. Rzepecka-Stojko, A.; Stojko, J.; Kurek-Górecka, A.; Górecki, M.; Kabała-Dzik, A.; Kubina, R.; Moździerz, A.; Buszman, E. Polyphenols from bee pollen: Structure, absorption, metabolism and biological activity. *Molecules* **2015**, *20*, 21732–21749. [CrossRef]
25. Wu, W.; Qiao, J.; Xiao, X.; Kong, L.; Dong, J.; Zhang, H. In vitro and in vivo digestion comparison of bee pollen with or without wall-disruption. *J. Sci. Food Agric.* **2021**, *101*, 2744–2755. [CrossRef] [PubMed]

26. Dong, J.; Gao, K.; Wang, K.; Xu, X.; Zhang, H. Cell wall disruption of rape bee pollen treated with combination of protamex hydrolysis and ultrasonication. *Food Res. Int.* **2015**, *75*, 123–130. [CrossRef]
27. Xiang, X.; Sun, S.; Dong, J.; Zhang, H. Breaking the cells of rape bee pollen and consecutive extraction of functional oil with supercritical carbon dioxide. *Innov. Food Sci. Emerg. Technol.* **2009**, *10*, 42–46. [CrossRef]
28. Adaškevičiūtė, V.; Kaškonienė, V.; Barčauskaitė, K.; Kaškonas, P.; Maruška, A. The impact of fermentation on bee pollen polyphenolic compounds composition. *Antioxidants* **2022**, *11*, 645. [CrossRef]
29. Kaškonienė, V.; Katilevičiūtė, A.; Kaškonas, P.; Maruška, A. The impact of solid state fermentation on bee pollen phenolic compounds and radical scavenging capacity. *Chem. Pap.* **2018**, *72*, 2115–2120. [CrossRef]
30. Kaškonienė, V.; Adaškevičiūtė, V.; Kaškonas, P.; Mickienė, R.; Maruška, A. Antimicrobial and antioxidant activities of natural and fermented bee pollen. *Food Biosci.* **2020**, *34*, 100532–100541. [CrossRef]
31. Zuluaga-Domínguez, C.; Castro-Mercado, L.; Cecilia Quicazán, M. Effect of enzymatic hydrolysis on structural characteristics and bioactive composition of bee-pollen. *J. Food Process.* **2019**, *43*, e13983. [CrossRef]
32. Damulienė, V.; Kaškonienė, V.; Kaškonas, P.; Maruška, A. The influence of enzymatic hydrolysis on bee pollen antioxidant and antibacterial activities. *Foods* **2023**, *12*, 3582. [CrossRef]
33. Acaroz, U.; Kurek-Gorecka, A.; Olczyk, P.; Tas, N.; Ali, A.; Paramanya, A.; Balyan, P.; Noor, A.; Kamaraj, S.; Malekifard, F.; et al. The role of bee products in the control of antimicrobial resistance and biofilm formation. *Kafkas Univ. Vet. Fak. Derg.* **2024**, *30*, 131–153. [CrossRef]
34. Al-Ani, I.; Zimmermann, S.; Reichling, J.; Wink, M. Antimicrobial activities of European propolis collected from various geographic origins alone and in combination with antibiotics. *Medicines* **2018**, *5*, 2. [CrossRef] [PubMed]
35. Hanafy, N.A.; Eltonouby, E.A.B.; Salim, E.I.; Mahfouz, M.E.; Leporatti, S.; Hafez, E.H. Simultaneous administration of bevacizumab with bee-pollen extract-loaded hybrid protein hydrogel NPs is a promising targeted strategy against cancer cells. *Int. J. Mol. Sci.* **2023**, *24*, 3548. [CrossRef] [PubMed]
36. Araque, M.; Vit, P. Evaluation of the potential synergistic effect of *Tetragonisca angustula* pot-pollen with amikacin and meropenem against extensively drug-resistant bacteria of clinical origin. *Med. Res. Arch.* **2024**, *12*, 1–8. [CrossRef]
37. Ilie, C.I.; Oprea, E.; Geana, E.I.; Spoiala, A.; Buleandra, M.; Gradisteanu Pircalabioru, G.; Badea, I.A.; Ficai, D.; Andronescu, E.; Ficai, A.; et al. Bee pollen extracts: Chemical composition, antioxidant properties, and effect on the growth of selected probiotic and pathogenic bacteria. *Antioxidants* **2022**, *11*, 959. [CrossRef] [PubMed]
38. Végh, R.; Csóka, M.; Sörös, C.; Sipos, L. Food safety hazards of bee pollen—A review. *Trends Food Sci. Technol.* **2021**, *114*, 490–509. [CrossRef]
39. Carrera, M.A.; Fernández-Alba, A.R.; Hernando, M.D. Unveiling bee pollen's contamination with pesticides and mycotoxins: Current analytical procedures, results and regulation. *TrAC Trends Anal. Chem.* **2024**, *180*, 117935. [CrossRef]
40. Regulation (EU) 2023/915 of 25 April 2023 on Maximum Levels for Certain Contaminants in Food and Repealing Regulation (EC) No 1881/2006. Available online: http://data.europa.eu/eli/reg/2023/915/2024-07-22 (accessed on 14 October 2024).
41. Regulation (EC) No 396/2005 of the European Parliament and of the Council of 23 February 2005 on Maximum Residue Levels of Pesticides in or on Food and Feed of Plant and Animal Origin and Amending Council Directive 91/414/EEC (Text with EEA relevance). Available online: http://data.europa.eu/eli/reg/2005/396/2024-11-06 (accessed on 14 October 2024).
42. Yatomi, R.; Nakamura, S.; Nakamura, N. Immunochemical and cytochemical detection of wall components of germinated pollen of gymnosperms. *Grana* **2002**, *41*, 21–28. [CrossRef]
43. Zhang, D.; Li, H. Exine export in pollen. In *Plant ABC Transporters*; Springer International Publishing: Cham, Switzerland, 2014; pp. 49–62. [CrossRef]
44. Elzain, A.M.; Elsanousi, S.M.; Ibrahim, M.A. Effectiveness of ethanol and methanol alcohols on different isolates of *Staphylococcus* species. *J. Bacteriol. Mycol. Open Access* **2019**, *7*, 71–73. [CrossRef]
45. Rutala, W.A.; Weber, D.J.; Guideline for Disinfection and Sterilization in Healthcare Facilities, 2008. Update: May 2019. 2019. Available online: https://www.cdc.gov/infection-control/hcp/disinfection-sterilization/chemical-disinfectants.html (accessed on 17 December 2024).
46. Xu, C.; Fu, Y.; Liu, F.; Liu, Z.; Ma, J.; Jiang, R.; Song, C.; Jiang, J.; Hou, J. Purification and antimicrobial mechanism of a novel bacteriocin produced by *Lactobacillus rhamnosus* 1.0320. *LWT* **2021**, *137*, 110338. [CrossRef]
47. Kacaniova, M.; Vukovic, N.; Chlebo, R.; Hascik, P. The antimicrobial activity of honey, bee pollen loads, and beeswax from Slovakia. *Arch. Biol. Sci.* **2012**, *64*, 927–934. [CrossRef]
48. Fatrcová-Šramková, K.; Nôžková, J.; Kacaniova, M.; Máriássyová, M.; Mikláŝová, K.; Stričík, M. Antioxidant and antimicrobial properties of monofloral bee pollen. *J. Environ. Sci. Health* **2013**, *48*, 133–138. [CrossRef]
49. Mohdaly, A.A.A.; Mahmoud, A.A.; Roby, M.H.H.; Smetanska, I.; Ramadan, M.F. Phenolic extract from propolis and bee pollen: Composition, antioxidant and antibacterial activities. *J. Food Biochem.* **2015**, *39*, 538–547. [CrossRef]
50. Stefanović, O.D. Synergistic activity of antibiotics and bioactive plant extracts: A study against Gram-positive and Gram-negative bacteria. In *Bacterial Pathogenesis and Antibacterial Control*; IntechOpen: London, UK, 2018; pp. 23–48. [CrossRef]

51. Reygaert, W.C. An overview of the antimicrobial resistance mechanisms of bacteria. *AIMS Microbiol.* **2018**, *4*, 482–501. [CrossRef] [PubMed]
52. Wiermann, R.; Gubatz, S. Pollen wall and sporopollenin. *Int. Rev. Cytol.* **1992**, *140*, 35–72. [CrossRef]
53. Amin, M.U.; Khurram, M.; Khattak, B.; Khan, J. Antibiotic additive and synergistic action of rutin, morin and quercetin against methicillin resistant *Staphylococcus aureus*. *BMC Complement. Altern. Med.* **2015**, *15*, 59. [CrossRef] [PubMed]
54. Borges, A.; Ferreira, C.; Saavedra, M.; Simões, M. Antibacterial activity and mode of action of ferulic and gallic acids against pathogenic bacteria. *Microb. Drug Resist.* **2013**, *19*, 256–265. [CrossRef]
55. Ibitoye, O.B.; Ajiboye, T.O. Ferulic acid potentiates the antibacterial activity of quinolone-based antibiotics against *Acinetobacter baumannii*. *Microb. Pathog.* **2019**, *126*, 393–398. [CrossRef]
56. Yougbare, S.; Chang, T.K.; Tan, S.H.; Kuo, J.C.; Hsu, P.H.; Su, C.Y.; Kuo, T.R. Antimicrobial gold nanoclusters: Recent developments and future perspectives. *Int. J. Mol. Sci.* **2019**, *20*, 2924. [CrossRef] [PubMed]
57. *ISO 24382:2023*; Bee Pollen—Specifications. International Organization for Standardization: Geneva, Switzerland, 2023.
58. Adaškevičiūtė, V.; Kaškonienė, V.; Maruška, A. Optimization of conditions for bee pollen lactic acid fermentation. In Proceedings of the CYSENI 2021: The 17th International Conference of Young Scientists on Energy Issues, Kaunas, Lithuania, 24–28 May 2021.

pharmaceuticals

MDPI

Article

Beeswax Alcohol (BWA, Raydel®) Improved Blood Oxidative Variables and Ameliorated Severe Damage of Zebrafish Kidneys, Testes, and Ovaries Impaired by 24-Week Consumption of a High-Cholesterol and High-Galactose Diet: A Comparative Analysis with Coenzyme Q_{10}

Kyung-Hyun Cho [1,*], Ashutosh Bahuguna [1], Ji-Eun Kim [1], Yunki Lee [1], Sang Hyuk Lee [1], Cheolmin Jeon [1] and Cheol-Hee Kim [2]

1 Raydel Research Institute, Medical Innovation Complex, Daegu 41061, Republic of Korea
2 Department of Biology, Chungnam National University, Daejeon 34134, Republic of Korea
* Correspondence: chok@raydel.co.kr; Tel.: +82-53-964-1990; Fax: +82-53-965-1992

Abstract: Objectives: The present study describes the comparative effect of 24-week supplementation of beeswax alcohol (BWA, Raydel®, 0.5% and 1.0%, wt/wt) and coenzyme Q_{10} (CoQ_{10}, 0.5% and 1.0%, wt/wt) on plasma oxidative variables and the prevention of organ injury in adult zebrafish subjected to a high-cholesterol (HC, 4%, wt/wt) and -D-galactose (Gal, 30%, wt/wt) diet. Methods: Adult zebrafish were fed various HC+Gal diets enriched with either BWA or CoQ_{10}. After 24 weeks of dietary intervention, blood and organs were harvested for subsequent biochemical and histological evaluations. Results: The HC+Gal-elevated plasma oxidative variables were reverted by the consumption of BWA, marked by the lowest plasma malondialdehyde (MDA) level and highest sulfhydryl content. The HC+Gal-impaired zebrafish swimming ability (staggering movement) was substantially recovered by BWA, manifested by a ~three-fold ($p < 0.001$) enhancement in swimming distance and speed. Also, the intake of BWA affected the morphology of HC+Gal-compromised kidney and induced histological changes by mitigating reactive oxygen species (ROS) production and cellular senescence, which was markedly more effective than the results seen in the CoQ_{10} group. Likewise, BWA proved effective in preventing HC+Gal-induced testis damage, apparent in the 48.3% ($p < 0.05$) higher spermatozoa and 26.3% ($p < 0.01$) reduced interstitial space between the seminiferous tubules. BWA substantially prevented HC+Gal-induced ovary damage by suppressing oxidative stress, lipid deposition and senescence, leading to the restoration of mature vitellogenic oocyte counts. Conclusion: BWA demonstrated a greater ability than CoQ_{10} to enhance plasma antioxidant status, suppress ROS generation, delay organ aging and alleviate HC+Gal-induced adversity in zebrafish.

Keywords: beeswax alcohol (BWA); coenzyme Q_{10} (CoQ_{10}); oxidative variables; senescence; oocytes; cholesterol; kidney; ovary; testis

1. Introduction

Many investigations have established that extensive consumption of D-galactose (Gal) is associated with severe damage in major organs such as the brain, liver, kidneys, ovaries, and testes via the formation of galactitol, which causes oxidative stress and mitochondrial dysfunction [1,2]. It is well known that the accumulation of galactitol leads to depletion of reduction power to defend against oxidative stress, consequently exacerbating neurotoxicity, hepatotoxicity, and cell aging [3,4]. Due to the build-up of reactive oxygen species (ROS)/free radicals and the hypertonic nature of galactitol, severe oxidative damage occurs in various cell membranes, proteins, and mitochondrial DNA [5,6]. In particular, the long-term consumption of D-galactose induces significant oxidative stress and the formation of advanced glycation end products (AGEs), which contribute to brain aging in animal models, closely resembling the aging process observed in the human brain and liver [7,8]. Besides the effect on the brain and liver, it was documented that D-galactose causes the aging of testicular tissue, the thymus, and the spleen, with severe oxidative damage in a murine model [3,9,10].

Beeswax alcohol (BWA) is a blend of long-chain aliphatic alcohol (LCAA) extracted from honey beeswax [11]. BWA is widely recognized for its potent antioxidants and anti-inflammatory properties, which enable it to exert hepatic and gastroprotective roles and prevent the oxidation of protein and lipids in the cell membrane [12–14]. Moreover, in vitro experiments highlighted BWA's role in inhibiting the oxidation of low-density lipoprotein (LDL) [15] while protecting the activity of high-density lipoprotein (HDL)-associated paraoxonase (PON) and reducing HDL glycation [16]. The administration of BWA intake demonstrated therapeutic potential against dyslipidemia by lowering the total cholesterol (TC) and triglyceride (TG) levels while increasing the HDL-C levels in hyperlipidemic zebrafish exposed to both mild [11] and high doses of D-galactose [17].

Like BWA, coenzyme Q_{10} (CoQ_{10}) is a hydrophobic substance known for its various activities, such as its anti-inflammatory, antioxidant, and hepatoprotective properties [18,19]. In addition, CoQ_{10} was reported to significantly contribute to the maintenance of the plasma lipoprotein profile in a study on dyslipidemic Chinese adults [20]. Despite the several benefits of BWA and CoQ_{10}, limited studies are available to precisely describe their comparative effect against high cholesterol- and high galactose-guided events. However, recently, we reported a substantially better effect of BWA over CoQ_{10} in protecting the brain and liver against high cholesterol and galactose (HC+Gal)-triggered oxidative stress, inflammation, and cellular senescence in adult zebrafish [17]. A potent protective effect was noticed in the brain, where BWA reduced ROS production, apoptosis, and senescence; protected the myelin sheath integrity; and restored cognitive changes in the zebrafish impaired by long-term dietary supplementation with HC+Gal [17]. In continuation of the previous study, the current study assessed the comparative pharmacological effect of BWA and CoQ_{10} on the plasma oxidative parameters and organs like the kidney, testis, and ovary of zebrafish consuming a high-cholesterol (HC, 4% wt/wt) and high-galactose (Gal, 30% wt/wt) diet. The zebrafish was chosen as the model species in light of its higher genetic similarity with higher vertebrates [21], which has been widely accepted as a suitable model for studying oxidative damage in the brain, liver, kidney, and reproduction systems and has a very similar lipid and lipoprotein metabolism to humans [22].

2. Results

2.1. Change in Motion Pattern and Swimming Behavior in Top-Down View Assay

The bird's-eye-view motion assay (Figure 1) revealed that zebrafish in the ND group showed the highest swimming distance, around 5.3 m, and the most comprehensive swimming pattern around the rim of the wall (of the round tank), while the zebrafish in the HC alone group showed a decreased swimming distance (~2.7m) with a narrow swimming pattern along the half-rim wall of the tank. Furthermore, the HC+Gal group showed the shortest swimming distance (1.5 m), which was highly restricted to the tank's center without approaching the tank's wall, suggesting that galactose consumption along with the HC diet causes severe loss of swimming ability and sense of direction. By contrast, the co-

consumption of 0.5% BWA and 1.0% BWA culminated in improved swimming distances of 4.7 m and 5.1 m, respectively, with a broader swimming pattern along the wall of the round tank. Precisely, the zebrafish in the 1.0% BWA group displayed swimming movements along the complete rim of the tank. The co-consumption of 0.5% and 1.0% CoQ_{10} also resulted in improved swimming distances of ~3.7 m and 3.3 m, respectively, which was remarkably ~2-fold more than the swimming distance noted in the HC+Gal group. Also, a much-improved swimming pattern was noticed in the CoQ_{10} group compared to the HC+Gal group; however, the swimming motion was almost restricted to half the rim of the tank. Compared to CoQ_{10}, zebrafish in the BWA group, specifically in the 1.0% group, showed free movement across the tank with a significantly ~1.5-fold ($p < 0.001$) higher swimming distance than that of the 0.5% and 1.0% CoQ_{10} groups, respectively.

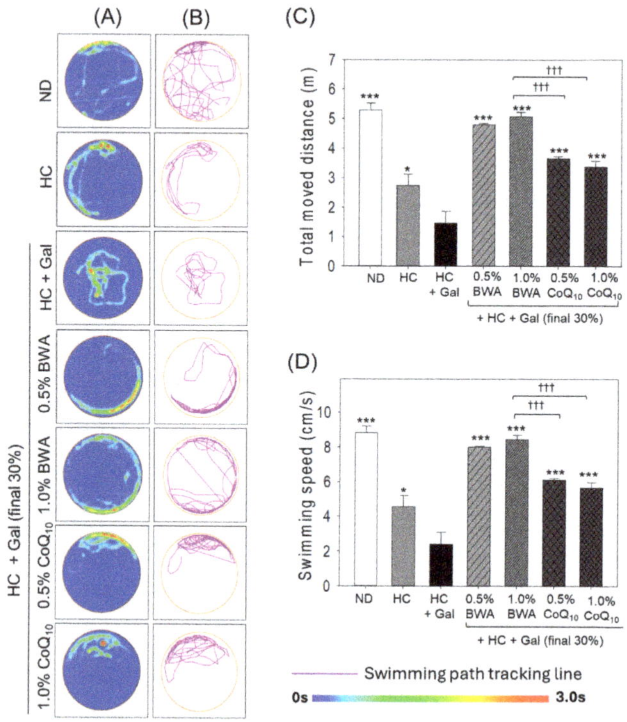

Figure 1. Overview of zebrafish motion captured from a top-down perspective (bird's eye view) at 24 weeks of dietary intervention with high cholesterol and D-galactose. (**A**) Heat map illustrating zebrafish swimming pattern. (**B**) Visual representation of swimming trajectory. (**C**) and (**D**) Quantification of mean swimming distance and speed (cm/s), respectively. Seven zebrafish (n = 7) from each group were examined for 1 min using software (Any-Maze version 7.0, Kim & friends, Seoul, Republic of Korea) to analyze average swimming distance and speed. ND, HC, Gal, BWA, and CoQ_{10} are abbreviations for normal diet, high cholesterol, galactose, beeswax alcohol, and coenzyme Q_{10}, respectively. * ($p < 0.05$) and *** ($p < 0.001$) depict statistical significance concerning the HC+Gal group, while ††† ($p < 0.001$) highlights statistical difference compared to the BWA 1.0% group.

Alongside swimming distance, the highest swimming speed (8.8 cm/s) was noticed in the ND group, which was significantly reduced to 4.6 cm/s in the HC group and further reduced to 2.4 cm/s in the HC+Gal group. In contrast, the swimming speed was substantially restored in the CoQ_{10} and BWA consumption groups. The zebrafish in the 0.5% and 1.0% BWA groups displayed a swimming speed of 7.9 and 8.5 cm/s, respectively, which was remarkably ~3-fold better than the swimming speed observed in the HC+Gal group. Similarly, the intake of CoQ_{10} resulted in a noticeable increase in swimming speed, reaching 6.1 cm/s and 5.6 cm/s in the 0.5% CoQ_{10} and 1.0% CoQ_{10} groups, respectively. Nevertheless, BWA demonstrated a more substantial impact on swimming speed, as reflected by the ~39% higher swimming speed in the 1.0% BWA group than that of the 1.0% CoQ_{10} group.

2.2. Oxidative Extent and Antioxidant Status of Plasma

The thiobarbituric acid reactive substance (TBARS) assay revealed the highest malondialdehyde (MDA) level in the HC+Gal group (11.7 μM), which was significantly 1.7-fold and 1.5-fold more compared to the MDA level quantified in the ND (4.0 μM) and HC (7.8 μM) consumption groups (Figure 2A). The consumption of BWA displayed a dose-dependent effect to reduce the HC+Gal-elevated MDA level, as evidenced by the 6.3 μM and 5.5 μM MDA levels in the 0.5% and 1.0% BWA groups, which was significantly 1.9-fold ($p < 0.01$) and 2.1-fold ($p < 0.01$) lower compared to the MDA level detected in the HC+Gal group. Similarly, a positive effect of CoQ_{10} supplementation, a reduction in the plasma MDA level was observed, which was ~1.4-fold ($p < 0.05$) lower compared to the MDA level in the HC+Gal group, while compared to 1.0% CoQ_{10}, the 1.0% BWA group displayed a ~33.2% ($p < 0.001$) reduced MDA level.

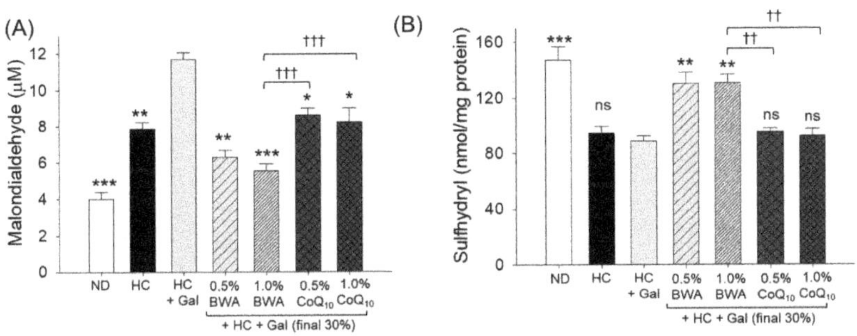

Figure 2. Oxidative variables in zebrafish plasma from different groups after 24 weeks of consumption of the specific diets along with high cholesterol and high galactose. (**A**) Quantification of the lipid peroxidation [assessed by thiobarbituric acid reactive substance (TBARS) assay using malondialdehyde (MDA) as the standard]. (**B**) Sulfhydryl content quantification. * ($p < 0.05$), ** ($p < 0.01$), and *** ($p < 0.001$) depict statistical significance concerning the HC+Gal group, while †† ($p < 0.01$) and ††† ($p < 0.001$) highlight statistical differences compared to the BWA 1.0% group; ns represents a non-significant difference between groups.

The plasma sulfhydryl content was significantly reduced by 39.5% in the HC+Gal group compared to that in the ND group (Figure 2B). The HC+Gal-diminished sulfhydryl content was restored in the BWA consumption group, evidenced by the significantly, ~32% ($p < 0.01$), elevated sulfhydryl content in the 0.5% and 1.0% BWA groups. In contrast, CoQ_{10} consumption displayed a non-significant effect on the plasma sulfhydryl content, disturbed by the consumption of HC+Gal. The combined results of the plasma analysis attested to BWA's greater efficacy compared to CoQ_{10} in diminishing HC+Gal oxidative stress markers.

2.3. Change in Organ Weight: Kidneys, Testes, and Ovaries

As shown in Figure 3B,E, the HC alone and HC+Gal groups displayed 1.4-times and 1.7-times augmented kidney weight compared to the ND alone group, suggesting that the HC+Gal diet exacerbates the kidney burden more than the HC alone diet. The BWA 0.5%

and 1.0% groups displayed 15% and 27% less kidney weight relative to the HC+Gal group, suggesting that supplementation with BWA alleviated enlargement of the kidneys and damage caused by the HC+Gal diet. Like the BWA group, the 1.0% CoQ_{10} group displayed a substantially, 29% ($p < 0.001$), reduced kidney weight compared to the HC+Gal group; however, 0.5% CoQ_{10} consumption displayed a non-significant effect.

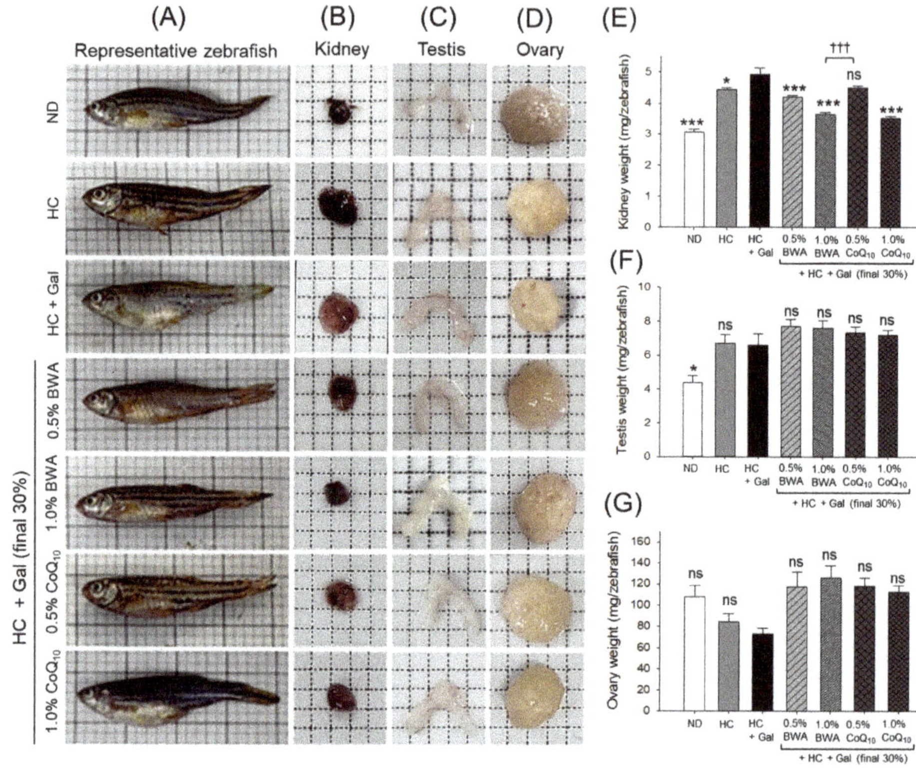

Figure 3. Images of different organs obtained from the zebrafish following 24 weeks of consumption of the designated diets under the influence of high-cholesterol and high-galactose diets. Representative images of (**A**) whole zebrafish, (**B**) kidney, (**C**) testis, and (**D**) ovary. The average weight of the (**E**) kidney, (**F**) testis, and (**G**) ovary. * ($p < 0.05$) and *** ($p < 0.001$) depict statistical significance concerning the HC+Gal group, while ††† ($p < 0.001$) highlights statistical difference compared to the BWA 1.0% group; ns represents a non-significant difference between groups.

As shown in Figure 3C,F, a non-significant change in the testes size and weight was observed between the groups compared to the HC+Gal group. Similar to the findings of the testis, no substantial change in the ovary weight was detected in different groups (Figure 3D,G). Nonetheless, the morphological analysis showed a slightly reduced ovary size in the HC+Gal consumed group compared to the other groups (Figure 3D).

2.4. Histological Examination and Senescence Assay in Kidney

As depicted in Figure 4A, a disorganized tubular structure was observed in the HC-group that substantially elevated with the co-consumption of Gal (HC+Gal). The HC+Gal group exhibited an enlarged tubular lumen (indicated by a blue arrowhead) at multiple locations, along with frequent degeneration and debris in the lumen. The BWA, mainly at 1.0%, significantly restored the HC+Gal-induced kidney impairment reflected by the well-organized distal and tubular structure; however, elevated space in the tubular lumen was noticed at some places. In contrast, the CoQ_{10}-supplemented groups showed limited preventive effect, where the occasional presence of the lumen debris and the dilated tubular lumen was noticed.

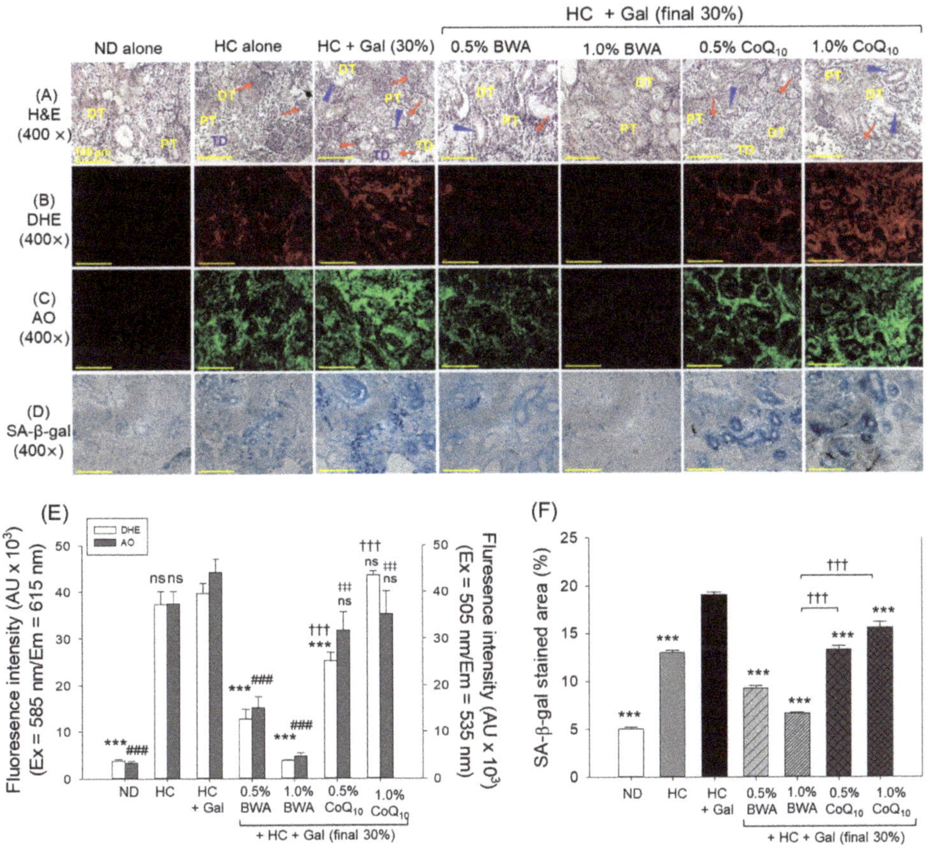

Figure 4. Histological analysis of zebrafish kidneys following 24 weeks of consumption of designated diets under the influence of high cholesterol and galactose supplementation. (**A**) Hematoxylin and eosin (H&E) staining; DT and PT depicting the distal and proximal tubules, respectively. The red arrow highlights the luminal debris, while the blue arrowhead indicates elevated tubular lumen. Scale bar = 100 µm. (**B**) Dihydroethidium (DHE) and (**C**) acridine orange (AO), fluorescent staining. (**D**) Senescent-associated β-galactosidase (SA-β-gal) staining. (**E**) Image J-based DHE and AO fluorescent staining quantification. (**F**) SA-β-gal-stained area. *** ($p < 0.001$) depicts statistical significance (for DHE and SA-β-gal-stained area), while ### ($p < 0.001$) depicts statistical significance (for AO fluorescent intensity) concerning the HC+Gal group. ††† ($p < 0.001$) highlights statistical difference (for DHE and SA-β-gal-stained area), and ‡‡‡ highlights statistical difference (for AO fluorescent intensity) compared to the BWA 1.0% group; ns represents a non-significant difference between groups.

DHE staining suggested abundant ROS generation in the HC+Gal group, which was significantly 10.4-fold more than the ROS level quantified in the ND group (Figure 4B,E). The supplementation of 0.5% and 1.0% BWA effectively reduced the HC+Gal-elevated ROS level, as reflected by the 3.2-fold ($p < 0.001$) and 10-fold ($p < 0.001$) diminished DHE fluorescent intensities, respectively, compared to that of the HC+Gal group. Like BWA, the 0.5% CoQ_{10} consumption group showed a substantial effect against HC+Gal-induced ROS generation. Surprisingly, 1.0% CoQ_{10} supplementation failed to prevent HC+Gal-induced ROS production.

AO staining revealed that the HC+Gal group exhibited the highest level of apoptosis, indicated by a 14-fold higher AO-stained area than the ND group (Figure 4C,E). Supplementation of BWA at both 0.5% and 1.0% concentrations efficiently counters HC+Gal-provoked apoptosis, evidenced by the 2.9-fold and 9.2-fold lower AO-stained areas in the 0.5% and 1.0% BWA groups, compared to those in the HC+Gal group (Figure 4C,E). Unlike BWA, the consumption of CoQ_{10} failed to prevent HC+Gal-induced apoptosis.

The SA-β-gal-stained area was significantly increased by 3.8-fold ($p < 0.001$) and 1.5-fold ($p < 0.001$) in the HC+Gal group compared to those in the ND and HC groups, respectively, indicating that HC+Gal consumption promotes cellular senescence in the kidneys (Figure 4D,F). Supplementation of BWA and CoQ_{10} at both doses (0.5% and 1.0%) adequately prevented HC+Gal-provoked cellular senescence. In the BWA, 0.5%, and 1.0% groups, notably 1.6-fold and 2.3-fold lower cellular senescence was quantified than in the 1.0% CoQ_{10} group, attesting to the substantially better impact of BWA over CoQ_{10} in restraining HC+Gal-triggered cellular senescence.

2.5. Histological Analysis and Senescence Assay in Testis Tissue

As depicted in Figure 5, the ND group displayed normal testis histology with an adequately arranged tubular structure that was substantially compromised by the consumption of HC and HC+Gal diets, as evident by the ~1.4-times ($p < 0.01$) elevated interstitial space between the seminiferous tubules and the ~1.5-times diminished spermatozoa area compared to the ND group (Figure 5A,B). The supplementation of BWA, mainly at 1.0%, significantly restricts HC+Gal-induced testis damage, as reflected by the 26.1%-reduced interstitial space between the seminiferous tubules and 48.3% ($p < 0.05$) higher spermatozoa than those in the HC+Gal group (Figure 5F,G). In contrast, CoQ_{10} consumption at 0.5% and 1.0% showed no significant therapeutic impact on the testis damage induced by HC+Gal.

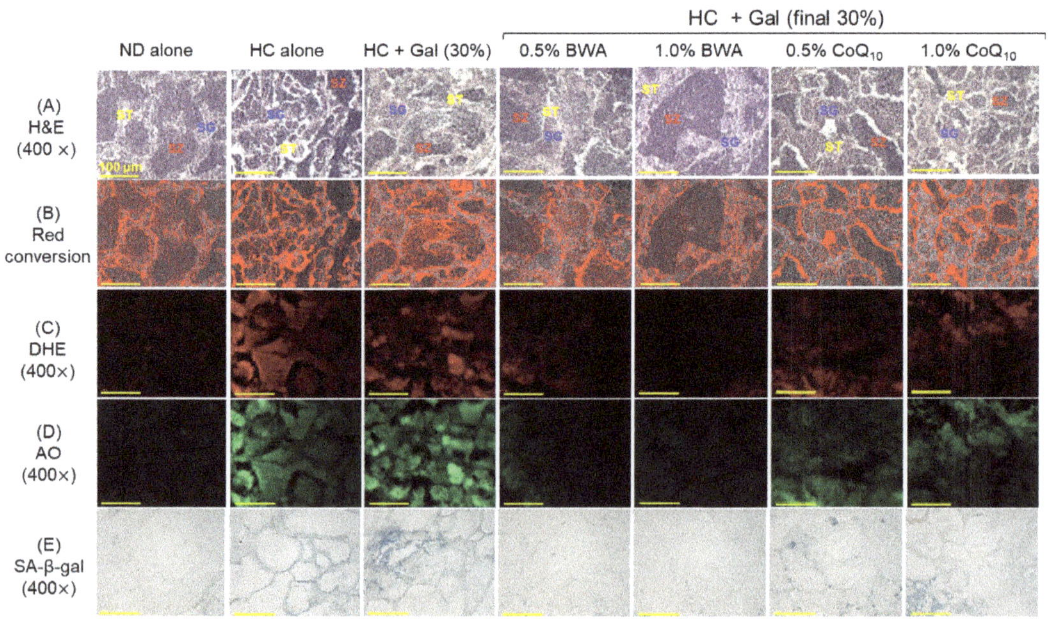

Figure 5. *Cont.*

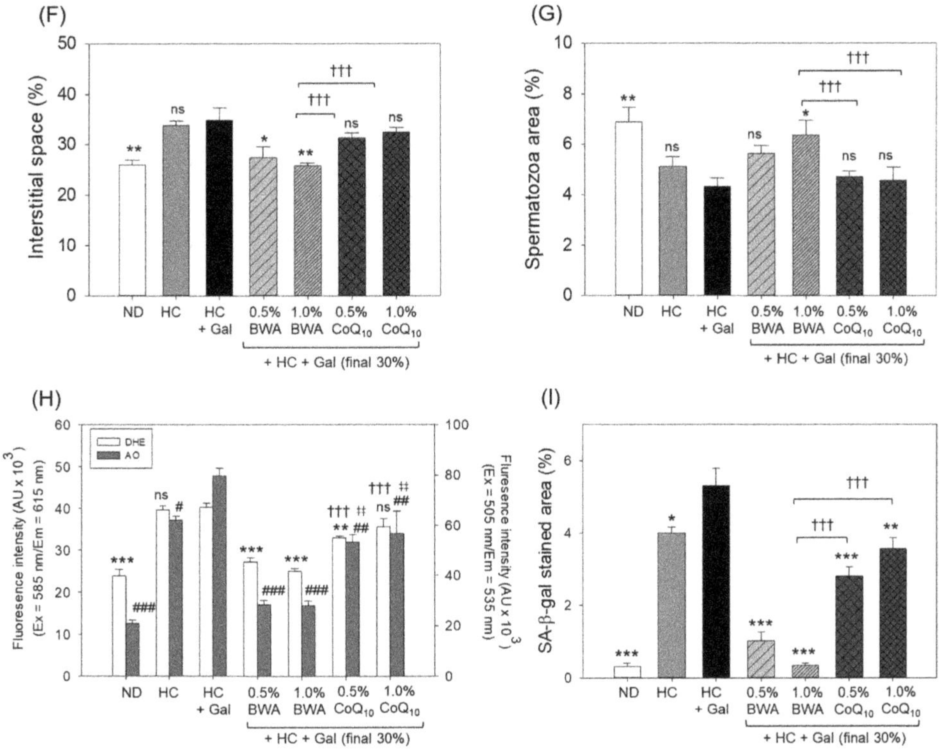

Figure 5. Histological analysis of testes obtained from zebrafish after 24 weeks of consumption of designated diets under the influence of high cholesterol and galactose supplementation. (**A**) Hematoxylin and eosin (H&E) staining; SG, ST, and SZ depicting the spermatogonia, spermatocytes, and spermatozoa, respectively. Scale bar = 100 μm. (**B**) Red conversion of the images of H&E staining to enhance visibility. The red conversion was performed using Image J-software (version 1.53, https://imagej.net/ij; accessed on 16 June 2023) at the white color threshold value (0-120). (**C**) Dihydroethidium (DHE) and (**D**) acridine orange (AO), fluorescent staining. (**E**) Senescent-associated β-galactosidase (SA-β-gal) staining. Quantification of (**F**) interstitial space between seminiferous tubules and (**G**) spermatozoa, (**H**) DHE and AO fluorescent intensity, and (**I**) SA-β-gal-stained area. * ($p < 0.05$), ** ($p < 0.01$), and *** ($p < 0.001$) depict statistical significance concerning the HC+Gal group (for interstitial space, spermatozoa area, DHE, and SA-β-gal area), while # ($p < 0.05$), ## ($p <$ 0.001) and ### ($p < 0.001$) depicts statistical significance (for AO fluorescent intensity) concerning the HC+Gal group. ††† ($p < 0.001$) highlight statistical differences (for interstitial space, spermatozoa area, DHE, and SA-β-gal area), and ‡‡ ($p < 0.01$) highlights statistical differences (for AO fluorescent intensity) compared with the BWA 1.0% group; ns represents a non-significant difference between groups.

DHE and AO staining revealed the heightened production of ROS and apoptosis in response to the consumption of HC+Gal, which was significantly 1.8-fold and 3.8-fold higher than the ROS and apoptosis detected in the ND group (Figure 5C,D,H). The supplementation of BWA and CoQ_{10} showed a substantial preventive role against the HC+Gal-triggered ROS generation and apoptosis in the testis. Notably, a substantially 1.4-fold and 2.0-fold lower DHE and AO-stained area was quantified in the 1.0% BWA group compared to the 1.0% CoQ_{10} group.

SA-β-gal staining (Figure 5E,I) suggests a 15.5-fold and 1.5-fold higher prevalence of the senescent-positive cells in the HC+Gal group compared to in the 1.0% BWA and 1.0%

CoQ_{10} groups, testifying to the protective role of BWA and CoQ_{10}. However, the BWA effect is much superior to that of CoQ_{10} to minimize the HC+Gal-triggered senescence, as reflected by an 8.4-fold and 10.5-fold reduced senescent-stained area in the 1.0% BWA consumption group compared to the 0.5% and 1.0% BWA groups, respectively.

2.6. Histological Analysis of Ovaries

The histological analysis of the ovaries revealed a significant detrimental effect of HC+Gal on the ovary cellular structure by elevating the pre-vitellogenic oocyte counts by 1.2-fold and reducing the early-vitellogenic oocyte counts by 3.4-fold those in the ND group (Figure 6A,F,G). BWA consumption prevents HC+Gal-triggered ovary damage, as reflected by the ~1.2-fold reduced pre-vitellogenic oocyte counts in response to 0.5% and 1.0% BWA compared to those in the HC+Gal group. Likewise, early and mature oocyte counts were ~2.0-fold and ~3.6-fold higher in the BWA groups compared to those in the HC+Gal group. In contrast, CoQ_{10} failed to demonstrate any restorative effect on the oocyte counts impacted by the HC+Gal consumption of HC+Gal.

The DHE staining showed the effect of BWA and CoQ_{10} in curtailing HC+Gal-triggered ROS generation. A noticeable ~1.5-times diminished ROS level was noticed in the 0.5% and 1.0% BWA groups compared to the HC+Gal group (Figure 6B,H). Also, CoQ_{10} (0.5% and 1.0%) substantially diminished HC+Gal-triggered ROS production; however, the ROS levels remained approximately 20% higher ($p < 0.001$) in these groups compared to those in the 1.0% BWA group.

The highest apoptosis indicated by AO staining was observed in the HC+Gal group, which was remarkably 1.6-fold and 1.9-fold reduced in response to the consumption of 0.5% and 1.0% BWA (Figure 6C,H). Likewise, CoQ_{10} (0.5% and 1.0%) reduced HC+Gal-triggered apoptosis, although their efficacy was ~1.4 fold lower compared to the effect exerted by 1.0% BWA.

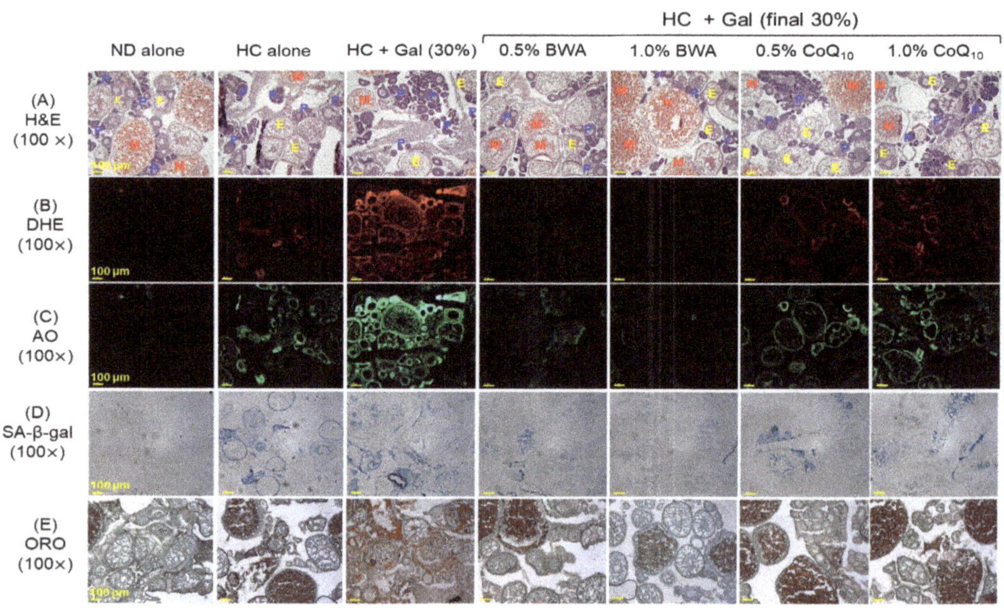

Figure 6. *Cont.*

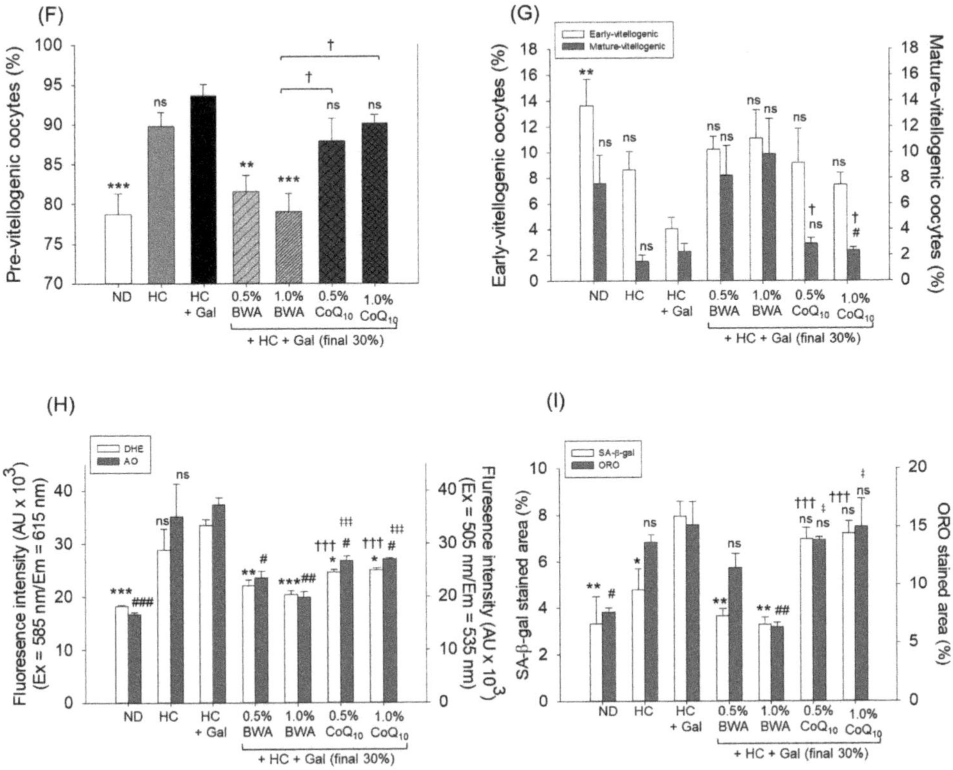

Figure 6. Histological analysis of the zebrafish ovaries after 24 weeks of consumption of designated diets under the presence of high cholesterol and galactose supplementation. (**A**) Hematoxylin and eosin (H&E) staining; P, E, and M depicting the pre-, early, and mature oocytes, respectively. Scale bar = 100 μm. (**B**) Dihydroethidium (DHE) and (**C**) acridine orange (AO), fluorescent staining. (**D**) Senescent-associated β-galactosidase (SA-β-gal) staining. (**E**) Oil red O (ORO) staining. Quantification of (**F**) pre-vitellogenic and (**G**) early and mature vitellogenic oocytes; five distinct sections for each group were examined for the quantitative estimation of pre-, early, and mature oocyte counts. (**H**) Image J-based DHE and AO fluorescent intensity quantification. (**I**) Quantification of SA-β-gal and ORO-stained areas. * ($p < 0.05$), ** ($p < 0.01$), and *** ($p < 0.001$) depict statistical significance (for pre-, early vitellogenic oocytes, DHE, and SA-β-gal area), while $^{\#}$ ($p < 0.05$), $^{\#\#}$ ($p < 0.001$) and $^{\#\#\#}$ ($p < 0.001$) depict statistical significance (for AO fluorescent intensity and ORO-stained area) concerning the HC+Gal group. † ($p < 0.05$) and ††† ($p < 0.001$) highlight statistical difference (for pre-vitellogenic oocytes, DHE, and SA-β-gal area) and ‡ ($p < 0.05$) and ‡‡‡ ($p < 0.001$) highlight statistical difference (for AO fluorescent intensity and ORO-stained area) compared to the BWA 1.0% group; ns represents a non-significant difference between groups.

The SA-β-gal staining results demonstrated that BWA (at concentrations of 0.5% and 1.0%) significantly reduced HC+Gal-induced senescence by ~2.0-fold ($p < 0.01$) (Figure 6D,I). In contrast, CoQ_{10} did not exhibit a significant effect in preventing HC+Gal-induced cellular senescence.

Additionally, BWA significantly reduced HC+Gal-provoked lipid accumulation, evidenced by 1.3-fold and 2.4-fold diminished ORO-stained areas in the 0.5% and 1.0% BWA-supplemented group, compared to the HC+Gal-group (Figure 6E,I). In contrast, CoQ_{10} exhibited no effect against HC+Gal-induced lipid accumulation.

3. Discussion

It has been well known that high cholesterol consumption has been associated with several detrimental effects [23–25] that enhance oxidative stress and alter antioxidant status [26]. Likewise, high sugar consumption has been reported to cause oxidative stress [27], inflammation [28], and adverse events that substantially affect different organs [27]. Furthermore, the combined intake of sugar and HC results in greater exacerbation than either substance alone, making it an ideal dietary model for inducing obesity and other disorders that mimic the pathophysiology and progression of the disease in humans [29].

Galactose displayed severe toxic effects in adult zebrafish [11,17], leading to altered swimming behavior marked by retard swimming speed and paths of movement that concentrated in a fixed space. The consumption of BWA and CoQ_{10} showed a substantial preventive impact on the recovery of HC+Gal-altered swimming behavior; however, a higher effect of BWA than CoQ_{10} on HC+Gal-inducted adversity was noticed. It has been well recognized that galactose-induced ROS generation [30] and impaired cellular antioxidants [31] are the key contributors to brain aging and cognitive changes [30,32,33]. Substances that have a positive impact on the brain's oxidative parameters and antioxidants, such as SOD, CAT, and glutathione peroxidase (GSH-px), lead to the recovery of brain damage and cognitive changes provoked by the galactose [31]. We believe that BWA has a better effect in restoring HC+Gal-hampered swimming behavior than CoQ_{10} due to its higher antioxidant impact [15]. Also, a direct positive modulatory effect of BWA on cellular antioxidants like superoxide dismutase (SOD), catalase (CAT), and glutathione peroxidase (GSH-px) has been documented [14,15,34] and strengthens the present finding that, owing to substantial antioxidant activity, BWA protects zebrafish against the HC+Gal-induced challenges. Besides the induction of oxidative stress, galactose consumption has been noticed to cause glycation, leading to the generation and accumulation of AGEs in the brain [30,35] and, consequently, brain damage and cognitive changes [36,37]. Therefore, a substance that can prevent protein glycation will have a definite effect on preventing glycation-induced detrimental effects. The accumulating literature suggests the inhibitory effect of BWA in preventing protein glycation, while CoQ_{10} was found ineffective [15]. Moreover, compared to CoQ_{10}, BWA displayed a substantial protective effect against carboxymethyllysine (CML, a typical AGE)-induced toxicity in zebrafish embryos [15]. These findings support the current results, suggesting that BWA, due to its antiglycation properties and significantly more vigorous antioxidant activity than CoQ_{10}, mitigates HC+Gal-induced swimming alterations in zebrafish.

The plasma analysis revealed substantially higher MDA levels in the HC+Gal group, along with a reduced plasma sulfhydryl content, underscoring the impact of HC+Gal on the induction of oxidative stress. The consumption of CoQ_{10} and BWA effectively mitigated the HC+Gal-induced MDA level. Similarly, plasma sulfhydryl is a crucial oxidative stress marker [38,39], and its diminished levels have been associated with different pathological conditions [40]. Following HC+Gal supplementation, a reduction in plasma sulfhydryl content was noticed, which was significantly elevated by the intake of BWA; however, CoQ_{10} consumption did not restore the HC+Gal-disrupted plasma sulfhydryl content. The collective results of the plasma analysis depict a low level of MDA and higher sulfhydryl content in BWA than the CoQ_{10} directed the higher antioxidant nature of BWA over CoQ_{10} that effectively prevents the HC+Gal induced oxidative stress. These results align with those of earlier studies documenting the impact of BWA on the plasma oxidative variables and its modulatory effect on cellular antioxidants [41,42].

Severe damage to the kidney, testis, and ovary have been noticed in response to HC+Gal consumption, which is consistent with the literature documenting the adverse effects of HC and Gal in different organs [11]. Consistent with the observations of the plasma analysis, BWA consumption showed a significant curative impact in preventing the HC+Gal-induced impairment of kidneys and reproductive organs. Notably, in all organs, a high generation of ROS was noticed in response to HC+Gal consumption, which has been recognized as a key culprit for the induction of apoptosis [43,44] and senescence [45,46]. It is apparent from the current study that the higher antioxidant efficacy of BWA counters the HC+Gal-provoked ROS generation, which leads to the inhibition of apoptosis and senescence and the prevention of organ damage. The results are supported by earlier reports documenting the protective effect of antioxidants against Gal-induced kidney damage by minimizing oxidative stress [47]. In addition, the higher plasma sulfhydryl content in the BWA group suggests better kidney health, as higher sulfhydryl content has been associated with a decreased risk of kidney disease [38]. A visible impact of high cholesterol and galactose has been described for testis damage by impairment of the testicular structures and interstitial area between the seminiferous tubules, altered spermatogenesis [48], and decreased sperm count [49]. Also, galactose consumption has been documented to elevate oxidative stress and the inhibition of cellular antioxidant activities such as those of SOD and GSH-px, leading to severe damage to the testis [48]. BWA, owing to its antioxidant nature, suppresses the HC+Gal-posed oxidative stress, preventing testicular damage. The results aligned with a previous study highlighting caffeic acid antioxidant properties, which countered Gal-induced oxidative stress and safeguarded the testes [48]. Similarly, oxidative stress impacts the physiology of the ovary and oocyte quality and causes female reproductive health disorders [50], while the substance reduces oxidative stress and improves antioxidant status to prevent ovary damage [50]. BWA, due to the inhibitory effect of ROS generation and its inductive effect on cellular antioxidants, improves the oxidative stress environment in different organs, protecting against HC+Gal-induced damage, alongside its established role in preventing gastrointestinal and joint health of humans [51]. The current findings decode BWA's efficacy in protecting vital organs and offer promising possibilities for the consumption of human and veterinary supplements to manage health issues linked to high cholesterol and sugar consumption. Further research and trials are essential to confirm its efficacy across different veterinary species.

4. Materials and Methods

4.1. Materials

Beeswax alcohol (BWA) (Cat#330020123) was extracted from the block beeswax of *Apis mellifera* (mainly mellifera lineage) and was complimentarily provided by Raydel® Australia Pty. Ltd. (Sydney, NSW, Australia). Detailed specification of the BWA is provided in Supplementary Table S1. All the other chemicals and reagents were of analytical grade. The list of chemicals used is listed in Supplementary Method S1.

4.2. Zebrafish Husbandry and Production of Embryos

Adult ~16-week-old zebrafish were cultured in an aerated water tank equipped with a circulated water supply. The water temperature was maintained at 28 ± 1 °C, and a 14 h light/10 h dark photoperiod was used. The animal experiments were performed according to the suggested guidelines of the Animal Care Committee and approved by the Raydel Research Institute (RRI, approval code RRI-23-007, approval date 27 July 2023). Zebrafish were fed the normal diet (ND, tetrabit, Gmbh D4930, Melle, Germany).

4.3. Different Diets' Preparation and Consumption by Adult Zebrafish

The normal diet (ND) of tetrabits was purchased from Tetrabit Gmbh (Melle, Germany). The ND was mixed with cholesterol (4%, wt/wt) to make the high-cholesterol (HC) diet following a previously described method [11]. The HC diet was blended with galactose (Gal, 30%, wt/wt) to form an HC diet infused with galactose (HC+Gal) [11,17]. The HC+Gal diet was blended with BWA (0.5% or 1.0% wt/wt) and CoQ_{10} (0.5% or 1.0% wt/wt) to make the four different HC+Gal diets supplemented with BWA and CoQ_{10}.

Zebrafish (16 weeks aged, n = 392) were allocated to the different cohorts, named Group I (n = 56, ND), Group II (n = 56, HC), Group III (n = 56, HC + Gal + 0.5% BWA), Group IV (n = 56, HC + Gal + 1.0% BWA), Group V (n = 56, HC + Gal + 0.5% CoQ_{10}), and Group VI (n = 56, HC + Gal + 1.0% CoQ_{10}). The zebrafish in Group I were fed ND, while the zebrafish in Group II were fed the HC diet. Zebrafish in Groups III and IV were fed HC + Gal + 0.5% BWA and HC + Gal + 1.0% BWA, respectively. Similarly, the zebrafish in Groups V and VI were fed HC + Gal + 0.5% CoQ_{10} and HC + Gal + 1.0% CoQ_{10}, respectively. Zebrafish in all groups (I–VI) were maintained on their respective diets for 24 weeks. Zebrafish in Groups II-VI were pre-fed with an HC diet for one month (before the experimentation) to induce hyperlipidemia. Figure 7 illustrates the experimental design for feeding across the groups.

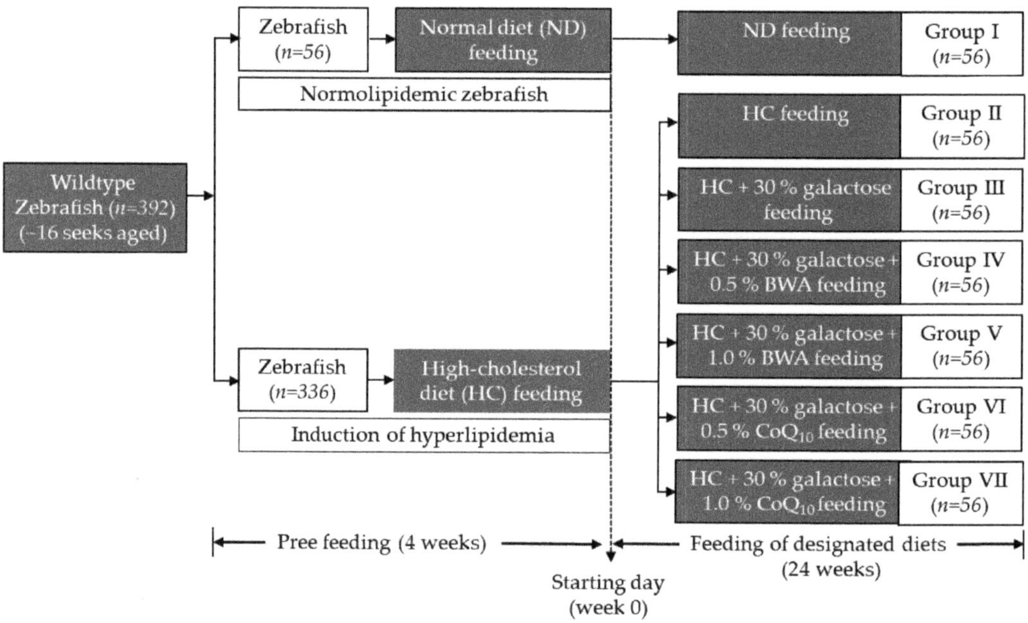

Figure 7. The experimental design involves zebrafish feeding on different diets: ND (normal diet), HC (high-cholesterol diet), BWA (beeswax alcohol), and CoQ_{10} (coenzyme Q_{10}).

4.4. Swimming Behavior Analysis

The swimming behavior of zebrafish following 24-week consumption of different diets was performed in a white circular water tank with a 35 cm diameter and a 11 cm height. The water tank was ~2/3 filled with water, and zebrafish from the different groups were allowed to swim in it. Before the swimming analysis, zebrafish were kept in the tank for 60 min to acclimate to the conditions. Afterward, zebrafish swimming activity was observed (1 min), and their swimming patterns were recorded using a digital camera (Canon EOS 90D, EFS 17-55 mm 1:2.8 IS-USM, ultrasonic lens, Tokyo, Japan) placed 100 cm above the water tank [as depicted in Supplementary Figure S1]. The recorded swimming activity was processed to analyze the path of motion, swimming distance, and speed using software (Any-Maze version 7.0, Kim & friends, Seoul, Republic of Korea).

4.5. Harvesting Blood and Tissues

Following 24 weeks of dietary intervention, zebrafish were euthanized via hypothermic shock [52]. Blood samples were promptly collected thereafter, and the organs (kidneys, testes, and ovaries) from the different groups were dissected and preserved separately in a 10% formalin solution for further analysis.

4.6. Estimation of Plasma Monoaldehyde (MDA) and Sulfhydryl Groups

The plasma MDA level was measured using the thiobarbituric acid reactive substance (TBARS) assay, following previously described methods with slight modifications [53]. Briefly, 50 μL of plasma (0.1 mg of equivalent protein) was mixed with 50 μL of trichloro acetic acid (TCA) and 100 μL of TBA. The mixture was subjected to 10 min at 95 °C, followed by an absorbance measurement at 560 nm.

The plasma sulfhydryl content was measured spectrophotometrically, following a previously established method with minor modifications [54]. In brief, 50 μL of plasma (0.1 mg of equivalent protein) was blended with 50 μL of 5,5-dithiol-bis-(2-nitrobenzoic acid) (DTNB) and incubated at room temperature. After 12 h of incubation, the absorbance at 412 nm was determined, and the sulfhydryl content was quantified using the DTNB molar extinction coefficient (ε) 1.36×10^4 M^{-1} cm^{-1}.

4.7. Histological Evaluation

The tissue sections (kidneys, testes, and ovaries) were sectioned (7 μm thick) using cryo-sectioning (Leica CM 1510S, Nussloch, Germany). The histological changes in the tissue section were investigated by hematoxylin and eosin (H&E) staining employing a previously outlined method [55]. Lipid accumulation in the tissue was determined by oil red O (ORO) staining [17]. Briefly, a 7 μm thick tissue section was submerged with the ORO stain followed by 5 min of heating at 60 °C and subsequent washing with 60% isopropanol and counter-stained hematoxylin (30 s). After washing with water, the section was observed under a microscope.

4.8. Staining for the Detection of Cellular Senescence, Reactive Oxygen Species, and Apoptosis

Cellular senescence in the tissue sections was assessed using the senescent-associated β-galactosidase (SA-β-gal) assay [17]. The tissue section, 7 μm thick, was coated with 250 μL of 5-bromo-4-chloro-3-indoly-β-D-galactopyranoside (X-gal, 5 mg/mL) and incubated in the dark for 16 h. It was washed two times with PBS and then examined under a microscope to identify blue-colored SA-β-gal-positive cells. The tissues' reactive oxygen species and apoptosis were determined by fluorescent staining following a previously described method [56,57]. A detailed methodology is provided in Supplementary Method S2.

4.9. Statistical Analysis

SPSS (version 29.0, Chicago, IL, USA) software was used to determine one-way ANOVA after Tukey's post hoc analysis to evaluate the statistical difference between the groups. For the pairwise statistical analysis, a Student's *t*-test was performed.

5. Conclusions

This comparative consumption study concludes BWA's substantially higher protective effect over CoQ_{10} against the HC+Gal-induced detrimental effect in zebrafish. BWA showed an affirmative impact on oxidative variables and restored sulfhydryl content hindered by the consumption of HC+Gal. BWA, owing to its antioxidant nature, impact on ROS generation, apoptosis, and cellular senescence paves a way to protect the kidney, testis, and ovary from the deleterious effects of HC+Gal. The findings suggest that incorporating BWA into the diet helps to improve antioxidant status and protects the kidney and reproductive organs from oxidative stress caused by excessive cholesterol and galactose intake.

Supplementary Materials: The following supporting information can be downloaded at https://www.mdpi.com/article/10.3390/ph18010017/s1, Supplementary Methods S1 and S2: List of chemicals and methodology for fluorescent staining. Supplementary Table S1: Certificate of analysis and composition of beeswax alcohol (BWA). Supplementary Figure S1: Ray diagram of zebrafish swimming activity analysis experimental system.

Author Contributions: Conceptualization, K.-H.C.; methodology, A.B., J.-E.K., Y.L., S.H.L., C.J. and C.-H.K.; data curation, writing—original draft preparation, K.-H.C.; writing—review and editing, K.-H.C., supervision, K.-H.C. All authors have read and agreed to the published version of the manuscript.

Funding: This research received no external funding.

Institutional Review Board Statement: The animal study protocol was approved by the Committee of Animal Care and Use of Raydel Research Institute (approval code RRI-23-001, approval date 27 July 2023).

Informed Consent Statement: Not applicable.

Data Availability Statement: The data used to support the findings of this study are available from the corresponding author upon reasonable request.

Conflicts of Interest: The authors declare no conflicts of interest.

References

1. Lai, K.; Elsas, L.J.; Wierenga, K.J. Galactose toxicity in animals. *IUBMB Life* **2009**, *61*, 1063–1104. [CrossRef] [PubMed]
2. Conte, F.; van Buuringen, N.; Voermans, N.C.; Lefeber, D.J. Galactose in human metabolism, glycosylation and congenital metabolic diseases: Time for a closer look. *Biochim. Biophys. Acta (BBA) Gen. Subj.* **2021**, *1865*, 129898. [CrossRef] [PubMed]
3. Uddin, M.N.; Nishio, N.; Ito, S.; Suzuki, H.; Isobe, K.I. Toxic effects of D-galactose on thymus and spleen that resemble aging. *J. Immunotoxicol.* **2010**, *7*, 165–173. [CrossRef]
4. Holden, H.M.; Thoden, J.B.; Timson, D.J.; Reece, R.J. Galactokinase: Structure, function and role in type II galactosemia. *Cell. Mol. Life Sci. CMLS* **2004**, *61*, 2471–2484. [CrossRef]
5. Bo-Htay, C.; Palee, S.; Apaijai, N.; Chattipakorn, S.C.; Chattipakorn, N. Effects of d-galactose-induced ageing on the heart and its potential interventions. *J. Cell. Mol. Med.* **2018**, *22*, 1392–1410. [CrossRef]
6. Murphy, M.P. How mitochondria produce reactive oxygen species. *Biochem. J.* **2009**, *417*, 1–13. [CrossRef] [PubMed]
7. Sadigh-Eteghad, S.; Majdi, A.; McCann, S.K.; Mahmoudi, J.; Vafaee, M.S.; Macleod, M.R. D-galactose-induced brain ageing model: A systematic review and meta-analysis on cognitive outcomes and oxidative stress indices. *PLoS ONE* **2017**, *12*, e0184122.
8. Shwe, T.; Pratchayasakul, W.; Chattipakorn, N.; Chattipakorn, S.C. Role of D-galactose-induced brain aging and its potential used for therapeutic interventions. *Exp. Gerontol.* **2018**, *101*, 13–36. [CrossRef]
9. Azman, K.F.; Zakaria, R. D-Galactose-induced accelerated aging model: An overview. *Biogerontology* **2019**, *20*, 763–782. [CrossRef]
10. Aydin, S.; Yanar, K.; Simsek, B.; Cebe, T.; Sitar, M.E.; Belce, A.; Cakatay, U. Galactose-induced Aging Model in Rat Testicular Tissue. *J. Coll. Physicians Surg. Pak.* **2018**, *28*, 501–504. [CrossRef]
11. Cho, K.-H.; Bahuguna, A.; Kim, J.-E.; Lee, Y.; Lee, S.H. Comparative Assessment of Beeswax Alcohol and Coenzyme Q_{10} (CoQ_{10}) to Prevent Liver Aging, Organ Damage, and Oxidative Stress in Hyperlipidemic Zebrafish Exposed to D-Galactose: A 12-Week Dietary Intervention. *Pharmaceuticals* **2024**, *17*, 1250. [CrossRef] [PubMed]
12. Menéndez, R.; Más, R.; Illnait, J.; Pérez, J.; Amor, A.M.; Fernández, J.C.; González, R.M. Effects of D-002 on lipid peroxidation in older subjects. *J. Med. Food* **2001**, *4*, 71–77. [CrossRef] [PubMed]
13. Illnait, J.; Rodríguez, I.; Mendoza, S.; Fernández, Y.; Mas, R.; Miranda, M.; Piñera, J.; Fernández, J.C.; Mesa, M.; Fernández, L.; et al. Effects of D-002, a mixture of high molecular weight beeswax alcohols, on patients with nonalcoholic fatty liver disease. *Korean J. Intern. Med.* **2013**, *28*, 439. [CrossRef]
14. Pérez, Y.; Oyárzabal, A.; Mas, R.; Molina, V.; Jiménez, S. Protective effect of D-002, a mixture of beeswax alcohols, against indomethacin-induced gastric ulcers and mechanism of action. *J. Nat. Med.* **2013**, *67*, 182–189. [CrossRef]
15. Cho, K.-H.; Baek, S.-H.; Nam, H.-S.; Bahuguna, A.; López-González, L.E.; Rodríguez-Cortina, I.; Illnait-Ferrer, J.; Fernández-Travieso, J.C.; Molina-Cuevas, V.; Pérez-Guerra, Y.; et al. Beeswax alcohol prevents low-density lipoprotein oxidation and

demonstrates antioxidant activities in zebrafish embryos and human subjects: A clinical study. *Curr. Issues Mol. Biol.* **2024**, *46*, 409–429. [CrossRef] [PubMed]
16. Cho, K.-H.; Baek, S.-H.; Nam, H.-S.; Bahuguna, A. Enhancement of antioxidant and anti-glycation properties of beeswax alcohol in reconstituted high-density lipoprotein: Safeguarding against carboxymethyllysine toxicity in zebrafish. *Antioxidants* **2023**, *12*, 2116. [CrossRef]
17. Cho, K.-H.; Bahuguna, A.; Kim, J.-E.; Lee, Y.; Lee, S.H. Consumption of beeswax alcohol (BWA, Raydel®) improved zebrafish motion and swimming endurance via protecting brain and liver from oxidative stress induced by 24 weeks supplementation of high cholesterol and D-galactose diets: A comparative analysis between BWA and coenzyme Q_{10}. *Antioxidants* **2024**, *13*, 1488.
18. Farsi, F.; Nezhad, P.A.; Morshedzadeh, N. The Hepatoprotective Effects of Coenzyme Q_{10} Against Oxidative Stress. In *The Liver*; Academic Press: Cambridge, MA, USA, 2018; pp. 281–294.
19. Sifuentes-Franco, S.; Sánchez-Macías, D.C.; Carrillo-Ibarra, S.; Rivera-Valdés, J.J.; Zuñiga, L.Y.; Sánchez-López, V.A. Antioxidant and anti-inflammatory effects of coenzyme Q_{10} supplementation on infectious diseases. *Healthcare* **2022**, *10*, 487. [CrossRef]
20. Zou, J.; Tian, Z.; Zhao, Y.; Qiu, X.; Mao, Y.; Li, K.; Shi, Y.; Zhao, D.; Liang, Y.; Ji, Q.; et al. Coenzyme Q_{10} supplementation improves cholesterol efflux capacity and antiinflammatory properties of high-density lipoprotein in Chinese adults with dyslipidemia. *Nutrition* **2022**, *101*, 111703. [CrossRef] [PubMed]
21. Poureetezadi, S.J.; Wingert, R.A. Little fish, big catch: Zebrafish as a model for kidney disease. *Kidney Int.* **2016**, *89*, 1204–1210. [CrossRef] [PubMed]
22. Stoletov, K.; Fang, L.; Choi, S.H.; Hartvigsen, K.; Hansen, L.F.; Hall, C.; Pattison, J.; Juliano, J.; Miller, E.R.; Almazan, F.; et al. Vascular lipid accumulation, lipoprotein oxidation, and macrophage lipid uptake in hypercholesterolemic zebrafish. *Circ. Res.* **2009**, *104*, 952–960. [CrossRef]
23. Han, Y.; Zee, S.; Cho, K.-H. Beeswax alcohol and fermented black rice bran synergistically ameliorated hepatic injury and dyslipidemia to exert antioxidant and anti-inflammatory activity in ethanol-supplemented zebrafish. *Biomolecules* **2023**, *13*, 136. [CrossRef] [PubMed]
24. Udomkasemsab, A.; Prangthip, P. High fat diet for induced dyslipidemia and cardiac pathological alterations in Wistar rats compared to Sprague Dawley rats. *Clin. Investig. Arterioscler.* **2019**, *31*, 56–62.
25. Puska, L.G.; Nagy, Z.B.; Giricz, Z.; Onody, A.; Csonka, C.; Kitajka, K.; Hackler, L., Jr.; Zvara, A.; Ferdinandy, P. Cholesterol diet-induced hyperlipidemia influences gene expression pattern of rat hearts: A DNA microarray study. *FEBS Lett.* **2004**, *562*, 99–104. [CrossRef] [PubMed]
26. Balkan, J.; Doğru-Abbasoğlu, S.; Aykaç-Toker, G.; Uysal, M. The effect of a high cholesterol diet on lipids and oxidative stress in plasma, liver and aorta of rabbits and rats. *Nutr. Res.* **2004**, *24*, 229–234. [CrossRef]
27. González, P.; Lozano, P.; Ros, G.; Solano, F. Hyperglycemia and Oxidative Stress: An Integral, Updated and Critical Overview of Their Metabolic Interconnections. *Int. J. Mol. Sci.* **2023**, *24*, 9352. [CrossRef]
28. Ma, X.; Nan, F.; Liang, H.; Shu, P.; Fan, X.; Song, X.; Hou, Y.; Zhang, D. Excessive intake of sugar: An accomplice of inflammation. *Front. Immunol.* **2022**, *13*, 988481. [CrossRef]
29. Bala, S.; Ganz, M.; Babuta, M.; Zhuang, Y.; Csak, T.; Calenda, C.D.; Szabo, G. Steatosis, inflammasome upregulation, and fibrosis are attenuated in miR-155 deficient mice in a high fat-cholesterol-sugar diet-induced model of NASH. *Lab. Investig.* **2021**, *101*, 1540–1549. [CrossRef] [PubMed]
30. Budni, J.; Pacheco, R.; da Silva, S.; Garcez, M.L.; Mina, F.; Bellettini-Santos, T.; de Medeiros, J.; Voss, B.C.; Steckert, A.V.; da Silva Valvassori, S.; et al. Oral administration of d-galactose induces cognitive impairments and oxidative damage in rats. *Behav. Brain Res.* **2016**, *302*, 35–43. [CrossRef] [PubMed]
31. Qu, Z.; Zhang, J.; Yang, H.; Huo, L.; Gao, J.; Chen, H.; Gao, W. Protective effect of tetrahydropalmatine against d-galactose induced memory impairment in rat. *Physiol. Behav.* **2016**, *154*, 114–125. [CrossRef]
32. Lei, M.; Su, Y.; Hua, X.; Ding, J.; Han, Q.; Hu, G.; Xiao, M. Chronic systemic injection of D-galactose impairs the septohippocampal cholinergic system in rats. *Neuroreport* **2008**, *19*, 1611–1615. [CrossRef] [PubMed]
33. Hsieh, H.-M.; WA, W.-M.; Hu, M.-L. Soy isoflavones attenuate oxidative stress and improve parameters related to aging and Alzheimer's disease in C57BL/6J mice treated with D-galactose. *Food Chem. Toxicol.* **2009**, *47*, 625–632. [CrossRef] [PubMed]
34. Molina, V.; Ledón, T.; Ravelo, Y.; Zamora, Z.; Mena, L. Effects of D-002 (Beeswax alcohols) on concentrations of prostaglandin E2 in rat gastric mucosa. *J. Pharm. Pharm. Res.* **2017**, *1*, 2.
35. Münch, G.; Westcott, B.; Menini, T.; Gugliucci, A. Advanced glycation endproducts and their pathogenic roles in neurological disorders. *Amino Acids* **2012**, *42*, 1221–1236. [CrossRef] [PubMed]
36. Yaffe, K.; Lindquist, K.; Schwartz, A.V.; Vitartas, C.; Vittinghoff, E.; Satterfield, S.; Simonsick, E.M.; Launer, L.; Rosano, C.; Cauley, J.A.; et al. Advanced glycation end product level, diabetes, and accelerated cognitive aging. *Neurology* **2011**, *77*, 1351–1356. [CrossRef]

37. D'Cunha, N.M.; Sergi, D.; Lane, M.M.; Naumovski, N.; Gamage, E.; Rajendran, A.; Kouvari, M.; Gauci, S.; Dissanayka, T.; Marx, W.; et al. The Effects of Dietary Advanced Glycation End-Products on Neurocognitive and Mental Disorders. *Nutrients* **2022**, *14*, 2421. [CrossRef]
38. Bourgonje, A.R.; Abdulle, A.E.; Bourgonje, M.F.; Binnenmars, S.H.; Gordijn, S.J.; Bulthuis, M.L.C.; la Bastide-van Gemert, S.; Kieneker, L.M.; Gansevoort, R.T.; Bakker, S.J.L.; et al. Serum free sulfhydryl status associates with new-onset chronic kidney disease in the general population. *Redox Biol.* **2021**, *48*, 102211. [CrossRef] [PubMed]
39. Bourgonje, A.R.; Bourgonje, M.F.; Post, A.; Gemert, S.L.B.-V.; Kieneker, L.M.; Bulthuis, M.L.; Gordijn, S.J.; Gansevoort, R.T.; Bakker, S.J.; Mulder, D.J.; et al. Systemic oxidative stress associates with new-onset hypertension in the general population. *Free Radic. Biol. Med.* **2022**, *187*, 123–131. [CrossRef]
40. Hu, M.-L. Measurement of protein thiol groups and glutathione in plasma. *Methods Enzym.* **1994**, *233*, 380–385.
41. Menéndez, R.; Más, R.; Amor, A.M.; Pérez, Y.; González, R.M.; Fernández, J.; Molina, V.; Jiménez, S. Antioxidant effects of D002 on the in vitro susceptibility of whole plasma in healthy volunteers. *Arch. Med. Res.* **2001**, *32*, 436–441. [CrossRef] [PubMed]
42. Lopez, E.; Illnait, J.; Molina, V.; Oyarzabal, A.; Fernandez, L.; Perez, Y.; Mas, R.; Mesa, M.; Fernandez, J.; Mendoza, S. Effects of D-002 (beeswax alcohol) on lipid peroxidation in middle-aged and older subjects. *Lat. Am. J. Pharm.* **2008**, *27*, 695–703.
43. Kannan, K.; Jain, S.K. Oxidative stress and apoptosis. *Pathophysiology* **2000**, *7*, 153–163. [CrossRef]
44. Lee, Y.-J.; Cho, H.-N.; Soh, J.-W.; Jhon, G.J.; Cho, C.-K.; Chung, H.-Y.; Bae, S.; Lee, S.-J.; Lee, Y.-S. Oxidative stress-induced apoptosis is mediated by ERK1/2 phosphorylation. *Exp. Cell Res.* **2003**, *291*, 251–266. [CrossRef]
45. Nousis, L.; Kanavaros, P.; Barbouti, A. Oxidative stress-induced cellular senescence: Is labile iron the connecting link? *Antioxidants* **2023**, *12*, 1250. [CrossRef]
46. Faraonio, R. Oxidative stress and cell senescence process. *Antioxidants* **2022**, *11*, 1718. [CrossRef]
47. Feng, Y.; Yu, Y.H.; Wang, S.T.; Ren, J.; Camer, D.; Hua, Y.Z.; Zhang, Q.; Huang, J.; Xue, D.L.; Zhang, X.F.; et al. Chlorogenic acid protects D-galactose-induced liver and kidney injury via antioxidation and anti-inflammation effects in mice. *Pharm. Biol.* **2016**, *54*, 1027–1034. [CrossRef]
48. Khoshdel, F.; Golmohammadi, M.G.; Dost, M.J.; Najafzade, N.; Salimnejad, R. Impact of caffeic acid on the testicular damages in D-galactose-induced aging model in mice. *Iran. J. Basic Med. Sci.* **2022**, *25*, 1190.
49. Salman, T.M.; Olayaki, L.A.; Alagbonsi, I.A.; Oyewopo, A.O. Spermatotoxic effects of galactose and possible mechanisms of action. *Middle East Fertil. Soc. J.* **2016**, *21*, 82–90. [CrossRef]
50. Pandey, A.K.; Gupta, A.; Tiwari, M.; Prasad, S.; Pandey, A.N.; Yadav, P.K.; Sharma, A.; Sahu, K.; Asrafuzzaman, S.; Vengayil, D.T.; et al. Impact of stress on female reproductive health disorders: Possible beneficial effects of shatavari (*Asparagus racemosus*). *Biomed. Pharmacother.* **2018**, *103*, 46–49. [CrossRef]
51. Korean Food and Drug Administration (KFDA). Available online: https://www.foodsafetykorea.go.kr/portal/healthyfoodlife/searchHomeHFDetail.do?prdlstReportLedgNo=2023021000330706 (accessed on 16 May 2023).
52. Cho, K.-H.; Kim, J.-E.; Bahuguna, A.; Kang, D.-J. Long-term supplementation of ozonated sunflower oil improves dyslipidemia and hepatic inflammation in hyperlipidemic zebrafish: Suppression of oxidative stress and inflammation against carboxymethyllysine toxicity. *Antioxidants* **2023**, *12*, 1240. [CrossRef]
53. Blois, M.S. Antioxidant determinations by the use of a stable free radical. *Nature* **1958**, *181*, 1199–1200. [CrossRef]
54. Cho, K.-H.; Kim, J.-E.; Lee, M.-S.; Bahuguna, A. Oral Supplementation of Ozonated Sunflower Oil Augments Plasma Antioxidant and Anti-Inflammatory Abilities with Enhancement of High-Density Lipoproteins Functionality in Rats. *Antioxidants* **2024**, *13*, 529. [CrossRef] [PubMed]
55. Fischer, A.H.; Jacobson, K.A.; Rose, J.; Zeller, R. Hematoxylin and eosin staining of tissue and cell sections. *Cold Spring Harb. Protoc.* **2008**, *2008*, prot4986. [CrossRef] [PubMed]
56. Owusu-Ansah, E.; Yavari, A.; Mandal, S.; Banerjee, U. Distinct mitochondrial retrograde signals control the G1-S cell cycle checkpoint. *Nat. Genet.* **2008**, *40*, 356–361. [CrossRef]
57. Umali, J.; Hawkey-Noble, A.; French, C.R. Loss of foxc1 in zebrafish reduces optic nerve size and cell number in the retinal ganglion cell layer. *Vis. Res.* **2019**, *156*, 66–72. [CrossRef]

pharmaceuticals

MDPI

Article

Evaluation of the Antioxidant Properties and Biological Effects of a Novel Combined Barberry Root–Propolis Extract on HEK293T Cells

Dana Marcinčáková [1], Nikola Hudáková [2,*], Michal Miłek [3], Mária Kolesárová [1], Małgorzata Dżugan [3], Dasa Cizkova [2,4] and Jaroslav Legáth [1]

1 Department of Pharmacology and Toxicology, University of Veterinary Medicine and Pharmacy in Kosice, Komenského 73, 041 81 Kosice, Slovakia; dana.marcincakova@uvlf.sk (D.M.); maria.kolesarova@uvlf.sk (M.K.); jaroslav.legath@uvlf.sk (J.L.)
2 Centre of Experimental and Clinical Regenerative Medicine, Small Animal Clinic, University of Veterinary Medicine and Pharmacy in Kosice, 041 81 Kosice, Slovakia; dasa.cizkova@uvlf.sk
3 Department of Chemistry and Food Toxicology, Institute of Food Technology and Nutrition, University of Rzeszow, Ćwiklińskiej 1a St., 35-601 Rzeszow, Poland; mmilek@ur.edu.pl (M.M.); mdzugan@ur.edu.pl (M.D.)
4 Institute of Neuroimmunology, SAS, 845 10 Bratislava, Slovakia
* Correspondence: nikola.hudakova@uvlf.sk

Abstract: Background/Objectives: The health benefits of honeybee products and herbs are well known, and their appropriate combination may enhance their biological efficacy. This study investigated the biological properties of a combined barberry root and propolis extract (PBE) in comparison to a propolis extract (PE), a barberry root extract (BE), and pure berberine (BN). **Methods:** The antioxidant properties were evaluated using DPPH and FRAP methods and total phenolic contents (TPC) were assessed by the Folin–Ciocalteu method. HPTLC was used to quantify the BE in the tested samples. Their effect on HEK293T cells was monitored in real-time by using the xCELLigence system which recorded changes in the proliferative activity (PA). The metabolic activity (MA) was evaluated using an MTS test and cell migration was analyzed via a scratch assay. **Results:** The PE exhibited a higher TPC (198.67 mg/g) than the BE (119.3 mg/g). The PBE exhibited a comparable antioxidant effect to that of the PE. In the cell assays, the PE, the BE, and BN significantly reduced the proliferative activity at higher concentrations ($p < 0.0001$) while the PBE demonstrated a lower cytotoxicity and proved to be safer for the tested cells. The highest IC_{50} value was determined for the PBE (130 μg/mL), suggesting that this combination has a reduced cytotoxicity. However, the scratch test did not confirm a significant supportive effect of the PBE on cell migration. **Conclusions:** Although the PBE did not show enhanced antioxidant properties, it may mitigate cytotoxicity and support proliferation at lower concentrations. This suggests that extraction of raw propolis with a previously prepared barberry extract results in a safer preparation, but its therapeutic potential requires further studies using biological models.

Keywords: propolis; barberry; berberine; antioxidant; HPTLC; cell proliferation; metabolic activity; migration

1. Introduction

In the era of many human diseases and the increasingly common phenomenon of drug resistance, new medicinal substances are constantly sought. In recent years, there has been a return to substances of natural origin isolated from natural sources of active substances or complex extracts [1]. Medicinal plants are the most commonly used; however, bee products such as honey, propolis, royal jelly, bee venom, bee pollen, and bee bread have also demonstrated great pharmaceutical potential [2,3]. Due to the unique properties of honey, the use of a combination of bee products with herbs is not a new idea; historical sources prove that the effectiveness of such combinations has been understood by humans since ancient times [4–6]. However, most of these recipe types and complex medicines involve combinations of herbs with honey; the idea of creating new formulations based on propolis and herbs is relatively new.

The general composition of propolis is as follows: the majority are resinous and balsamic substances (up to 70%), the wax content ranges from a few to a dozen or so percent (less frequently over 20%), and volatile substances usually constitute up to 1% (in the case of specific types of propolis there may be even up to 8.5%) [7]. The detailed phytochemical profile depends on the botanical sources used by bees and includes numerous compounds from the groups of polyphenols (phenolic acids, flavonoids, phenylpropanoids, stilbenes), terpenoids, esters, fatty acids, and hydrocarbons [8,9]. The chemical profile of propolis extracts depends on the extraction solvent type, solvent ratio, and extraction procedure [10]. The main biological effects of propolis and its extracts include antioxidant, antimicrobial, antiviral, anti-inflammatory, and anticancer effects [8,9]. Possible mechanisms of the anticancer effect of propolis and its constituents include induction of apoptosis, induction of autophagy, anti-proliferative action and cell cycle arrest, inhibition of angiogenesis and metastasis, suppression of the immune response, and epigenetic mechanisms [11,12].

Among the numerous medicinal plants used in the pharmaceutical industry, the genus *Berberis* has recently become very popular. This genus includes several hundreds of species of shrubs distributed mainly in Asia, Europe, North Africa, and North America [13,14]. Various species of barberry are cultivated worldwide for decorative purposes but also as a source of pharmaceutical raw materials which include almost all parts of the plant such as the roots, root bark, twigs, leaves, and fruit [13]. The main barberry species of pharmacognostic importance is *B. vulgaris* L. which is a typical alkaloid raw material. It contains a full set of isoquinoline alkaloids including berberine, oxyberberine, lambertine, magniflorine, berbamine, palmatine, columbamine, and jatrorrhizine [13,14]. Additionally, secondary metabolites of barberry include flavonoids, anthocyanins, and carotenoids [13]. The dominant alkaloid of barberry is berberine which is also present in other plants mainly from the *Ranunculaceae*, *Rutaceae*, and *Berberidaceae* families [15]. Literature reviews have described a wide spectrum of biological effects of berberine: antioxidant, anti-inflammatory, anticancer, antidiabetic, and antimicrobial [15,16]. Studies on cancer cells have shown the possibility of including berberine as a part of cancer therapy due to the inhibition of telomerase, induction of apoptosis, involvement in reactive-oxygen-species-mediated mechanisms, and antimetastatic, antiproliferative, and anti-invasive effects [16].

The main aim of this work was to evaluate the biological properties of a unique combined extract; propolis extracted using a previously prepared aqueous-ethanolic extract of barberry root. The antioxidant properties, polyphenol contents, and in vitro effect of a novel extract (propolis–barberry root extract; PBE) on a cell model were compared with propolis extract (PE), barberry root extract (BE), and pure berberine (BN). The research hypothesis assumes that propolis extraction using a plant extract will allow for the obtainment of preparation with enhanced positive effects due to the interactions of the propolis and barberry components.

2. Results and Discussion

2.1. TPC and Antioxidant Capacity

TPC and the antioxidant capacity were assessed for freeze-dried extracts. The results are shown in Table 1.

Table 1. TPC and antioxidant capacity of the tested extracts.

	TPC [mg GAE/g]	FRAP [µmol TE/g]	DPPH [µmol TE/g]
PE	198.67 ± 11.51 [b]	618.70 ± 20.88 [b]	398.22 ± 8.17 [b]
BE	119.30 ± 21.24 [a]	450.72 ± 23.25 [a]	243.80 ± 65.75 [a]
PBE	194.31 ± 8.12 [b]	626.81 ± 30.94 [b]	366.42 ± 24.71 [b]

PE—propolis extract, BE—barberry root extract, PBE—propolis–barberry root extract. [a,b]—means that the columns marked with different superscript letters are significantly different ($p < 0.05$). The data is presented as the mean ± SD.

The prepared PE contained 198.67 mg/g of phenolic contents expressed as gallic acid equivalents which is a typical value for extracts of Polish poplar propolis prepared in this manner. Similarly, slightly higher results (252.38–326.34 mg/g) were obtained earlier for nine propolis samples from the same region of Poland [17]. The composition and activity of propolis are strongly influenced by its quality as well as environmental factors such as climate, flora composition, and harvest time [9]. The quantity of phenolic contents in ethanol extracts of Polish propolis determined earlier by Moskwa et al. was also comparable (137.19 to 275.79 mg/g) [18,19]. In addition, the antioxidant properties tested via two different methods using two different mechanisms are similar to the levels obtained for the previously tested ethanolic propolis extracts [17]. In the BE, 119.3 ± 21.24 mg GAE/g of phenolic content per gram was determined. This value is higher than that provided in the literature, e.g., for the roots of *B. vulgaris* collected in Croatia where a content of 7.29–10.34 mg/g was reported [20]. In this case, discrepancies may result from the use of different extraction conditions or the quality of the raw material itself. Surprisingly, after the extraction of propolis, the use of BE did not result in the enhancement of the antioxidant effect nor the polyphenol content in the obtained PBE preparation. The obtained results did not differ significantly ($p > 0.05$) from the values for the PE extract obtained using 70% ethanol instead of BE. The lack of at least an additive effect can be explained by interactions between the components of BE and raw propolis. Due to the resinous structure of propolis, it can be assumed that some of the BE components were adsorbed by propolis which in turn reduced the extraction efficiency of the bioactive components of propolis.

2.2. HPTLC Berberine Determination

Barberry root (like all other parts of the plant) is a typical alkaloid raw material [14,21]. The tested extracts were analyzed by High-Performance Thin Layer Chromatography (HPTLC) to estimate the content of the main alkaloid BN. An assessment of the berberine content is usually performed by HPLC; however, HPTLC has been used more recently [22–24]. This technique is less cost- and time-consuming; moreover, it allows for the direct comparison of samples during a single analysis. Figure 1 shows images of the HPTLC tracks and chromatograms for the tested extracts.

Chromatographic separation conducted on an HPTLC plate revealed two main bands which fluoresced yellow under a 366 nm UV light at Rf 0.14 and 0.19. The second of these bands, based on a comparison with the standard, was assigned to BN. Moreover, blue bands were also visible which may have come from other unidentified compounds; it is particularly visible in the case of the PE for which the blue bands remained unresolved in the high Rf range. The pattern of two main bands originating from alkaloids is typical for extracts from barberry root [25–27]. Thanks to calibrating for berberine sulfate, the content of this alkaloid in the extracts was determined. The BE contained 111.06 mg/g of BN (11.1%) which is consistent with the literature that reports the content of this alkaloid in *B. vulgaris* root extracts to be at a level of 7–12% [20,28]. The BN content in the PBE was much lower and amounted to 1.48 mg/g. These results confirm our previous speculations about the absorption of BE components in the resinous propolis matrix.

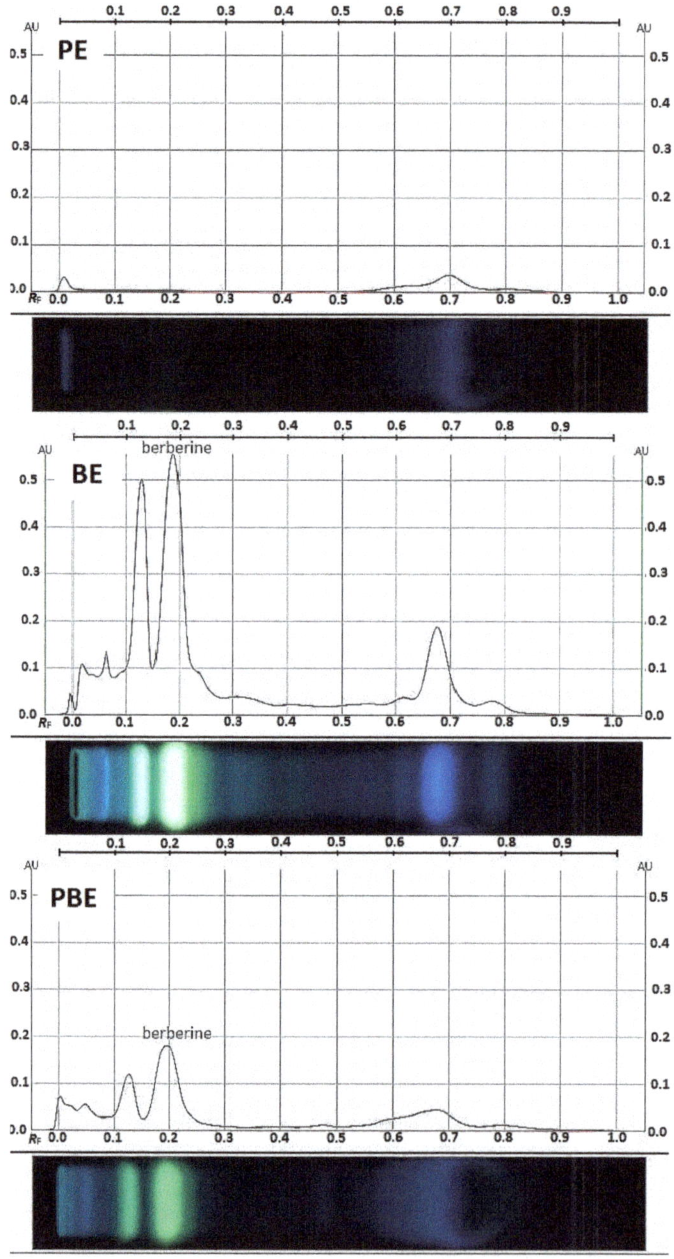

Figure 1. HPTLC profiles of the tested extracts (50 mg/mL) visualized in UV 366 nm. PE—propolis extract, BE—barberry root extract, PBE—propolis–barberry root extract.

2.3. The In Vitro Functional Effect on HEK293T Cells

2.3.1. Monitoring the Cell Response via the Real-Time–xCELLigence System

The biological effect of the tested substances was evaluated using an analyzer of cell behavior in real-time, the xCELLigence system (real-time cell analyzer; RTCA, Acea Bioscience, CA, USA). This system allows the continuous observation of cell behavior, adherence, and proliferative activity (PA) through impedance measurements that are expressed as cell index values (CI) and recorded into curves. This enables the tracking of cellular responses dynamically over time, providing insights into substance effects at multiple time points rather than relying solely on endpoint analyses [22]. RTCA has been previously used by many authors for drug screening [23], toxicology studies [24,29], and virology research [30].

The functional effect of the tested samples of PE, BE, PBE, and BN on normal epithelial HEK293T cells was evaluated during a 72 h treatment. The PA of the treated cells was recorded in real-time via the xCELLigence system (shown in Figure 2). At all tested concentrations, the PE, the BE, and BN caused a significant dose-dependent drop in the PA during the entire experiment ($p < 0.05$; $p < 0.0001$). On the other hand, the PA was not reduced by the PBE combination at lower concentrations (6.25 and 12.5 µg/mL) after 24 h of exposition ($p > 0.05$). The decline in the PA was weaker but significant ($p < 0.001$) in comparison to the PA of cells treated with other tested substances after 48 and 72 h of treatment with the PBE combination.

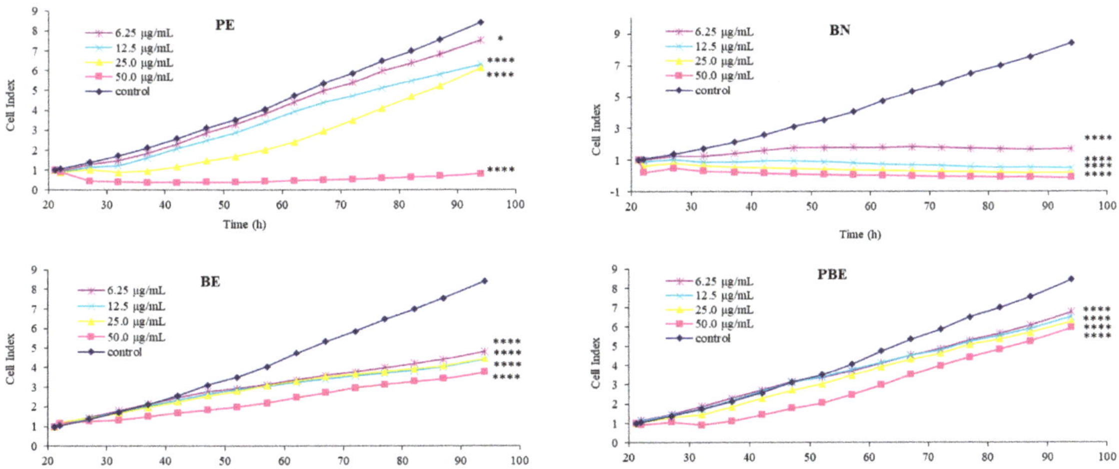

Figure 2. Changes in cell index after treatment with PE—propolis extract, BE—barberry root extract, BN—berberine, PBE—propolis–barberry root extract at tested concentrations (6.25, 12.5, 25.0, and 50.0 µg/mL) in comparison to a control group without treatment. Statistical processing of the results at the end of treatment (72 h) is shown as significance compared to the control group (one-way ANOVA followed by post hoc Dunnett's test: * $p < 0.05$, **** $p < 0.0001$).

In our experiment, no significant increase in cell proliferation was observed for any of the tested samples and concentrations compared to the control. The effect of propolis on the PA was marginally demonstrated in cells treated with PE at lower concentrations (6.25 and 12.5 µg/mL) where the trend of the PA was similar to that of the control until 48 h of the experiment ($p > 0.05$). The higher concentrations (25.0 and 50.0 µg/mL) caused a drop in the CI ($p < 0.0001$). This finding is consistent with Garcia et al. [31], who found that lower concentrations of propolis can promote the viability and proliferation of human adipose-derived stem cells (ADSC) but that higher concentrations can lead to cytotoxic effects. The cytotoxicity is supposedly attributed to the pro-apoptotic effects and oxidative stress induced by natural extracts when used in excess [32].

Similarly, barberry exerts strong antioxidant properties which, except for positive effects, can also induce cytotoxic effects in various cells. An in vitro study conducted by Ivan et al. [33] showed that barberry extract as well as berberine exerted cytotoxic effects and inhibited the growth of cancer cells (MCF-7, HepG2, and Caco-2) dependent on time and concentration. In addition to *Berberis vulgaris*, extracts from ornamental varieties of *Berberis thunbergii* have recently been tested for their effect on cell viability (HaCaT, A375, and Caco-2) in vitro, demonstrating differences between varieties as well as a dose-dependent effect. However, no clear link between the studied effects of the extracts and their berberine content has been established [34].

Except for monitoring the effects of the tested substances in real-time, the xCELLigence software (vs. 1.2.1) can also calculate the IC_{50} (half-maximal inhibitory concentration) which is a crucial metric in pharmacology indicating the amount of a substance needed to inhibit a biological process by 50%. The *Berberis vulgaris* root extract has been studied for its chemopreventive properties and the IC_{50} value against LS180 cells was 4.31 μg/mL and 46.06 μg/mL against HT-29 cells [35]. It indicates varying degrees of effectiveness dependent on the cell line [36,37]. Similarly, propolis extracts exert different IC_{50} values depending on the specific cell line tested. Teerasripreecha et al. [38] found that the IC_{50} values ranged between 41.3 to 52.4 μg/mL for normal human fibroblast cells (Hs27). These findings are consistent with our results: the IC_{50} for the PE was 63 μg/mL, for the BE 45 μg/mL, and for BN 6.5 μg/mL (48 h). However, we found that the IC_{50} for the combination PBE was even higher (130 μg/mL). These results indicate the mitigation of propolis's and barberry's cytotoxicity when combined (PBE).

2.3.2. Evaluation of the Metabolic Activity via an MTS Test

The effect of the PE, BE, BN, and PBE on the metabolic activity (MA) of HEK293T cells was evaluated via a standard colorimetric MTS test after 24, 48, and 72 h of application of the extracts (Figure 3).

The results show that BN had the strongest effect on the MA of the cells. Compared to the control, we recorded a significant decrease in metabolic activity (MA) at concentrations of 50 μg/mL ($p < 0.001$) at 24 h, 6.25 ($p < 0.001$), 12.5 ($p < 0.01$), and 50.0 μg/mL ($p < 0.01$) after 48 h and at all observed concentrations of BN ($p < 0.0001$) after 72 h. Regarding BN, experimental studies focusing on the toxic effect of BN reported that exposure of 10 and 30 μM BN to PC12 cells increased the cytotoxicity which was manifested as an increase in apoptotic cell death. In vitro and in vivo studies (10 and 30 μM up to 48 h) with BN against 6-hydroxydopamine (6-OHDA) induced neurotoxicity in rats and PC-12 cells [39]. Moreover, BN has been reported to cause cytotoxicity and adversely influence the synthesis of DNA [39]. Several authors also focused on the in vitro cytotoxicity of propolis; Lopez et al. placed great emphasis on the limited data regarding the cytotoxicity of propolis preparations against non-cancerous human cells. He stated that safe use of red propolis requires reduction in the dose to below 50 μg/mL [37,40]. In our study, the tested PE significantly improved ($p < 0.01$) the MA of the HEK293T cells compared to the control at a concentration of 12.5 μg/mL after 24 h.

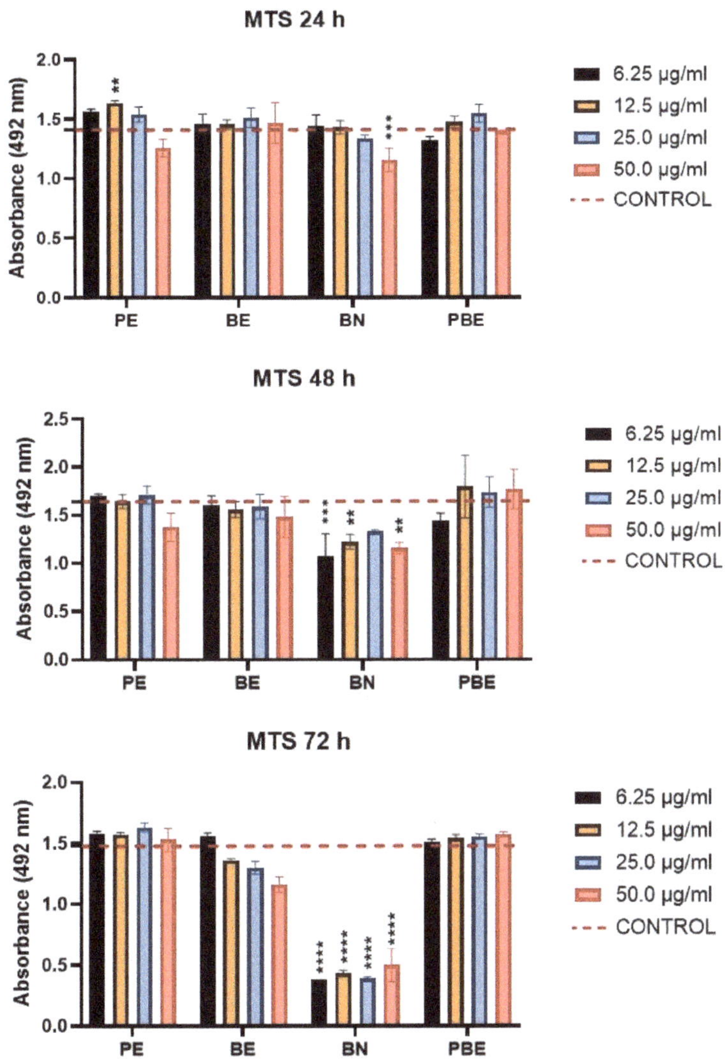

Figure 3. Results of the MTS assay on HEK293T cells after 24, 48, and 72 h. Cells were cultured in media supplemented with PE—propolis extract, BE—barberry root extract, BN—berberine, PBE—propolis–barberry root extract at various concentrations (6.25, 12.5, 25.0, and 50.0 µg/mL) and a standard culture medium in the case of the control. Statistical processing of the results is shown as a significance compared to the control group (one-way ANOVA followed by post hoc Dunnett's test: ** $p < 0.01$, *** $p < 0.001$, **** $p < 0.0001$). The data is presented as the mean ± SD (n = 3).

Interestingly, the PBE combination at 12.5 ($p < 0.05$) and 25.0 µg/mL ($p < 0.01$) significantly increased the MA compared to the BE after 72 h of exposure. However, we were more interested in studying whether the combined extract (PBE) affects the MA of cells or not. The beneficial effect of propolis combined with several substances has been described in more detail. For example, the combined application of propolis and honey to aid in the healing process of an open wound in rats exhibited a synergistic effect [37]. The combination of propolis nanoparticles (NPro) and photodynamic therapy based on nanocurcumin (NCur-PDT) in the remineralization of WSL ex vivo was also described [41].

Concerning barberry root, a recent study demonstrated that the combination of galangin, one of the flavonoids found in propolis, with berberine synergistically led to the inhibition of cell growth, apoptosis, and cell cycle arrest in the G2/M phase with increased levels of intracellular reactive oxygen species (ROS) in esophageal carcinoma cells [42].

The results quoted, however, refer to the combination of propolis extract with plant extracts immediately before application. In our study, a different approach was used. We combined the bioactive components during propolis extraction using barberry extract (BE). As shown by HPTLC, the bioactive fraction of the PBE is different from the expected additive effect of the PE + the BE. Already in the evaluation of the antioxidants, it is clearly visible that there is no additive effect as the activity of the PBE is comparable to that of the PE and higher than that of the BE. In the evaluation of the biological activity, the effect is BE > PBE > PE which confirms that the PBE extract contains fewer barberry components than BE and the barberry components enhance the effect of the PE. We have, therefore, obtained a preparation better than the PE and the BE which is especially visible in the scratch test.

2.3.3. Comparison of the RTCA and MTS Results

For better visualization and evaluation of the results obtained by the xCELLigence system (CI values) and MTS test (absorbance in nm), all the data obtained were expressed as percentages compared to control cells without treatment (100%). Values are summarized in Table 2.

Table 2. A table summarizing the changes in the proliferative and metabolic activity of HEK293T cells treated with the tested substances expressed as percentages.

	24 h		48 h		72 h	
	PA (%)	MA (%)	PA (%)	MA (%)	PA (%)	MA (%)
PE (µg/mL)						
6.25	91.20 ± 5.29	110.48 ± 1.66	92.47 ± 2.71	102.53 ± 1.58	89.61 ± 1.37 *	103.56 ± 1.52
12.5	79.97 ± 3.71 ****	115.79 ± 1.49 **	80.89 ± 0.27 ****	99.37 ± 4.30	75.04 ± 0.13 ****	103.15 ± 1.35
25.0	46.08 ± 5.77 ****	109.01 ± 4.50	56.09 ± 2.33 ****	103.42 ± 5.74	72.27 ± 4.37 ****	107.27 ± 2.39
50.0	13.14 ± 4.35 ****	89.13 ± 5.12	9.27 ± 2.78 ****	83.27 ± 8.77	9.61 ± 3.14 ****	100.54 ± 6.35
BE (µg/mL)						
6.25	91.74 ± 4.98	103.44 ± 5.76	66.01 ± 4.86 ****	97.19 ± 5.69	57.34 ± 4.83 ****	102.75 ± 1.45
12.5	86.38 ± 4.82 **	103.06 ± 2.83	62.32 ± 4.56 ****	94.19 ± 5.00	51.94 ± 4.51 ****	89.26 ± 1.06
25.0	83.32 ± 4.21 **	107.05 ± 5.83	64.00 ± 2.84 ****	96.15 ± 7.65	52.29 ± 1.49 ****	85.34 ± 3.32 *
50.0	61.68 ± 1.24 ****	110.57 ± 4.14	50.81 ± 1.48 ****	89.51 ± 12.90	44.35 ± 0.34 ****	76.29 ± 4.17
BN (µg/mL)						
6.25	59.25 ± 6.19 ****	102.18 ± 6.55	32.20 ± 4.92 ****	65.22 ± 9.71 ***	20.27 ± 3.39 ****	24.97 ± 0.00 ****
12.5	33.20 ± 4.95 ****	101.22 ± 3.90	11.87 ± 1.41 ****	73.95 ± 3.27 **	5.70 ± 0.13 ****	28.32 ± 1.31 ****
25.0	15.46 ± 1.15 ****	94.88 ± 1.81	4.92 ± 0.61 ****	80.45 ± 0.57	1.69 ± 0.34 ****	25.69 ± 0.53 ****
50.0	4.69 ± 0.28 ****	81.71 ± 6.91 ***	0.70 ± 0.72 ****	69.81 ± 2.51 **	1.58 ± 0.82 ****	32.92 ± 6.44 ****
PBE (µg/mL)						
6.25	102.74 ± 9.42	93.26 ± 2.35	84.27 ± 9.57 ***	87.12 ± 4.70	79.61 ± 8.38 ****	99.38 ± 1.30
12.5	100.29 ± 2.44	104.36 ± 3.46	83.20 ± 3.97 ***	108.48 ± 19.68	77.02 ± 4.77 ****	101.42 ± 1.85
25.0	87.08 ± 2.41 *	109.51 ± 5.35	79.23 ± 3.29 ****	105.01 ± 9.56	73.63 ± 3.32 ****	102.12 ± 1.48
50.0	56.25 ± 2.02 ****	98.88 ± 0.55	66.27 ± 3.00 ****	106.83 ± 12.46	69.75 ± 4.60 ****	103.17 ± 1.50
control	100.00 ± 4.74	100.00 ± 4.50	100.00 ± 6.79	100.00 ± 1.73	100.00 ± 8.18	100.00 ± 7.73

PE—propolis extract, BE—barberry root extract, BN—berberine, PBE—propolis–barberry root extract. Results are expressed in % in comparison to a control group without treatment (100%). Statistical processing of the results is shown as a significance compared to the control group (one-way ANOVA followed by post hoc Dunnett's test: * $p < 0.05$, ** $p < 0.01$, *** $p < 0.001$, **** $p < 0.0001$). Data is presented as the mean ± SD (n = 3).

The results obtained by the xCELLigence system and MTS test were in correlation as indicated by the Pearson correlation coefficient. The value after 24 h was r = 0.507 (moderate correlation), after 48 h r = 0.745 (moderate correlation), and 0.850 (strong correlation) was observed after 72 h of treatment. Overall, in all mentioned time intervals, the value of the Pearson test was 0.518 indicating a moderate positive linear correlation.

2.3.4. Cell Migration

Since cell migration is an important factor involved in many biological processes such as embryological development, new tissue formation, immune response or inflammation, and oncological diseases [43], the study of the migratory response of cells to substances of various origins is important. Using the scratch test, we determined whether the tested extracts could alter the migration of HEK293T cells.

The results shown in Figure 4 represent the changes in the percentage of the empty area (that is, the area not occupied by cells) at 0, 24, 48, and 72 h after mechanical damage was conducted. In our measurements, we did not notice a significant difference between the control and the experimental groups (PE, BE, PBE) in which the cells were cultured in media with the addition of PE, BE, and PBE. In the BN group, we noticed a significant decrease in cell adhesion after 24 h which made it impossible to quantitatively and statistically evaluate the data from this experimental group. On the other hand, as shown in Figure 4 in the case of the BE and the PBE, we observed an improvement in cell migration into the area not covered by cells after 24, 48, and 72 h compared to the control group despite it not being statistically significant. This difference, however, was not observed in cells treated with the PE. The samples with the best capacity to influence cell migration were the PBE after 24 and 72 h and the BE after 48 h (Figure 4). Many authors have investigated the role of bee products in wound healing at a cellular level. When investigating the effect of propolis on keratinocyte migration, Martinotti et al. proposed H_2O_2 as the main mediator of the regenerative properties of propolis [44]. On the other hand, when analyzing the promotion of cell migration of human fibroblasts, Afonso et al. stated that the effect of the combination of propolis and honey is not synergistic and there is only an additive effect of propolis and honey [45]. In our experiment, the positive effect of propolis on cell migration was not confirmed. Interestingly, we recorded the combined PBE as the sample with the best cell migration despite it not being significant ($p > 0.05$).

Several authors describe propolis as a natural substance with nephroprotective properties mediated by several mechanisms. Propolis improves kidney function and reduces the retention of uremic toxins in plasma. It inhibits α-SMA expression and collagen deposition, and disrupts fibrotic epithelial–mesenchymal transition and TGF-β signaling pathways, thereby alleviating fibrosis [46]. Propolis can also improve kidney function thanks to its antioxidant, anti-inflammatory, and anti-apoptotic properties as it modulates oxidative stress, inflammation, and DNA damage [47]. Specifically, studies have demonstrated that propolis possesses strong antioxidant properties which reduce oxidative damage of renal tissues by decreasing lipid peroxidation and oxidative stress markers such as malondialdehyde and reactive oxygens species (ROS) [48–50].

As for berberine, the positive effect on kidneys is due to its antifibrotic, anti-inflammatory, and antioxidant properties [51]. It can activate the PI3K/Akt signaling pathway, reduce oxidative stress by increasing antioxidant enzymes (GSH and SOD), and inhibit apoptosis by modulating the expression of Nrf2 and HO-1 [52].

Wound healing is another critical area where propolis exerts beneficial effects. Its anti-inflammatory and antimicrobial properties contribute significantly to the wound-healing process. Al-Waili states that propolis enhances the immune response and reduces inflammation, which is vital for effective wound healing [53].

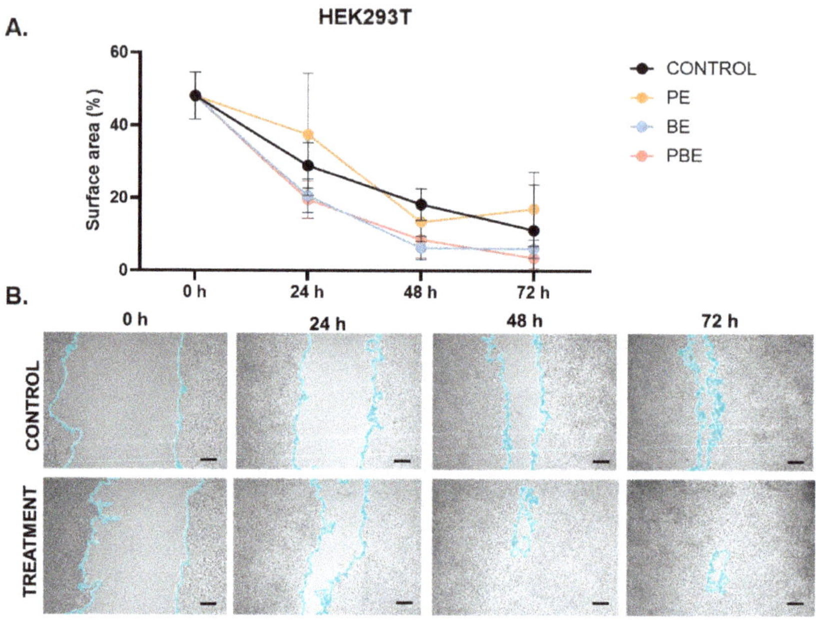

Figure 4. The effects of barberry root and propolis extracts on HEK293T cell migration. Results of the scratch assay on HEK293T cells during which mechanical damage was followed by culturing cells in PE, BE, PBE, and DMEM (control). Photos were taken after 24, 48, and 72 h. (**A**) The graph shows the time-dependent profile of the % of the area not occupied by cells ± SD. (**B**) Representative photos of the scratch test after 0, 24, 48, and 72 h in the control group and in the groups with the largest difference in the area not covered by cells compared to the control group which was the PBE after 24 h, BE after 48 h, and PBE after 72 h. Scale bar: 100 µm.

In conclusion, the innovative combined extract of propolis and barberry root (PBE) demonstrates a higher safety for renal cells. The antioxidant and anti-inflammatory properties of this preparation along with the potential to promote cellular migration suggest that this combination could be beneficial in the management of renal injuries and diseases. However, due to the great variability of raw materials (propolis and barberry root), the results should be considered preliminary, and the research should be repeated with emphasis on the analysis of the phytochemical composition of the obtained preparation. Further research should aim to elucidate the specific mechanisms underlying these effects and to explore the potential clinical applications of this combined propolis–barberry extract.

3. Materials and Methods

3.1. Materials

Propolis for the study was purchased from a local apiary (Sieklówka, Poland) and barberry root (*Berberis vulgaris*) was purchased from Nat Vita (Długołęka, Poland). All reagents used were of at least analytical grade.

3.2. Preparation of Extracts

Barberry root extract (BE) was prepared as follows: 20 g of ground barberry root was mixed with 200 mL of 70% aqueous ethanol (Stanlab, Lublin, Poland) and then sonicated in an ultrasonic bath (Sonic-10, Polsonic, Warsaw, Poland) in two cycles (20 min each, 700 W, max. 50 °C). Part of this crude extract was used to prepare propolis–barberry root extract (PBE): 10 g of crushed propolis was poured into 100 mL of the extract, shaken for half an hour (400 rpm, Benchmark OrbiShaker MP, Benchmark Scientific, Sayreville, NJ, USA), and then left to macerate for 5 days with occasional shaking. Afterward, the extract was filtered through a filter paper. Propolis extract (PE) was prepared analogously using 70% aqueous ethanol as the solvent. Fifteen mL of each crude extract was subjected to ethanol evaporation using a centrifugal evaporator (RVC 2–18 CDPlus, Martin Christ, Osterode am Harz, Germany) and then lyophilized to obtain dry extracts (Alpha 1–2 LD plus, Martin Christ, Osterode am Harz, Germany).

3.3. *Total Phenolic Content and Antioxidant Capacity*

To determine the phenolic content and antioxidant properties, extracts were reconstituted in 70% aqueous ethanol at a concentration of 500 μg/mL. TPC, DPPH antiradical potential, and FRAP-reducing power were determined as described by Miłek et al. [54].

3.4. *HPTLC Berberine Profile*

Berberine content in the tested extracts was determined by the HPTLC method according to Alam et al. [55] with a slight modification [34]. HPTLC Silica Gel 60 F254 plates (20 cm × 10 cm) (Merck, Darmstadt, Germany) were used. Quantitative analysis was performed based on software-generated chromatograms (Vision CATS 3.2, Camag, Muttenz, Switzerland) for plate visualization at UV 366 nm. Berberine sulfate (Aliness, Ostrówiec, Poland) methanolic solution (HPLC-grade methanol, Honeywell, Charlotte, NC, USA) (250 μg/mL) was used for calibration (0.5 to 2 μg per band).

3.5. *Cultivation of HEK293T Cells*

An immortalized human embryonic kidney cell line HEK293T (ATCC CRL-11268) was purchased and kindly provided by the Institute of Neuroimmunology of the Slovak Academy of Sciences in cooperation with the Small Animal Clinic, Veterinary Hospital at the University of Veterinary Medicine and Pharmacy in Košice. The cell culture was maintained in cultivation conditions of 37 °C and 5% CO_2 in DMEM high-glucose medium (Dulbecco's Modified Eagle's Medium High glucose, Sigma Aldrich, Darmstadt, Germany) supplemented with 10% fetal bovine serum (FBS, Sigma, Aldrich, Germany) and 2% antibiotics (Penicillin/Streptomycin/Amphotericin; ATB/ATM, Sigma Aldrich, Darmstadt, Germany). The medium was replaced by a fresh one every 2–3 days.

3.6. *xCELLigence Real-Time Cell Analysis*

The xCELLigence system (Roche Applied Science, Mannheim, Germany) is a commercial microfluidic system that enables continuous monitoring of cell adherence in vitro. In this work, xCELLigence 1.2.1 software was used. This system is based on an established electronic impedance (relative resistance). The wells in which the cells are cultured are equipped at the bottom with microelectrodes that connect to the cultured cells through sensors and record resistance changes. Microelectrodes are embedded in special 16-well E-plates (Acea Bioscience, Mannheim, Germany). The measured impedance changes are evaluated as the so-called cell index (CI), which represents differences in the number of cells, adherence, morphology, viability, and proliferation [23]. In the absence of live or proliferating cells, CI values are close to zero. Shortly, the first step was the addition of 100 μL of medium to the wells of three E-plates for a background measurement. After equilibration at 37 °C and 5% CO_2, the E-plates were inserted into the xCELLigence impedance measurement system. After ensuring that all junctions function within the specified measurement range, cells were seeded (5×10^3 cells per well). After the initial 22 h of cell cultivation, solutions of PE, BE, BN, and PBE at final concentrations of 6.25, 12.5, 25.0, and 50.0 μg/mL were added to the cells. Cells without treatment served as the control. The xCELLigence software recorded CI values every hour (94 h) and displayed them in curves. IC_{50} values for the tested extracts were determined using the xCELLigence software for the 48th hour of treatment.

3.7. MTS Test

To determine the effect of the tested substances on the MA, a colorimetric MTS assay using an MTS kit (Invitrogen Inc, Carlsbad, CA, USA) was used. This test was performed simultaneously with RTCA monitoring and the cells from the same passage were used. Cells were seeded into three 96-well plates (Greiner-bio-one, Kremsmünster, Austria) at a density of 8×10^3 cells/well and cultured in a standard culture medium (DMEM High Glucose + 10% FBS + 2% ATB/ATM) at 37 °C and 5% CO_2. After 24 h, the medium was replaced with 100 µL of media with PE, BE, BN, and PBE at final concentrations of 6.25, 12.5, 25.0, and 50.0 µg/mL. Cells in the standard medium were used as a negative control. After 24, 48, and 72 h, 10 µL of MTS reagent was added. At the end of the incubation period, the absorbance was measured at 450 nm using a Synergy HT spectrophotometer (Biotek, Winooski, VT, USA). The data was statistically evaluated and recorded into graphs.

3.8. Scratch Assay

A scratch assay was used to determine the rate of cell migration. Briefly, cells were seeded into a 24-well tissue culture plate at a density of 400,000 cells/well in DMEM culture medium. After the cells reached ~80–90% confluence as a monolayer, the medium was removed from each well. A 200 µL pipette tip was used to scrape the cell monolayer in a straight line to create a scratch. Cell debris was removed by washing the cells with phosphate buffered saline (PBS, Sigma Aldrich, Darmstadt, Germany) and replaced by DMEM (Dulbecco's Modified Eagle Medium) for the control group and PE, BE, and PBE solutions for the experimental groups. The scratch assay was performed in triplicate wells. Seven pictures per group were taken after 0, 24, 48, and 72 h after scraping the cells. Pictures were taken by an inverted microscope Zeiss Axiovert 200 (Zeiss, Oberkochen, Germany) and the ImageJ FIJI Wound Healing Tool was used to measure the surface area of the wounds.

3.9. Statistical Evaluation

Statistical analyses were performed using GraphPad Prism software 10.3.1 (GraphPad, La Jolla, CA, USA) with the statistical significance set at $p < 0.05$. To compare the continuous variables between group means, we used ANOVA with Tukey's and Dunnett's post hoc corrections. The results obtained were expressed as the mean ± standard deviation (n = 3). The intensity of the correlation between the results of the RTCA analysis and the MTS test was determined using the Pearson correlation coefficient.

Author Contributions: Conceptualization, D.M., M.M. and N.H.; methodology, M.M., D.C., D.M. and N.H.; software, D.M., M.M. and N.H.; validation, J.L., D.C. and M.K.; formal analysis, D.M., M.M. and N.H.; investigation, M.M., M.K. and N.H.; resources, D.M., M.M. and N.H.; data curation, M.K., D.M. and N.H.; writing—original draft preparation, D.M., D.C. and N.H.; writing—review and editing, D.M.; visualization, N.H.; supervision, M.D., D.C. and J.L.; project administration, N.H.; funding acquisition, M.D. and J.L. All authors have read and agreed to the published version of the manuscript.

Funding: This work was supported by the Polish Ministry of Science and Higher Education research project within the University of Rzeszów PB/ZCHTZ/2024, by National Reference Laboratory for Pesticides of the University of Veterinary Medicine and Pharmacy in Kosice and project VEGA 1/0122/24.

Institutional Review Board Statement: Not applicable.

Informed Consent Statement: Not applicable.

Data Availability Statement: Data is contained within the article.

Acknowledgments: We would like to thank Peter Filipčík and the Institute of Neuroimmunology of the Slovak Academy of Sciences for the kind provision of the HEK293T cell line used for this work. Especially we would like to express our gratitude to Serena Faith Amrit a native speaker, and an excellent student at the University of Veterinary Medicine and Pharmacy in Kosice, Slovakia for the linguistic revision of the text.

Conflicts of Interest: The authors declare no conflicts of interest.

References

1. Atanasov, A.G.; Zotchev, S.B.; Dirsch, V.M.; Supuran, C.T. Natural Products in Drug Discovery: Advances and Opportunities. *Nat. Rev. Drug Discov.* **2021**, *20*, 200–216. [CrossRef] [PubMed]
2. Münstedt, K.; Bogdanov, S. Bee Products and Their Potential Use in Modern Medicine. *J. ApiProd. ApiMed. Sci.* **2009**, *1*, 57–63. [CrossRef]
3. Szabat, P.; Poleszak, J.; Szabat, M.; Boreński, G.; Wójcik, M.; Milanowska, J. Apitherapy—The Medical Use of Bee Products. *J. Educ. Health Sport.* **2021**, *9*, 384–396.
4. Kuropatnicki, A.K.; Szliszka, E.; Krol, W. Historical Aspects of Propolis Research in Modern Times. *Evid.-Based Complement. Altern. Med. ECAM* **2013**, *2013*, 964149. [CrossRef] [PubMed]
5. Arawwawala, M.; Hewageegana, S. Health Benefits and Traditional Uses of Honey: A Review. *J. Apitherapy* **2017**, *2*, 9. [CrossRef]
6. Naqvi, S.A.R.; Mahmood, N.; Naz, S.; Hussain, Z.; Sherazi, T.A.; Khan, Z.A.; Shahzad, S.A.; Yar, M.; Bukhari, I.H.; Ahmad, M.; et al. Antioxidant and Antibacterial Evaluation of Honey Bee Hive Extracts Using in Vitro Models. *Mediterr. J. Nutr. Metab.* **2013**, *6*, 247–253. [CrossRef]
7. Salatino, A.; Salatino, M.L.F. Scientific Note: Often Quoted, but Not Factual Data about Propolis Composition. *Apidologie* **2021**, *52*, 312–314. [CrossRef]
8. Wieczorek, P.P.; Hudz, N.; Yezerska, O.; Horčinová-Sedláčková, V.; Shanaida, M.; Korytniuk, O.; Jasicka-Misiak, I. Chemical Variability and Pharmacological Potential of Propolis as a Source for the Development of New Pharmaceutical Products. *Molecules* **2022**, *27*, 1600. [CrossRef]
9. Hossain, R.; Quispe, C.; Khan, R.A.; Saikat, A.S.M.; Ray, P.; Ongalbek, D.; Yeskaliyeva, B.; Jain, D.; Smeriglio, A.; Trombetta, D.; et al. Propolis: An Update on Its Chemistry and Pharmacological Applications. *Chin. Med.* **2022**, *17*, 100. [CrossRef] [PubMed]
10. Šuran, J.; Cepanec, I.; Mašek, T.; Radić, B.; Radić, S.; Tlak Gajger, I.; Vlainić, J. Propolis Extract and Its Bioactive Compounds—From Traditional to Modern Extraction Technologies. *Molecules* **2021**, *26*, 2930. [CrossRef] [PubMed]
11. Forma, E.; Bryś, M. Anticancer Activity of Propolis and Its Compounds. *Nutrients* **2021**, *13*, 2594. [CrossRef] [PubMed]
12. Altabbal, S.; Athamnah, K.; Rahma, A.; Wali, A.F.; Eid, A.H.; Iratni, R.; Al Dhaheri, Y. Propolis: A Detailed Insight of Its Anticancer Molecular Mechanisms. *Pharmaceuticals* **2023**, *16*, 450. [CrossRef]
13. Rajasekaran, A.; Pant, J.; Pant, J. The Genus Berberis Linn.: A Review. *Pharmacogn. Rev.* **2008**, *2*, 369–385.
14. Salehi, B.; Selamoglu, Z.; Sener, B.; Kilic, M.; Kumar Jugran, A.; de Tommasi, N.; Sinisgalli, C.; Milella, L.; Rajkovic, J.; Flaviana B. Morais-Braga, M.; et al. Berberis Plants—Drifting from Farm to Food Applications, Phytotherapy, and Phytopharmacology. *Foods* **2019**, *8*, 522. [CrossRef] [PubMed]
15. Ai, X.; Yu, P.; Peng, L.; Luo, L.; Liu, J.; Li, S.; Lai, X.; Luan, F.; Meng, X. Berberine: A Review of Its Pharmacokinetics Properties and Therapeutic Potentials in Diverse Vascular Diseases. *Front. Pharmacol.* **2021**, *12*, 762654. [CrossRef]
16. Song, D.; Hao, J.; Fan, D. Biological Properties and Clinical Applications of Berberine. *Front. Med.* **2020**, *14*, 564–582. [CrossRef] [PubMed]
17. Miłek, M.; Ciszkowicz, E.; Tomczyk, M.; Sidor, E.; Zaguła, G.; Lecka-Szlachta, K.; Pasternakiewicz, A.; Dżugan, M. The Study of Chemical Profile and Antioxidant Properties of Poplar-Type Polish Propolis Considering Local Flora Diversity in Relation to Antibacterial and Anticancer Activities in Human Breast Cancer Cells. *Molecules* **2022**, *27*, 725. [CrossRef]
18. Moskwa, J.; Naliwajko, S.K.; Markiewicz-Żukowska, R.; Gromkowska-Kępka, K.J.; Nowakowski, P.; Strawa, J.W.; Borawska, M.H.; Tomczyk, M.; Socha, K. Chemical Composition of Polish Propolis and Its Antiproliferative Effect in Combination with Bacopa Monnieri on Glioblastoma Cell Lines. *Sci. Rep.* **2020**, *10*, 21127. [CrossRef] [PubMed]
19. Wezgowiec, J.; Wieczynska, A.; Wieckiewicz, W.; Kulbacka, J.; Saczko, J.; Pachura, N.; Wieckiewicz, M.; Gancarz, R.; Wilk, K.A. Polish Propolis—Chemical Composition and Biological Effects in Tongue Cancer Cells and Macrophages. *Molecules* **2020**, *25*, 2426. [CrossRef] [PubMed]

20. Zovko Koncić, M.; Kremer, D.; Karlović, K.; Kosalec, I. Evaluation of Antioxidant Activities and Phenolic Content of *Berberis vulgaris* L. and Berberis Croatica Horvat. *Food Chem. Toxicol. Int. J. Publ. Br. Ind. Biol. Res. Assoc.* **2010**, *48*, 2176–2180. [CrossRef] [PubMed]
21. Sarraf, M.; Beig Babaei, A.; Naji-Tabasi, S. Investigating Functional Properties of Barberry Species: An Overview. *J. Sci. Food Agric.* **2019**, *99*, 5255–5269. [CrossRef]
22. Yan, G.; Sun, W.; Pei, Y.; Yang, Z.; Wang, X.; Sun, Y.; Yang, S.; Pan, J. A Novel Release Kinetics Evaluation of Chinese Compound Medicine: Application of the xCELLigence RTCA System to Determine the Release Characteristics of Sedum Sarmentosum Compound Sustained-Release Pellets. *Saudi Pharm. J.* **2018**, *26*, 445–451. [CrossRef] [PubMed]
23. Martinez-Serra, J.; Gutierrez, A.; Muñoz-Capó, S.; Navarro-Palou, M.; Ros, T.; Amat, J.C.; Lopez, B.; Marcus, T.F.; Fueyo, L.; Suquia, A.G.; et al. xCELLigence System for Real-Time Label-Free Monitoring of Growth and Viability of Cell Lines from Hematological Malignancies. *OncoTargets Ther.* **2014**, *7*, 985–994. [CrossRef] [PubMed]
24. Milek, M.; Marcinčáková, D.; Csank, T.; Kšonžeková, P.; Falis, M.; Legáth, J.; Pistl, J. Real-Time Monitoring of Cadmium Toxicity in Rabbit Kidney Cells. *Acta Vet. Brno* **2015**, *84*, 351–356. [CrossRef]
25. Bhatt, I. Analysis of Berberine Content Using HPTLC Fingerprinting of Root and Bark of Three Himalayan Berberis Species. *Asian J. Biotechnol.* **2010**, *2*, 239–245.
26. Development and Validation of an HPTLC Method for Estimation of Berberine in Berberis Aristata. Available online: https://scialert.net/abstract/?doi=rjphyto.2021.58.65 (accessed on 26 November 2024).
27. Chaudhary, M.K.; Misra, A.; Shankar, U.; Agnihotri, P.; Srivastava, S. Intra-Specific Variation of Alkaloid Content in Berberis Lycium from the Western Himalaya. *J. Herbs Spices Med. Plants* **2021**, *27*, 386–395. [CrossRef]
28. Ahmad, S.; Hussain, A.; Hussain, A.; Abdullah, I.; Ali, M.S.; Froeyen, M.; Mirza, M.U. Quantification of Berberine in *Berberis vulgaris* L. Root Extract and Its Curative and Prophylactic Role in Cisplatin-Induced In Vivo Toxicity and In Vitro Cytotoxicity. *Antioxidants* **2019**, *8*, 185. [CrossRef] [PubMed]
29. Marcinčáková, D.; Schusterová, P.; Mudroňová, D.; Csank, T.; Falis, M.; Fedorová, M.; Marcinčák, S.; Hus, K.K.; Legáth, J. Impact of Zinc Sulfate Exposition on Viability, Proliferation and Cell Cycle Distribution of Epithelial Kidney Cells. *Pol. J. Environ. Stud.* **2019**, *28*, 3279–3286. [CrossRef]
30. Goh, V.S.L.; Ang, C.C.W.; Low, S.L.; Lee, P.X.; Setoh, Y.X.; Wong, J.C.C. Evaluation of Three Alternative Methods to the Plaque Reduction Neutralizing Assay for Measuring Neutralizing Antibodies to Dengue Virus Serotype 2. *Virol. J.* **2024**, *21*, 208. [CrossRef]
31. Garcia, C.S.C.; Garcia, P.M.C.; Santos, O.B.A.F.; Steffens, D.; Martins, S.T.; Pranke, P.; Crespo, J.S.; Henriques, J.A.P.; Roesch-Ely, M. Red Propolis Extract Associated to Platelet-Rich Plasma and Stromal Cells with Focus in Cell Therapy and Functional Tissue Regeneration. *An. Acad. Bras. Cienc.* **2024**, *96*, e20240100. [CrossRef]
32. Jiang, X.; Xie, H.; Li, C.; You, M.; Zheng, Y.; Li, G.Q.; Chen, X.; Zhang, C.; Hu, F. Chinese Propolis Inhibits the Proliferation of Human Gastric Cancer Cells by Inducing Apoptosis and Cell Cycle Arrest. *Evid. Based Complement. Alternat. Med.* **2020**, *2020*, 2743058. [CrossRef]
33. Ivan, I.M.; Olaru, O.T.; Popovici, V.; Chițescu, C.L.; Popescu, L.; Luță, E.A.; Ilie, E.I.; Brașoveanu, L.I.; Hotnog, C.M.; Nițulescu, G.M.; et al. Antioxidant and Cytotoxic Properties of *Berberis vulgaris* (L.) Stem Bark Dry Extract. *Molecules* **2024**, *29*, 2053. [CrossRef]
34. Miłek, M.; Dżugan, M.; Pieńkowska, N.; Galiniak, S.; Mołoń, M.; Litwińczuk, W. Ornamental Barberry Twigs as an Underexploited Source of Berberine-Rich Extracts—Preliminary Research. *Curr. Issues Mol. Biol.* **2024**, *46*, 13193–13208. [CrossRef] [PubMed]
35. Och, A.; Lemieszek, M.K.; Cieśla, M.; Jedrejek, D.; Kozłowska, A.; Pawelec, S.; Nowak, R. *Berberis vulgaris* L. Root Extract as a Multi-Target Chemopreventive Agent against Colon Cancer Causing Apoptosis in Human Colon Adenocarcinoma Cell Lines. *Int. J. Mol. Sci.* **2024**, *25*, 4786. [CrossRef]
36. El Khalki, L.; Tilaoui, M.; Jaafari, A.; Ait Mouse, H.; Zyad, A. Studies on the Dual Cytotoxicity and Antioxidant Properties of *Berberis vulgaris* Extracts and Its Main Constituent Berberine. *Adv. Pharmacol. Sci.* **2018**, *2018*, 3018498. [CrossRef] [PubMed]
37. Campoccia, D.; Ravaioli, S.; Santi, S.; Mariani, V.; Santarcangelo, C.; De Filippis, A.; Montanaro, L.; Arciola, C.R.; Daglia, M. Exploring the Anticancer Effects of Standardized Extracts of Poplar-Type Propolis: In Vitro Cytotoxicity toward Cancer and Normal Cell Lines. *Biomed. Pharmacother.* **2021**, *141*, 111895. [CrossRef]
38. Teerasripreecha, D.; Phuwapraisirisan, P.; Puthong, S.; Kimura, K.; Okuyama, M.; Mori, H.; Kimura, A.; Chanchao, C. In Vitro Antiproliferative/Cytotoxic Activity on Cancer Cell Lines of a Cardanol and a Cardol Enriched from Thai Apis Mellifera Propolis. *BMC Complement. Altern. Med.* **2012**, *12*, 27. [CrossRef] [PubMed]
39. Singh, N.; Sharma, B. Toxicological Effects of Berberine and Sanguinarine. *Front. Mol. Biosci.* **2018**, *5*, 21. [CrossRef]
40. Lopez, B.G.-C.; de Lourenço, C.C.; Alves, D.A.; Machado, D.; Lancellotti, M.; Sawaya, A.C.H.F. Antimicrobial and Cytotoxic Activity of Red Propolis: An Alert for Its Safe Use. *J. Appl. Microbiol.* **2015**, *119*, 677–687. [CrossRef]

41. Zaleh, A.-A.; Salehi-Vaziri, A.; Pourhajibagher, M.; Bahador, A. The Synergistic Effect of Nano-Propolis and Curcumin-Based Photodynamic Therapy on Remineralization of White Spot Lesions: An Ex Vivo Study. *Photodiagn. Photodyn. Ther.* **2022**, *38*, 102789. [CrossRef] [PubMed]
42. Ren, K.; Zhang, W.; Wu, G.; Ren, J.; Lu, H.; Li, Z.; Han, X. Synergistic Anti-Cancer Effects of Galangin and Berberine through Apoptosis Induction and Proliferation Inhibition in Oesophageal Carcinoma Cells. *Biomed. Pharmacother. Biomed. Pharmacother.* **2016**, *84*, 1748–1759. [CrossRef] [PubMed]
43. Pijuan, J.; Barceló, C.; Moreno, D.F.; Maiques, O.; Sisó, P.; Marti, R.M.; Macià, A.; Panosa, A. In Vitro Cell Migration, Invasion, and Adhesion Assays: From Cell Imaging to Data Analysis. *Front. Cell Dev. Biol.* **2019**, *7*, 107. [CrossRef] [PubMed]
44. Martinotti, S.; Pellavio, G.; Laforenza, U.; Ranzato, E. Propolis Induces AQP3 Expression: A Possible Way of Action in Wound Healing. *Molecules* **2019**, *24*, 1544. [CrossRef]
45. Afonso, A.M.; Gonçalves, J.; Luís, Â.; Gallardo, E.; Duarte, A.P. Evaluation of the In Vitro Wound-Healing Activity and Phytochemical Characterization of Propolis and Honey. *Appl. Sci.* **2020**, *10*, 1845. [CrossRef]
46. Chang, J.-F.; Hsieh, C.-Y.; Lu, K.-C.; Chen, Y.-W.; Liang, S.-S.; Lin, C.-C.; Hung, C.-F.; Liou, J.-C.; Wu, M.-S. Therapeutic Targeting of Aristolochic Acid Induced Uremic Toxin Retention, SMAD 2/3 and JNK/ERK Pathways in Tubulointerstitial Fibrosis: Nephroprotective Role of Propolis in Chronic Kidney Disease. *Toxins* **2020**, *12*, 364. [CrossRef] [PubMed]
47. Geyikoglu, F.; Koc, K.; Colak, S.; Erol, H.S.; Cerig, S.; Yardimci, B.K.; Cakmak, O.; Dortbudak, M.B.; Eser, G.; Aysin, F.; et al. Propolis and Its Combination with Boric Acid Protect Against Ischemia/Reperfusion-Induced Acute Kidney Injury by Inhibiting Oxidative Stress, Inflammation, DNA Damage, and Apoptosis in Rats. *Biol. Trace Elem. Res.* **2019**, *192*, 214–221. [CrossRef]
48. Fadel, M.A.; Abdullah, M.A.; Al-Mahmood, S.S.; Thanoon, I.A. Protective Effect of Propolis on Liver and Kidney Injury Caused by Methotrexate in Chicks. *Iraqi J. Vet. Sci.* **2022**, *36*, 1061–1067. [CrossRef]
49. Sameni, H.R.; Ramhormozi, P.; Bandegi, A.R.; Taherian, A.A.; Mirmohammadkhani, M.; Safari, M. Effects of Ethanol Extract of Propolis on Histopathological Changes and Anti-Oxidant Defense of Kidney in a Rat Model for Type 1 Diabetes Mellitus. *J. Diabetes Investig.* **2016**, *7*, 506–513. [CrossRef]
50. Anvarifard, P.; Anbari, M.; Ostadrahimi, A.; Ardalan, M.; Ghoreishi, Z. A Comprehensive Insight into the Molecular and Cellular Mechanisms of the Effects of Propolis on Preserving Renal Function: A Systematic Review. *Nutr. Metab.* **2022**, *19*, 6. [CrossRef] [PubMed]
51. Hu, S.; Wang, J.; Liu, E.; Zhang, X.; Xiang, J.; Li, W.; Wei, P.; Zeng, J.; Zhang, Y.; Ma, X. Protective Effect of Berberine in Diabetic Nephropathy: A Systematic Review and Meta-Analysis Revealing the Mechanism of Action. *Pharmacol. Res.* **2022**, *185*, 106481. [CrossRef] [PubMed]
52. Zhang, X.; Liang, D.; Lian, X.; Jiang, Y.; He, H.; Liang, W.; Zhao, Y.; Chi, Z.-H. Berberine Activates Nrf2 Nuclear Translocation and Inhibits Apoptosis Induced by High Glucose in Renal Tubular Epithelial Cells through a Phosphatidylinositol 3-Kinase/Akt-Dependent Mechanism. *Apoptosis* **2016**, *21*, 721–736. [CrossRef] [PubMed]
53. Al-Waili, N. Mixing Two Different Propolis Samples Potentiates Their Antimicrobial Activity and Wound Healing Property: A Novel Approach in Wound Healing and Infection. *Vet. World* **2018**, *11*, 1188–1195. [CrossRef] [PubMed]
54. Miłek, M.; Franke, G.; Tomczyk, M.; Górecki, M.; Cwiková, O.; Jarošová, A.; Dżugan, M. The Influence of Geographical Origin on Poplar Propolis Composition and the Impact of Human Microbiota. *Pharmaceuticals* **2024**, *17*, 768. [CrossRef] [PubMed]
55. Alam, S.D.; Beg, M.A.; Bagadi, M.; Locatelli, M.; ALOthman, Z.A.; Mustaqeem, M.; Ali, I. Facile Extraction of Berberine from Different Plants, Separation, and Identification by Thin-Layer Chromatography, High-Performance Liquid Chromatography, and Biological Evaluation against Leishmaniosis. *J. Sep. Sci.* **2023**, *46*, 2300582. [CrossRef]

pharmaceuticals

MDPI

Article

Topical Application of Manuka Honey for the Treatment of Non-Healing Venous Leg Ulcers

Marek Kucharzewski [1,2], Kinga Spyrka [1], Ewa Rojczyk [1,3,*] and Jakub Brela [1]

1 Wladyslaw Bieganski Collegium Medicum, Jan Dlugosz University in Czestochowa, 42-200 Czestochowa, Poland; kucharzewskimarek@poczta.onet.pl (M.K.); ikingaxd@gmail.com (K.S.); j.brela@ujd.edu.pl (J.B.)

2 Surgical Outpatient Clinic, John Paul II District Hospital in Włoszczowa, 29-100 Włoszczowa, Poland

3 Faculty of Medicine, Academy of Silesia in Katowice, 40-555 Katowice, Poland

* Correspondence: ewarojczyk@gmail.com; Tel.: +48-60-546-6076

Abstract: Background/Objectives: Issues related to the chronic venous leg ulcer (VLU) treatment and prevention of recurrences remain the subject of research, but so too do common clinical problems in daily medical practice. Due to its medicinal properties, Manuka honey is increasingly used in the treatment of wounds of various origins. The aim of the study was to investigate the effectiveness of Manuka honey for the topical treatment of non-healing, chronic, venous leg ulcers. **Methods**: Eighty patients with chronic VLU participated in the study and were randomized into two equinumerous groups. In group 1, patients were treated with topical Manuka honey application and short stretch bandage compression, whereas, in group 2, antimicrobial calcium alginate wound dressing + Ag was used instead of Manuka honey. The efficacy of both treatment methods was compared. **Results**: The ulcerations in patients from group 1 have healed completely after up to seven weeks of therapy in all cases. In contrast, in all patients from group 2, the healing process was longer but completed successfully after up to 14 weeks of the therapy. The process of wound cleaning from microorganisms was also faster in group 1, as well as the reduction in ulcer area during treatment. **Conclusions**: It was found that the topical administration of Manuka honey may be a promising alternative to traditional methods of non-healing VLU treatment.

Keywords: Manuka honey; venous leg ulcer; wound healing; microorganisms

1. Introduction

Venous leg ulcer (VLU) has become a common medical problem among elderly patients. Non-healing VLU is defined as a chronic wound of the lower limb that does not heal after 3 months of therapy or is still not fully healed after 12 months of treatment. Chronic leg ulcers of various origin (70% of which are VLUs) cause long-term illness in older adults and the condition places a significant burden on health service resources. It affects 0.6–3% of those aged over 60 years, increasing to over 5% of those aged over 80 years, whereas the overall prevalence of chronic leg ulcers in the community ranges from 1.9% to 13.1%. Moreover, the patients suffer from multiple comorbidities and the illness has a remarkable impact on life quality [1–3].

It is estimated that the annual incidence of leg ulcers is 3.5 per 1000 individuals in the UK and 0.2 per 1000 in Switzerland. In the USA, the prevalence of VLU is between 500,000 and 600,000 and increases with age [1]. Jawień et al. reported that active or healed leg ulcers are found in 1.53% of patients visiting primary care institutions in Poland [4].

https://doi.org/10.3390/ph18020149

As found in previous studies and practice, compression therapy and local therapy are helpful ulcer treatment methods. However, the rate of wound healing complications after their application is still very high. As such, TIME strategy (Tissue debridement, Infection/Inflammation, Moisture balance, Edge effect) and proper wound dressing are of great importance and various hydrogels and hydrocolloids, as well as alginates and foams help in proper treatment [5].

Honey has been used in wound care since ancient times. It was found in scriptures from Sumer (from about 2000 BC) and in Smith papyrus (1700 BC) as a prescription for treating wounds. According to the Ebers papyrus (1550 BC), it was included in 147 prescriptions for external applications. Similarly, Chinese and Indian ayurvedic medicine used honey for many purposes, not only for wound healing but also against different internal and external infections. The ancient Greeks and Romans, represented by thinkers like Homer, Hippocrates, Dioscorides, and Pliny, gave honey much attention, emphasizing that it is a product that should be regularly used to preserve health and vigor [6]. Honey is now being rediscovered by modern medicine as a topical agent for wound treatment, especially where conventional modern therapeutic agents fail. It is one of the most complex and valuable natural biological products that has been widely used for its therapeutic effects.

Honey is a mixture of sugars prepared by honey bees from the natural sugar solutions—called nectar. The bee performs an inversion of the sucrose in the nectar, which increases the attainable density of the final product. Then, thanks to the addition of enzymes and the evaporation of water, honey bees transform it into a sweet liquid. There are two main types of honey: apiary honey and forest honey. Apiary honeys are produced in apiaries by Indian *Apis cerana indica* bees and the European *Apis millifera* bees, they are transparent and free from foreign materials. In contrast, forest honeys are produced by the rock bee, *Apis dorsata*, or from wild nests of *Apis cerana indica* in forests, and they are turbid owing to the abundant presence of pollen, wax, brood (bee larvae), and plant materials [7].

Natural honey is mainly made up of sugar and water, with sugar accounting for over 95% of the dry matter. Generally, it is a complex of carbohydrates; however, over 200 health-promoting substances have been found in natural honey, including various vitamins, flavonoids, minerals, and enzymes, as well as amino acids, organic acids, and volatile chemicals. It is important to note that numerous factors affect the quality of honey, including plant type, location, and season, as well as processing method and microbiological characteristics. Thus, such factors also influence the medicinal properties of honey [8–10].

Honey has numerous health-promoting properties (like antioxidant and anti-inflammatory properties), it contains a wide range of vitamins, amino acids, and minerals, glucose oxidase producing hydrogen peroxide (H_2O_2) in diluted honey, and also gluconic acid (inhibited in undiluted honey) resulting in the pH level of honey ranging from 3.2 to 4.5. Moreover, honey is known to have strong antibacterial properties because of high osmolarity—it was shown, that in undiluted honey, bacterial growth is prevented. Furthermore, honey is non-toxic, non-allergenic, does not stick to wounds, and helps rapid wound healing because of its moisture content. Most importantly, honey is cheap and, therefore, the application of honey as a topical treatment is very beneficial in regard to infection control and wound management [5,11–17].

Manuka honey (the Maori name for the New Zealand/Australian tea tree/bush *Leptospermum scoparium*) is a monofloral honey derived from the tea tree by honey bees *Apis melifera* [18]. It has antibacterial properties and, as stated by Moore, it has "very special healing properties", which makes it "the best natural antibiotic in the world". Medical-grade Manuka honey is prepared very purely and undergoes very specific and rigorous quality control [6,19,20].

Due to its properties, Manuka honey has many applications, including the treatment of burns as well as the treatment of external ulcers. It was shown that not only does honey produce a clean, granulating wound bed, but it also has a positive impact on wound repair because of its nutritional activity. Such activity includes supporting the osmotic flow of lymph towards the wound, the intake of carbohydrates (which are easily metabolized) as well as amino acids, vitamins, and minerals, all of which support wound healing. The high osmotic property of honey results in interstitial fluid drainage, promoting tissue regeneration, which (observed in areas of angiogenesis) is seen as granulation [21–25]. Honey may also have an influence on whether surgical debridement or adherence of dressing to the wound is necessary, as osmotic flow impacts the removal of waste and debris from the wound. As honey forms a fluid layer on wound surfaces after application, wounds may be rinsed, resulting in painless dressing changes, which do not involve reparative tissue damage [13,14,16,17,20,26].

After applying Manuka honey to wounds, healing time decreases, wound surface decreases, and tissue repair is accelerated [13,16,27]. What is more, Manuka honey dressings can be applied directly to dry and also to moist wounds. They are frequently used instead of modern antibacterial wound dressings containing ionic silver, especially in critically colonized wounds, i.e., those with a bacterial load that exceeds the host's defense capabilities [18,26,27]. An example of such a wound is a diabetic foot ulcer (DFU). It was shown that honey is a cost-effective and safe option for DFU management that reduces the time of healing, as well as amputation or hospitalization rates [21,28–30]. However, another type of difficult-to-heal wound—VLU—is not so widely described in the literature in the context of using honey for its treatment. There are only some promising case series describing less than ten patients with VLUs, who were successfully treated with Manuka honey within several weeks [31,32]. On the other hand, a systematic review of the literature concerning medical-grade honey used in patients with VLUs gives contradictory results [33].

Thus, in order to complete data on this topic, the aim of the study was to determine the effectiveness of Manuka honey in a topical dressing for the treatment of non-healing VLUs, as well as to assess the impact of such dressing on the wound bacterial microbiota. Despite extensive knowledge about the healing effects of honey, our study is the first one that concerns only one, specific type of wound—VLUs. This study is a kind of continuation of an earlier experiment on the effect of propolis on VLU healing [34].

2. Results

In the course of the study, none of the patients rejected the proposed treatment in both groups.

2.1. Complete Healing Time

In all 40 patients in group 1, the ulcers healed successfully (i.e., completely) within the first 7 weeks of treatment by topical Manuka honey application. Ulcer healing was also observed in all the cases in group 2 (antimicrobial calcium alginate wound dressing + Ag). However, within the first 7 weeks of treatment, complete healing was found only in 12 out of 40 patients in this group and the time up to the complete healing of the last two cases was significantly longer—14 weeks. (Table 1). The maximum time of the ulcer healing in group 1 was significantly shorter (49 days) than in group 2 (98 days); $p < 0.05$.

Table 1. The number of new patients with completely healed ulcers depending on the duration of treatment (group 1—Manuka honey, group 2—standard treatment).

Group	Duration of Treatment (Weeks)													
	1	2	3	4	5	6	7	8	9	10	11	12	13	14
1		4	10	8	7	7	4							
2				6		6		7		7	5	4	3	2

2.2. Ulceration Area and a Rate of Wound Area Reduction

The mean ulceration area in groups 1 and 2 in the course of the treatment is presented in Figure 1, whereas Figure 2 presents changes in the rate of wound area reduction over time.

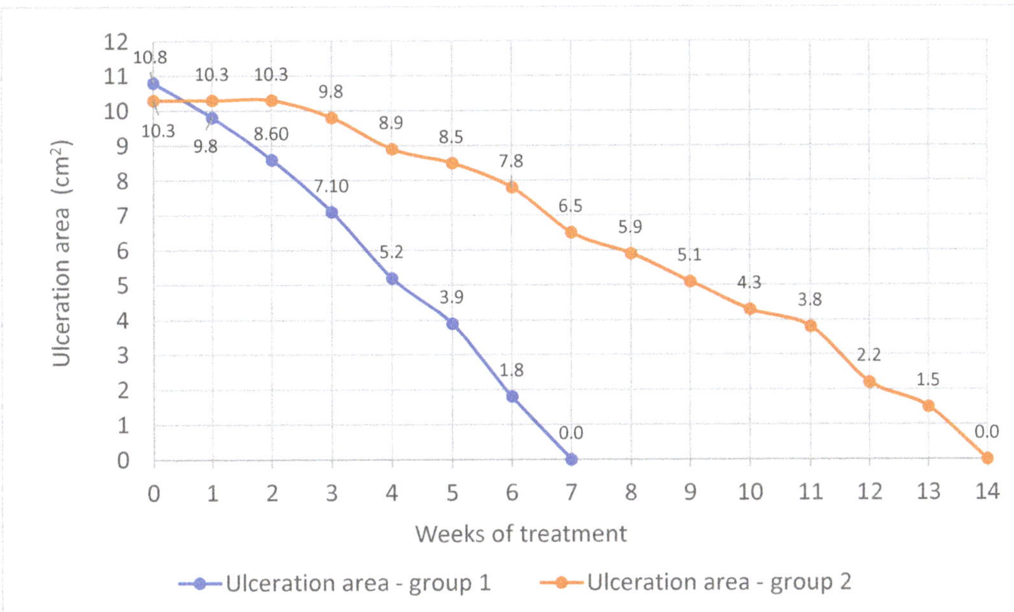

Figure 1. Changes in ulceration area in subsequent weeks of treatment. Group 1—Manuka honey; group 2—standard treatment.

In group 1, the mean ulceration area at the beginning of the study was 10.8 cm^2. After 7 days of treatment, the average ulceration area diminished by 1.0 cm^2 and the rate of reduction of the wound area (v_1) was 0.142 cm^2/day. After another 7 days, the rate with which the ulcer area was decreasing equaled 0.171 cm^2/day, and the mean area of the wound decreased by 1.2 cm^2. By this time, the ulcers in four patients have been healed. After the following 14 days of using the Manuka honey dressing, the ulcers of a further 12 women and 6 men healed completely, and the mean wound area of the remaining patients decreased by 3.4 cm^2. The rate at which the wound area decreased was 0.214 cm^2/day (first week) and 0.271 cm^2/day (second week). After a further 7 days, the ulcers of 7 more patients healed, the rate of wound area reduction was 0.186 cm^2/day and the mean area of the wound decreased by 1.3 cm^2. In the next 7 days of treatment, the mean ulceration area diminished by 2.1 cm^2, and the rate of wound area reduction was 0.3 cm^2/day. The ulcers of four women and three men healed completely. The healing of the ulcers in the last patients was completed after the next 7 days of treatment. The rate of decrease in the wound area in that period was 0.257 cm^2/day.

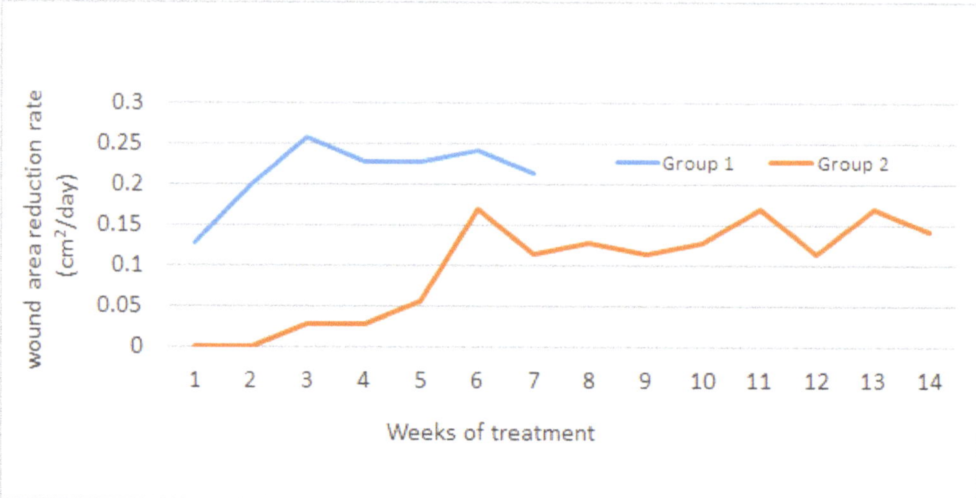

Figure 2. The rate of wound area reduction depending on the treatment time. Group 1—Manuka honey; group 2—standard treatment.

Group 2 consisted of 40 patients with a mean ulceration area of 10.3 cm^2. Over the following 2 weeks of treatment, the surface area of the ulcers did not change and was 10.3 cm^2. After a further 7 days of treatment, the mean wound area decreased by only 0.5 cm^2 and the rate at which it decreased (v_2) was 0.071 cm^2/day. After a further 7 days, the rate of ulceration area reduction was also 0.129 cm^2/day and the mean wound area was 8.9 cm^2. The ulcers of four women and two men healed completely. After the following 14 days of treatment, the mean ulcer area decreased by 1.1 cm^2 and the rate with which the wound surface decreased was 0.057 cm^2/day (first week) and 0.1 cm^2/day (second week). The mean ulcer area of the other patients decreased (7.8 cm^2). After a further 7 days, the rate of the ulceration surface reduction was 0.186 cm^2/day and the mean wound area was 6.5 cm^2. The ulcers in seven patients were healed. After a further 7 days of treatment, the mean wound area decreased by 0.6 cm^2 and the rate at which it decreased was 0.086 cm^2/day. After a further 14 days, the mean wound area was 1.6 cm^2 and the reduction in the wound area was 0.114 cm^2/day for both weeks. The ulcers of eight women and four men healed completely. After the following 14 days of treatment, the mean ulcer area was 2.1 cm^2, and the rate of wound area reduction was 0.071 cm^2/day (first week) and 0.229 cm^2/day (second week). The ulcers of seven patients healed completely. The ulcerations of the remaining five patients in this group healed after a further 14 days of treatment and the rate at which the ulceration area decreased was 0.1 cm^2/day (first week) and 0.214 cm^2/day (second week).

Thus, a significantly faster rate of wound area reduction was observed in group 1 (treated with Manuka honey). In group 2, the healing process accelerated only from the sixth week of treatment. However, even after such a long time, the rate of wound area reduction was comparable to the value for group 1 in the first week of treatment (Figure 2).

2.3. *Microbiota Analysis*

The qualitative analysis of microbiota isolated from the surface of venous leg ulcers is shown below. Diagnostic cultures performed before treatment indicated that all wounds in both patient groups were infected. After three weeks of wound therapy, bacterial cultures were detected in 18 patients from group 1 and in 35 patients from group 2. After five weeks of treatment, the cultures made from ulcer swabs were positive for bacteria in six patients of group 2. All ulcerations in patients of group 1 treated with Manuka honey dressing did not support culturable microorganisms. Generally, 12 species of bacteria were grown from all samples taken before treatment, but only seven of the most common ones are presented in Table 2. In ulcers of the patients treated with calcium alginate wound dressing + Ag the incidence of individual isolates did not differ substantially from the results obtained in patients in group 1 (treated with Manuka honey). In both groups, the most common isolated microorganisms were *Staphylococcus aureus, Echerichia coli, Pseudomonas aeruginosa,* and *Proteus mirabilis*, whereas *Streptococcus β-haemoliticus, Enterococcus faecalis,* and *Klebsiella pneumoniae* were rarely isolated species. Before treatment, 182 strains of different bacteria were isolated from the wounds of patients in group 1, whereas, in group 2, there were 194. The application of Manuka honey dressing for three weeks resulted in reducing the number of bacterial strains to 40, and, after 5 weeks, no bacterial strain was isolated. In swabs from the wounds of patients treated with topical antimicrobial calcium alginate wound dressing, 131 strains were cultured after 3 weeks, and 78 after 5 weeks (Table 2).

Table 2. The incidence of chosen 7 bacteria species in tested ulcerations, measured as a number of patients with particular species being isolated from wounds.

Isolated Bacteria Species	Before Treatment		After 3 Week Treatment		After 5 Week Treatment	
	Group 1	Group 2	Group 1	Group 2	Group 1	Group 2
Staphylococcus aureus	35	36	18	29	0	15
Escherichia coli	33	32	11	21	0	12
Pseudomonas aeruginosa	25	26	10	17	0	11
Proteus mirabilis	23	25	11	15	0	12
Streptococcus β-haemoliticus	23	26	13	18	0	11
Enterococcus faecalis	22	22	10	17	0	9
Klebsiella pneumoniae	21	22	12	14	0	8

3. Discussion

Despite the vast improvement in epidemiological and pathophysiological knowledge, one of the largest clinical concerns in phlebology includes VLUs. The number of patients suffering from this complication remains high; therefore, there is a need to search for more effective treatment strategies [34].

Both systemic and local factors affect the wound-healing process. That is why it is highly important that topical medications have a positive effect on healing. One of the promising natural products supporting wound healing is Manuka honey. In recent years, the molecular mechanisms of its activity in the context of healing promotion have become increasingly better understood. Leukocyte stimulation greatly affects the healing rate by the release of cytokines and growth factors, stimulating keratinocyte transcription of TNF-α, IL-1β and TGF-β genes resulting in tissue repair activation [35,36]. Apart from interactions with the immune system, honey induces Ca^{2+} entry into keratinocytes as a result of H_2O_2 release in a reaction mediated by glucose oxidase. Consequently, wound closure is triggered [22,23]. Another interesting mechanism of anti-inflammatory honey activity is the inhibition of the nuclear factor kappa B (NF-κB) pathway, which decreases inflammatory mediators, such as cyclooxygenase-2 (COX-2) and cyclooxygenase-1 (COX-1) [21,24].

The most important molecular factors modulated by honey in the context of wound healing promotion are summarized in Figure 3.

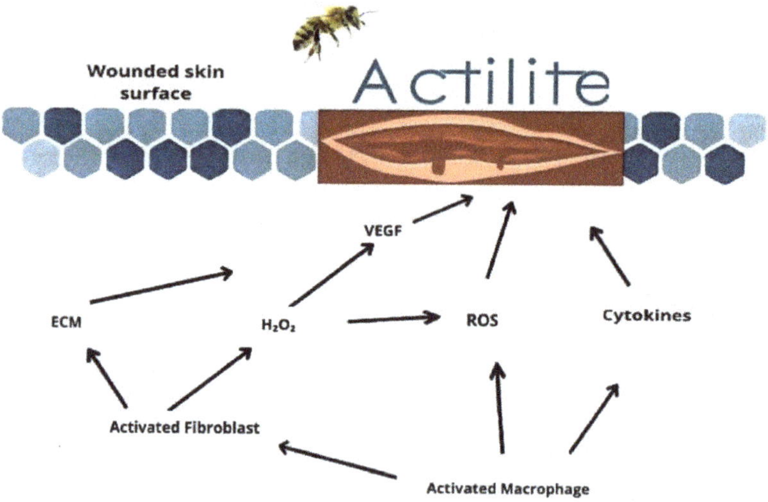

Figure 3. Most important molecular changes in wound area after honey dressing Actilite application [21,22,24].

All these physical and chemical factors give honey unique properties as a wound dressing. Indeed, it is probably due to the abovementioned properties that, in our study, faster healing of VLUs was observed in patients treated with Manuka honey than in patients from the group receiving calcium alginate wound dressing + Ag. Honey contributed to wound healing within a maximum of 7 weeks as compared to a maximum of 14 weeks in patients treated with calcium alginate wound dressing + Ag.

Other research groups observed similar results. For example, the healing outcomes of relatively small, short-duration venous ulcers, treated with multi-layer compression and calcium alginate dressings impregnated with Manuka honey (n = 187) or primary dressings according to "usual care" changed as needed (n = 181) were compared by Jull et al. Within a 12-week period, 55.6% of patients belonging to the Manuka honey group and 49.7% of "usual care" patients ($p = 0.258$) experienced fully healed wounds [35]. Similarly, the case series of nine patients with wounds of various aetiologies confirmed that medical-grade honey can be an effective alternative for antibiotics in locally infected wound treatment [37].

Conflicting results were presented by Ingle et al. in a prospective, randomized, double-blind study. In this study, the effects of honey and IntraSite gel were compared. It was observed that even after adjusting for wound size, the healing time of shallow wounds treated with honey did not significantly differ from the healing time of shallow wounds treated with IntraSite gel. In the case of shallow wounds, those treated with honey healed 2.8 days sooner, while, in regard to abrasions, there was no significant difference. It was concluded that there was no significant difference between IntraSite gel and honey when used as treatment agents [38].

Du Toit and Page used an in vitro tissue explant culture model to examine how honey and silver-impregnated dressings influence the morphology of two key cellular components of the wound bed, i.e., keratinocytes and fibroblasts. It was shown that the honey-impregnated dressings promoted new tissue regeneration [39]. Another study, which compared silver-sulphadiazine with the honey gel provided similar results—the honey gel significantly stimulated re-epithelialization, whereas silver sulphadiazine significantly reduced it [40].

Wounds are exposed to a number of microbes found on the skin and in the external environment. If the repair process does not run properly and wounds do not heal, they may become infected, which leads to the formation of biofilm in the wound. The biofilm contains many species of bacteria, which strongly adhere to the wound bed and to each other [41]. Topical application of the dressing with Manuka honey maintains a moist environment in the wound and shows antibacterial activity against a broad range of pathogens, such as aerobic and anaerobic bacteria, fungi, and viruses [42–44]. Another advantage (over antibiotics) is also the long-lasting antibacterial effect and a significantly lower tendency to induce bacterial resistance.

Numerous studies [43–49] have shown that Manuka honey inhibits more than 60 species of bacteria, including anaerobic Gram-positive bacteria and Gram-negative bacteria, and even a few yeast species of the *Aspergillus* and *Penicillium* genus. The antibacterial properties of honey are due to its high osmolarity and the production of H_2O_2. Its secretion from the dressing is slow and continuous, which results in the elimination of microorganisms; however, it is not cytotoxic to the tissues surrounding ulceration. The acidic environment in the wound produced by honey also inhibits the growth of pathogens in the skin loss. The low pH increases the release of oxygen from hemoglobin in the wound, which stimulates angiogenesis and cytokine secretion and consequently increases the rate of granulation [21–25]. Cooper et al. studied the antibacterial effectiveness of three honeys (including artificial honeys) on 17 strains of *Pseudomonas aeruginosa* isolated from the wounds of patients. Manuka honey showed antibacterial properties at a concentration of 6.8–7.5%, and two other (artificial) honeys required a concentration of 17% and 22%, respectively, to inhibit the development of all 17 strains [50]. Similar results were obtained by many other authors [27,51–53], concerning many types of chronic wounds, including VLUs.

Our results confirm the high effectiveness of Manuka honey in combating bacterial colonization of the wound: after 5 weeks of treatment, there were no culturable bacterial strains isolated in the group receiving honey dressings (as opposed to the traditionally treated group). It is worth mentioning that Manuka honey successfully eradicated *Enterococcus faecalis*, which is a non-pathogenic commensal when isolated from the healthy skin of a healthy subject. However, in patients with VLUs, it is highly pathogenic and seriously delays wound healing. It can be a source of local wound infection leading to sepsis.

To sum up, there are many studies comparing various applications of Manuka honey with other methods for the topical treatment of burns and DFUa. However, few studies examine the treatment of VLUs with honey. Thus, in one of our experimental groups, we used the Manuka honey dressing to determine how it affects the treatment of VLUs. Despite the encouraging effects achieved using Manuka honey therapy of non-healing VLUs, further, more detailed studies concerning honey implementation should be performed, including randomized controlled trials, comparisons with other methods of treatment, and involving larger experimental groups.

4. Materials and Methods

4.1. Patients

The study was conducted at the Surgical Outpatient Clinic of the John Paul II District Hospital in Włoszczowa in the period from February 2022 to September 2024.

The experiment comprised 80 patients with non-healing venous leg ulcer (VLU) and a history of active crural ulcer $\geq$12 months as well as a lack of complete healing despite previous non-surgical treatment. Each patient provided information about ulcer treatment and other significant medical problems. All patients were previously treated by a general practitioner with elastic bandage compression stocking along with wound antiseptic lavage and local application of traditional dressing, like hydrogel and hydrocolloid.

However, none of these methods led to the complete healing of the wound within the pre-randomization period.

After clinical examination, the venous origin of the ulcer was confirmed with the help of the venous duplex Doppler sonography and ankle-brachial index (ABI) measurement (in all the cases the ABI was $\geq$0.8). Patients with previous or active deep vein thrombosis were excluded from the study. Additional exclusion criteria were diabetes, chronic or critical leg ischemia, contraindications to compression therapy, orthosis immobilization or plastic cast, paresis related to stroke or paraplegia, chronic cardiac failure with peripheral swelling, systemic infection, clinically significant peripheral atherosclerotic occlusive disease, and previous honey implementation. Moreover, patients treated pharmacologically with sulodexide or other anticoagulants as well as patients on pentoxifylline or prostaglandins were not included in the study.

The patients qualified for the study were divided into two groups using a randomized method. Similarly, randomized numbers were given to patients according to the order of inclusion into the study (group 1 included the patients with odd numbers, and group 2 those with even numbers).

Group 1 included 27 women and 13 men aged 49–79 years (mean 56.5 years). Their ulceration area varied from 6.8 cm^2 to 17.4 cm^2 (mean 10.8 cm^2). The ulcer location of 14 patients was on the left crus, and, for 26 patients, it was on the right one. The wound persisted at the start of therapy for 17–29 months (mean 21 months). Thirty patients were fully mobile, and ten women had limited mobility. Body mass index (BMI) ranged from 23.6 to 39.7 kg/m^2 (mean 31.2 kg/m^2). It was >30 kg/m^2 in 10 women and 6 men (Table 3).

Table 3. Characteristics of the research groups; (group 1—Manuka honey; group 2—standard treatment).

	Group 1	Group 2
Number of patients	40	40
Women	27	26
Men	13	12
Age (years)	49–79	51–75
Ulcer location—left crus	14	16
Ulcer location—right crus	26	24
Ulcer area at the beginning (cm^2)	6.8–17.4	6.6–17.8
Duration of ulceration (months)	17–29	18–31
Full mobility	30	29
Limited mobility	10	11
Ankle-brachial index (ABI)	0.92–1.11	0.96–1.12
Body mass index (BMI) (kg/m^2)	23.6–39.7	24.8–40.2

Group 2 included 28 women and 12 men aged from 51 to 75 years (mean 58.1 years). The ulceration area varied from 6.6 to 17.8 cm^2 (mean 10.3 cm^2), the duration of wound occurrence from 18 months to 31 months (mean 22 months). In 16 patients, the ulcers were located on the left crus, and, in 24 patients, they were on the right one. Full mobility was possible in 29 patients and limited mobility in 11 patients. BMI ranged from 24.8 to 40.2 kg/m^2 (mean 29.8 kg/m^2). It was >30 kg/m^2 in 9 women and 8 men (Table 3).

Importantly, there were no statistically significant differences between groups in the parameters presented in Table 3.

Each ulcer was classified by wound morphology, severity, and location. A systematic description of wound and limb appearance was recorded, including edema, erythema, exudation, granulation, and the presence of fibrin or eschar. Moreover, based on clinical and sonographic results, the chronic venous disease of each patient was classified according to CEAP classification (Table 4).

Table 4. Classification of venous dysfunction (according to the CEAP classification); (group 1—Manuka honey, group 2—standard treatment).

CEAP Class	Group 1	Group 2
$C_6E_PA_{S2,3}P_R$	19	17
$C_6E_PA_{S3D18}P_R$	11	13
$C_6E_PA_{S3D18P18}P_R$	5	6
$C_6E_PA_{S4}P_R$	5	4

4.2. Procedures

All patients underwent ambulatory treatment and were examined by a physician every week until the complete healing of the ulceration. The drug therapy in both groups followed a standard regimen. All patients received micronized flavonoid fraction (450 mg diosmin, 50 mg hesperidin), and 2 tablets of 500 mg once a day.

The ulcers were thoroughly debrided together with the removal of fibrin, eschar, and, if necessary, necrotic tissue. The necrotic tissues were removed from ulcerations through surgery or with the help of enzyme-containing ointment and antiseptic lavage.

For the local treatment in group 1, a topical application of Manuka honey dressing (Activon Honey, Advancis Medical, Nottingham, UK) was used. The ulcers were rinsed with physiological sodium chloride solution and then the Manuka honey dressing was applied. Gauze pads were then placed on the ulcer and the leg was bandaged with a non-elastic supportive bandage. The compression short-stretch bandages were applied to all patients in this group. Specifically, it was a spiral two-layer bandaging technique with a 10 cm wide bandage applied from toe to knee. Manuka honey dressing was changed every day until the ulcer was healed. For the proper measurement of compression pressure, the Kikuhime device pressure sensor was used and a pressure of 25–35 mm Hg was applied.

The patients in group 2 were treated with antimicrobial calcium alginate wound dressing + Ag (Suprasorb® A + Ag, Lohmann and Rausche, Pabianice, Poland). After rinsing the wound with physiological sodium chloride solution, the above-mentioned wound dressing was used. Then, as in group 1, gauze pads were placed on the ulcer, the limb was bandaged with a non-elastic supportive bandage and the compression short-stretch bandages were used. The Suprasorb® A + Ag dressing was changed every day until the ulcer was healed. As in group 1, 25–35 mm Hg compression pressure was precisely applied with the help of the Kikuhime device pressure sensor.

At the baseline, and after 3 and 5 weeks of treatment, the wounds (from both groups) were swabbed for microbiological assessment. The tested material was inoculated onto a medium for selective bacterial culture and incubated for 24–48 h at 37 °C.

The culture for aerobic bacteria was performed with the following media: Columbia agar with 5% sheep blood, Chapman medium, selective-differentiating MacConkey medium (Becton, Dickinson and Company, Franklin Lakes, USA), and D-coccosel medium. Incubation was performed under aerobic conditions at a temperature between 35 and 37 °C and the bacteria growth was assessed after 48 h. Anaerobic bacteria were incubated for 4 to 5 days in an anaerobic atmosphere using Genoboxanaer (Bio Merieux, Warsaw, Poland) at 35–37 °C. In order to culture these bacteria Schaedlerbase (Neo) and Vanco substrate (Bio Merieux, Warsaw, Poland) were used.

The identification of isolated microorganisms was performed using standard microbiological methods, and the following were assessed: morphology using Gram-stained preparation, growth on selective media, morphology of colonies, and their biochemical and serological properties. To perform this, an ATB system with reagent kits (Bio Merieux) was used.

Prior to the treatment and during wound dressing and compression changes, the area of ulcers was measured. It was performed once a week until the wound healed completely. The procedure was carried out as follows: firstly, homothetic congruent projections of the ulcers were plotted onto transparent foil, after which planimetric measurements of the wounds were taken with the use of digitizer Mutoh Kurta XGT-1218A3 (Mutoh, Phoenix, AZ, USA) [54–56]. The speed with which the ulceration area was decreasing daily was calculated for each patient according to the formula:

$$v_s = (S_{i-1} - S_i)/t$$

s (subscript): group number (1 or 2);
S_i: ulceration area at the time of the previous measurement (one week earlier);
S_{i-1}: ulceration area on the day of a given measurement;
t: time (in days) in which the ulceration area changed from S_{i-1} to S_i (7 days).

4.3. Statistical Analysis

Statistical characteristics of the continuous variables have been presented as arithmetic means and their standard deviations (SD) or as medians and interquartile ranges. The results were analyzed using the Mann–Whitney U-test; p-values < 0.05 were considered statistically significant. All calculations were carried out using Statistica 8 (software version 8, StatSoft, Cracow, Poland).

5. Conclusions

1. The application of Manuka honey in the treatment of non-healing, chronic VLUs is beneficial, as it significantly shortens the healing time of such wounds.
2. Manuka honey dressings reduce the surface of VLUs and, thus, shorten the time of treatment.
3. The use of Manuka honey dressings results in the faster removal of bacterial microbiota from VLUs

Author Contributions: Conceptualization, M.K. and K.S.; methodology, M.K.; validation, M.K., E.R. and J.B.; formal analysis, K.S. and J.B.; investigation, M.K.; literature search, J.B. and E.R.; data curation, M.K.; writing—original draft preparation, M.K. and K.S.; writing—review and editing, E.R.; visualization, M.K. and E.R.; supervision, M.K.; project administration, M.K. and K.S. All authors have read and agreed to the published version of the manuscript.

Funding: This research received no external funding.

Institutional Review Board Statement: The study was conducted in accordance with the Declaration of Helsinki. Manuka honey dressing is registered in Poland and commonly used for treating wounds (leg ulcers, burns). Therefore, the use of this dressing in our study does not require approval from the Bioethics Committee.

Informed Consent Statement: Informed consent was obtained from all subjects involved in the study.

Data Availability Statement: The original contributions presented in this study are included in the article. Further inquiries can be directed to the corresponding author.

Conflicts of Interest: The authors declare no conflicts of interest.

References

1. Agale, S.V. Chronic Leg Ulcers: Epidemiology, Aetiopathogenesis, and Management. *Ulcers* **2013**, *2013*, 1–9. [CrossRef]
2. Sopata, M.; Kucharzewski, M.; Tomaszewska, E. Antiseptic with modern wound dressings in the treatment of venous leg ulcers: Clinical and microbiological aspects. *J. Wound Care* **2016**, *25*, 419–426. [CrossRef] [PubMed]

3. Szewczyk, M.T.; Moscicka, P.; Jawien, A.; Cwajda-Bialasik, J.; Cierzniakowska, K.; Slusarz, R.; Hancke, E. Quality of life in patients with leg ulcers or skin lesions—A pilot study. *Postep. Dermatol. Alergol.* **2015**, *32*, 465–469. [CrossRef] [PubMed]
4. Jawień, A.; Grzela, T.; Ochwat, A. Prevalence of chronic venous insufficiency in men and women in Poland: Multicentre cross-sectional study in 40,095 patients. *Phlebology* **2003**, *18*, 110–122. [CrossRef]
5. Molan, P.C. Re-introducing honey in the management of wounds and ulcers—Theory and practice. *Ostomy Wound Manag.* **2002**, *48*, 28–40.
6. Bogdanov, S. Honey in Medicne. *Bee Prod. Sci.* **2014**. [CrossRef]
7. Subrahmanyam, M. Topical application of honey for burn wound treatment—An overview. *Ann. Burn. Fire Disasters* **2007**, *20*, 137–139. [PubMed] [PubMed Central]
8. Kingsley, A. The use of honey in the treatment of infected wounds: Case studies. *Br. J. Nurs.* **2001**, *10*, S13–S20. [CrossRef]
9. Mandal, M.D.; Mandal, S. Honey: Its medicinal property and antibacterial activity. *Asian Pac. J. Trop. Biomed.* **2011**, *1*, 154–160. [CrossRef]
10. Moniruzzaman, M.; Khalil, M.I.; Sulaiman, S.A.; Gan, S.H. Physicochemical and antioxidant properties of Malaysian honeys produced by Apis cerana, Apis dorsata and Apis mellifera. *BMC Complement. Altern. Med.* **2013**, *13*, 43. [CrossRef]
11. Cutting, K.F. Honey and contemporary wound care: An overview. *Ostomy Wound Manag.* **2007**, *53*, 49–54.
12. Jull, A.B.; Rodgers, A.; Walker, N. Honey as a topical treatment for wounds. *Cochrane Database Syst. Rev.* **2008**, CD005083. [CrossRef]
13. Jull, A.B.; Walker, N.; Deshpande, S. Honey as a topical treatment for wounds. *Cochrane Database Syst. Rev.* **2013**, CD005083. [CrossRef]
14. Lee, D.S.; Sinno, S.; Khachemoune, A. Honey and wound healing: An overview. *Am. J. Clin. Dermatol.* **2011**, *12*, 181–190. [CrossRef]
15. Lusby, P.E.; Coombes, A.; Wilkinson, J.M. Honey: A potent agent for wound healing? *J. Wound Ostomy Cont. Nurs.* **2002**, *29*, 295–300. [CrossRef]
16. Tashkandi, H. Honey in wound healing: An updated review. *Open Life Sci.* **2021**, *16*, 1091–1100. [CrossRef]
17. Yaghoobi, R.; Kazerouni, A.; Kazerouni, O. Evidence for Clinical Use of Honey in Wound Healing as an Anti-bacterial, Anti-inflammatory Anti-oxidant and Anti-viral Agent: A Review. *Jundishapur J. Nat. Pharm. Prod.* **2013**, *8*, 100–104. [CrossRef]
18. White, R. Manuka honey in wound management: Greater than the sum of its parts? *J. Wound Care* **2016**, *25*, 539–543. [CrossRef]
19. Alvarez-Suarez, J.M.; Gasparrini, M.; Forbes-Hernandez, T.Y.; Mazzoni, L.; Giampieri, F. The Composition and Biological Activity of Honey: A Focus on Manuka Honey. *Foods* **2014**, *3*, 420–432. [CrossRef]
20. Moore, O.A.; Smith, L.A.; Campbell, F.; Seers, K.; McQuay, H.J.; Moore, R.A. Systematic review of the use of honey as a wound dressing. *BMC Complement. Altern. Med.* **2001**, *1*, 2. [CrossRef]
21. Bezerra, A.; Fonseca, H.; Rodrigues, F.; Delerue-Matos, C.; Gouvinhas, I.; Garcia, J. Honey Therapy in Diabetic Foot Ulcers: A Promising Strategy for Effective Wound Healing. *Appl. Sci.* **2023**, *13*, 12820. [CrossRef]
22. Martinotti, S.; Bonsignore, G.; Ranzato, E. Applications of Beehive Products for Wound Repair and Skin Care. *Cosmetics* **2023**, *10*, 127. [CrossRef]
23. Martinotti, S.; Laforenza, U.; Patrone, M.; Moccia, F.; Ranzato, E. Honey-Mediated Wound Healing: H_2O_2 Entry through AQP3 Determines Extracellular Ca^{2+} Influx. *Int. J. Mol. Sci.* **2019**, *20*, 764. [CrossRef] [PubMed]
24. Scepankova, H.; Combarros-Fuertes, P.; Fresno, J.M.; Tornadijo, M.E.; Dias, M.S.; Pinto, C.A.; Saraiva, J.A.; Estevinho, L.M. Role of Honey in Advanced Wound Care. *Molecules* **2021**, *26*, 4784. [CrossRef] [PubMed]
25. Yupanqui Mieles, J.; Vyas, C.; Aslan, E.; Humphreys, G.; Diver, C.; Bartolo, P. Honey: An Advanced Antimicrobial and Wound Healing Biomaterial for Tissue Engineering Applications. *Pharmaceutics* **2022**, *14*, 1663. [CrossRef] [PubMed]
26. Davies, P. Recent clinical usage of honey in the treatment of wound—A review. *Wounds* **2005**, *5*, 14–22.
27. Al-Waili, N.; Salom, K.; Al-Ghamdi, A.A. Honey for wound healing, ulcers, and burns; data supporting its use in clinical practice. *Sci. World J.* **2011**, *11*, 766–787. [CrossRef]
28. Kamaratos, A.V.; Tzirogiannis, K.N.; Iraklianou, S.A.; Panoutsopoulos, G.I.; Kanellos, I.E.; Melidonis, A.I. Manuka honey-impregnated dressings in the treatment of neuropathic diabetic foot ulcers. *Int. Wound J.* **2014**, *11*, 259–263. [CrossRef]
29. Teobaldi, I.; Stoico, V.; Perrone, F.; Bruti, M.; Bonora, E.; Mantovani, A. Honey dressing on a leg ulcer with tendon exposure in a patient with type 2 diabetes. *Endocrinol. Diabetes Metab. Case Rep.* **2018**, *2018*, 18–117. [CrossRef]
30. Tsang, K.K.; Kwong, E.W.; Woo, K.Y.; To, T.S.; Chung, J.W.; Wong, T.K. The Anti-Inflammatory and Antibacterial Action of Nanocrystalline Silver and Manuka Honey on the Molecular Alternation of Diabetic Foot Ulcer: A Comprehensive Literature Review. *Evid. Based Complement. Altern. Med.* **2015**, *2015*, 218283. [CrossRef]
31. Gethin, G.; Cowman, S. Case series of use of Manuka honey in leg ulceration. *Int. Wound J.* **2005**, *2*, 10–15. [CrossRef]
32. Papanikolaou, G.E.; Gousios, G.; Cremers, N.A.J.; Peters, L.J.F. Treating Infected Non-Healing Venous Leg Ulcers with Medical-Grade Honey: A Prospective Case Series. *Antibiotics* **2024**, *13*, 614. [CrossRef] [PubMed]

33. Holland, L.C.; Norris, J.M. Medical grade honey in the management of chronic venous leg ulcers. *Int. J. Surg.* **2015**, *20*, 17–20. [CrossRef] [PubMed]
34. Kucharzewski, M.; Kozka, M.; Urbanek, T. Topical treatment of nonhealing venous leg ulcer with propolis ointment. *Evid. Based Complement. Altern. Med.* **2013**, *2013*, 254017. [CrossRef]
35. Jull, A.; Walker, N.; Parag, V.; Molan, P.; Rodgers, A. Randomized clinical trial of honey-impregnated dressings for venous leg ulcers. *Br. J. Surg.* **2008**, *95*, 175–182. [CrossRef]
36. Majtan, J.; Bohova, J.; Garcia-Villalba, R.; Tomas-Barberan, F.A.; Madakova, Z.; Majtan, T.; Majtan, V.; Klaudiny, J. Fir honeydew honey flavonoids inhibit TNF-alpha-induced MMP-9 expression in human keratinocytes: A new action of honey in wound healing. *Arch. Dermatol. Res.* **2013**, *305*, 619–627. [CrossRef]
37. Holubova, A.; Chlupacova, L.; Cetlova, L.; Cremers, N.A.J.; Pokorna, A. Medical-Grade Honey as an Alternative Treatment for Antibiotics in Non-Healing Wounds-A Prospective Case Series. *Antibiotics* **2021**, *10*, 918. [CrossRef]
38. Ingle, R.; Levin, J.; Polinder, K. Wound healing with honey—A randomised controlled trial. *S. Afr. Med. J.* **2006**, *96*, 831–835.
39. Du Toit, D.F.; Page, B.J. An in vitro evaluation of the cell toxicity of honey and silver dressings. *J. Wound Care* **2009**, *18*, 383–389. [CrossRef]
40. Boekema, B.K.; Pool, L.; Ulrich, M.M. The effect of a honey based gel and silver sulphadiazine on bacterial infections of in vitro burn wounds. *Burns* **2013**, *39*, 754–759. [CrossRef] [PubMed]
41. Kołwzan, B. Analysis of Biofilms—Their Formation and Functioning. *Ochr. Srodowiska* **2011**, *33*, 3–14.
42. Campeau, M.E.; Patel, R. Antibiofilm Activity of Manuka Honey in Combination with Antibiotics. *Int. J. Bacteriol.* **2014**, *2014*, 795281. [CrossRef] [PubMed]
43. Cooper, R.A.; Molan, P.C.; Harding, K.G. Antibacterial activity of honey against strains of Staphylococcus aureus from infected wounds. *J. R. Soc. Med.* **1999**, *92*, 283–285. [CrossRef] [PubMed]
44. Cooper, R.A.; Molan, P.C.; Harding, K.G. The sensitivity to honey of Gram-positive cocci of clinical significance isolated from wounds. *J. Appl. Microbiol.* **2002**, *93*, 857–863. [CrossRef]
45. Al-Waili, N.S.; Salom, K.; Butler, G.; Al Ghamdi, A.A. Honey and microbial infections: A review supporting the use of honey for microbial control. *J. Med. Food* **2011**, *14*, 1079–1096. [CrossRef]
46. Cooper, R.A.; Halas, E.; Molan, P.C. The efficacy of honey in inhibiting strains of Pseudomonas aeruginosa from infected burns. *J. Burn. Care Rehabil.* **2002**, *23*, 366–370. [CrossRef]
47. Okhira, O.A.; Henriques, A.F.M.; Burton, N.F.; Peters, A.; Cooper, R.A. Honey modulates biofilms of Pseudomonas aeruginosa in a time and dose dependent manner. *J. ApiProduct ApiMedical Sci.* **2009**, *1*, 6–10. [CrossRef]
48. Olaitan, P.B.; Adeleke, O.E.; Ola, I.O. Honey: A reservoir for microorganisms and an inhibitory agent for microbes. *Afr. Health Sci.* **2007**, *7*, 159–165.
49. Rajeswari, T.; Venugopal, A.; Viswanathan, C.; Kishmu, L.; Venil, C.K.; Sasikumar, J.M. Antibacterial activity of honey against Staphylococcus aureus from infected wounds. *Pharmacol. Online* **2010**, *1*, 537–541.
50. Cooper, R.A.; Jenkins, L. A comparison between medical grade honey and table honeys in relation to antimicrobial efficacy. *Wounds A Compend. Clin. Res. Pract.* **2009**, *21*, 29–36.
51. Alcaraz, A.; Kelly, J. Treatment of an infected venous leg ulcer with honey dressings. *Br. J. Nurs.* **2002**, *11*, 859–866. [CrossRef] [PubMed]
52. Oluwatosin, O.M.; Olabanji, J.K.; Oluwatosin, O.A.; Tijani, L.A.; Onyechi, H.U. A comparison of topical honey and phenytoin in the treatment of chronic leg ulcers. *Afr. J. Med. Med. Sci.* **2000**, *29*, 31–34. [PubMed]
53. Visavadia, B.G.; Honeysett, J.; Danford, M.H. Manuka honey dressing: An effective treatment for chronic wound infections. *Br. J. Oral. Maxillofac. Surg.* **2008**, *46*, 55–56. [CrossRef]
54. Kucharzewski, M.; Franek, A.; Koziołek, H. Treatment of venous leg ulcer with sulodexide. *Phlebologie* **2003**, *32*, 115–120. [CrossRef]
55. Kucharzewski, M.; Mieszczanski, P.; Wilemska-Kucharzewska, K.; Taradaj, J.; Kuropatnicki, A.; Sliwinski, Z. The application of negative pressure wound therapy in the treatment of chronic venous leg ulceration: Authors experience. *Biomed. Res. Int.* **2014**, *2014*, 297230. [CrossRef]
56. Kucharzewski, M.; Ślęzak, A.; Franek, A. Topical treatment of non-healing leg ulcers by cellullose membrane. *Phlebologie* **2003**, *32*, 147–151. [CrossRef]

MDPI AG
Grosspeteranlage 5
4052 Basel
Switzerland
Tel.: +41 61 683 77 34

Pharmaceuticals Editorial Office
E-mail: pharmaceuticals@mdpi.com
www.mdpi.com/journal/pharmaceuticals